MW01099182

LASIK

Edited by
Ioannis G. Pallikaris, MD, and
Dimitrios S. Siganos, MD

SLACK Incorporated, 6900 Grove Road, Thorofare, NJ 08086-9447

Publisher: John H. Bond

Editorial Director: Amy E. Drummond

Senior Associate Editor: Jennifer J. Cahill

Creative Director: Linda Baker

The procedures and practices described in this book should be implemented in a manner consistent with the professional standards set for the circumstances that apply in each specific situation. Every effort has been made to confirm the accuracy of the information presented and to correctly relate generally accepted practices. The authors, editors, and publisher cannot accept responsibility for errors or exclusions or for the outcome of the material presented herein. There is no expressed or implied warranty of this book or information imparted by it.

Care has been taken to ensure that drug selection and dosages are in accordance with currently accepted/recommended practice. Due to continuing research, changes in government policy and regulations, and various effects of drug reactions and interactions, it is recommended that the reader carefully review all materials and literature provided for each drug, especially those that are new or not frequently used.

LASIK/edited by Ioannis Pallikaris and Dimitrios Siganos.

p. cm.

Includes bibliographical references and index.

ISBN 1-55642-323-3

1. Cornea--Laser surgery. I. Pallikaris, Ioannis. II. Siganos, Dimitrios.

[DNLM: 1. Cornea--surgery. 2. Keratectomy, Photorefractive, Excimer Laser--methods. 3. Keratectomy, Photorefractive, Excimer Laser--adverse effects. 4. Refractive Errors--surgery. WW 220 L344 1997]

RE336.L27 1997

617.7'19059--dc21

DNLM/DLC

for Library of Congress 97-37263

Printed in the United States of America

Published by: SLACK Incorporated

6900 Grove Road

Thorofare, NJ 08086-9447 USA

Telephone: 609-848-1000

Fax: 609-853-5991

WWW: http://www.slackinc.com

Contact SLACK Incorporated for more information about other books in this field or about the availability of our books from distributors outside the United States.

Last digit is print number: 10 9 8 7 6 5 4 3 2 1

DEDICATION

To vision beyond optics.

CONTENTS

ACKNOWLEDGMENTS

It is with pleasure and gratitude that we acknowledge people who deserve credit for the evolution of this work. The book in hand represents a cumulative effort by our distinguished colleagues in the wide field of refractive surgery, our associates, and our students. We would like to thank them all for their response, their time, their offer of expertise, and their brilliant work.

We would like to thank the people at SLACK Incorporated, especially Amy Drummond, John Bond, and Jennifer Cahill for the motivation and numerous deadline extensions.

Last, but by no means least, we would like to thank our wives and children. It is true that they have no connection with ophthalmology, but they are unfortunate enough to be related to and to have to deal with crazy ophthalmologists!

Without the support of all the above, it would have never been possible to realize this huge work, a work to come out of our beloved island of Crete—a tiny part of the world, but also a land that has witnessed one of the earliest and greatest civilizations on earth, the Minoan civilization. We are proud to be their ancestors and we wish they would have been proud of their successors.

CONTRIBUTORS

Pietro Airaghi, MD
Monza, Italy

Till Anschuetz, MD
Gaggenau, Germany

Maria-Clara Arbelaez, MD
Cali, Colombia

Andrea Ascari, MD
Modena, Italy

Guillermo Avalos, MD
Guadalajara, Mexico

Marco Azzolini, MD
Monza, Italy

Carmen Barraquer C., MD
Bogota, Colombia

Perry S. Binder, MD
San Diego, California

Brian S. Boxer Wachler, MD
St. Louis, Missouri

Stephen F. Brint, MD, FACS
New Orleans, Louisiana

Jonathan D. Carr, MD, MA, FRCOphth
Atlanta, Georgia

J. Charles Casebeer, MD
Scottsdale, Arizona

Alice Chuang, PhD
Houston, Texas

Patrick I. Condon, MCh, FRCOphth
Waterford, Ireland

Klaus Ditzen, MD
Weinheim, Germany

John F. Doane, MD
Independence, Missouri

Mark W. Doubrava, MD
New Orleans, Louisiana

Daniel Durrie, MD
Kansas City, Missouri

Alexander Dybbs, PhD
Cleveland, Ohio

Mohammad Akef El-Maghraby, MD
Jeddah, Saudi Arabia

Kyriaki Evangelatou, MD
Crete, Greece

David W. Evans, PhD
Indianapolis, Indiana

Donald C. Fiander, MD, FRCSC
Southgate, Michigan

Laurent Gauthier-Fournet, MD
Saint Jean de Luz, France

Marc A. Goldberg, MD
New York, New York

Eugene I. Gordon, PhD
Edison, New Jersey

Jose L. Güell, MD
Barcelona, Spain

Alice Handzel, MD
Frankfurt, Germany

Greg Hanson, PA
Scottsdale, Arizona

Tibor Juhasz, PhD
Ann Arbor, Michigan

Petros V. Kapoulas, BSc
Crete, Greece

Vikentia I. Katsanevaki, MD
Crete, Greece

Guy M. Kezirian, MD, FACS
Scottsdale, Arizona

Asma T. Khan
Houston, Texas

Mohammed N. Khan, MD
Houston, Texas

Stephen D. Klyce, PhD
New Orleans, Louisiana

Michael C. Knorz, MD
Mannheim, Germany

Russell G. Koepnick, MS
Scottsdale, Arizona

Ronald R. Krueger, MD, MSE
St. Louis, Missouri

Richard L. Lindstrom, MD
Minneapolis, Minnesota

Vincenzo Marchi, MD
Rome, Italy

António Marinho, MD
Porto, Portugal

Carlos E. Martínez, MD, MS
New Orleans, Louisiana

Marguerite B. McDonald, MD, FACS
New Orleans, Louisiana

Antonio Mendez G., MD
Tijuana Baja California, Mexico

Antonio Mendez Noble, MD
Tijuana Baja California, Mexico

Francesco Nizzola, MD
Modena, Italy

Guido Maria Nizzola, MD
Modena, Italy

Irini I. Naoumidi, PhD
Crete, Greece

Ioannis G. Pallikaris, MD
Crete, Greece

Sophia I. Panagopoulou, BSc
Crete, Greece

Thekla G. Papadaki, MD
Crete, Greece

Barbara Parolini, MD
Edison, New Jersey

Paola Radice, MD
Monza, Italy

Narayanan Ramesh, MBBS
Houston, Texas

Jeffery B. Robin, MD
Cleveland, Ohio

Tarek Salah, MD, FRCS
Jeddah, Saudi Arabia

Dimitrios S. Siganos, MD
Crete, Greece

Stephen G. Slade, MD, FACS
Houston, Texas

Mark Speaker, MD, PhD
New York, New York

Holger K. Steiner, MD
Ludwigshafen, Germany

Pavel Stodulka, MD
Zlin, Czech Republic

R. Doyle Stulting, MD, PhD
Atlanta, Georgia

Keith P. Thompson, MD
Atlanta, Georgia

Stephen A. Updegraff, MD
St. Petersburg, Florida

Paolo Vinciguerra, MD
Monza, Italy

George O. Waring III, MD, FACS, FRCOphth
Atlanta, Georgia

Bettina B. Wiesinger, MD
Mannheim, Germany

Richard W. Yee, MD
Houston, Texas

PREFACE

It is an unattainable dream no more. We travel in space. We walk on the moon. We play games with Halley's comet. We are planing to change Mars' atmosphere in order to render it habitable.

It is the amazing nature of that miraculous thing called "the human mind." It is the continuous, relentless wondering that spurs us on and is constantly renewing itself, guiding us into the sphere of fantasy. It is the subsequent landing of this fantasy that provides that vital spark of light, stimulating the need to realize and to wonder all the time: "How can this be achieved?"

The answer is Science. The process of observing, experimenting, and always asking "What's next?" And there is always something "next" to be revealed from an endless store of secrets, thus forming a circle of new conflicts and settlements between imagination and reality, giving birth to a marvelous symphony in which every scientist adds a note here, removes a note there, in an attempt to perfect it.

LASIK. Is it good? Is it here to stay? For good? We hope not. LASIK should be only the current step, no matter how long this step lasts, in the long ladder of refractive surgery, started many years ago by its father of recent refractive surgery, Jose I. Barraquer. That which we consider to be modern, hopefully will end up out of fashion in a few years. This is what a true scientist would expect: an inspiration that adds triumphant notes to the symphony, only to yield with time, giving way to new, improved, and more impressive features.

Ioannis G. Pallikaris, MD
Dimitrios S. Siganos, MD

SECTION 1

BACKGROUND

Chapter 1

HISTORICAL EVOLUTION OF LASIK

Ioannis G. Pallikaris, MD

Refractive corneal lamellar surgery began in the late 1940s and has its roots in the ingenious work of Dr. Jose I. Barraquer. He was the first to understand that the refractive power of the eye could be altered by subtraction or addition of corneal tissue.[1] The term keratomileusis, which is derived from the Greek roots "keras" (hornlike = cornea) and "smileusis" (carving), was introduced in order to describe lamellar techniques.[2]

Barraquer's initial technique consisted of performing a free-hand lamellar dissection of the anterior half of the cornea using a Paufique knife or a keratome to create a corneal lamellar disc. He then attempted the refractive cut by removing stroma from either the bed (keratomileusis in situ) or the stromal surface of the corneal lamellar disc. The many technical difficulties of keratomileusis in situ could not be overcome with the instrumentation available at that time, and the procedure had, therefore, to be temporarily abandoned. Barraquer focused his research on refining lamellar resection and carving of the resected corneal disc.[3] His efforts for more accurate, predictable, and reproducible cuts led to the development of applanator lenses, suction rings of various diameters, and various heights of microkeratome tracks.[3] The cryolathe was used to sculpture the lamellar corneal disc, and so myopic keratomileusis (MKM) was introduced.[4-6] The many disadvantages of the procedure (ie, complex instrumentation, steep learning curve, high rate of complications, such as irregular astigmatism or corneal scarring[4]) shadowed the initial enthusiasm. Other techniques including epikeratophakia,[7-13] incisional keratotomy,[14-16] and IOL implantation[17] for the correction of refractive errors began to develop.

However, lamellar refractive surgery did not cease to evolve. It was revealed that freezing procedures were often complicated with corneal haze and induced irregular astigmatism[18-22] and, therefore, had to be replaced by non-freezing ones. A manual microkeratome was initially used to perform a second cut on the stromal side of the resected lamellar disc. Despite their technical difficulty, non-freezing techniques proved to have a major advantage: the rapid and comfortable recovery of patients.[3,18,19,21] Dr. Luis Ruiz turned to keratomileusis in situ in an effort to overcome the technical difficulties of MKM. The second pass of the microkeratome was performed on the bed and not on the disc. In 1987, Dr. Leo Bores performed the first keratomileusis in situ in the United States.[3] Keratomileusis in situ with the use of manual microkeratomes, however, was reported as being not technically safe, precise, or predictable and failed to be adopted by a large number of surgeons.[23] In the 1980s, development of the automated microkeratome by Ruiz introduced automated lamellar keratoplasty (ALK) in the field of lamellar refractive corneal surgery.

The first clinical trials on ALK revealed its advantages: ease of use, rapid recovery and stability of refraction, and efficacy in the correction of high myopias. Major disadvantages, however, were the relative high rate of irregular astigmatism (2%) and the reduced predictability of the procedure (within 2 D).[24]

Trokel et al suggested photorefractive keratectomy (PRK) in 1983.[25] An earlier attempt to remove corneal tissue using CO_2 laser had failed because of considerable tissue coagulation and scarring.[26] Other lasers, such as erbium: yttrium-aluminum-garnet (Er:YAG), were reported as successful in modifying the corneal curvature by ablation of stromal tissue.[27] As the use of 193-nm excimer laser in refractive surgery was generated, it was revealed quickly that for myopias greater than 6 D, PRK resulted in significant central corneal haze, regression of the refractive effect, and poor predictability.[28] It was then that we thought of combining the precision of PRK with the technique of ALK.

LASIK was introduced, designed, and developed at the University of Crete and the Vardinoyannion Eye Institute of Crete (VEIC).[29] We suggested the term "laser in situ keratomileusis," or LASIK, as we thought it best describes a combination of lamellar refractive corneal surgery and excimer laser photo-ablation of the cornea under a hinged corneal flap.[1] The first animal studies began in 1987, using a Lamda Physik excimer laser and a microkeratome that was specially designed to produce a 150-µm flap instead of a total cap. These studies aimed at determining wound healing reactions after LASIK.[30]

ALKs so far were performed by resecting a total lamellar corneal disc, which was sutured in place at the end of the procedure. The original idea of creating a corneal cap and removing central tissue from the bed was first described by Pureskin in 1966.[31] He attempted to perform the cut manually and cut out the in situ part with a trephine. Fairly crude by today's standards, but the idea was there. The breakthrough in my philosophy was the thought to create a corneal flap and to combine it with the excimer laser submicron accuracy of stromal tissue removal. My initial theory was that a flap would ensure better fitting of tissues after removing the intrastromal tissue with laser, and would not affect the anatomic relations of corneal layers mainly by two ways: by preserving Bowman's layer and by ensuring better integrity of the superficial nerve plexus of the cornea, as the latter follows at a great length its route through the base of the flap.

In 1992, Buratto et al[32] used excimer laser for intrastromal keratomileusis of the corneal button. He suggested the term "laser intrastromal keratomileusis." One disadvantage over the Buratto's intrastromal keratomileusis technique[1] (where the button is ablated) is that perforation into the anterior chamber is possible. However, the advantages over the same technique are the following: it is a sutureless technique, a flap being produced instead of a button that requires only a mere reapposition. The flap, being returned and fit exactly to its original place without sutures, does not induce any operative (healing or sutural) astigmatism.

Other advantages were the reduction of maneuvers and total time required for the operation. During the 1993 American Academy of Ophthalmology Meeting, Dr. George O. Waring III gave LASIK the temporary name "Flap & Zap" in order to emphasize the alacrity of the procedure. The first papers on LASIK were presented at the 7th European Congress of the European Society of Cataract and Refractive Surgeons in Zurich in August 1989 and were published in 1990.[30] The first LASIK on a blind human eye was performed in June 1989 as a part of an unofficial blind eye protocol.

To date, we have published several articles concerning

healing of partially sighted eyes,[33,34] results on partially sighted eyes,[35] a comparative study between LASIK and PRK in partially sighted eyes,[36] and a series of normal sighted eyes with varying follow-up.[37]

References

1. Barraquer JI. Queratoplastia Refractiva. *Estudios Inform*. 1949;10:2-21.
2. Bores L. Lamellar refractive surgery. In: Bores L, ed. *Refractive Eye Surgery*. Boston, Mass: Blackwell Scientific Publications; 1993:324-392.
3. Barraquer JI. Keratomileusis. *Int Surg*. 1967;48:103-117.
4. Barraquer JI. Results of myopic keratomileusis. *J Refract Surg*. 1987;3:98-101.
5. Littman H. Optic of Barraquer's keratomileusis. *Arch Oftal Optom*. 1966;6:1.
6. Barraquer JI. Method for cutting lamellar grafts in frozen corneas: new orientations for refractive surgery. *Arch Soc Am Ophthalmol*. 1958;1:237.
7. Kaufmann HE. The correction of aphakia. *Am J Ophthalmol*. 1980;89:1-10.
8. Werblin TP, Klyce SD. Epikeratophakia: the correction of aphakia. I. Lathing of corneal tissue. *Curr Eye Res*. 1981-1982;1:591-597.
9. Barraquer JI. Modification of refraction by means of intracorneal inclusions. *Int Ophthalmol Clin*. 1966;6:53-78.
10. Baumgartner SD, Binder PS, Deg JK, et al. Epikeratophakia: clinical and histopathologic evaluation in non-human primates. *Invest Ophthalmol Vis Sci*. 1983;24:148.
11. Werblin TP, Kaufmann HE, Friedlander MH, et al. A prospective study of the use of hyperopic epikeratophakia grafts for the correction of aphakia in adults. *Ophthalmology*. 1981;88:1137-1140.
12. Kaufmann HE, Werblin TP. Epikeratophakia. A form of lamellar keratoplasty for the treatment of keratoconus. *Am J Ophthalmol*. 1982;93:342-347.
13. Werblin TP, Blaydes JE, Kaufman HE. Epikeratophakia. The correction of astigmatism—preliminary experimental results. *CLAO J*. 1983;9:61-63.
14. Bores LD, Myers W, Cowden J. Radial keratotomy: an analysis of the American experience. *Ann Ophthalmol*. 1981;13:941-948.
15. Arrowsmith PN, Sanders DR, Marks RG. Visual, refractive and keratometric results of radial keratotomy. *Arch Ophthalmol*. 1983;101:873-881.
16. Deitz MR, Sanders DR, Marks RG. Radial keratotomy: an overview of the Kansas City study. *Ophthalmology*. 1984;91:467-478.
17. Shearing SP. Posterior chamber lens implantation. *Int Ophthalmol Clin*. 1982;22:135-153.
18. Swinger CA, Barker BA. Prospective evaluation of myopic keratomileusis. *Ophthalmology*. 1984;91:785-792.
19. Nordan LT, Fallor MK. Myopic keratomileusis: 74 consecutive non-amblyopic cases with one year follow-up. *J Refract Surg*. 1986;2:124-128.
20. Maquire LJ, Klyce SD, Sawelson H, et al. Visual distortion after myopic keratomileusis: computer analysis of keratoscope photographs. *Ophthalmic Surg*. 1987;18:352-356.
21. Nordan LT. Keratomileusis. *Int Ophthalmol Clin*. 1991;31:7-12.
22. Barraquer C, Guitierrez A, Espinoza A. Myopic keratomileusis: short term results. *Refract Corneal Surg*. 1989;5:307-313.
23. Arenas-Archila E, Sanchez-Thorin JC, et al. Myopic keratomileusis in situ: a preliminary report. *J Cataract Refract Surg*. 1991;17:424-435.
24. Slade SG, Updegraff SA. Complications of automated lamellar keratectomy (comment). *Arch Ophthalmol*. 1995;113(9):1092-1093.
25. Trokel S, Srinivasan R, Braren B. Excimer laser surgery of the cornea. *Am J Ophthalmol*. 1983;94:125.
26. Peyman GA. Modification of rabbit corneal curvature with the use of carbon dioxide laser burns. *Ophthalmic Surg*. 1980;11:325-329.
27. Peyman GA, Badaro RM, Khoobehi B. Corneal abaltion in rabbits using an infrared (2.9 microns) erbium: YAG laser. *Ophthalmology*. 1989;96:1160-1170.
28. Seiler T, McDonnell PJ. Excimer laser photorefractive keratectomy. *Surv Ophthalmol*. 1995;40(2):89-118.
29. Pallikaris I, Papatzanaki M, Stathi EZ, Frenschock O, Georgiadis A. Laser in situ keratomileusis. *Lasers Surg Med*. 1990;10:463-468.
30. Pallikaris I, Papatzanaki M, Georgiadis A, Frenschock O. A comparative study of neural regeneration following corneal wounds induced by argon fluoride excimer laser and mechanical methods. *Lasers Light Ophthalmol*. 1990;3:89-95.
31. Pureskin N. Weakening ocular refraction by means of partial stromectomy of the cornea under experimental conditions. *Vestn Oftalmol*. 1967;8:1-7.
32. Buratto L, Ferrari M, Rama P. Excimer laser intrastromal keratomileusis. *Am J Ophthalmol*. 1992;113:291-295.
33. Pallikaris IG, Papatzanaki ME, Siganos DS, Tsilimbaris MK. A corneal flap technique for laser in situ keratomileusis. *Arch Ophthalmol*. 1991;109(12):1699-1702.
34. Pallikaris IG, Papatzanaki ME, Siganos DS, Tsilimbaris MK. Tecnica de colajo corneal para la queratomileusis in situ mediane laser. Estudios en Humanos. *Arch Ophthalmol* (Ed Esp). 1992;3(3):127-130.
35. Siganos DS, Pallikaris IG. Laser in situ keratomileusis in partially sighted eyes. *Invest Ophthalmol Vis Sci*. 1993;34(4):800.
36. Pallikaris IG, Siganos DS. Excimer laser in situ keratomileusis and photorefractive keratectomy for the correction of high myopia. *J Refract Corneal Surg*. 1994;10(15):498-510.
37. Pallikaris IG, Siganos DS. Laser in situ keratomileusis to treat myopia: early experience. *J Cataract Refract Surg*. 1997;23(1):9-49.

Chapter 2

NEW DEVELOPMENTS IN EXCIMER LASER

Marguerite B. McDonald, MD, FACS,
Mark W. Doubrava, MD

Since the mid 1980s, we have seen the expansion of excimer technology throughout the world. The number of excimer-based refractive surgeries performed to date continues to increase: so far an estimated 1 million procedures have been performed internationally and 100,000 procedures in the United States (Michael Moretti, personal communication, February 1997). Updated software, new delivery systems, and tracking systems are all making a dramatic impact in the surgical treatment of myopia, astigmatism, and hyperopia. Commensurate with the technological advancements, the clinical data and visual results have improved over the past 8 years. This has prompted the refractive surgery market to grow (Figure 2-1, Table 2-1) and the number of excimer lasers to increase around the world.

Regarding the excimer laser status in the United States, Summit Technology and VisX Inc received regulatory approval for phototherapeutic keratectomy (PTK) on March 13, 1995 and September 25, 1995, respectively. Approval for photorefractive keratectomy (PRK) was granted on October 20, 1995 for Summit and on March 27, 1996 for the VisX lasers. Several laser companies have entered Phase III clinical studies for regulatory approval: Chiron Vision Corp, Nidek Inc, and Autonomous Technologies Corp. The other companies pursuing US approval are LaserSight Technologies Inc, Aesculap-Meditec, Novatec Laser Systems Inc, and Kera Technology Inc.

TABLE 2-1

Photorefractive Delivery Systems

Broad Beam (Wide Area Ablation)

Advantages

1. More forgiving of decentrations
2. Shorter procedure time
3. Lower repetition rate
4. No eyetracking necessary

Disadvantages

1. High output energy requirements
2. More complex delivery system (increased number of optical elements/homogenization systems required)
3. Higher maintenance
4. Higher beam uniformity required
5. Increased incidence of central islands
6. Limited ablation patterns (eg, asymmetric astigmatism not possible to correct)
7. Greater acoustic shockwave

Models	SUMMIT ExciMed, OmniMed, Apex, SVS Apex Plus	VISX 20/20 Model B, 20/15 (Taunton), Star	CHIRON TECHNOLAS Keracor 116	COHERENT-SCHWIND Keratom I/II	
Fluence (mJ/cm²)	180	160	130	Variable <250	
Pulse Frequency (Hz) [Maximum]	10	6 [30]	10 [40]	13	
Maximum Pulse Area	6.5 mm	8.0 mm	7.0 mm	8.0 mm	
Myopic Ablation Pattern	Iris diaphragm or erodible mask	Iris diaphragm	Iris diaphragm	Enlarging circular apertures	
Astigmatic Ablation Pattern	Emphasis erodible mask	Sequential and elliptical programs, iris diaphragm, rotatable slit	Linear scanning	Enlarging oval apertures	
Hyperopic Ablation Pattern	Emphasis erodible mask	Rotating scanning slit	Annular scanning spot	Annular apertures	
Eyetracker	None	None	Active	Passive	
Miscellaneous		Automated calibration	Oscillating beam joystick		

Adapted with permission from Machat JJ. *Excimer laser refractive surgery.* Thorofare, NJ: Slack Inc; 1996.

TABLE 2-1 (CONTINUED)

PHOTOREFRACTIVE DELIVERY SYSTEMS

Scanning	
Slit	Spot
1. Intermediate energy output requirements 2. Improved beam uniformity 3. No central islands 4. Reduced acoustic shockwave 5. Smoother ablative surfaces 6. No optical zone limitations for PRK/PTK	1. Small energy output requirements 2. More complex ablation patterns possible, including hyperopia 3. Lower beam homogeneity requirements 4. Lowest maintenance and fewest optics 5. No optical zone limitations for PRK/PTK 6. Reduced acoustic shockwave 7. No central islands
1. Eyetracker more important 2. Eye mask awkward 3. Slower procedure	1. Eyetracker necessary 2. Slowest procedure 3. Higher repetition rate necessary 4. Unknown/evolving algorithms

AESCULAP-MEDITEC MEL 60	**NIDEK** EC-5000	**AUTONOMOUS TECHNOL-OGIES CORP** Tracker-PRK	**LASERSIGHT** Compak-200 Mini Excimer	**CHIRON TECHNOLAS** Keracor 117	**CHIRON TECHNOLAS** Keracor 217	**NOVATEC** LightBlade (non-excimer)	**KERA TECH-NOLOGY** IsoBeam
250	130	180	160 to 300	130	130	100	150
20	30 [46]	100	100	20 to 40	50	>200	400
1.5 x 10 mm	2 x 7 mm, optical zone 7.5 mm maximum, TZ 9.0 mm maximum	<1 mm	<1 mm	1 to 2 mm	2 mm (TZ 14.0 mm maximum)	<0.3 mm	0.7 x 0.9 mm
Rotating eye mask	Iris diaphragm, scanning slit rotates 120°/pass	Spiral scanning program	Rotating linear scanning spot	Spiral/random scanning spot	Scanning spot using PlanoScan alogorithms	Spiral scanning spot	Two fractal scanning spot
Rotating (variable) eye mask	Rotatable scanning slit beam	Meridional scanning	Meridional scanning	Meridional scanning	Annular scanning spot	Elliptical scanning spot	Two fractal scanning spot
Rotating (inverse) eye mask	Annular scanning slit beam	Annular scanning spot	Annular scanning spot	Annular scanning spot		Annular scanning spot	Two fractal scanning spot
None	Passive	Active dual axis	None	Active	Active	Active	None
		Laser radar= LADAR eyetracking			Ceramic head lowers main-tenance costs	Solid-state tunable titanium sapphire	

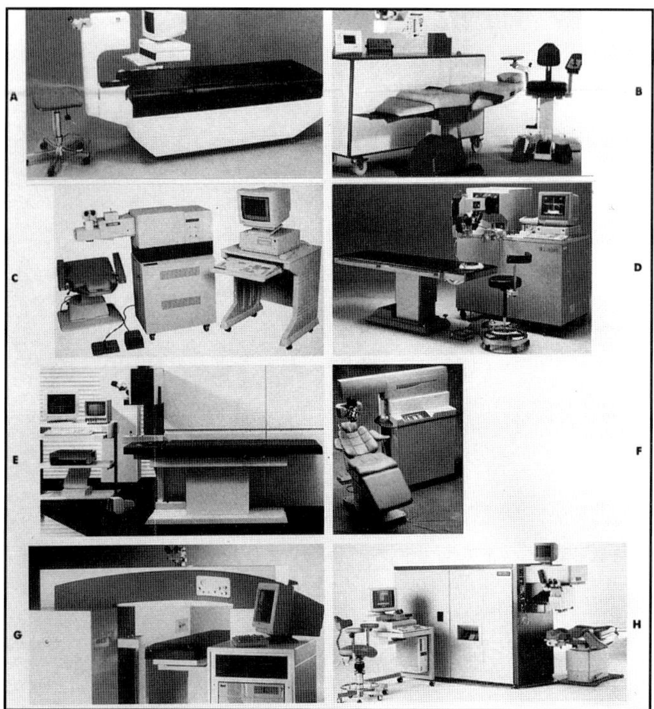

Figure 2-1.
Excimer lasers manufactured by (a) Autonomous Technologies Corp, (b) Aesculap-Meditec, (c) LaserSight Technologies Inc, (d) Nidek Inc, (e) Coherent Medical, (f) Summit Technology, (g) Chiron Vision Corp, and (h) VisX Inc. Not pictured: Kera Technology Inc. Reprinted with permission from Krachmer, Mannis, Holland. *Cornea*. Vol 3. St. Louis, Mo: Mosby-Yearbook; 1997.

WIDE FIELD LASERS

The wide beam, first-generation excimer laser from Summit Technology included the early ExciMed model with a 5.0-mm maximum ablation diameter. The smaller ablation zone diameter and gaussian beam profile led to greater hyperopic overshoot in the early healing phase. Currently, the OmniMed, Apex, and Apex Plus systems are capable of 6.5-mm ablations and much less hyperopic overshoot when treating myopia with surface PRK or laser in situ keratomileusis (LASIK). When used in conjunction with an erodible mask, astigmatism can also be treated. The Apex Plus utilizes the axicon prism to split the broad beam to treat hyperopia at an optical zone of 9.4 mm. Future developments include a customized mask designed from corneal topography to treat irregular astigmatism. Summit has 250 international lasers and 200 units in the United States.

Early lasers from VisX, such as the 20/20 A and 20/20 B, fall into the wide beam, first-generation category. The Taunton laser (20/15 laser) was an investigational, wide beam, first-generation laser that was discontinued when Taunton and VisX merged. The VisX Star is still a wide beam laser, but it qualifies for second-generation status because of its large selection of treatment options for myopia, astigmatism, and hyperopia. The Star uses an iris diaphragm to shape optical zones up to 8.0 mm in diameter. Astigmatism correction is possible with sequential and elliptical programs. Hyperopic ablation is possible with a rotating slit, and, as of this writing, VisX has placed approximately 200 lasers internationally and 100 lasers in the United States.

Schwind Keratom, distributed by Coherent Medical, uses a rotating disc with enlarging apertures to treat myopia and astigmatism. Annular apertures are used to treat hyperopia. The beam diameter ranges from 0.6 to 8.0 mm and operates at 10 Hz. Coherent is exploring the application of solid-state technology to its refractive lasers. Coherent has placed approximately 110 lasers internationally, but there are no lasers as yet in the United States.

SCANNING SLIT LASERS

The Nidek EC-5000, a second-generation laser that uses both a diaphragm and a rotating, scanning slit, is capable of treating myopia, astigmatism, and hyperopia. The optical zone for myopia is a maximum of 6.5 mm in diameter, and has a transition zone which allows the total diameter to be as large as 9.0 mm. The Nidek has an optional passive eyetracker that will automatically stop laser treatment if the eye moves more than 5 mm. Nidek has entered Phase III FDA clinical trials; it has eight lasers in the United States and 191 lasers in other countries. Current research includes treatment for presbyopia and customized ablations based on corneal topography.

The Aesculap-Meditec MEL 60 uses a scanning slit and a rotating hourglass aperture to treat myopia, astigmatism, and hyperopia. The ablation zone ranges from 7.0 to 8.0 mm for myopia and is created by rotation of a 1.5 x 10.0 mm slit at a rate of 20 Hz. There are four US units and approximately 200 international units.

FLYING SPOT LASERS

The LaserSight Compak-200 Mini Excimer utilizes a

scanning spot less than 1 mm in size and can perform surface PRK, hyperopic PRK, photoastigmatic refractive keratectomy (PARK), and LASIK. In the early 1990s, the LaserSight Laser Harmonic system was solid state, but it was expensive and slow at 10 to 50 Hz. Using the same scanning spot delivery system as the Laser Harmonic, the Compak-200 is less expensive and faster at 100 Hz. There are currently 120 international units and seven US units. Current research projects include the correction of presbyopia, customized ablations, and a return to solid-state technology and faster ablation rates. Active eyetracking is contemplated for future models.

The Autonomous Technologies Corp laser also utilizes a moving or flying spot delivery system to perform myopic, astigmatic, and hyperopic PRK. The spot size is less than 1.0 mm and operates at up to 100 Hz. The laser uses the Ladar Vision tracking system, which is centered first on the undilated, then dilated, pupil to ensure proper spot placement. Autonomous Technologies Corp's research includes development of a "smart" laser guided by a refractive map of the eye to give customized ablations that can correct irregular astigmatism. There are currently five laser sites in the United States and three internationally.

The first-generation laser from Chiron Technolas is the wide beam Keracor 116, which utilizes an iris diaphragm and has a maximum ablation of 7.0 mm; it operates at 10 Hz. The Keracor 117 operates a 1- to 2-mm spiral or random scanning spot at 20 to 40 Hz using an active tracker; it is considered a third-generation laser (flying spot, large menu of treatment options). The Keracor 217C has a flying 2.0-mm spot that can create a 14.0-mm ablation zone. Myopia, astigmatism, and hyperopia are treated with a random scanning spot at 50 Hz. PlanoScan is a new ablation pattern that utilizes a small, fixed diameter beam that has the ability to correct myopia, hyperopia, and myopic and hyperopic astigmatism. An advantage of the PlanoScan algorithm is a smoother ablated surface. The 217C has a ceramic head that accommodates the 50 Hz and lessens optic degradation and lowers maintenance costs. Chiron Technolas has placed 18 US units and 160 international units.

Kera Technology Inc has developed a new argon-fluoride flying spot excimer laser that generates a 193-nm ultraviolet beam. The IsoBeam D200 splits the source beam into two surgical beams that are identical and measure 0.3 x 0.9 mm in diameter. These beams ablate the cornea simultaneously in a random pattern, as opposed to other flying spot lasers which execute a linear or circular series of overlapping ablations. The two beams also shorten ablation time by effectively doubling the frequency from 200 to 400 Hz. There is no tracking device, although aiming beams are utilized for centration. The ablation pattern is executed using the "fractal" method. (Fractal geometry is the branch of mathematics concerned with irregular patterns. Fractal geometry has been applied to such diverse fields as the stock market, chemistry, meteorology, and computer graphics.) The laser can treat myopia, hyperopia, and both myopic and hyperopic astigmatism. There are two units in the United States and six international units.

The Novatec LightBlade is a solid-state crystal laser; it is not an excimer laser. Using a wavelength of 210 nm and a 0.3 mm scanning spot operating at 200 Hz, the LightBlade corrects myopia, astigmatism, and hyperopia. Corneal trephination and intrastromal cavitation are also possible with the Novatec LightBlade. Since the laser is solid state, excimer gas refill or disposal is not necessary. The LightBlade optics have a lifetime of approximately 2500 procedures which compares favorably with excimer laser optics lasting about 350 procedures. There are 13 international units and nine US units.

The "custom built" excimer lasers are utilized by approximately 20 physicians in the United States and by an unknown number of physicians internationally. Considered a custom laser expert, Edward J. Sullivan, BSEE, of Drexel Hill, Pa, has served as an engineering consultant to many of the US surgeons who are building their own lasers. According to Sullivan, these lasers are all wide beam and utilize an iris diaphragm to treat myopia (personal communication, March 1997). Astigmatism and hyperopia treatments are possible with slit apertures. A perceived advantage of custom lasers is the ability to perform the diameter, shape, and depth of ablation that the surgeon desires, including the multipass/multizone technique. As of this writing, custom lasers are also free of the Pillar Point royalty in the United States. In the United States, custom built laser owners have been told to operate only under an investigational device exemption (IDE) from the FDA, and several of these lasers (without IDEs) have recently been seized.

Chapter 3

CORRECTION OF AMETROPIAS BY FREEZING REFRACTIVE LAMELLAR SURGERY: FREEZING KERATOMILEUSIS

Carmen Barraquer C., MD

The cornea is the lens with the highest refractive power in the eye's optical system. In 1949, Jose I. Barraquer proposed the surgical modification of the eye's refraction by changing the curvature radii of the cornea's anterior surface.[1]

The required research in order to accomplish this objective led him to establish the principles listed below, known today in ophthalmology as "The Thicknesses Law."

- "In order to change the anterior corneal surface to attain applanation of the optic zone by means of a *change in thickness*, it is necessary to remove corneal parenchyma at the center or to add it at the periphery; in order to steepen the optical zone, parenchyma has to be added at the center or removed at the periphery."
- "Action should be in one sense, either at the center or at the periphery, because if both zones are modified, one action will totally or partially cancel the other out."

Therefore, two surgical approaches were designed:

1. Alloplastic materials, homo or heteroplastic tissue addition techniques requiring the intracorneal inclusion of a lenticle, were called "keratophakias" by association of ideas.
2. Autoplastic tissue removal techniques that do not require the use of elements alien to the cornea. Since their goal is to reshape the cornea, they were called "keratomileusis." These are easier techniques that have come to dominate the field of refractive lamellar surgery as it is known today.

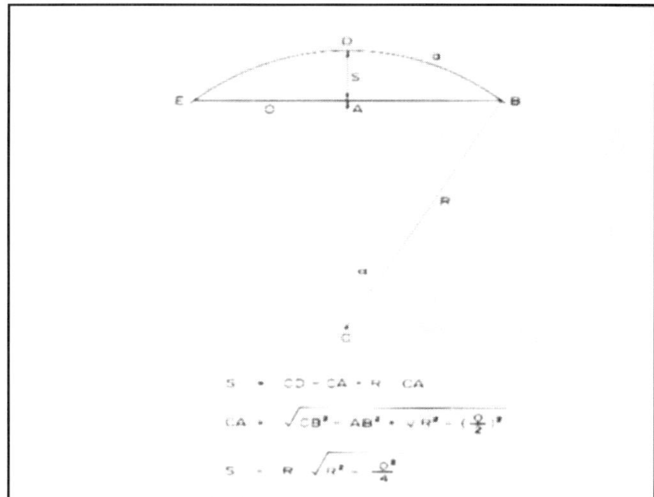

Figure 3-1.
Geometrical scheme. Explains the geometrical principles of lamellar refractive surgery.

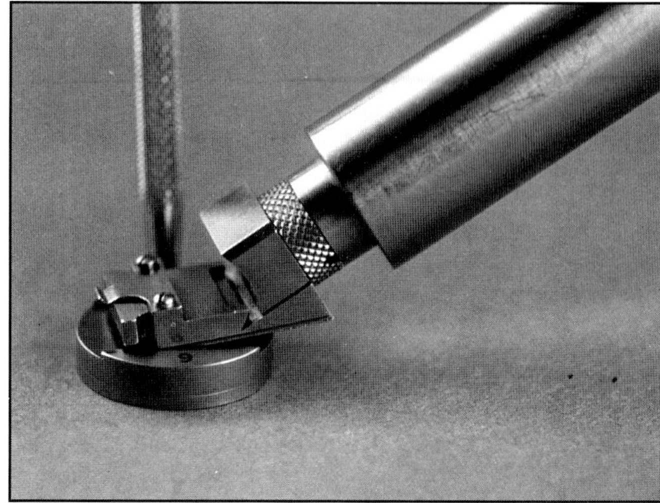

Figure 3-2.
The third-generation Barraquer microkeratome. It is placed over a suction ring.

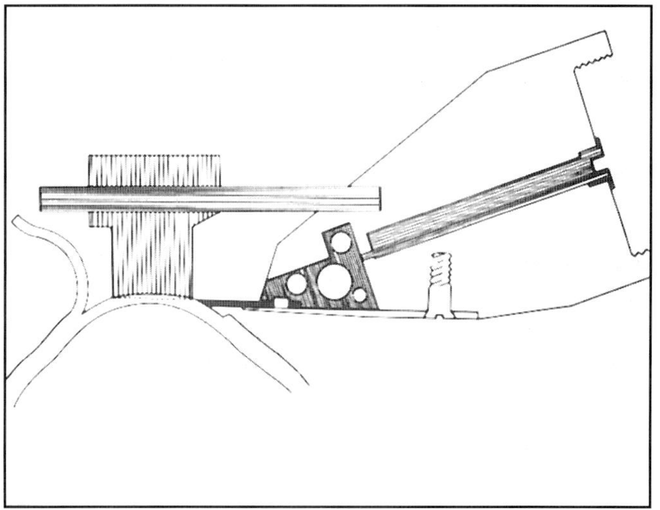

Figure 3-3.
The first microkeratome prototype based on Castroviejo's microkeratome. Performing an autoplastic refractive correction; now it is known as in situ keratomileusis. Reprinted with permission from Barraquer JI. *Cirugia Refractiva de la córnea.* Bogotá, Colombia: Instituto Barraquer de América; 1989.

Tissue removal techniques designed to reduce corneal power are used at present to correct ametropias due to excess power as is the case with myopia. Techniques designed to increase corneal power are used to correct default ametropias, namely, hyperopia. These reshaping procedures also allow the reduction of the cornea's asphericity and eccentricity, correcting defects such as astigmatism (Figure 3-1).

In order to accomplish the goals proposed in his Thicknesses Law, Barraquer designed multiple instruments and tried many approaches until 1954 when, following Eascott's discoveries about the viability of the frozen cornea, a new horizon opened for him, leading to the establishment of the surgical techniques that have been perfected over the years and are in current use. It is worth mentioning a few of the many instruments Barraquer designed during the development of lamellar refractive surgery.

THE MICROKERATOME

The microkeratome is designed to perform circular lamellar resections of a predetermined diameter and thickness in corneas of regular thickness (Figure 3-2). It is based on the principle of the carpenter's plane and consists of a plane through the center of which a cutting blade emerges. This blade has a 2.5-mm amplitude swinging motion, driven by a motorized foot pedal.

All of the instrument's dimensions were carefully studied in relation to the eyeball, the most frequent corneal curvatures, the palpebral fissure, and the mechanical needs.

The resection diameter is selected by means of the height of the pneumatic fixation ring, and its thickness by means of a plate located on the anterior plane of the microkeratome and the width of the blade. The maximum diameter that can be obtained with the microkeratome is 9.00 mm; as this size is approached, disc edges tend to become irregular. After several trials (Figure 3-3), Barraquer chose a 26° slope for the blade, like the

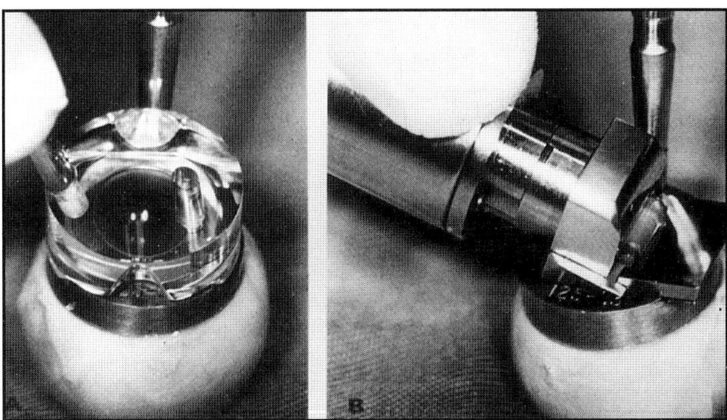

Figure 3-4.
Eye bank globe, suction ring, and applanation lens in place to measure the diameter of the disc resection (left). Second-generation microkeratome resecting a corneal disc (right). Reprinted with permission from Barraquer JI. *Cirugia Refractiva de la córnea.* Bogotá, Colombia: Instituto Barraquer de América; 1989.

one in the microtome used for histopathology (Figure 3-4).

The instrument was developed with all its ancillary parts, including the pneumatic fixation rings, the applanation lenses for measuring diameters, and the surgical tonometers, not to mention the theoretical foundation for the instrument's performance.

THE CRYOLATHE

This instrument began as a simple clockmaker's lathe and attained significant technological development, becoming the current prototype of the computerized lathe (Figure 3-5). With this prototype, tissue was frozen on the basis of the Peltier effect which allows one to program temperature reductions and to obtain great freezing time uniformity in all cases. The tool had a CO_2 cooling device. A steel tip was used to shape the base and the frozen corneal tissue because of its greater hardness compared to other materials. Moreover, it could be sharpened without dismounting. Standard tools must have a curvature radius of 2.5 at 0.5 mm at their tip in order to obtain good consistency in bicurved cuts.

Frozen lamellar refractive surgery was performed over 27 years and the clinical and surgical results of this experience have set the basis for the present excimer laser technology. Between 1963 and 1990, 4500 eyes were operated, 34 calculation programs were developed for correcting myopia and hyperopia, instruments were modified with three generations of microkeratomes and four generations of spherical cutting lathes, and the surgical technique was disseminated through lectures and 17 training courses conducted personally by Prof. Barraquer. Three books were published on the subject. With frozen lamellar refractive surgery, an organ was modified outside the body using a programmed computer for the first time in medicine.

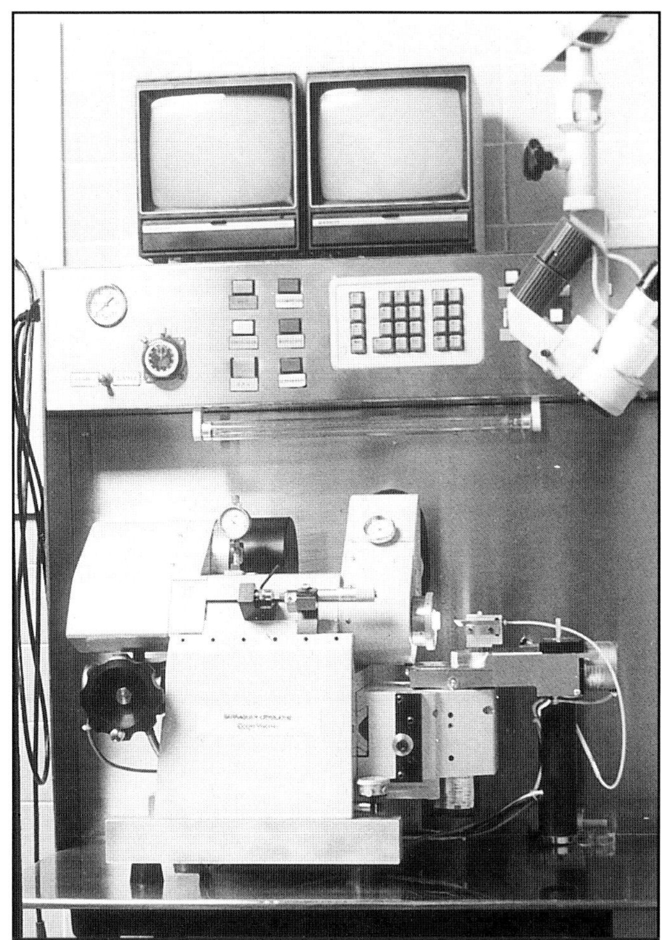

Figure 3-5.
The automatic computerized lathe.

FROZEN MYOPIC KERATOMILEUSIS

This procedure is performed resecting a corneal disc of parallel faces with predetermined diameter and thickness; consequently, it is optically neutral. The disc taken from the cornea to be operated comprises the epithelium, Bowman's layer, and part of the corneal parenchyma. The

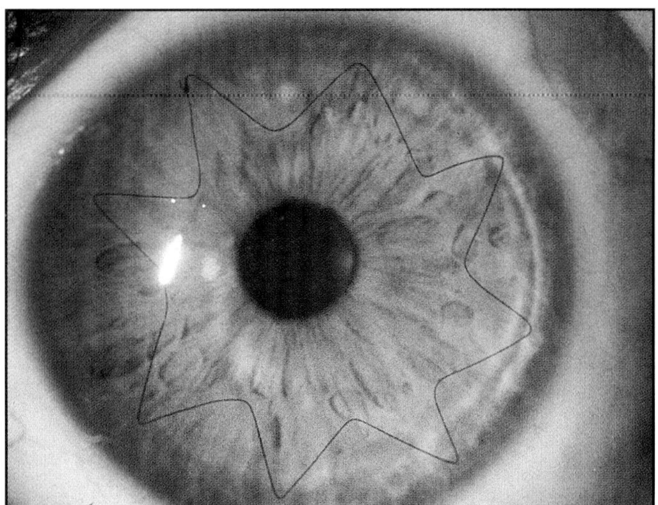

Figure 3-6.
Frontal view. Suture in place.

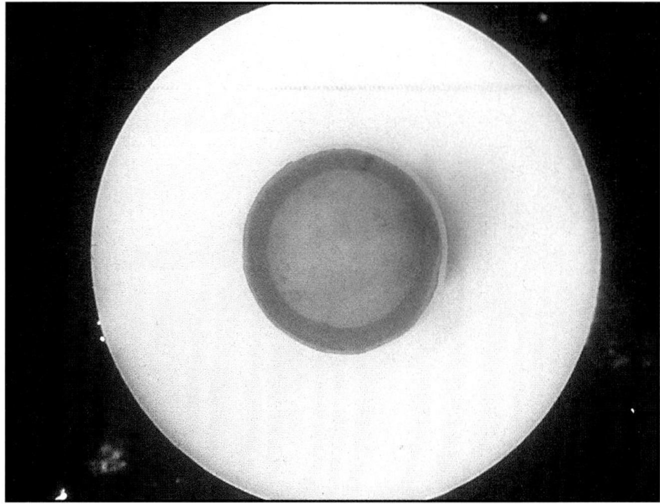

Figure 3-7.
Myopic lenticle.

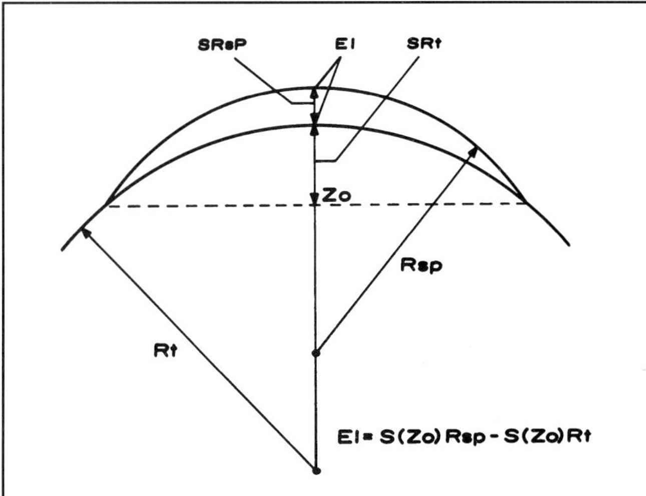

Figure 3-8.
Positive resection lenticle for myopia correction. Formula of tissue resection.

disc is placed on the lathe and frozen while in rotary motion for 2 minutes, before the optical cutting is started. Once the procedure is completed, the lenticle is thawed in Ringer's solution and sutured back onto the corneal bed with uninterrupted, eight-pass, antitorsion sutures (Figure 3-6).

As a matter of explanation in refractive terms, the corneal resection with the microkeratome that has no optical power is called "disc"; after lathing and already with a dioptric power it is called "lenticle" (Figure 3-7).

The precalculated surgical action of resecting a positive lens is performed on the exposed parenchyma of the corneal disc. For myopia correction, the central cornea is thinned and the anterior surface is flattened, causing it to lose refractive power.

Geometry formulas are applied in order to calculate frozen keratomileusis, and the tissue to be resected is calculated on the basis of sagittal values. These include initial radii, final radii, base radii, cutting radii, optical zones, freezing contraction factors, etc. Hence the use of a computer to help with fast calculation and minimal error possibilities.

Figure 3-8 shows the formula for myopic keratomileusis.

Between 1970 and 1990, 2686 eyes were operated on. As expected, this was a period of constant change, and the results obtained, although difficult and tedious to analyze and describe, are very satisfactory and speak for themselves. The analysis of the results led to the conclusion that the ideal parameters were the following:

- Disc diameter: 7.00 to 7.25 mm
- Disc thickness: 300 to 350 µm
- Lenticle central thickness: 160 to 200 µm
- Optical zone: 5.0 to 6.0 mm for any degree of ametropia (Figures 3-9a and 3-9b)

The average values of the variables used for performing the freezing surgical technique were:

Preoperative

Correction diopters: -11.70 D
Spherical equivalent: -10.80 D
Corneal thickness: 550 µm
Axial length: 26.91 mm
Initial radius: 7.74 mm

TABLE 3-1

DISTRIBUTION OF INITIAL DEFECT

Myopia	Requested Diopters	No.	%
Medium-Low	-4.50 to -7.00	399	14.86
Medium-High	-7.01 to -12.00	1.255	46.72
High	-12.01 to -17.00	678	25.24
Very High	-17.01 or more	354	13.18
Total		**2.686**	**100.00**

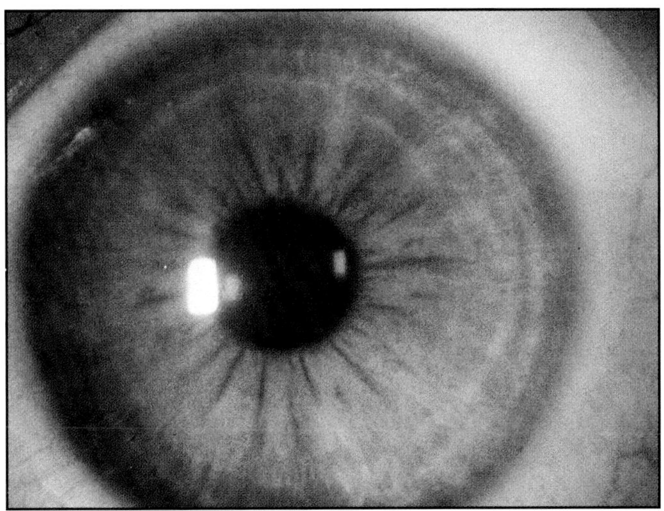

Figure 3-9a.
Frontal view of patient eye with myopic keratomileusis 15 years.

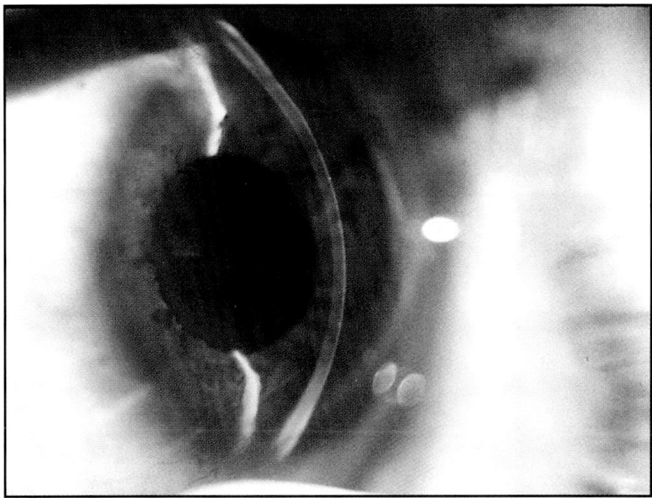

Figure 3-9b.
Slit lamp view of patient eye with myopic keratomileusis 15 years.

Intraoperative
Disc diameter: 7.27 ± 0.35 mm
Disc thickness: 300 ± 40 µm
Optical zone: 5.66 ± 0.58 mm
Final central thickness: 160 ± 50 µm
Freezing time: 120 seg
Resection thickness: 140 ± 50 µm

Initial Defect

According to the initial defect, 86.1% of patients had myopias above -7.01 D (Table 3-1).

Age and Sex

Of the total number of patients operated, 66.4% were females, 73.6% with ages between 15 to 35 years. The age range was 14 to 50 years.

Refractive Outcomes

Patients undergoing only myopic keratomileusis and who never were reoperated (1606 eyes) are the records we used for analyzing the percentage of correction and stability in time. There was loss of correction in all cases, but never down to the preoperative levels of ametropia (Figure 3-10 and Table 3-2). Corneas that went on to develop postoperative ectasia were considered deviant from normal corneal behavior, and more will be said about this under the section Complications.

Frozen keratomileusis used spherical lathing up until

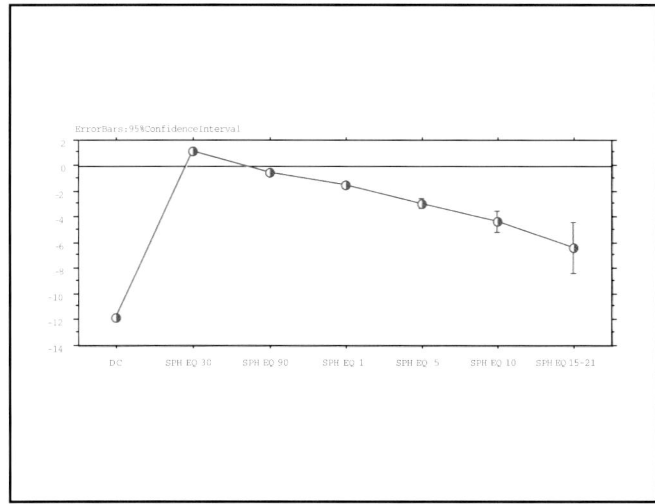

Figure 3-10.
Twenty-one years of evolution of the mean spherical equivalent (error bars: 95% confidence interval). There is a loss of correction with time.

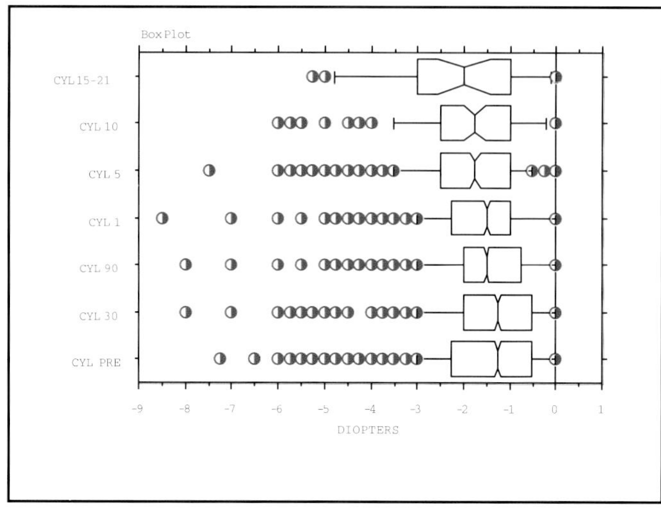

Figure 3-11.
Box plot. Cylinder evolution. The frozen myopic keratomileusis technique was being performed in spherical lathes. There was no astigmatic correction.

TABLE 3-2

Results of Myopic Keratomileusis

Pure Myopic Keratomileusis 1-Year Postoperative (938 eyes)

Spherical equivalent between	± 0.50 D	223 eyes	24%
	± 1.00 D	325 eyes	35%
	± 2.00 D	548 eyes	58%
	± 2.25 D	586 eyes	62%
	± 2.50 D	619 eyes	66%

Pure Myopic Keratomileusis 5-Years Postoperative (445 eyes)

Spherical equivalent between	± 0.50 D	68 eyes	15%
	± 1.00 D	110 eyes	25%
	± 2.00 D	197 eyes	44%
	± 2.25 D	218 eyes	48%
	± 2.50 D	238 eyes	53%

Pure Myopic Keratomileusis 10-Years Postoperative (99 eyes)

Spherical equivalent between	± 0.50 D	12 eyes	12%
	± 1.00 D	19 eyes	19%
	± 2.00 D	27 eyes	27%
	± 2.25 D	31 eyes	31%
	± 2.50 D	36 eyes	36%

Spherical equivalent in those patients who were never reoperated at 1, 5, and 10 years.

the 1980s, when the computerized lathe allowed the performance of parabolic cuts. Consequently, astigmatism was one of the residual defects influencing the refractive outcome (Figure 3-11).

The obtained correction improved with time, although it was always above 80% of the requested correction during the immediate postoperative period (Table 3-3). Efforts were made at simplifying and increasing predictability and stability of the results. This led to the establishment of relationships between depth, thickness, and diameter of the resections and correction stability (Figure 3-12).

The correction was found to be more predictable and stable when the resection was performed on the anterior corneal layers, that is, when leaving a central thickness of 160 to 200 µm after lathing, with a total minimal corneal thickness of two thirds the initial corneal thickness.

A relationship was found to exist among the optical zone diameter, stability, and visual quality, and for this reason we always worked with optical zones larger than 5.00 mm, with an average of 5.66 ± 0.58 mm in diameter.

Results showing a higher correlation coefficient were obtained with disc thickness ranging between 300 and 360 µm, in which 78.4% of the intended correction was maintained after 5 years with R2 = 0.64. The average of the central thickness of the lenticle was 180 µm (140 to 200) and the correlation between central thickness of the lenticle and achieved diopters at 5 years (R2 = 0.53) was significant, with P = < .001.

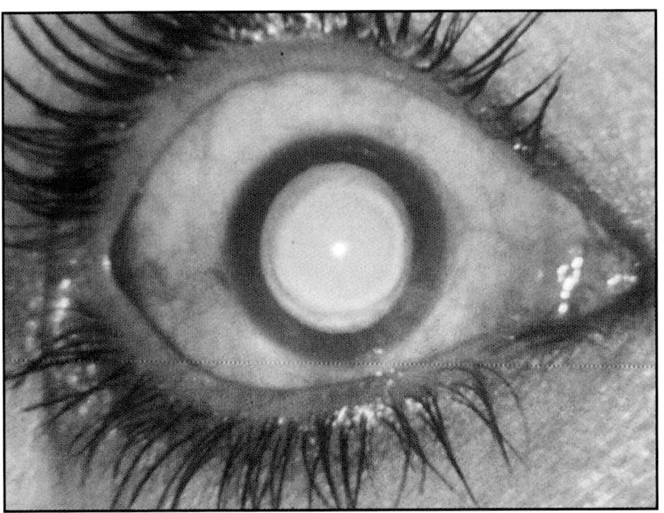

Figure 3-12.
Frontal view. Myopic keratomileusis with fundus reflex.

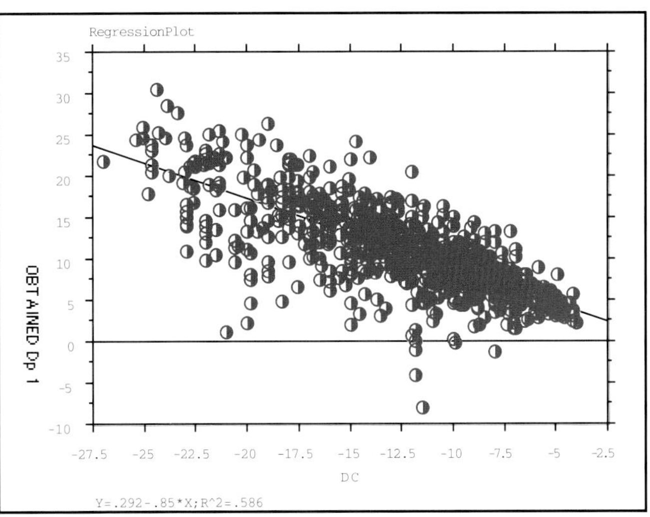

Figure 3-13.
Regression plot. Postoperative 1 year, myopic keratomileusis patients who were never reoperated.

TABLE 3-3

Percentage of Correction in Time According to the Computer Programs Developed

	COR 90		COR 1		COR 5		COR 10		COR 15	
Computer Program	*Mean*	*SD*	*Mean*	*SD*	*Mean*	*SD*	*Mean*	*SD*	*Mean*	*SD*
Olivetti	83.4	31.49	78.4	31.13	66.6	32.45	49.7	38.20	33.8	50.04
Texas Instruments 3180	99.8	29.16	88.8	36.04	74.4	34.47	90.9	32.34	44.9	48.87
Programs 80	100.5	22.93	91.1	23.31	87.5	27.53	66.0	39.01	—	—
Automatic (81 to 83)	86.5	33.34	83.7	32.43	65.0	48.89	56.2	23.18	—	—
Programs 84	102.2	19.48	92.0	20.03	79.2	29.63	—	—	—	—
Programs 86	94.6	20.95	84.3	23.75	68.5	30.74	—	—	—	—
Programs 87	91.1	26.51	83.0	28.18	77.6	28.42	—	—	—	—
Automatic (87-89-90)	95.4	27.44	91.2	20.36	86.4	9.68	—	—	—	—
Total	**96.0**	**25.95**	**87.6**	**26.43**	**75.0**	**33.21**	**63.4**	**38.21**	**35.7**	**49.19**

The statistical analysis began in 1991. Also noteworthy is the loss of correction with time.

A relationship among age, refractive outcomes, and long-term stability was determined. Patients who underwent myopic keratomileusis only and who were never reoperated showed that the older the age, the more stable the correction. In 1986, a correction factor was introduced into the programs on the basis of the refraction index used in the calculations.

This factor varies according to the age of the patient.

Fx 1.3 when n = 1.376

Fx = 1.3 for people under 30 years
= 1.2 over 30 years
= 1.1 over 40 years
= 1.0 over 50 years
= 0.9 over 60 years

TABLE 3-4

Percentage of Correction According to Age

	COR 90		COR 1		COR 5		COR 10		COR 15-21	
Age (years)	*Average*	*SD*	*Average*	*SD*	*Average*	*SD*	*Average*	*SD*	*Average*	*SD*
14 or under	93.1	31.1	83.8	35.7	60.9	35.8	46.0	41.4	14.8	44.1
15 to 24	95.2	24.4	85.3	24.3	67.7	29.9	53.4	41.6	38.8	30.0
25 to 34	98.5	24.7	85.9	24.9	70.1	36.0	59.3	20.5	32.6	30.4
35 to 44	98.5	26.7	85.5	30.1	78.1	26.5	78.0	48.9	76.4	22.5
45 or over	98.6	41.6	92.9	30.4	90.7	23.3	—	—	—	—
Total	**96.3**	**26.3**	**85.3**	**26.9**	**68.4**	**33.2**	**53.4**	**39.5**	**22.6**	**41.2**

The best stability is found in patients older than 35 years.

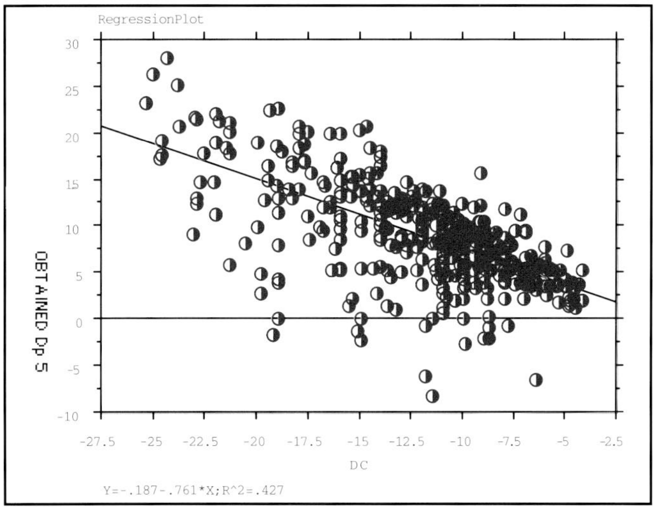

Figure 3-14.
Regression plot. Postoperative 5 years, myopic keratomileusis patients who were never reoperated.

Despite the correction factor, results show better correction and stability in older patients (Table 3-4).

Correlation coefficients between requested and achieved diopters for the group of patients operated only once were as follows:

30 days = R2 0.679
90 days = R2 0.646
1 year = R2 0.589 (Figure 3-13)
5 years = R2 0.437 (Figure 3-14)
10 years = R2 0.411
21 years = R2 0.106

having a very low significance the 21 year coefficients, due to myopia progression and the smaller number of patients analyzed.

Visual Acuity

As a whole, uncorrected visual acuity improved significantly in all patients during the first 5 years and remained stable in time. Not so the best corrected vision, which never recovered the preoperative averages (Figures 3-15a and 3-15b). Controls at 10 and 21 years are not very reliable because of the reduction in patient numbers (Table 3-5).

Ninety-four percent of the patients showed on average a 4 Snellen line gain on the uncorrected visual acuity during the first postoperative year. Best corrected vision remained the same as the preoperative or was better in 60% of cases, whereas 40% had lost two or more lines.

Five years into the postoperative period, uncorrected vision was maintained with a noticeable gain—three lines on average in 98% of patients (Figures 3-16a and 3-16b), although 64% showed a loss of best corrected visual acuity by one or more lines, owing to the progression of myopia (Figures 3-17a and 3-17b).

The group of patients was divided into five subgroups according to requested diopters, as follows:

-2.05 D to -5.90 D, 101 eyes
-6.00 D to -9.90 D, 533 eyes
-10.00 D to -15.90 D, 648 eyes
-16.00 D to -19.90 D, 196 eyes
-20.00 D to -25.00 D, 126 eyes

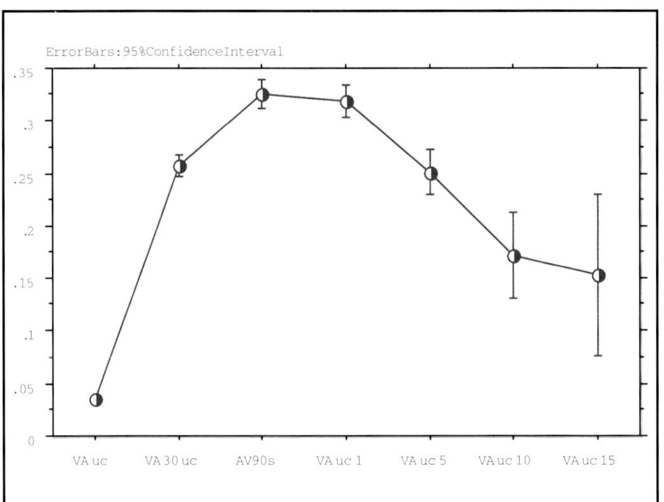

Figure 3-15a.
Line plot showing the mean uncorrected visual acuity in different stages of the postoperative. The confidence interval clearly shows low value at 21 years. Vision decreases with myopia progression.

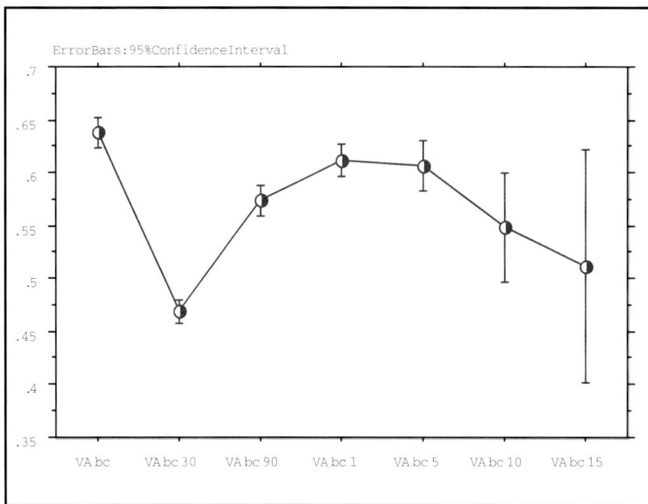

Figure 3-15b.
Line plot showing the mean best corrected visual acuity.

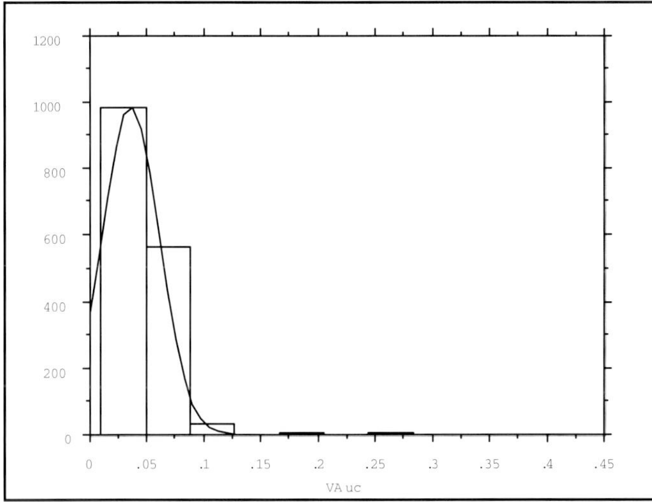

Figure 3-16a.
Uncorrected visual acuity. One hundred percent of eyes had less than 0.10 (20/200).

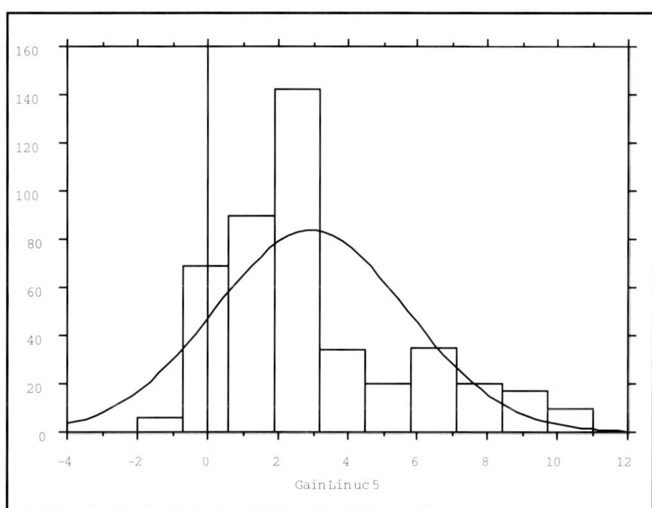

Figure 3-16b.
At 5 years, the Snellen line gain shows a mean gain of three lines.

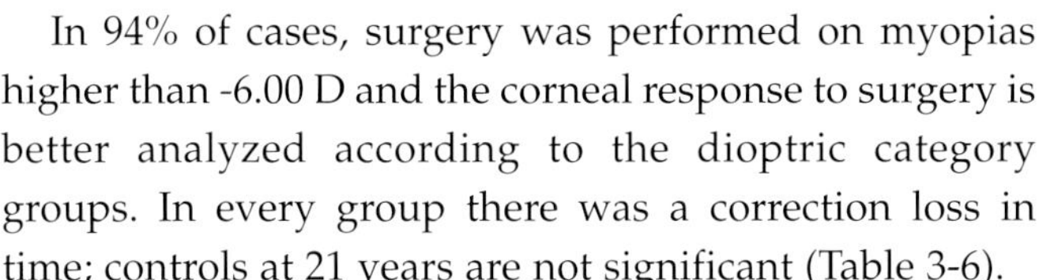

In 94% of cases, surgery was performed on myopias higher than -6.00 D and the corneal response to surgery is better analyzed according to the dioptric category groups. In every group there was a correction loss in time; controls at 21 years are not significant (Table 3-6).

The calculation programs were modified according to the results obtained in small series. A total of 17 programs for myopia correction were developed in the course of 20 years. Patients were regrouped considering the similarities among some programs and their use in just a few patients (Table 3-7).

The descriptive analysis was made by arranging the results by groups of programs of a single series, whose nomenclatures reflect the various years of evolution. From the scientific standpoint, we thought it was the only way to compare results, considering the differences derived from improvements in each of the groups as time passed.

Radii Behavior According to the Calculation Program

These radii were measured with the Zeiss keratometer; as we have already understood, these instruments take average measurements of a central area that is larger in

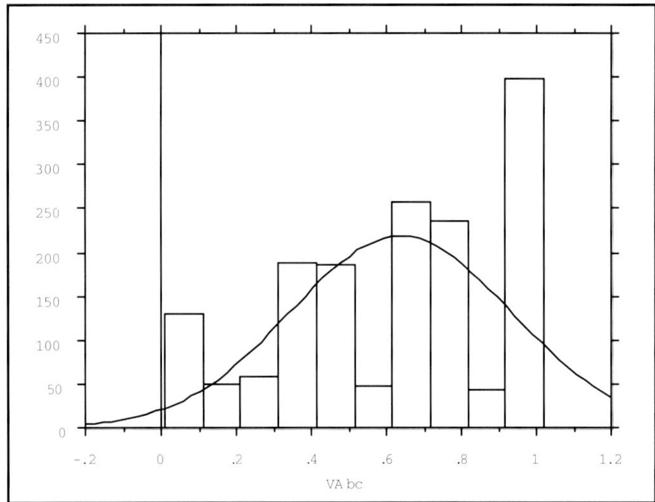

Figure 3-17a.
Best corrected visual acuity shows a normal distribution with a mean of 0.67 (20/30) preoperatively.

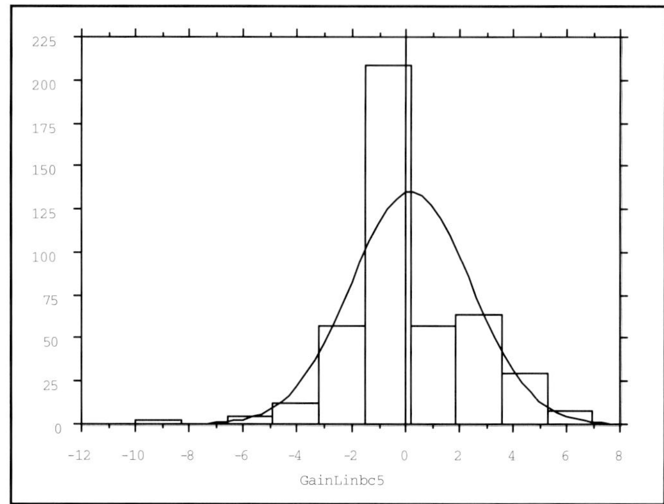

Figure 3-17b.
At 5 years, the Snellen line gain shows a normal distribution with a mean that explains no gain of vision, but there are a few cases with loss of more than one line.

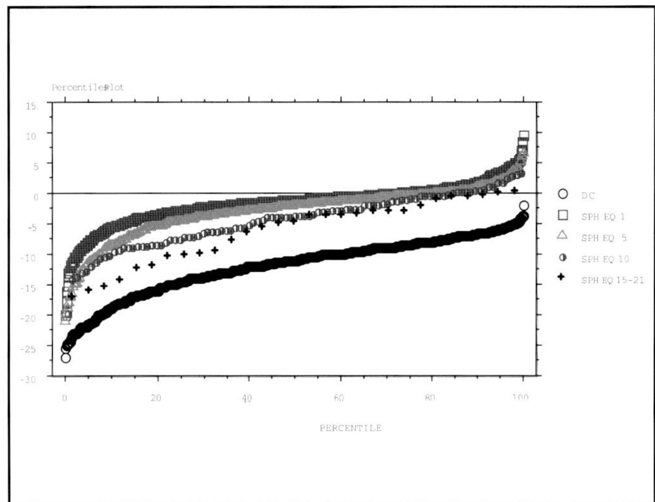

Figure 3-18.
Percentile plot. Stability of correction does not exist in myopic eyes.

TABLE 3-5

RANGE OF VISUAL ACUITY

	Preoperative		1 Year		5 Years	
	UC%	*BC%*	*UC%*	*BC%*	*UC%*	*BC%*
20/200	100	3.01	18.53	1.09	29.95	2.04
20/80		17.98	46.70	16.97	44.82	14.74
20/40		38.35	28.34	51.14	21.85	51.02
20/25		17.48	3.52	18.17	2.48	18.37
20/20		23.18	1.51	12.62	0.90	13.83

There is a maintained improvement in uncorrected and best corrected vision up to 5 years postoperatively. There is a decrease in best corrected vision at 1 and 5 years.

flattening surgeries giving in consequence a less accurate measurement. The cornea steepened in all patients as time elapsed with all programs (Table 3-8). The steepening is a loss of correction cause, but we were unable to determine reliably to what extent it serves as an explanation of the manifest myopic progression observed in all patients.

Axial Growth of the Eyeball

Eyeball growth analysis based on the measurement of the axial length was difficult considering the inconsistencies of clinical history data:

- Technological changes in 20 years led to the use of various instruments for measuring axial lengths.
- Many different operators performed measurements in the course of 20 years.
- Patient examinations show inaccurate objective data directly affecting the results obtained.

In view of these difficulties, a simple regression was applied between vertex diopters and axial length preoperatively, in order to obtain new adjusted values for preoperative axial length. The next step was to relate cases of axial length at 3 years postoperatively with the initial axial length, using a simple regression which revealed a

TABLE 3-6

Category Groups According to Intended Diopters

	1 Year				5 Years			10 Years		
Category Groups	*Preop Sph Eq*	*Obtained D*	*UCVA*	*BCVA*	*Obtained D*	*UCVA*	*BCVA*	*Obtained D*	*UCVA*	*BCVA*
-2.05 to -5.90	-4.98	4.77	0.52	0.86	3.76	0.42	0.9	3.00	0.46	0.98
-6.00 to -9.90	-7.50	7.18	0.41	0.74	6.27	0.14	0.72	4.40	0.12	0.63
-10.00 to -15.90	-11.72	11.06	0.27	0.52	9.33	0.23	0.55	7.64	0.18	0.51
-16.00 to -19.90	-16.31	15.54	0.2	0.43	13.02	0.16	0.44	12.31	0.14	0.44
-20.00 to -27.00	-20.21	19.32	0.21	0.44	17.98	0.18	0.45	16.00	0.11	0.45

TABLE 3-7

Calculation Programs Regrouped

Olivetti	234 eyes
Texas Instruments 3180	170 eyes
Programs 3280-3380	261 eyes
Programs 4284-24284-246841-246840	972 eyes
Programs (Auto 82-83)	313 eyes
Programs (Auto 87-89-90)	220 eyes
Programs 862-863	173 eyes
Programs 871-872-876-8750	324 eyes
Without information	19 eyes

0.78 mm growth coefficient for those 3 years, with significance for P =.0001.

Stability

Spherical equivalent percentiles were compared in order to find the correction stability during the postoperative period (Figure 3-18). They showed undercorrection in 60% of the cases at 1 year, and increasing loss of correction with every control up to 21 years. The loss of correction is consistent in time, thus confirming the myopic progression.

Therefore, there are factors such as age and axial growth that are responsible for myopic evolution. Moreover, we also found progressive corneal steepening in all cases, which can be explained on the basis of surgical technique, biomechanical consequences related to the corneal thinning, and/or chronic trauma to the cornea. What is the influence of each of these elements on the final stability of myopic correction? There are no answers to this question.

Complications

Without forgetting all those mechanical, relevant errors that happened in those early years, the most interesting complication and useful to analyze a corneal response that we could not easily explain at the beginning is "corneal ectasia."

This occurred in 45 of the 1606 operated eyes. We analyzed the problem and observed a relationship between ectasia and preoperatively steep corneas. At that time, and without having found any scientific explanation, it was decided to avoid refractive surgery in corneas steeper than 7.4-mm radius. The development of corneal topography has shown us the existence of subclinical keratoconus, and during the frozen myopic keratomileusis statistical study, we could demonstrate in the early keratographies an important incidence of subclinical conus in those eyes that underwent corneal ectasia after myopic keratomileusis.

At the same time, clinical postoperative observa-

TABLE 3-8

Average Corneal Radius of Curvature

	Initial	Requested	30 D	90 D	3 to 12 m	5 Years	10 Years	21 Years
Olivetti	7.6	9.7	9.0	8.7	8.8	8.6	8.6	8.5
Texas Instruments 3180	7.8	10.4	9.5	9.3	9.5	9.0	9.1	8.8
Programs 80	7.8	11.0	10.0	9.8	9.6	9.4	8.8	—
Automatic (81 to 83)	7.7	10.3	9.5	9.2	9.1	8.9	8.6	—
Programs 84	7.7	10.2	9.7	9.3	9.2	8.9	—	—
Programs 86	7.7	9.8	9.2	9.0	8.8	8.6	—	—
Programs 87	7.7	10.0	9.4	8.9	8.8	8.9	—	—
Automatic (87-89-90)	7.8	10.3	9.6	9.3	9.2	9.1	—	—
Total	**7.7**	**10.2**	**9.5**	**9.2**	**9.1**	**8.9**	**8.6**	**8.6**

tion led to another conclusion: very deep resections of the disc led to undercorrections and thick tissue resections led to postoperative thin corneas and subsequent ectasia. With that concept in mind, the lenticle thickness at the center was limited by the computer program to 120 µm, never thinner; the 6.0-mm optical zone was reduced to 5.0 mm to reduce the depth of resection, and the microkeratome plate was recommended to be 300 µm in myopic surgery.

After radial keratotomy (RK) experience, another clinical observation led us to conclude that ectasia in many cases is due to chronic corneal trauma (eye rubbing).

FROZEN HYPEROPIC KERATOMILEUSIS

Surgical correction of hyperopia as an autoplastic intervention, namely, freeze hyperopic keratomileusis, was developed after keratophakia and myopia correction. It was a slow development because of the modifications required in order to obtain a stable correction. The resection of a negative lenticle of greater thickness at the edge created a peripheral step that gave rise to instability and epithelialization of the disc edge because of poor coadaptation. Eventually, after smoothing the curve on the periphery of the optical zone, it was possible to attain an adequate readaptation of the anterior corneal layers to the desired curvature, with long-term stability.

The geometric elements that must be taken into account in order to solve the formula of freeze hyperopic correction are: the requested diopters to correct, the thickness and diameter of the disc obtained with the microkeratome, the diameter of the desired optical zone, and the thickness of the intersection zone. This latter thickness is the lowest that must remain in the maximum resection area at the periphery. (It is equivalent to the central thickness of the lenticle in myopia correction.) Resection thicknesses can be obtained with these elements (Figures 3-19 and 3-20).

This procedure is performed by resecting a corneal disc of parallel surfaces and predetermined diameter and thickness; consequently, it is optically neutral. The disc taken from the cornea to be operated comprises the epithelium, Bowman's layer, and part of the corneal parenchyma. It is placed on the lathe and frozen while in rotary motion for 2 minutes, before the optical cut is performed (Figure 3-21). Once the procedure is completed, the lenticle is thawed in Ringer's solution at 28° and sutured back onto the corneal bed with continuous, eight-pass, anti-torsion sutures.

The precalculated surgical action of resecting a nega-

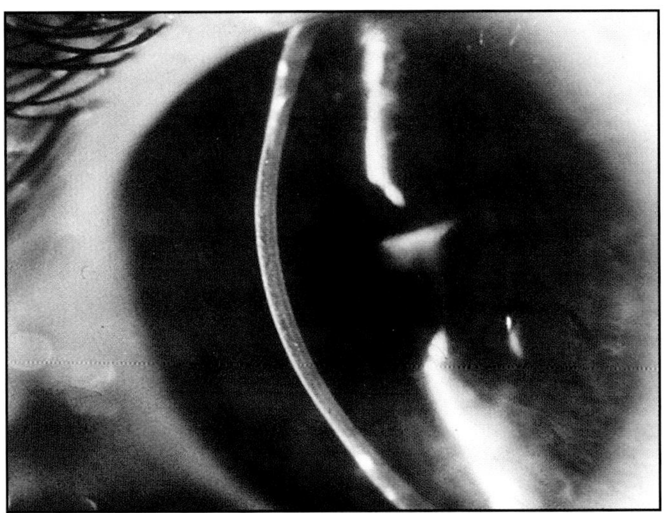

Figure 3-19.
Frontal view of hyperopic keratomileusis.

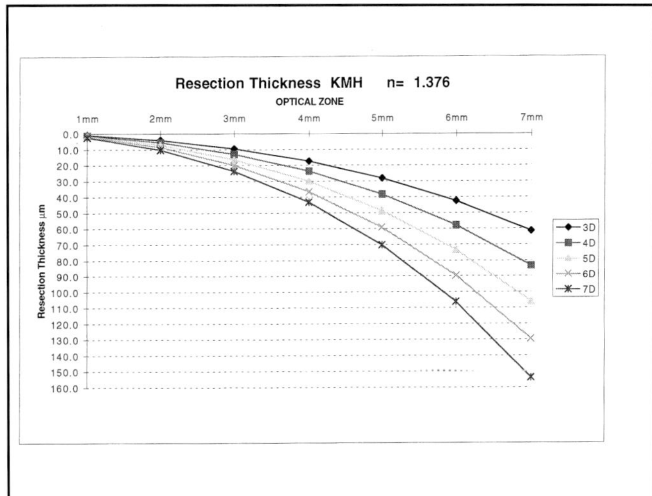

Figure 3-20.
Resection thickness hyperopic keratomileusis. Shows the amount of resection needed (calculated with refractive index 1.376), according to the diameter of the optical zone, for the correction of 3, 4, 5, 6, and 7 D of hyperopia.

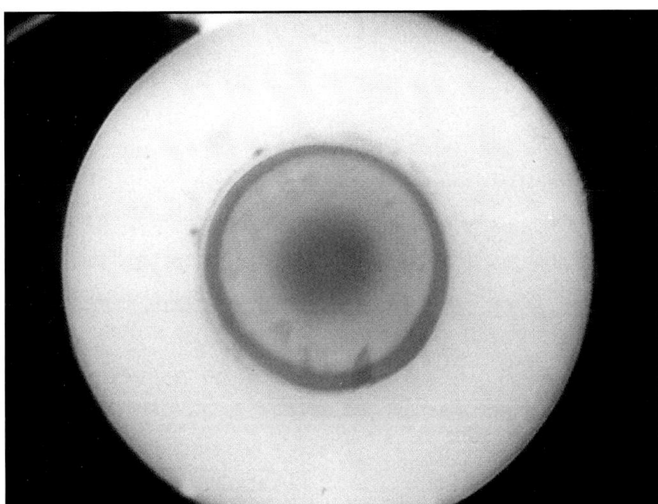

Figure 3-21.
Frontal view. Positive lenticle to correct hyperopia.

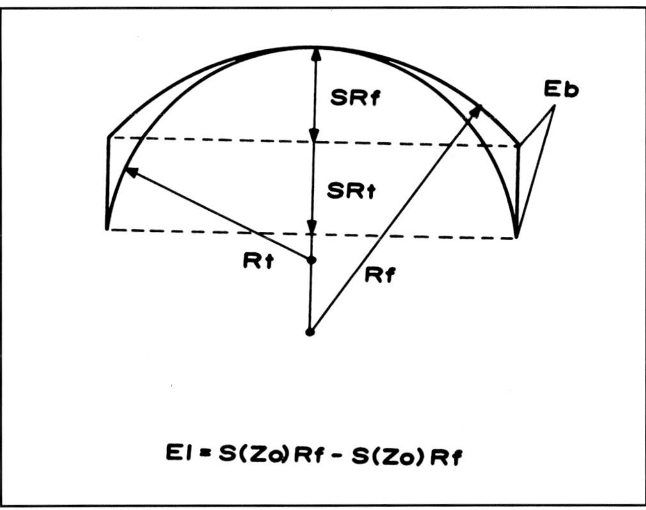

Figure 3-22.
Negative resection that has to be performed at the corneal periphery to correct hyperopia. The resection formula is written.

tive lens is performed on the exposed parenchyma of the corneal disc. For hyperopia correction, the peripheral cornea is thinned and the anterior surface steepens, causing an increase in refractive power.

The formula for hyperopic keratomileusis is shown in Figure 3-22.

Hyperopic keratomileusis started in 1976. Seventeen computer programs had been developed up until 1994, the last one in 1988. During this period, 1550 eyes were operated.

Retrospective analysis led to the conclusion that the ideal parameters were the following:

- Diameter of the disc: 8.25 to 8.50 mm
- Disc thickness: 360 to 490 µm
- Intersection zone: 140 to 160 µm
- Optical zone: 5.85 to 6.50 mm for any degree of ametropia.

We made a statistical analysis of 126 eyes with a 5-year follow-up that were performed following the ideal parameters. In this group of patients, the averages for the most important variables in congenital hyperopia were:

TABLE 3-9A

Spherical Equivalent Dioptric Defect

Hyperopia	Spherical Equivalent (D)	No.	%
Medium-Low	1.50 to 3.50	4	3.18
Medium-High	3.50 to 5.50	41	32.54
High	5.50 to 7.50	58	46.03
Very High	7.50 to 9.50	23	18.25
Total		**126**	**100.00**

TABLE 3-9B

Vertex Requested Diopters

Hyperopia	Vertex Requested (D)	No.	%
Medium-Low	4.00 to 5.75	4	3.18
Medium-High	5.75 to 7.50	47	37.30
High	7.50 to 9.25	54	42.85
Very High	9.25 to 11.00	21	16.66
Total		**126**	**100.00**

Preoperative

Spherical equivalent: 6.029 ± 1.64 D
Initial radius: 7.91 ± 0.24 mm
Corneal thickness: 560 ± 0.03 µm
Axial length: 20.64 ± 0.77 mm

Intraoperative

Requested diopters: 7.79 ± 1.34 D
Disc thickness: 430 ± 46 µm
Disc diameter: 8.30 ± 0.153 mm
Optic zone: 6.47 ± 0.56 mm
Intersection zone: 140 ± 10 µm
Resection thickness: 290 ± 50 µm

Initial Defect

The average spherical equivalent was 6.029, with a range between 1.50 and 9.25 D (Table 3-9a), but requested correction diopters were more than 4.00 D in 100% of cases (Table 3-9b). The calculation for resection was done by multiplying the requested vertex diopters by an increase factor of 2.01 in order to achieve the desired correction.

Age and Sex

Of a total of 126 eyes, 75.0% were patients between 16 and 37 years of age, with ages ranging from 8 to 50 years. Only 36.7% were females.

Refractive Outcome

Twelve months after surgery, achieved diopters were 5.606 D (0.375 to 11.750 D) with an average spherical equivalent of 0.44 ± 1.98 D (-6.00 to 6.00 D) (Figures 3-23 and 3-24). At 5 years, obtained diopters were 5.055 D (-0.50 to 9.250 D), with an average postoperative spherical equivalent of 1.44 ± 1.96 D (-2.25 to 5.87 D).

At 12 months, 60% of cases were between ± 1.50 D and 90% of cases between ± 3.00 D. At 5 years, 72.5% of cases were at ± 2.00 D with a tendency to hyperopia.

Passage of time (Figure 3-25) revealed a loss of 1.50 correction diopters in 5 years, meaning that at the end of that period, patients retained 84% of their initial correction. (Figures 3-26a and 3-26b show an eye with hyperopic keratomileusis.)

Correction was analyzed by groups based on the requested diopters of correction.

Requested Diopters	Achieved Diopters 12 months	5 years
From 4.00 D to 7.75 D 5.18 (± 1.11)	5.22 (± 1.63)	4.22 (± 2.61)
From 8.00 D to 11.00 D 6.94 (± 1.27)	6.01 (± 2.14)	5.39 (± 2.04)

From 4.00 to 7.75 D (64 eyes): 70% of cases between ± 1.00 D and 90% of cases between ± 2.00 D at 5 years. From 8.00 to 11.00 D (61 eyes): 50% of cases between ± 1.00 D and 70% of cases between ± 2.00 D at 5 years.

Visual Acuity

The mean preoperative uncorrected and best corrected visual acuities were 0.22 (20/100) (0.02 to 1.00) and 0.65 (20/30) (0.02 to 1.00), respectively.

Uncorrected 0.37 (20/55) (0.02 to 1.00) and best corrected 0.56 (20/35) (0.02 to 1.00) at 12 months. Uncorrected 0.32 (20/60) (0.08 to 0.80) and best corrected

TABLE 3-10

Visual Acuity in Category Dioptric Groups

	Preoperative		Postoperative			
			12 Months		5 Years	
	UC	BC	UC	BC	UC	BC
From 4.00 D to 7.75 D (64 eyes)	0.27	0.65	0.35	0.57	0.33	0.56
From 8.00 D to 11.00 D (61 eyes)	0.16	0.65	0.38	0.53	0.32	0.58

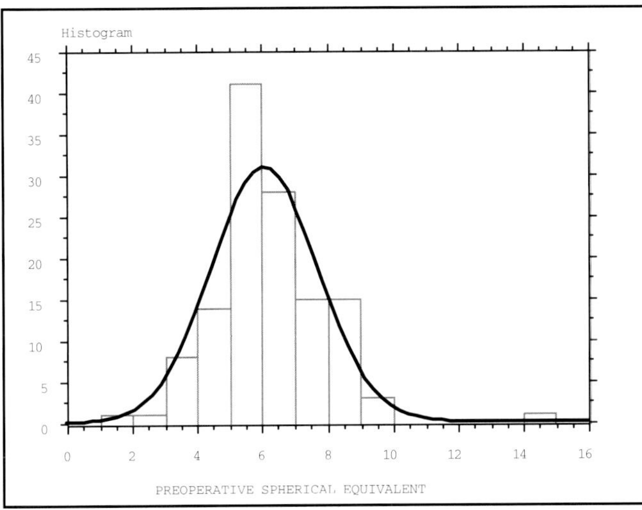

Figure 3-23.
Preoperative distribution of hyperopic spherical equivalent.

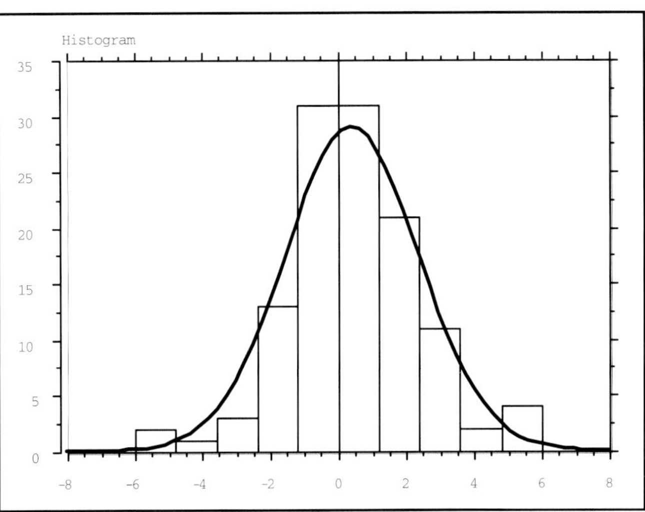

Figure 3-24.
Postoperative distribution of hyperopic spherical equivalent (12 months).

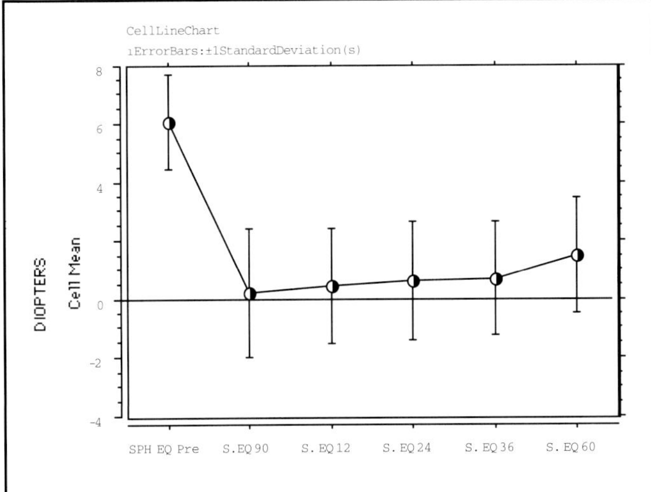

Figure 3-25.
Evolution shows a loss of 1.50 D of correction in 5 years. At the end of this period, the patients maintained 83.84% from the initial achieved correction.

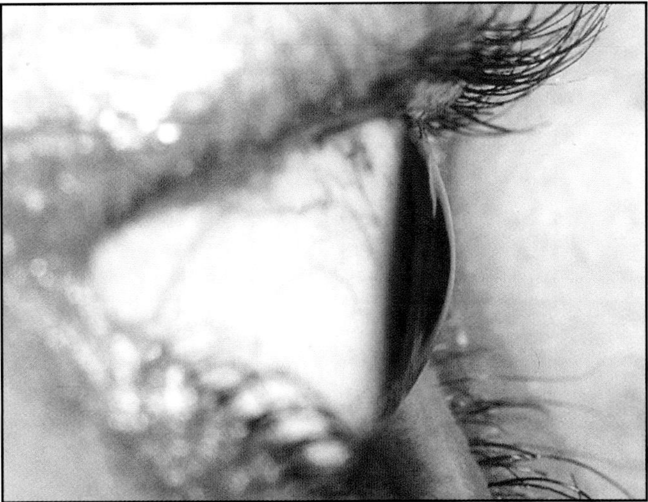

Figure 3-26a.
Lateral view of an eye with hyperopic keratomileusis.

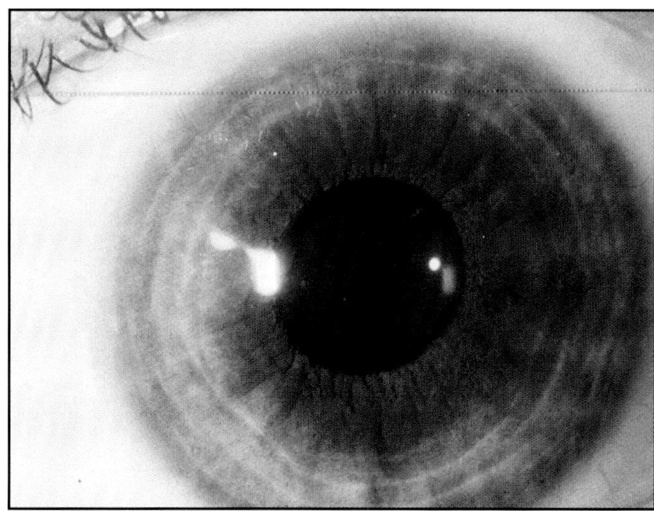

Figure 3-26b.
Frontal view of an eye with hyperopic keratomileusis.

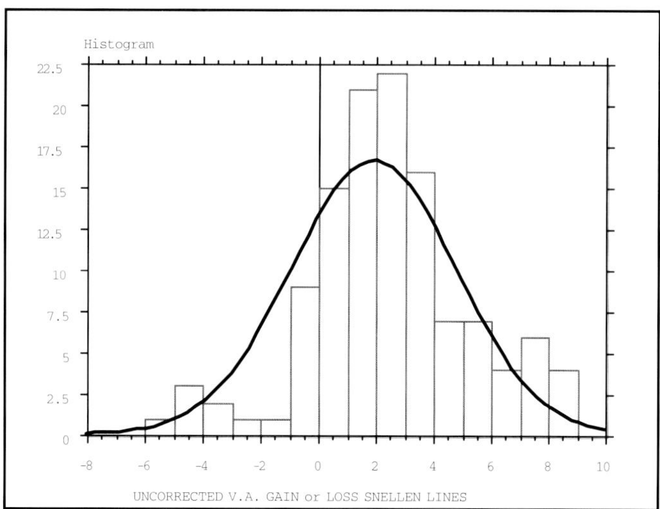

Figure 3-27a.
Gain or loss in Snellen lines of uncorrected visual acuity at 1 year.

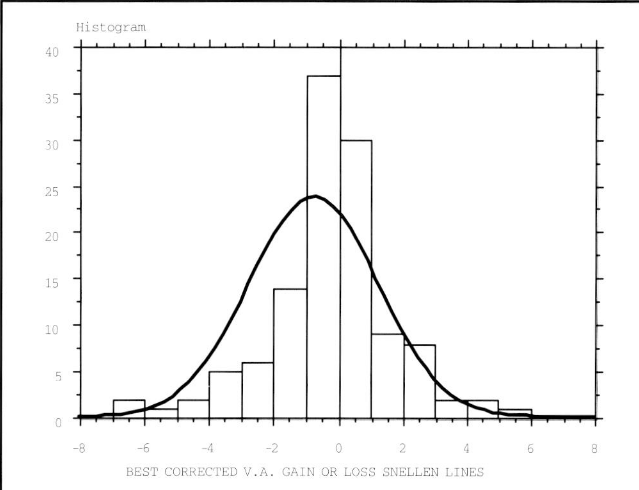

Figure 3-27b.
Gain or loss in Snellen lines of best corrected visual acuity at 1 year.

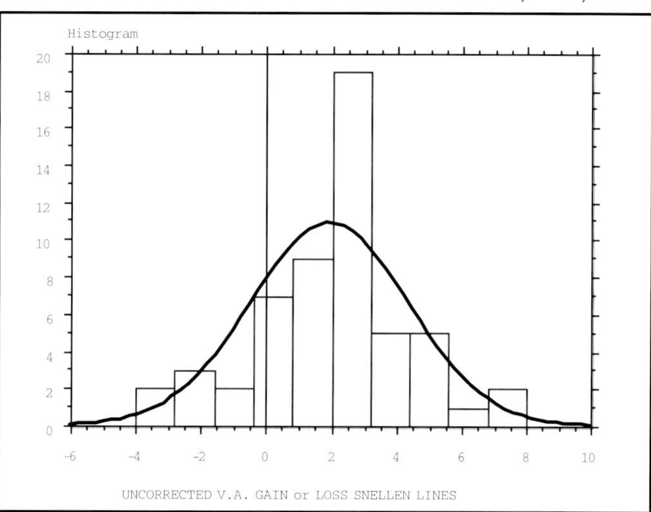

Figure 3-28a.
Gain or loss in Snellen lines of uncorrected visual acuity at 5 years.

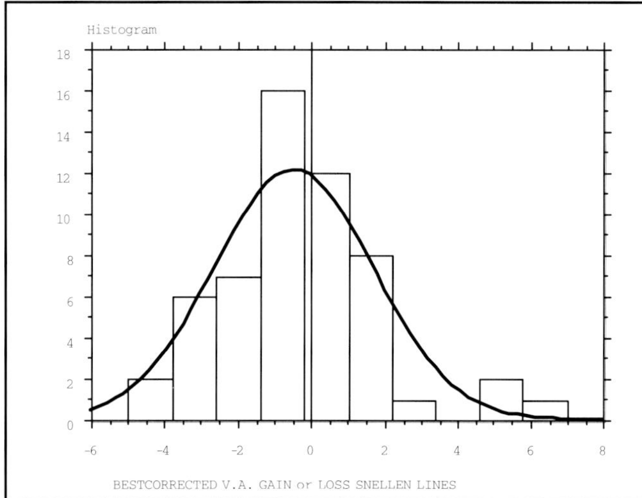

Figure 3-28b.
Gain or loss in Snellen lines of best corrected visual acuity at 5 years.

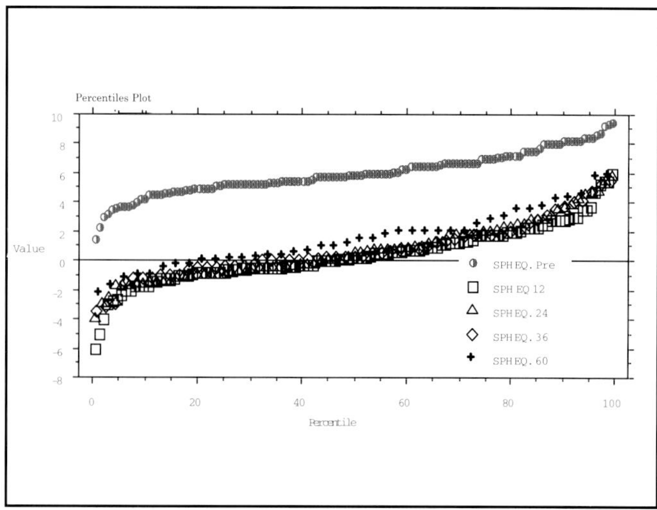

Figure 3-29.
Stability of correction. The coincidence of the achieved spherical equivalent percentiles for each period of time is observed.

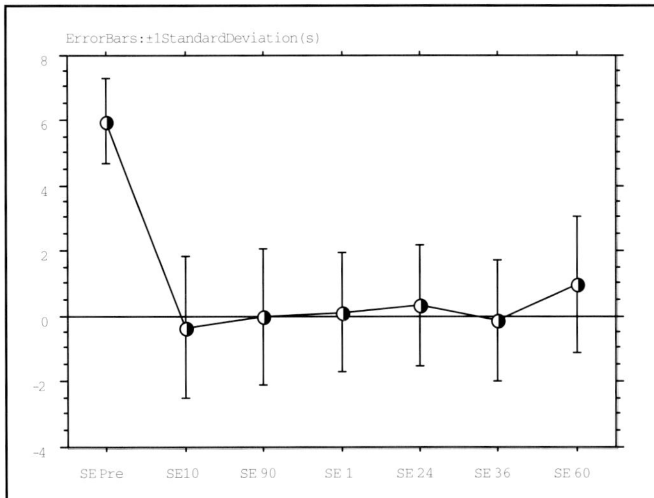

Figure 3-30a.
Program 1-88, computerized lathe. Results at 5 years postoperative evolution. Comparison of the results with two different lathes.

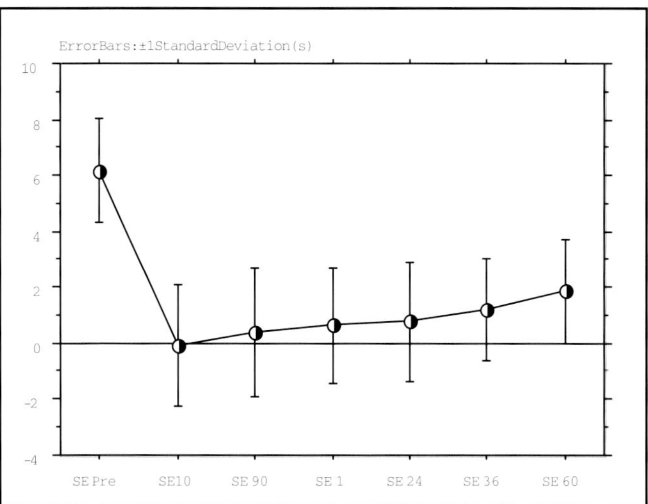

Figure 3-30b.
Program 42-84, turbine lathe. Results at 5 years postoperative evolution. Comparison of the results with two different lathes.

0.57 (20/35) (0.10 to 1.00) at 5 years. Seventy-five percent of uncorrected eyes gained two or more lines of vision, and this gain was maintained for 5 years. Sixty-five percent of the corrected eyes lost lines of vision, 35% losing one line and 30% two or more at 12 months. At 4 years, 46% of eyes maintained their loss of lines, 13% with a loss of one line, and 33% two or more (Figures 3-27a through 3-28b).

The absence of astigmatic correction together with involuntary decentrations of the disc resection or of the optic cut in relation to the patient's visual axis were the main causes found clinically to explain these visual results.

Visual acuity by group of requested diopters was similar to the previous results (Table 3-10).

Stability

Spherical equivalent percentiles of whole group were compared in order to find the correction stability during the postoperative period (Figure 3-29). They showed consistency in time, thus confirming its stability. The 2.0 D interval in the overall results between the 15th and 80th percentiles was maintained through time, and the loss of 1.0 D in achieved correction, remained stable between the first and fifth years.

As of 1988, the computerized lathe contributed to a further improvement of the results (Figures 3-30a and 3-30b). Result comparisons clearly reflect technological improvements in time, and were especially favorable for the computerized lathe.

Complications

- Intraoperative: These complications were associated with disc resection and the use of the microkeratome, carving on the lathe, and disc suturing.
- Postoperative: Alterations of the corneal epithelium (spiral keratitis) from the action of the upper lid as a result of excess steepening because of the failure of the tarsus to adapt to the new corneal curvature. Best visual results are obtained with final radii not steeper than 6.00 mm.
- Inclusion epithelial cysts in the interphase: in hyperopia, these are always found at the periphery, in the resection area.
- Residual and/or induced astigmatism due to decentering of the disc resection or the optic cut.
- Undercorrection due to inadequate disc thickness for the desired correction.

References

1. Barraquer JI. *Cirugia Refractiva de la córnea*. Bogotá, Colombia: Instituto Barraquer de América; 1989.

SECTION 2

LASIK HISTOLOGY

Chapter 4

INTRASTROMAL EXCIMER LASER—CORNEAL INTERACTION

Michael C. Knorz, MD, Holger K. Steiner, MD, Bettina B. Wiesinger, MD

Of the many different refractive surgical procedures that have evolved in the past century,[1] excimer laser corneal treatment holds the greatest promise to achieve accurate and predictable refractive results. This is because the laser can theoretically create any anterior radius of curvature in the central cornea by removing very small amounts of tissue without significantly changing the biomechanics of the cornea. There are two major areas that must be developed and controlled for excimer laser treatment of the cornea to be successful: technical aspects of the laser and delivery system and biological responses of the cornea. In contrast to the histological changes after photorefractive keratectomy (PRK), little is known about alterations associated with laser in situ keratomileusis (LASIK). In addition to experimental results from pig and human cadaver eyes, we also had the opportunity to investigate the corneal changes 1 week after LASIK was performed on human patients.

HISTOLOGY IN PRK

The fascination of the excimer laser is the minimal thermal energy effect produced by the 193-nm wavelength that limits the degree of collateral damage to the surrounding tissue and provides the characteristic smooth ablation surface. Minimal disruption of the lasered bed is observed with a well-contoured surface,[2] but PRK treatment of the anterior corneal stroma causes a modified healing process by

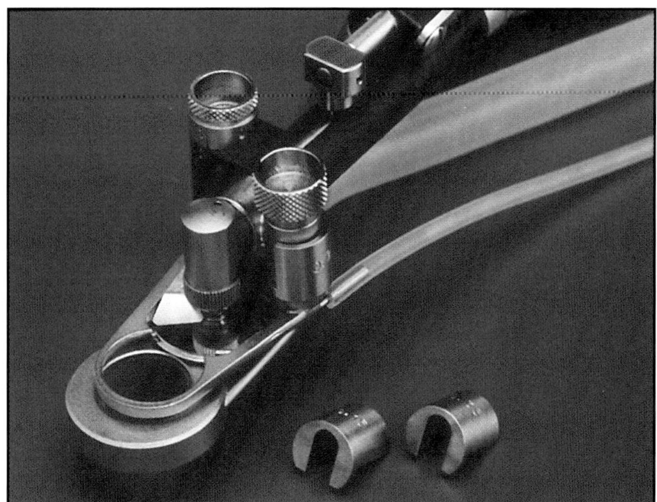

Figure 4-1.
The Draeger keratome, rotating blade.

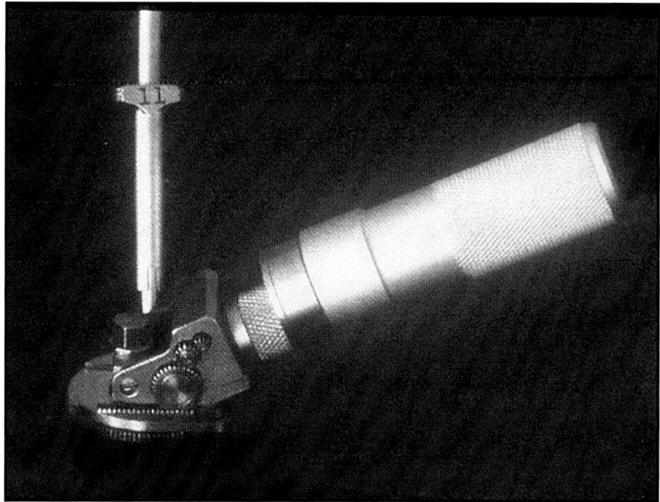

Figure 4-2.
The Ruiz keratome, oscillating blade.

expression of different collagens[3,4] as well as a transient thickening of the epithelium and hypercellularity in the anterior stroma.[4,5] There is a marked reduction in the number of keratocytes and presence of damaged keratocytes in the anterior 40 µm of the stroma. One can also find discontinuity of the basement membrane which is typically seen with an epithelial healing over bare stroma.[6] Irregularities in the basal epithelial cells, increased numbers of fibroblasts, and production of extracellular matrix cause light scattering and corneal haze.[7] The loss of Bowman's layer during PRK treatment is probably responsible for this reaction. The severity is dependent on several factors including ablation rate, repetition rate, repeated PRK treatments on the same eye, and other case-dependent variables.

HISTOPATHOLOGICAL AND ULTRASTRUCTURAL FINDINGS IN LASIK

Mechanical Alterations

LASIK is the combination of a surgical technique, which is the cutting of a hinged corneal flap with a microkeratome, followed by an intrastromal laser treatment. The intrastromal application of the excimer laser enables the refractive surgeon to correct even high myopia without removal of Bowman's layer. Looking at histopathological findings of the cornea after excimer laser treatment, one can find changes due to laser treatment combined with mechanical alterations due to the use of a microkeratome.

We investigated the histological changes in human eyes after LASIK as well as the effect of different keratomes on the quality of the stromal surface in pig corneas.

Keratotomies on 10 consecutive pig eyes were performed using the Draeger (rotating blade, Figure 4-1) and the Ruiz keratomes (oscillating blade, Figure 4-2). In another instance, 12 pig eyes received, a keratotomy done with either the Draeger or Ruiz keratome first, and then a laser ablation was performed. After fixation, light and scanning electron microscopy (SEM) were performed.

The use of a microkeratome and cutting the corneal flap led to characteristic changes. In light microscopy, the structure of the stromal collagen of the lenticle was more undulating (Figure 4-3), probably due to the turning of the lenticle and an increased dehydration in the exposed position. This also led to a minimal, step-like epithelial layer (see Figure 4-3) at the lenticle rim. We believe that these changes are temporary and therefore do not have a lasting effect on optic quality.

SEM revealed no differences of the corneal surface using the different keratomes, but characteristic keratotomy-induced changes of the corneal surface could still be noticed. Wave-like ridges were found perpendicular to the sectional plane (Figures 4-4 and 4-5). The average distance between any two folds was 30 µm with an average

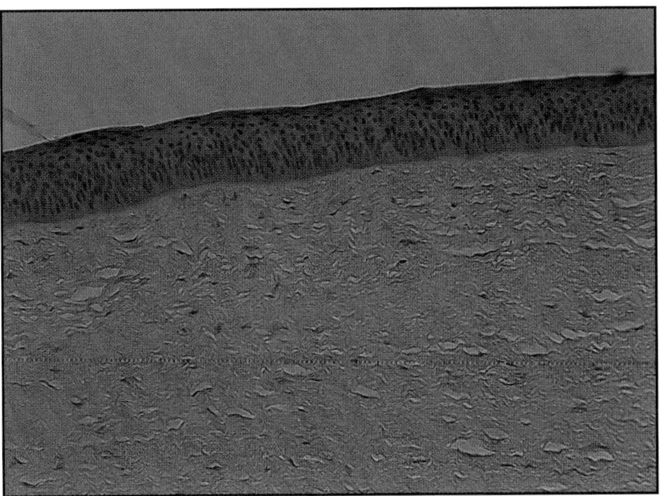

Figure 4-3.
Light microscopy, pig cornea. Microtome used for the first time. Stepwise epithelium at the lenticle rim. Plain cut through Bowman's layer. More pronounced distortion of lenticle collagens. No laser effects visible. Original magnification 120x.

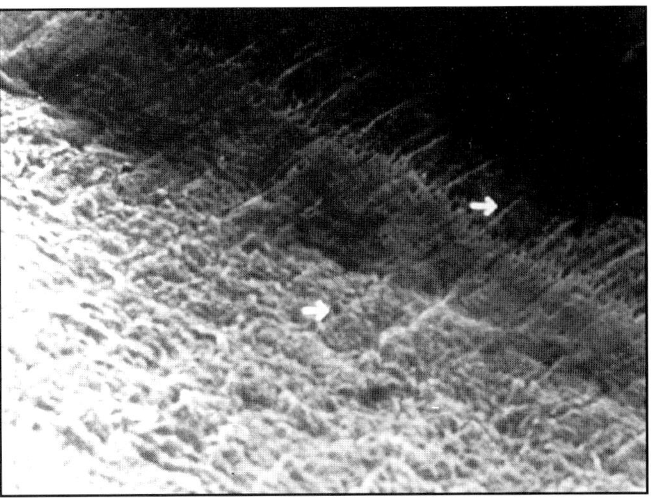

Figure 4-4.
SEM. Corneal surface at the lenticle rim. Perpendicular to the sectional plane typical ridges (arrowheads) by microtome movement (Ruiz keratome, oscillating blade). Original magnification 200x.

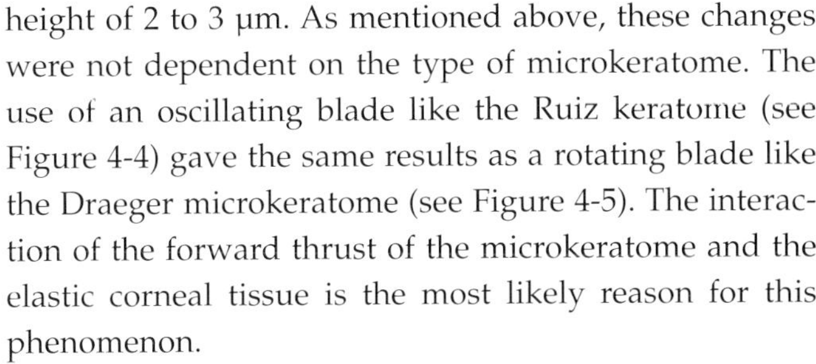

height of 2 to 3 µm. As mentioned above, these changes were not dependent on the type of microkeratome. The use of an oscillating blade like the Ruiz keratome (see Figure 4-4) gave the same results as a rotating blade like the Draeger microkeratome (see Figure 4-5). The interaction of the forward thrust of the microkeratome and the elastic corneal tissue is the most likely reason for this phenomenon.

Complete flattening of the ridges was obtained by laser treatment (Figure 4-6). Although these folds are still present on the back side of the lenticle surface, impairment of optical quality is unlikely. Present clinical data support this theory.

In further experiments, we showed that repeated use of a single blade as many as 10 times to create the corneal flap does not affect the quality of the corneal surface. Regularity and proportions of the wave-like ridges were not different from the first to the 10th treatment. Nevertheless, for safety reasons the blade should not be used more than once in clinical work.

Laser Effects

SEM revealed no difference in the corneal surface between PRK and LASIK (Figures 4-6 and 4-7). The same degree of surface "irregularity" after laser treatment is present in both methods. The typical ridges due to the use of the microkeratome were no longer visible after ablation. One author[8] has found that excimer laser ablation using humidified gases leaves an even smoother corneal surface. In addition, scanning electron micrographs of freshly ablated rabbit corneas with and without nitrogen blowing indicated that the no-blow technique also led to much smoother post-ablation surfaces.[9]

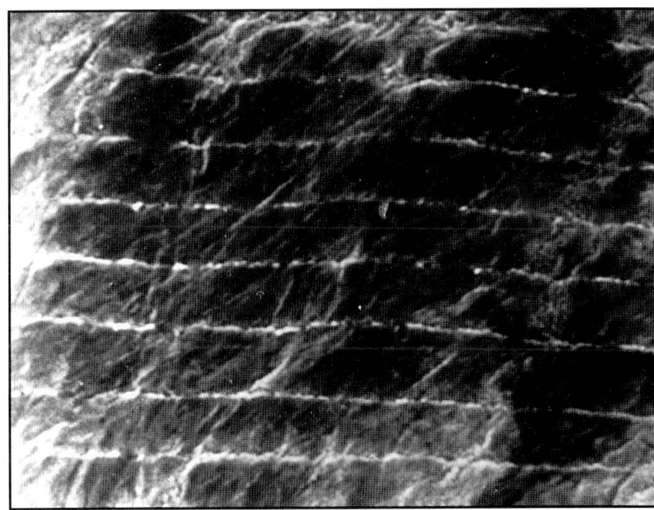

Figure 4-5.
SEM. Stromal surface of untreated area. Note the typical ridges produced by a rotating blade (Draeger keratome). Height: 2 to 3 µm. Distance: about 30 µm. Original magnification 200x.

Short-Time Changes After LASIK

We had the opportunity to perform LASIK on two eyes that were scheduled to undergo enucleation due to intraocular disorders.[10] In these cases, LASIK was per-

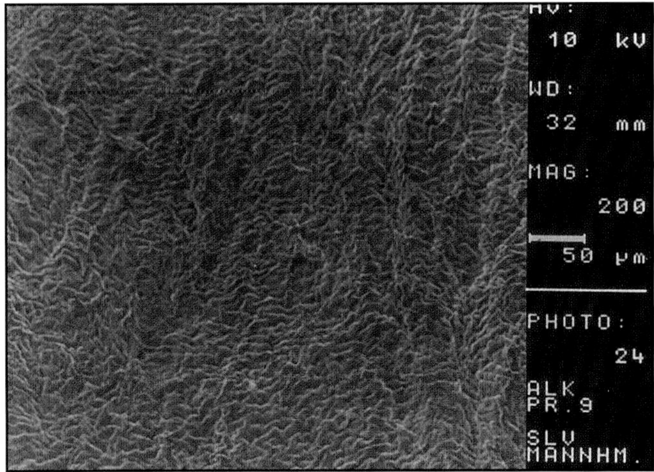

Figure 4-6.
Stromal surface after laser treatment. Irregular surface, sharp demolition of collagen bundles. Original magnification 200x.

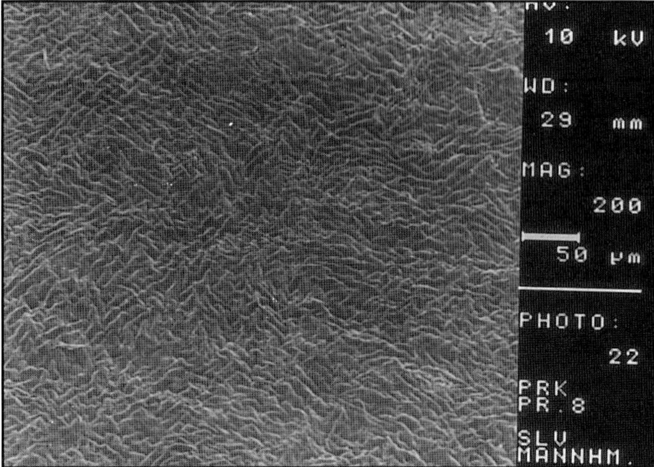

Figure 4-7.
Stromal surface after PRK. No difference to surface after LASIK. Original magnification 200x.

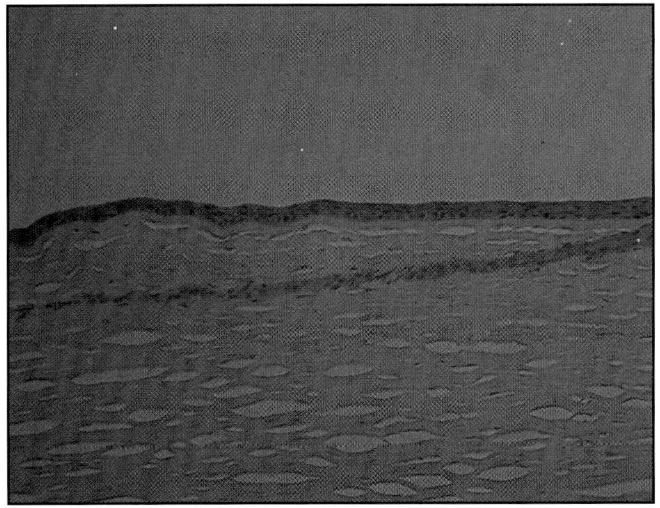

Figure 4-8a.
Light microscopy. Peripheral epithelial ingrowth at the lenticle rim. Maximum ingrowth up to 0.5 mm.

formed 1 week before enucleation. The histopathological findings were as follows in their anatomical order.

EPITHELIUM AND BOWMAN´S LAYER

The most prominent feature was the peripheral ingrowth of epithelium which could be seen to be almost circular at the edge of the flap. The maximum distance from the edge of the flap was up to 0.5 mm (Figures 4-8a and 4-8b). However, this specimen was cut at the superior edge of the flap which resulted in a seemingly larger area of ingrowth. At the rim, the epithelium was slightly thickened at some locations but otherwise entirely unaffected and of normal thickness. Bowman's layer was cut clean through at the lenticle rim (Figure 4-9). There, Bowman's layer, as well as the stroma, was separated by a two- to three-cell layer of basal epithelial cells (Figure 4-10).

STROMA

The anterior and the posterior stroma revealed no abnormalities. There was no hypercellularity nor any inflammatory reaction in the anterior stromal part as described in PRK.[4] Also, no decline in the number of keratocytes has been noticed. Ultrastructurally, no signs of cell death of the keratocytes were found either (Figure 4-11). The entire collagen structure of the corneal stroma was unaffected. The undulations of the collagen fibers of the flap, as seen immediately after LASIK in the study with porcine corneas (see above), had disappeared. The corneal-lenticular interface was detectable due to some fine deposits consisting of cellular debris only, mainly erythrocyte fragments and non-cellular fragments (Figure 4-12). In some parts of the central interface, a minimal condensation of collagen was present.

DESCEMET´S MEMBRANE AND ENDOTHELIUM

The long-term concern of photoablation upon the epithelium and endothelium in PRK has been studied by several investigators and has failed to demonstrate any clinically significant alterations in these structures to date.[11] Although long-term effects are not known, there is no evidence to suggest that problems will surface in the

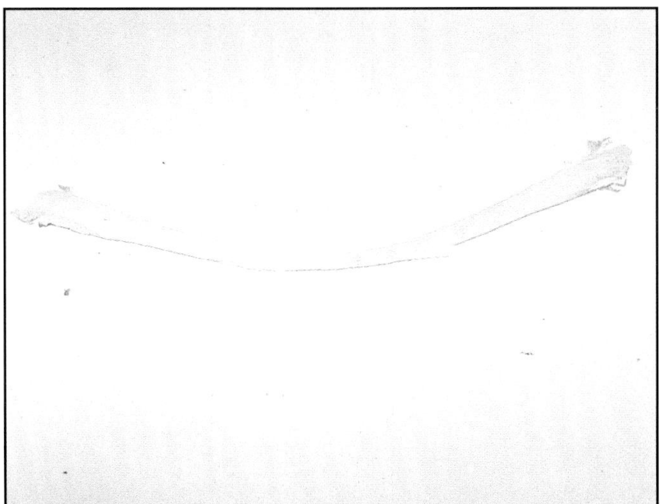

Figure 4-8b.
Light microscopy. Overview of central ablated cornea.

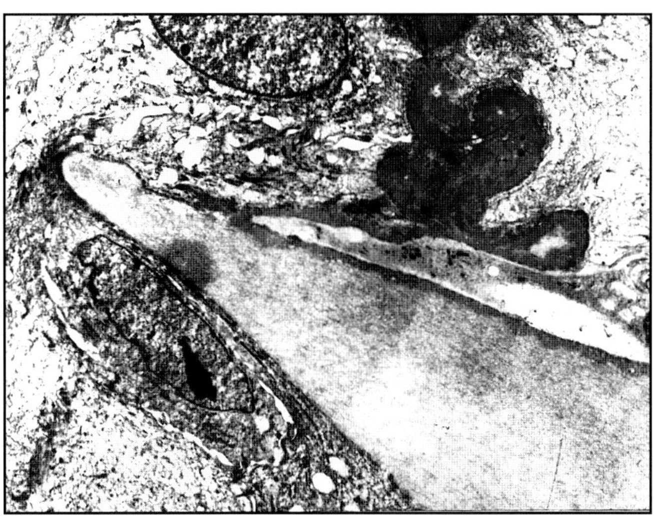

Figure 4-9.
Transmission electron microscopy (TEM). Epithelial cells bowing around Bowman's layer. Clear cut Bowman's layer. Anterior stroma. Original magnification 1800x.

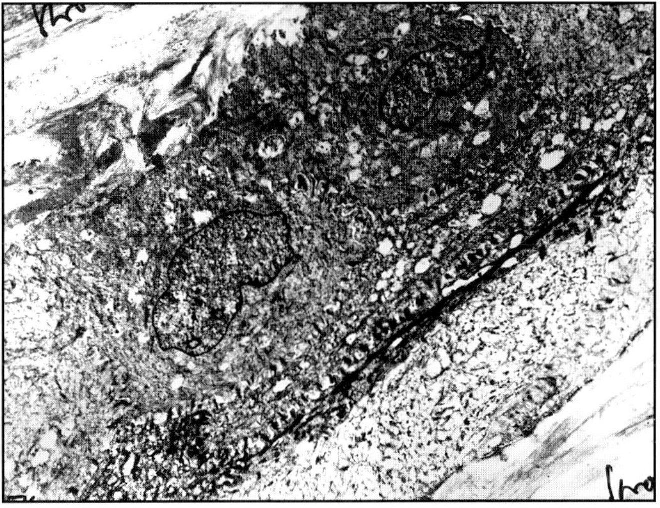

Figure 4-10.
TEM. Two to three layers of basal epithelial cells enclosed by corneal stroma. Original magnification 1800x.

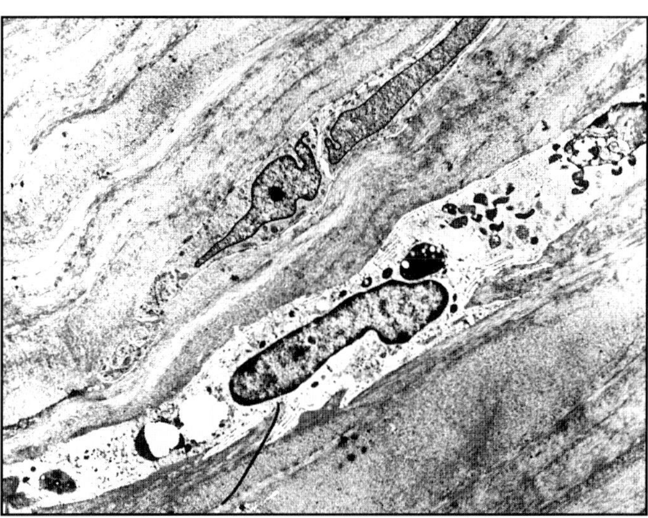

Figure 4-11.
TEM. Two keratocytes in the anterior stroma, about 0.05 mm below the central laser applanation zone. Collagen fibers of normal structure. Original magnification 900x.

future. In vitro clinical studies demonstrated that no endothelial changes were induced unless the ultraviolet radiation penetrated to within 50 µm of the endothelium.[11] Minimizing the depth of ablation is important not only to protect the endothelium, but to maintain long-term corneal stability. The residual corneal pachymetry in LASIK should ideally exceed 360 µm, to allow for a 160-µm flap and an at least 200-µm stromal bed. In our study, we had corrected 14 D in one eye and 16 D in the second eye which left a stromal bed according to these rules. Descemet's membrane and the endothelium were unaffected as expected, and endothelial cell counts after LASIK showed no significant cell loss up to 6 months postoperatively (Knorz et al, unpublished data).

Immunohistochemical Findings After LASIK

Although immunohistochemical analysis of healing in human corneas after PRK was done,[3,4,12] immunohistochemical studies following LASIK have not been performed to date to the best of our knowledge. A comparison of effects on the extracellular matrix and on collagen

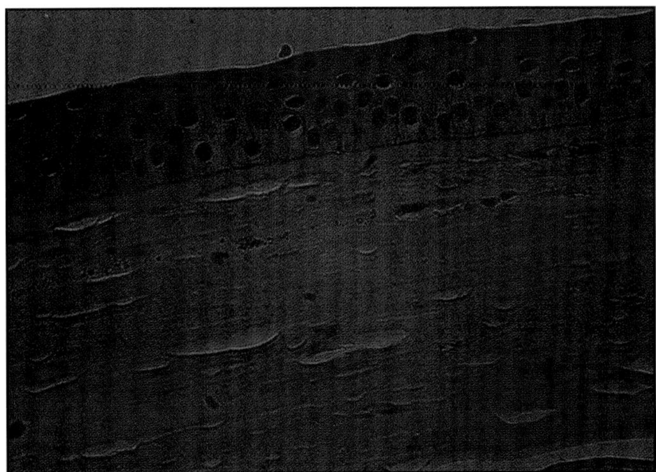

Figure 4-12.
Light microscopy. Central part of anterior cornea. The epithelium is of normal thickness, the lenticle and the corneal stroma are unremarkable. No loss in keratocytes nor any inflammatory reaction is detectable. The interface is marked by a fine layer of cellular and acellular debris. No laser affection of the collagen is detectable at light microscopic level.

structure between PRK and LASIK is therefore not possible.

CONCLUSION

The clinical results of LASIK are impressive and so are the results of histopathological research. Histologically, LASIK affects the corneal tissue dramatically less than PRK. LASIK reduces the effects of wound healing as the deeper stroma is less reactive. Only a negligible, self-limiting epithelial ingrowth occurs around the edges of the flap. Major changes were not observed. The most prominent reason for different cellular reactions to laser treatment is the preservation of Bowman's layer in LASIK. Results are therefore more predictable and less dependent upon topical steroid usage. Thus, although more technically challenging than PRK, the rapid and virtually painless visual rehabilitation combined with reduced risk of stromal scarring and progressive wound healing will allow LASIK to develop as the predominant refractive procedure of the next decade.

References

1. Waring GO III. Making sense of keratospeak: a classification of refractive corneal surgery. *Arch Ophthalmol*. 1986;103:1472-1477.
2. Machat JJ. *Excimer Laser Refractive Surgery*. Thorofare, NJ: SLACK Inc; 1996:11.
3. SundarRaj N, Geiss MJ, Fantes F, et al. Healing of excimer laser ablated monkey corneas. *Arch Ophthalmol*. 1990;108:1604-1610.
4. Malley DS, Steinert RF, Puliafito CA, Dobi ET. Immunofluorescence study of corneal wound healing after excimer laser anterior keratectomy in the monkey eye. *Arch Ophthalmol*. 1990;108:1316-1322.
5. Shieh E, Moreira H, D'Arcy J, Clapham TN, McDonnell PJ. Quantitative analysis of wound healing after cylindrical and spherical excimer laser ablations. *Ophthalmology*. 1992;99(7):1050-1055.
6. Taylor DM, L'Esperance FA, Del Pero RA, et al. Human excimer laser lamellar keratectomy. *Ophthalmology*. 1989;96:654-663.
7. Fantes FE, Hanna KD, Waring GO III, Pouliquen Y, Thompson KP, Savoldelli M. Wound healing after excimer laser keratomileusis (photorefractive keratectomy) in monkeys. *Arch Ophthalmol*. 1990;108:665-675.
8. Krueger RR, Campos M, Wang XW, Lee M, McDonnell PJ. Corneal surface morphology following excimer laser ablation with humidified gases. *Arch Ophthalmol*. 1993;111:1131-1137.
9. Campos M, Cuevas K, Garbus J, Lee M, McDonnell P. Corneal wound healing after excimer laser ablation. *Ophthalmology*. 1992;99:893-897.
10. Steiner H, Knorz MC, Seiberth V, Liesenhoff H. Histological and ultrastructural findings in laser in situ keratomileusis. *Ger J Ophthal*. 1995;4(suppl 1):117.
11. Machat JJ. *Excimer Laser Refractive Surgery*. Thorofare, NJ: SLACK Inc; 1996:53.
12. Anderson JA, Binder PS, Rock ME, Vrabec MP. Human excimer laser keratectomy. Immunohistochemical analysis of healing. *Arch Ophthalmol*. 1996;114:54-60.

Scanning Electron Microscopic Pictures

PAVEL STODULKA, MD

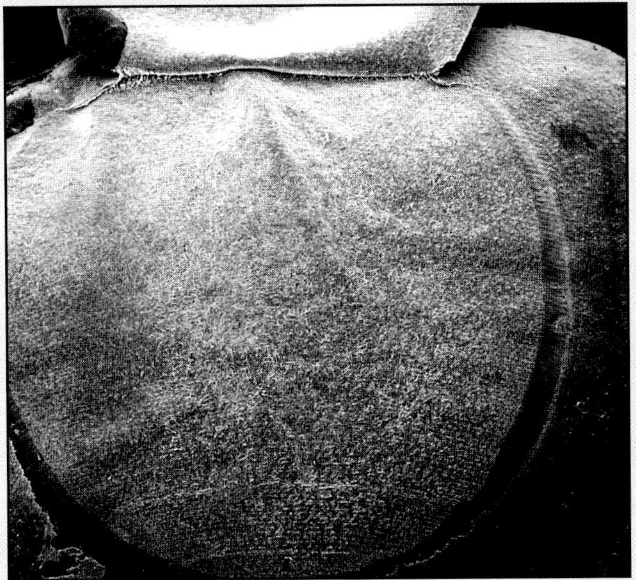

Figure 1.

The cornea after microkeratome cut with the lamella folded at the upper part. Notice the darker inside edge of the microkeratome cut—Bowman's membrane and the transversal grooves spreading over the whole stromal surface. The grooves are depicted at higher magnification on Figures 3 through 5. The ridge on the stromal surface going down from the hinge is artificial due to the shrinkage caused by fixation procedure before scanning electron microscopy (SEM). (Human cornea, original magnification 13x.)

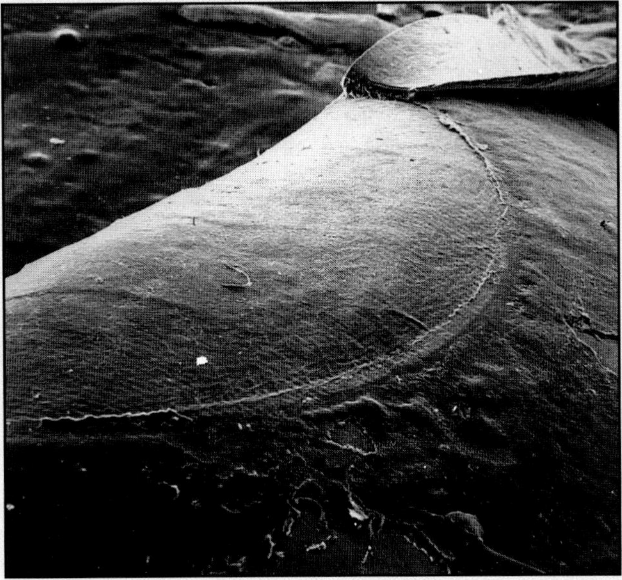

Figure 2.

One half of the human cornea after laser in situ keratomileusis (LASIK) with the lamella at the right upper part. Epithelial defects are artificial after the fixation procedure for SEM. (Human eye, original magnification, 20x.)

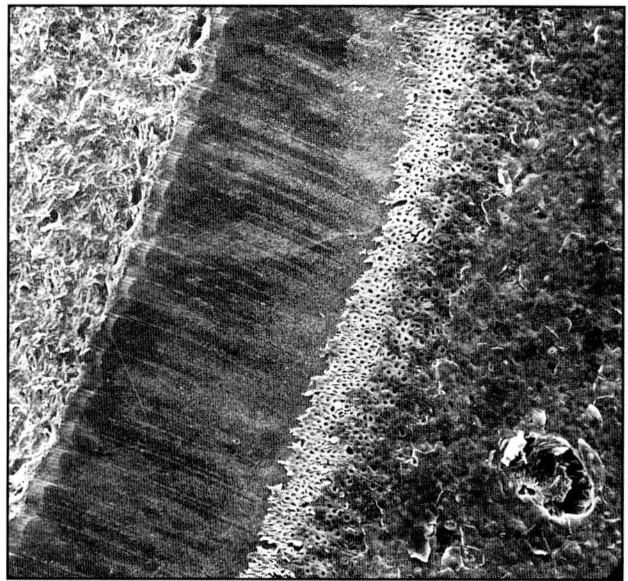

Figure 3.
Microkeratome cut border. There is epithelium on the right hand side, then the microkeratome cuts tangentially through the epithelial cell layers, then slices for about 0.25 mm on Bowman's membrane, and finally cuts the stroma. The transversal grooves are 0.056 (+0.0018) mm apart. Similar grooves are associated with both oscillating and rotating blades. They are depicted at higher magnification in Figures 4 and 5. (Human cornea, original magnification 100x.)

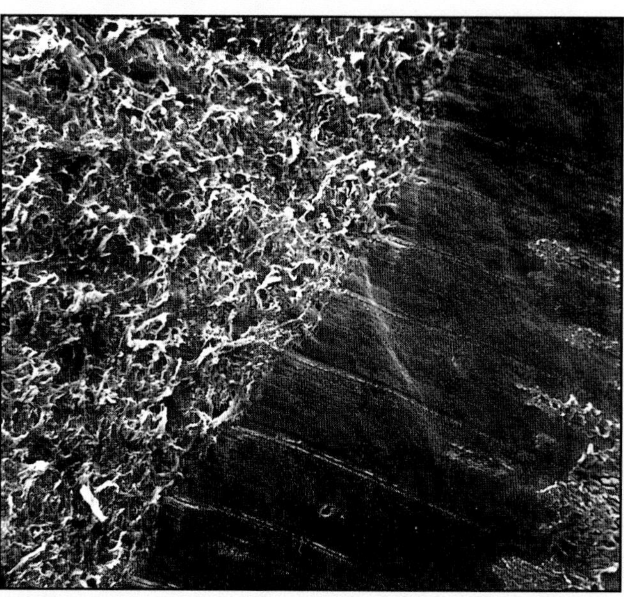

Figure 4.
Semi-detail of the border of the microkeratome cut shown in Figure 3. Transversal grooves are 0.056 mm apart on average. (Human cornea, original magnification 200x.)

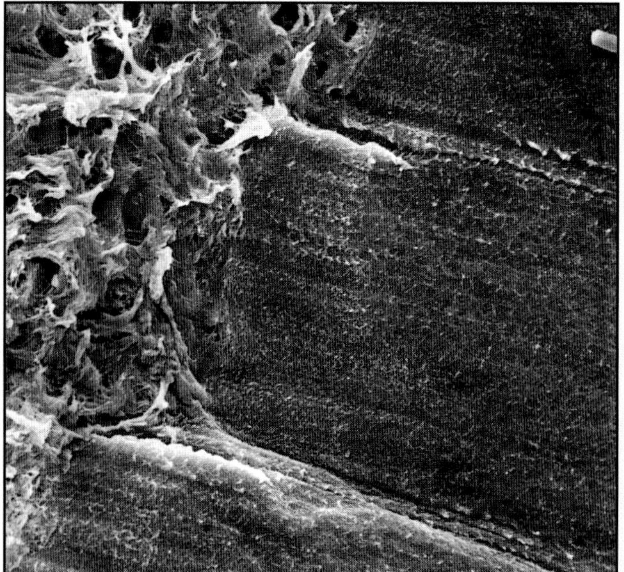

Figure 5.
Detail of the border of the microkeratome cut with the transversal grooves on Bowman's membrane and stromal surface. Both grooves are 0.05 mm apart. Detail from the area shown in Figures 3 and 4. (Human cornea, original magnification 1000x.)

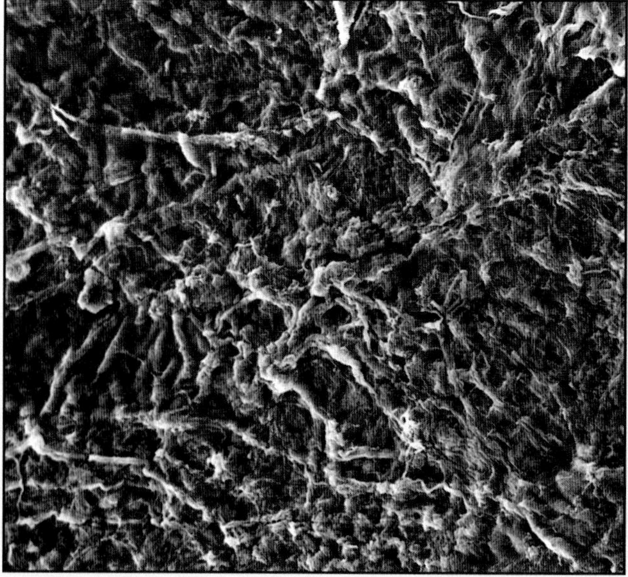

Figure 6.
Corneal surface after the excimer laser photoablation on the stromal bed. This surface has a very uniform pattern. (Rabbit cornea, magnification 390x.)

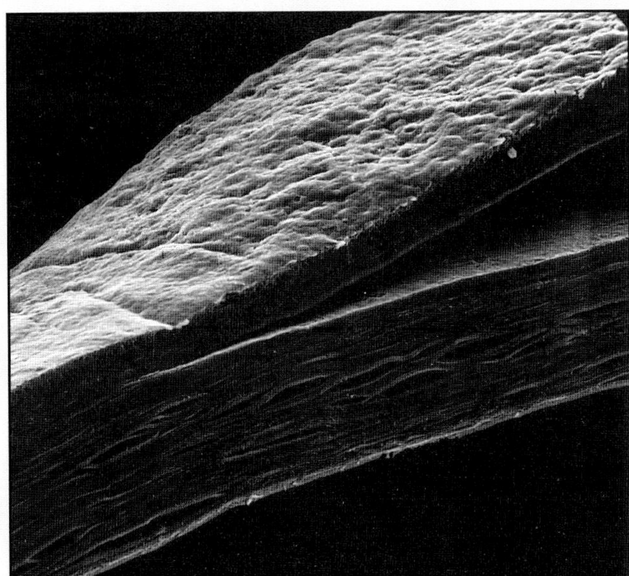

Figure 7.
Partially elevated lamella and the hinge on the corneal cross-section. Lamella is one third to one fourth of the corneal thickness. (Rabbit cornea, magnification 100x.)

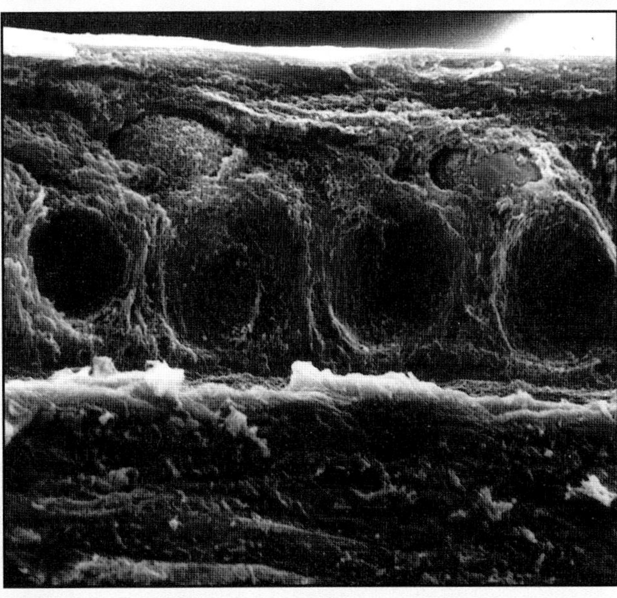

Figure 8.
Cross-section of the corneal epithelium and Bowman's membrane, which remain intact over the visual axis after LASIK. There is stroma under Bowman's membrane at the bottom of the photograph. There is a nice layer of basal columnar cells above the basement membrane and one can see several wing cells above the columnar cells. (Rabbit cornea, magnification 4000x.)

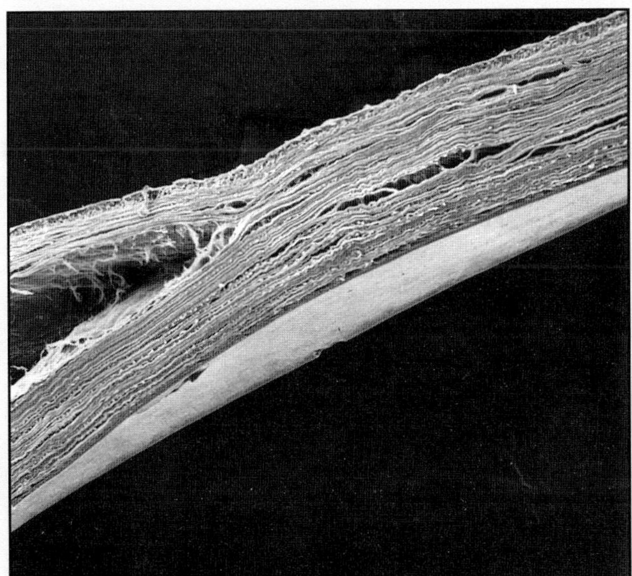

Figure 9.
Artificially partially elevated flap on the left hand side with completely joined corneal lamellae on the right hand side, which is the healed side after LASIK. We can hardly detect any corneal stromal tissue alteration by SEM on the corneal cross-section at the magnification up to 400 times 3 weeks after the procedure. This photograph demonstrates the healing process 3 weeks after LASIK. (Rabbit cornea, magnification 10x.)

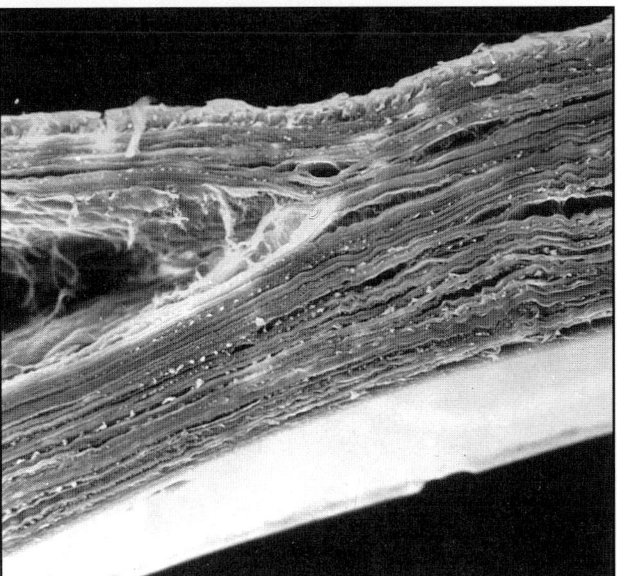

Figure 10.
Semi-detail of the junction of the flap and stromal bed. The same area as shown in Figures 9 and 11. (Rabbit eye, magnification 200x.)

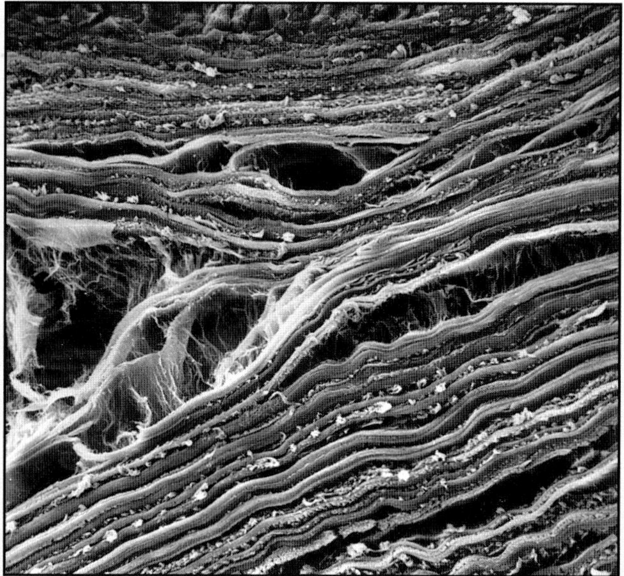

Figure 11.
Detail of the junction of the flap and the stromal bed after their separation by force. This picture shows precise apposition of the corneal lamellae after LASIK at the healed cornea 3 weeks after the procedure. Detail from the area shown in Figures 9 and 10. (Rabbit cornea, magnification 600x.)

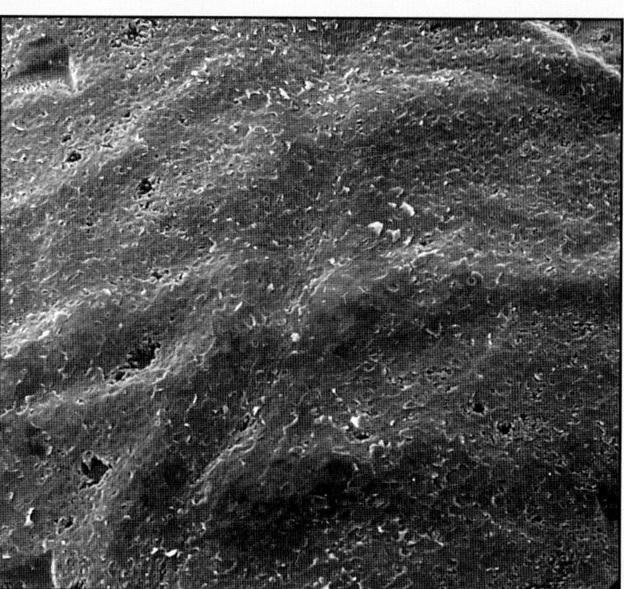

Figure 12.
Epithelium at the border of the lamella 3 weeks after LASIK. There is a flat, round sulcus with no significant surface irregularities marking the edge of the lamella. The sulcus goes from the middle of the upper side of the picture to the left lower corner. (Rabbit cornea, magnification 600x.)

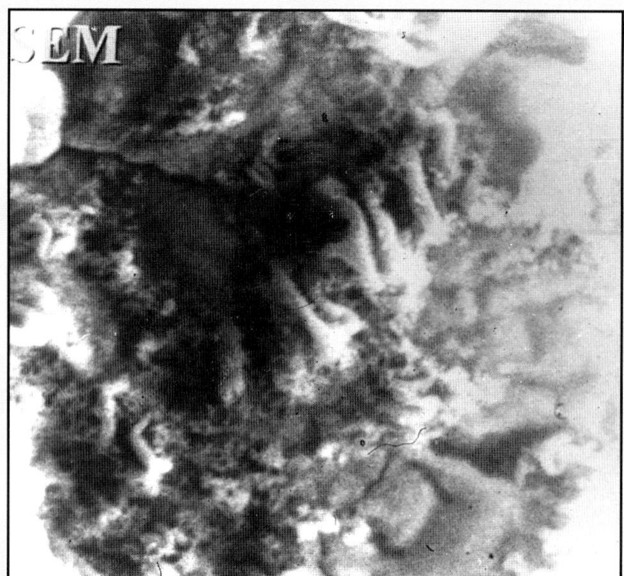

Figure 13.
AQUASEM: Different SEM method without previous drying of the water containing tissue. We can observe the stromal surface after the microkeratome cut on this picture. This method is limited mostly by the small diameter of the observation field, which is just 0.3 mm.

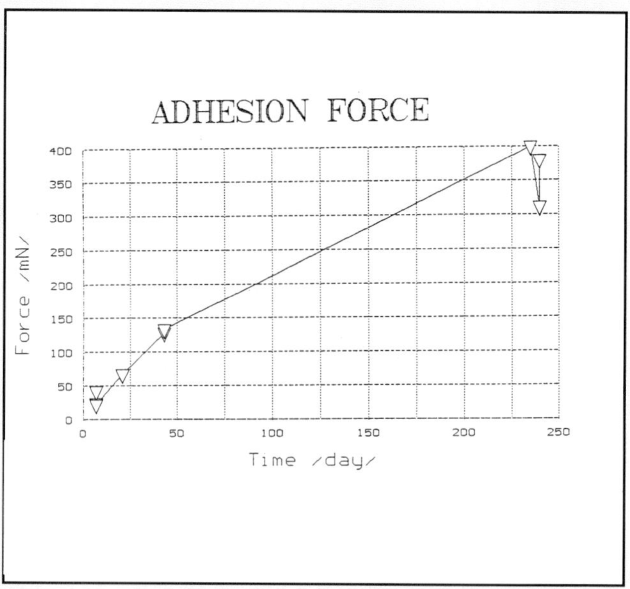

Figure 14.
Adhesion force graph. The lamella to stroma adhesion rose from 25 mN 1 week postoperative to 125 mN 6 weeks postoperative. (Preliminary rabbit cornea measurements.)

Chapter 5

HISTOLOGICAL OBSERVATIONS IN LASIK

Irini I. Naoumidi, PhD, Dimitrios S. Siganos, MD

CASE REPORT

A 41-year-old man underwent laser in situ keratomileusis (LASIK) on his left eye (attempted correction: -11.5 D). Two days after LASIK, the corneal flap was lost. It was decided to wait for epithelialization to be completed, as epithelialization was proceeding slowly. Lamellar keratoplasty was performed on the 10th postoperative day. The donor flap transplant was smaller in diameter (7.5 mm) in comparison with the original flap (8.5 mm), so the uncovered peripheral part of the original flap area underwent epithelialization of "PRK type" (photorefractive keratectomy type). Twenty months later, corneal haze grade IV compelled the surgeon to perform penetrating keratoplasty, which allowed histological examination of the removed central part of the cornea.

PREPARATION OF HISTOLOGICAL SPECIMENS

The explant was prefixed in cold glutaraldehyde 2.5% in 0.1 M cacodylate buffer (pH 7.4). After short prefixation, it was placed in the same fresh fixative. Postfixation was performed in 2% osmium tetroxide in 0.1 M cacodylate buffer (pH 7.4) for 1 hour at 4°C, dehydrated in a series of alcohols and in propylene oxide, and then embedded in epoxy resin. For light microscopic examination, 1 to 3 μm sections were pre-

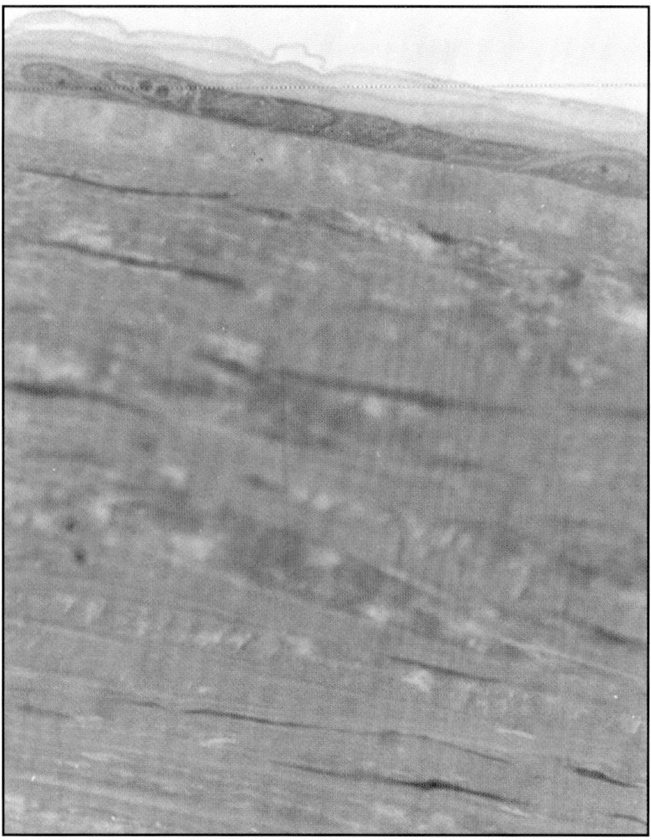

Figure 5-1.
Thinning of the central part of donor flap epithelium. Toluidine blue, original magnification 250x.

pared and stained with 1% toluidine blue, as well as with a modified trichrome stain.[1] For electron microscopic examination, the selected areas were thin-sectioned and stained with uranyl acetate and lead citrate.

SURVEY OF HISTOLOGICAL FINDINGS

The described clinical case allows us to perform a histological survey of the most frequent complications of LASIK:

- Misaligned or lost flap.
- Irregular reepithelialization.
- New collagen and proteoglycans production following stimulation of keratocytes during healing.
- Epithelial ingrowth.

The first complication is described clinically in other chapters. Histological characterization of other complications, which in this particular case was actually caused by the first one, is summarized below.

During the normal healing process after LASIK, the small circular defect around the flap margin is usually totally re-epithelialized by the first postoperative visit (ie, less than 24 hours after surgery). In the described case, however, the lost flap as well as the succeeding lamellar keratoplasty allows histological analysis of two principally different zones:

1. The central zone that was covered by the flap transplant, in which the postoperative healing does not have any significant differences with histological observations after standard LASIK procedures
2. The peripheral part of the original flap area, which was not covered by the flap transplant; the healing process within this zone followed the general course that is characteristic for PRK.

In the first (central) zone, the structure of the epithelium is close to normal. Preservation of Bowman's layer provided a typical histological appearance of interaction of epithelial layers with basal lamina and Bowman's layer. Right below Bowman's layer, the corneal stroma and keratocytes demonstrate normal morphological structure. Only slight epithelial thinning may be noticed in the center of this zone. Minimal thickness of the epithelium is presented in Figures 5-1 through 5-2b, and does not exceed two to three cell layers. In this area, the structure of superficial epithelial cells and wing cells is close to normal. However, the basal cell layer, in its normal appearance, is practically absent. Normally, these cells represent the germinative layer of epithelium, and allow for the straight contact of the epithelial layer with basal lamina, to which these cells are attached through hemidesmosomes.

It is clear from the microphotographs of Figures 5-2a and 5-2b that the number of hemidesmosomes is significantly reduced with respect to normal, and their structure differs from the normal by a notable decrease of a number of anchoring filaments, which secure the attachment.

It seems reasonable to suppose that such a pronounced basal epithelial layer may explain the noticed epithelial thinning.

Contacts between wing cells, structure of their organoids, as well as of Bowman's layer, are close to normal (see Figures 5-2a and 5-2b).

In the peripheral part (Figure 5-3) of the original flap

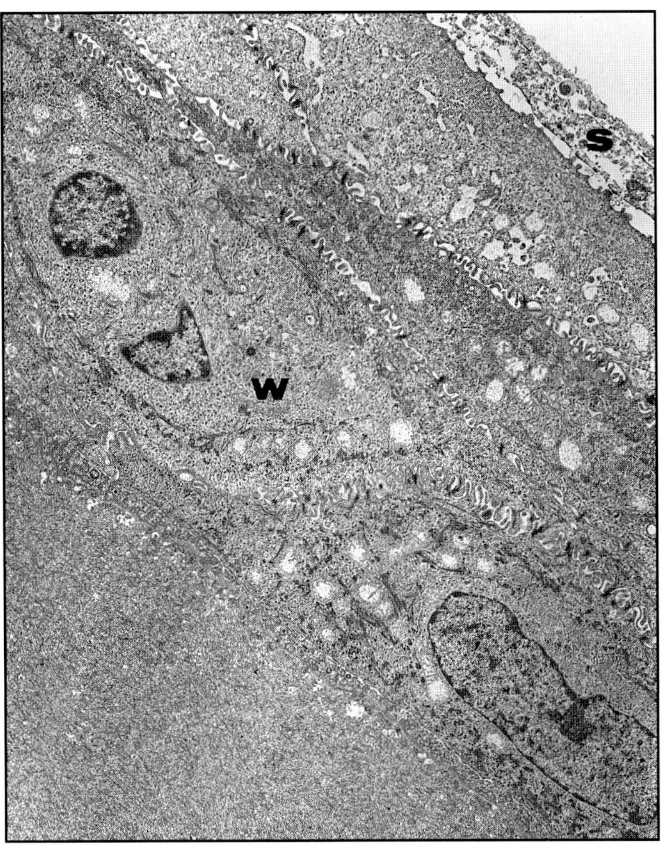

Figure 5-2a.
Epithelium in central flap area is extremely thin. Basal cells in their classical appearance are almost absent. Structure of superficial (S) and wing (W) cells is close to normal. Original magnification 6600x.

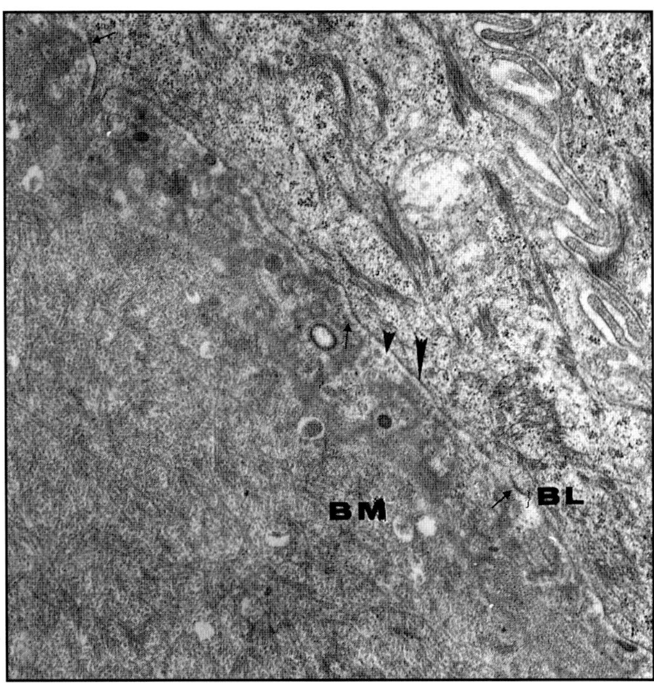

Figure 5-2b.
Magnified fragment (40,000x): Basal lamina (BL) has typical appearance. (Lamina lucida indicated by small arrowhead, Lamina densa indicated by big arrowhead.) Note that mechanical junctions (hemidesmosomes) have diminished amount of anchoring filaments (arrows). Randomly oriented cell fibers of Bowman's membrane have normal appearance.

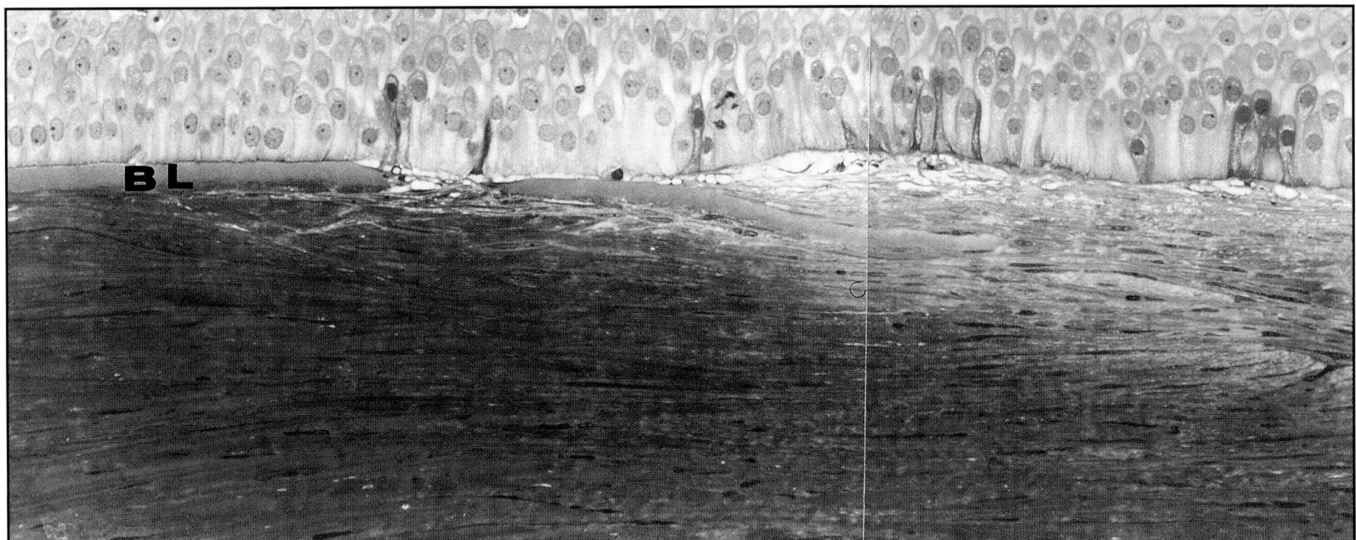

Figure 5-3.
The border of the flap transplant may be clearly seen as a wide gap in Bowman's layer. Hyperplasia of the epithelial layer is significant within this zone. Trichrome stain, original magnification 250x.

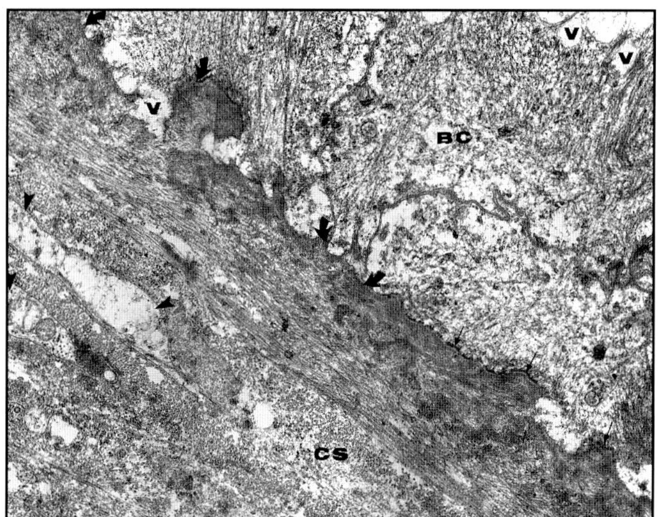

Figure 5-4.
In the peripheral flap area, within the zones where Bowman's membrane is absent, some basal epithelial cells (BC) demonstrate typical hemidesmosome contacts (small arrows). At the same time, other basal epithelial cells (between curved arrows) do not have any specialized contacts with basal lamina. Hypervacuolization (V) may be observed in most of the basal epithelial cells. Remodeling corneal stroma (CS) under epithelial basal lamina has abnormal structure, part of stromal cells are degrading (arrowheads). Original magnification 10,000x.

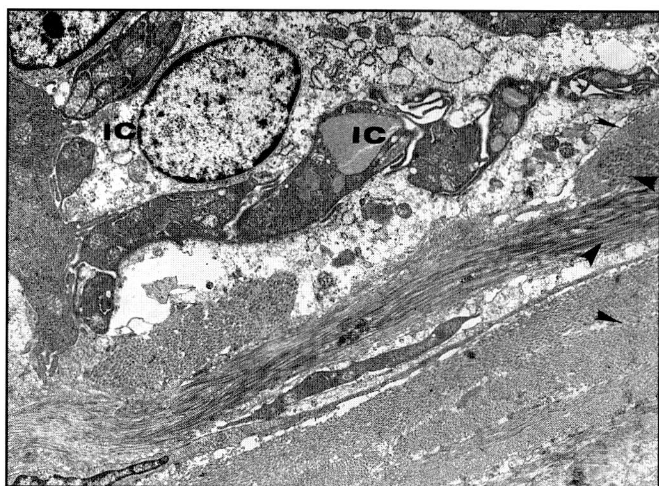

Figure 5-5a.
Cell islands under donor flap consist of cells (IC) whose morphology differs significantly from both stromal and epithelial cells. Original magnification 5000x.

area, which was not covered by the flap transplant, the thickness of the epithelial layer is gradually increasing in a centrifugal direction. At the outer border of the peripheral zone, the thickness of the epithelial layer reaches the level of eight to nine epithelial cells. Morphological appearance of superficial epithelial cells, wing cells, and basal cells may be characterized as normal.

The border of the flap transplant may be clearly seen as a wide gap in Bowman's layer (Figure 5-4). The condition of the epithelium in this zone may serve as further evidence of the essential role of the Bowman's layer in maintaining epithelial recovery.

In the peripheral zone, a significant increase of epithelial cell layers—hyperplasia of the corneal epithelium—may be noticed. Increase of total epithelial thickness is due to both the increase in number of epithelial layers and hyperpolarization of basal cells.

Both in the light and electron microphotographs, among basal cells one can clearly distinguish cells with picnotic nuclear changes, overvacuolization and destroyed cytoskeletal structure, as well as cells with a significantly reduced number of intercellular contacts and contacts with basal lamina (hemidesmosomes). At the same time, neighboring cells may demonstrate a well-developed system of mechanical contacts (hemidesmosomes), with a typical amount of anchoring filaments (see Figure 5-4).

One should notice the significant irregularity of corneal stroma structure at the contact with the zone with interrupted basal lamina. This may serve as more evidence of the importance of preservation of the Bowman's layer for corneal healing. The healing response of keratocytes is obviously more pronounced in the zone where Bowman's layer is absent. Activated keratocytes take an active part in stromal remodeling that involves extracellular matrix deposition, mainly in the subepithelial stroma (see Figures 5-3 and 5-4). Occurrence of a relatively large number of degrading fibrocyte-like cells in the remodeling tissue is, probably, evidence of the gradual returning of stromal cells back to their normal quantities.

Immunohistochemical studies[2-4] suggest that newly formed collagen could be type III collagen, as well as type VII (anchoring filaments), type IV (basal lamina), and some other type of immature collagen. These types of collagen comprise the main component of the extracellular matrix, which fills the zone of corneal defect. Except for collagen, this extracellular matrix also includes newly-synthesized proteoglycans and fibronectin.[2-4]

Since the spatial organization and structure of collagen fibrils, as well as composition of proteoglycans, are

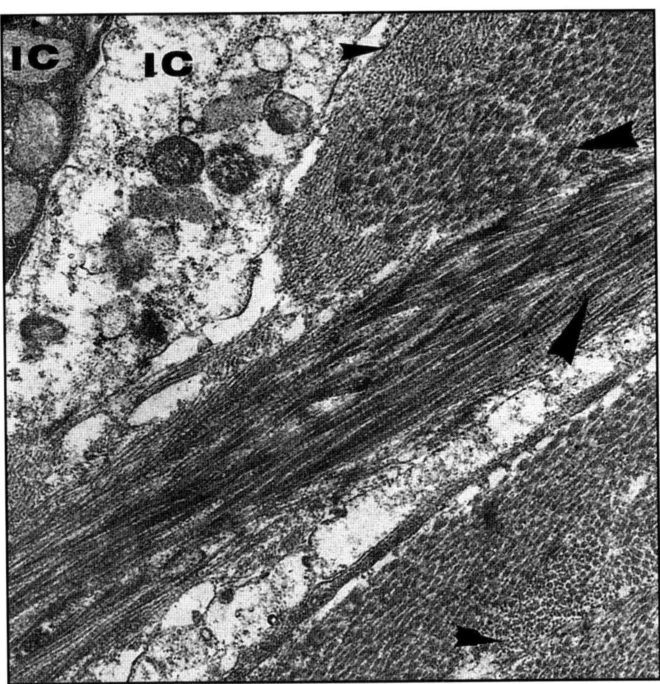

Figure 5-5b.
Magnified fragment (20,000x). Collagen fibrils (big arrowheads) around these cell islands differ from the cells of surrounding stroma (small arrowheads) in both their diameter and spatial orientation.

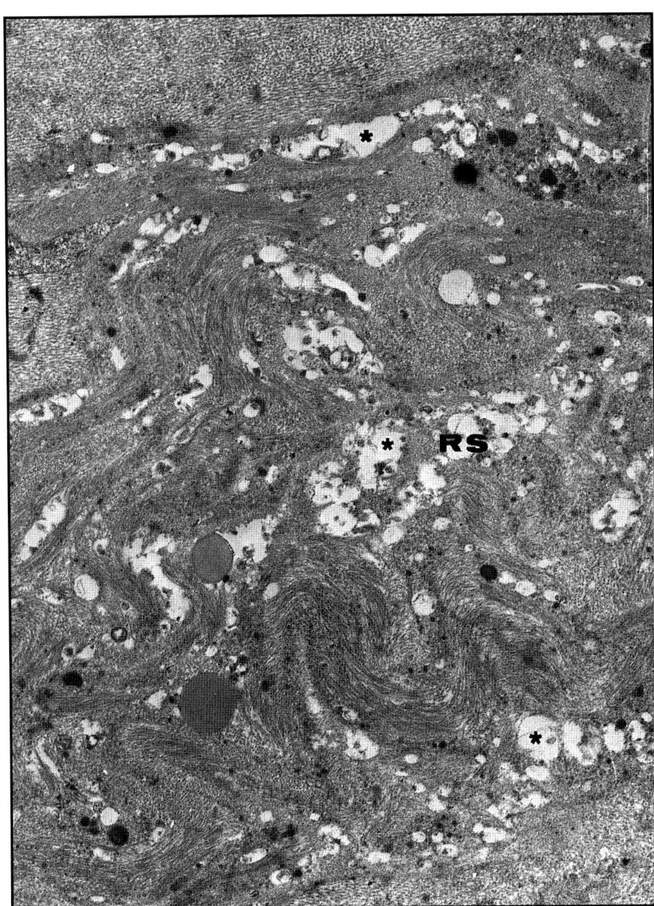

Figure 5-6.
Typical appearance of remodeling corneal stroma (RS). The collagen fibers have a characteristic wavy appearance, with multiple electronically transparent areas (asterisks) between the fibers. Original magnification 6600x.

substantially different in respect to normal (Figures 5-5a through 5-6), these new collagen fibrils, and other extracellular matrix components in the healing zone, are often characterized by increased light scattering.

The trichrome stain is staining the regions where the new extracellular matrix is deposited differently.[1] In Figure 5-3, the zone of flap transplant, the zone of corneal remodeling, and that of the remaining cornea are stained differently in light microscopic specimens, whereas in the electron microscopic specimens these zones can be distinguished by the difference in structure and spatial orientation of corneal stroma fibrils (see Figure 5-6).

In the incision area, keratocytes and stromal fibrils are randomly oriented. Intrastromal cavities with cells representing different phases of degradation may be observed.

Epithelial ingrowth in this case may also be responsible for corneal haze, since multiple, though small, cell groups were found under the flap transplant (Figure 5-7). Electron microscopic examination of these cell islands shows that part of the cells constituting these islands structurally resemble fibroblast-type cells, while other cells could be epithelial cells that were significantly altered morphologically. It should be noticed that the possibility for a more detailed morphological analysis was significantly reduced, owing to the remote (20 months) postoperative phase. An interesting observation is that most of the collagen fibrils surrounding these islands differ significantly from the collagen of intact stroma in their diameter, which is 2 to 2.5 times bigger with respect to stromal collagen.

Descemet's membrane does not differ from normal, either in the banded or the nonbanded regions. Endothelial cells have practically normal structure, with the exception of just a small number of cells under the central ablation zone. In this zone, endothelial cells have electronically dense intracytoplasmic condensations of a round shape. However, endothelial cells with such condensations appear to be functionally normal (Figure 5-8).

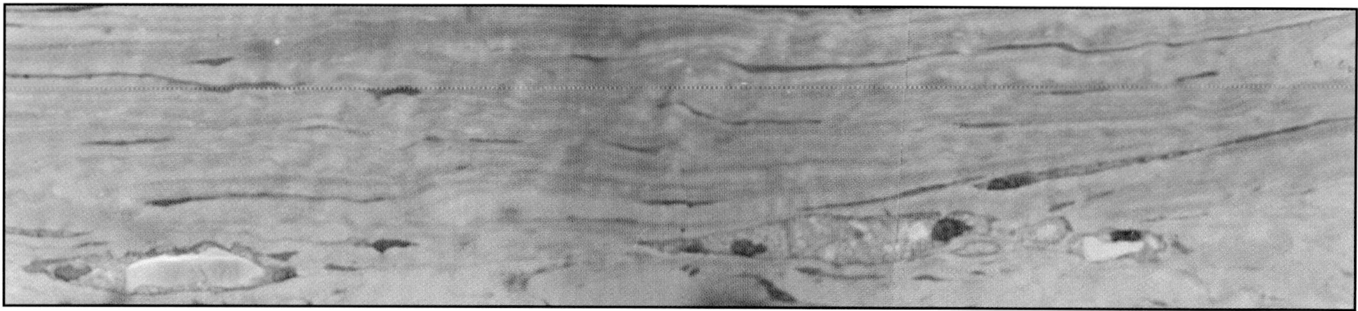

Figure 5-7.
Cell islands under the flap transplant. Trichrome stain, original magnification 250x.

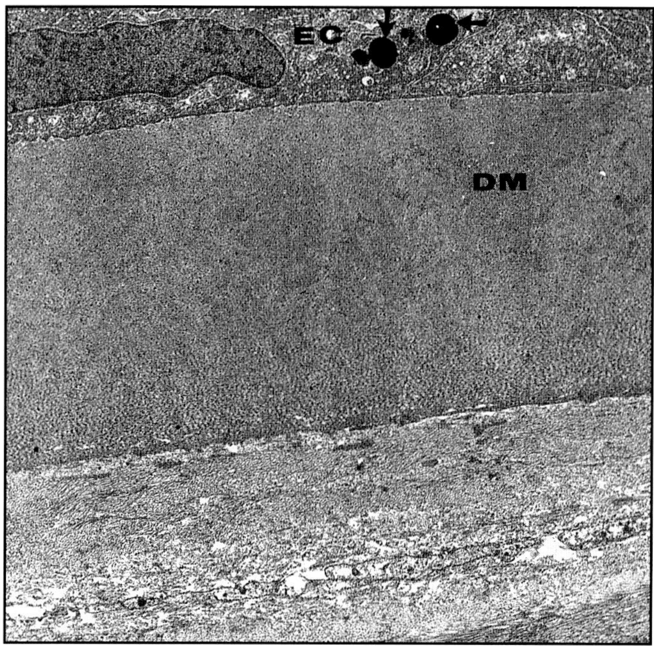

Figure 5-8.
Descemet's membrane (DM) and endothelial cells (EC) do not show any significant pathological abnormalities, with the exception of the occurrence of roundly shaped, electronically dense intracytoplasmic concentrations (arrows) in the central part of cornea. Original magnification 6600x.

References

1. Rock ME, Anderson J, Binder PS. A modified trichrome stain for light microscopic examination of plastic-embedded corneal tissue. *Cornea.* 1993;12(3):255-260.
2. Zimmerman DR, Fischer RW, Winterhalter KH, Witmer R, Vaughan L. Comparative studies of collagens in normal and keratoconus corneas. *Exp Eye Res.* 1988;46:431-442.
3. Nakayasu K, Tanaka M, Konomi H, Hayashi T. Distribution of types I, II, III, IV collagen in normal and keratoconus corneas. *Ophthalmic Res.* 1986;18:1-10.
4. Tsuchiya S, Tanaka M, Konomi H, Hayashi T. Distribution of specific collagen types and fibronectin in normal and keratoconus corneas. *Jpn J Ophthalmol.* 1986;30:14-31.

SECTION 3

KERATOMES

Chapter 6

AN ADVANCED MICROKERATOME DESIGN FOR LASIK AND KERATOMILEUSIS IN SITU

Perry S. Binder, MD, Russell G. Koepnick, MS

CURRENT KMIS AND LASIK

Several microkeratomes are currently available to perform keratomileusis in situ (KMIS) or laser in situ keratomileusis (LASIK) (Table 6-1). They all excise a corneal cap between 7.2 and 8 mm in diameter with a planned cap thickness of 130 to 160 µm.[1-5] The cap is now reflected nasally (whereas when the procedure was introduced it was totally excised)[6] and the microkeratome is passed across the host's stromal surface to excise tissue at a planned diameter between 4.2 and 5.0 mm at thicknesses between 30 to 120 µm to correct myopia up to -20 D. The shape of this "power cut" has parallel faces (ie, the anterior and posterior surfaces are parallel and therefore do not have any optical power). This is in contrast to the original cryolathe keratomileusis procedures that excised an optically correct lenticle from the posterior surface of the host excised corneal cap.[7] The cap is then reflected back into its in situ position and allowed to "adhere" by endothelial dehydration and epithelial surface dehydration.

In contrast, LASIK uses cap diameters between 8.5 and 9.2 mm of the same attempted cap thickness.[8-10] The diameter of the attempted power cut removed with the excimer laser exceeds 6.0 mm; attempted central excision thickness varies from 50 to 110 µm. The shape of the excised tissue is lenticular (ie, it has optical power). Clearly, LASIK is not the same procedure as currently performed KMIS.

Of the currently available microkeratomes (see Table 6-1), three are advanced

TABLE 6-1

Comparison of Current Microkeratome Systems

	UK	ACS	MLK	SCMD	Draeger	Berlin
Blade oscillation (cycles per sec)	14,000	8000	16,000	20,000	NA	1750
Applanation heads	PMMA	Multiple	Multiple	Multiple	NA	NA
Suction ring	Single	Adjustable	Multiple	Multiple	Single	NA
Blade direction	Oscillatory	Sideways	Sideways	Sideways	Rotation	Sideways
Blade angle approach	0°	25°	9°	25°	0°	0°
Single unit	Yes	No	No	No	Yes	No
Surgeon view of surgery	Yes	No	No	No	Yes	No
Power source	Electric	Electric	Pneumatic	Electric	Electric	Electric

UK=Phoenix Keratek Inc UniversalKeratome, ACS=Chiron Automated Corneal Shaper, MLK=Eye Technology Inc Microlamellar Keratome, SCMD=Microtech Inc, Draeger=Storz Instruments Inc, Berlin=Coherent Inc.

mechanically across a dove-tail suction ring and three are manually advanced. The planned diameter and thickness of tissue excision depends on an applanation ring placed in the suction fixation ring and a mechanical "spacer" in the microkeratome head. The IOP achieved with each suction system cannot be adjusted. In one system, the spacer consists of a series of plates designed to create a predictable gap. In two systems, a qualitative or quantitative micrometer head replaces the plates to provide a better approximation of the gap. Most of the current systems represent a significant improvement over the microkeratomes used in the early 1980s,[11] but in spite of the advances, each has certain drawbacks.

One major difficulty is the determination of the gap between the microkeratome blade and the spacer element. Even with a quantitative micrometer adjustment of the plate, a special micrometer gauge is required to confirm a base setting; subsequent micrometer settings for the same eye are dependent on this setting. If a micrometer-measured gap is not satisfactory with the systems that use plates, then the plates are exchanged until a reasonably close reading is obtained.

A second problem is the measurement of the thicknesses of the excised tissues which may be measured on either an inaccurate strain gauge or by the difference in ultrasonic pachymetry before and after the microkeratome pass. A third concern is the poor correlation of clinical outcome with planned gap and/or the measured thicknesses of excised tissues. All but one current system blocks the surgeon's view of the procedure as it is being performed. If there is a problem with the resection, the surgeon is unable to detect the complication until the resection process is complete. All but one of the current systems approach the corneal surface at an angle of 9° to 25°, which adversely impacts the achieved diameters of resection.[12] Poor predictability of refractive outcome, often exceeding the range of ± 2.00 D, loss of two or more lines of best spectacle corrected visual acuity due primarily to irregular astigmatism, and enhancement rates exceeding 50% have frustrated surgeons and patients alike.[2,5,13-20] Multiple pieces for the assembly of the microkeratomes and/or the suction rings have discouraged surgeons and their technicians. Postoperative patient complaints of glare and monocular diplopia are associated with small functional optical zones. The IOP cannot be adjusted with any current system. The current problems that presently exist have been addressed with the development of the UniversalKeratome of Phoenix Keratek Inc (Table 6-2).

INSTRUMENT DESIGN

The main components of the UniversalKeratome are shown in Figure 6-1. The suction ring pulls a vacuum in

TABLE 6-2

The Advantages of the Phoenix Keratek Inc UniversalKeratome

- Ease of use. The four-piece unit is easily assembled, is simple to operate, and is easily disassembled and cleaned.
- The unit is automated so that the advance across the cornea 0.50 to 1.5 mm/sec is uniform and controlled by the console unit.
- The diameters of resection are controlled by the optics that are ground into the PMMA inserts.
- One single suction ring system is used. There is no adjustment required during surgery.
- The instrument incises the cornea parallel to the iris. The blade oscillates at 14,000 cycles per second. The blade speed combined with a controlled advance parallel to the iris creates the smoothest possible tissue resection.
- The surgeon is able to visualize the entire procedure through the optically clear PMMA insert.
- The corneal tissue is not bent during the resection of the primary cap reducing the incidence of breaks in Bowman's layer commonly seen with instruments that approach (and resect) corneal tissue at angles between 9° and 25°.
- The blade stop position is controlled by the console unit.
- The diameter of the corneal cap is controlled by the PMMA insert. The hinge location is controlled by the electronics control on the console.
- The UK is the only microkeratome system to permit adjustment of IOP during surgery.
- The UK is the only microkeratome system to resect optically correct lenticular tissue or parallel-faced tissue, compared to current technology that resects only parallel-faced tissue.

an annulus around the sclera. By pulling this vacuum, the IOP of the eye is increased from a normal pressure of 10 to 21 mmHg to 65 mmHg or greater. Whereas all microkeratome systems use one vacuum setting, the IOP can range between 60 to 90 mmHg. It is this rise in pressure that is utilized by all microkeratomes to force the cornea up through an aperture and against a flat plate.

In existing microkeratomes, it is the geometry of the aperture and plate that determines the thickness and diameter of the lamellar tissue to be removed. With the UniversalKeratome, the clear, polymethylmethacrylate (PMMA) optical inserts (Figure 6-2) and the ability of the system to adjust the vacuum level until an exact IOP of 65 mmHg is reached directly control the thickness and diameter of the corneal cap. The keratome body (Figure 6-3) houses the optical insert. A track is formed between the suction ring and keratome body, in which a blade oscillating at 14,000 cycles per second rides from 0.50 mm/sec to 1.5 mm/sec as it excises the tissue forced up into the insert. The reciprocating motor (Figures 6-4a and 6-4b) rotates as it reciprocates the blade, which is trapped between the suction ring plate and the keratome body.

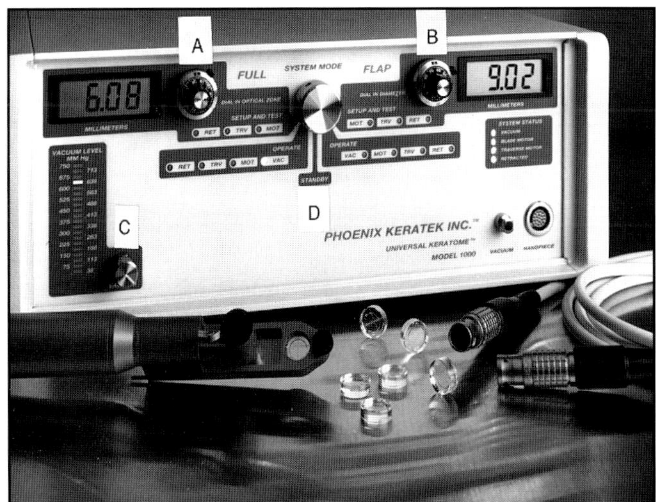

Figure 6-1.
Phoenix Keratek Inc control console. The two micrometers determine the traverse extent during the myopic power cut (A) and the cap (B). The vacuum dial (C) permits adjustment of the IOP to ensure predictable cuts at a standard IOP. The dial (D, inset) determines which part of the procedure (set-up and test, cap, power cut) is to be per-

The linear actuator (see Figure 6-3) drives the reciprocating motor forward, causing the blade to traverse over

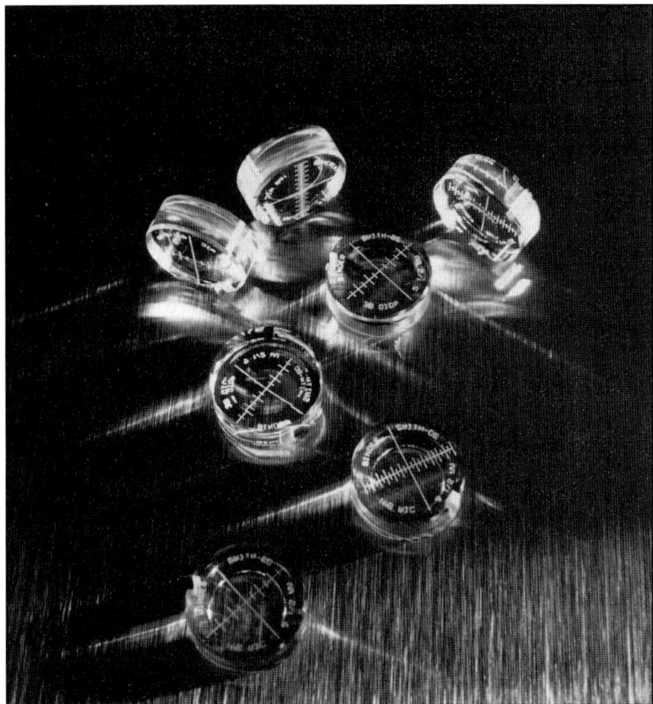

Figure 6-2.
PMMA optical inserts used in the UniversalKeratome. For the corneal cap for LASIK or KMIS, a diameter of 8.5 mm and a thickness (depth) is created in the PMMA disk. A second PMMA disk 6.0 mm in diameter with a concave depression whose depth determines the central thickness of the power cut is used in the suction ring piece.

the bottom surface of the optical insert, excising the entrapped tissue at an approach of 0°. This angle of approach creates a wound configuration at the edge of the cornea similar to that created with other microkeratomes; the 0° approach creates surface excisions parallel to the iris surface within this cap edge. The surgeon controls the vacuum, reciprocating motor, and linear actuator via foot pedals which are attached to a console unit (see Figure 6-1). Either an automatic flap or full excision of corneal tissue may be specified on the console micrometer dial (see Figure 6-1). Most importantly, the UniversalKeratome excises tissue dimensions in the power cut that are lenticular (ie, the shape of the excised tissue is shaped like a lenticle just like the tissue excised with the excimer laser, unlike the parallel surfaces excised with current microkeratomes [see Figures 6-4a and 6-4b]). For a review of the optical principles of the UniversalKeratome, the reader is referred to a recent reference.[21]

This design addresses all of the current concerns of current microkeratome technology. The simplicity of the unit in four pieces (microkeratome head, suction plate, PMMA optical insert, and blade) are easy to assemble and clean. There are no gears to get stuck. All microkeratome advance and suction is controlled by the computer console. The surgeon is able to observe the tissue as it is excised. The IOP may be adjusted using the Barraquer tonometer to set the pressure to exactly 65 mmHg for every eye. The dimensions of the tissue to be excised are predetermined by the optical PMMA insert. The excised tissue for the power cut is lenticular, unlike the parallel face tissue excised with all other microkeratomes.

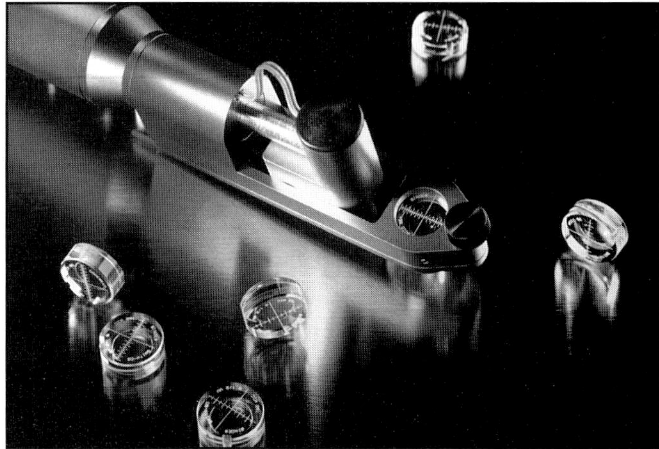

Figure 6-3.
Overview of UniversalKeratome microkeratome handpiece.

RESULTS OF COMPARATIVE LABORATORY EXPERIMENTS

The UniversalKeratome was initially tested on human cadaver eyes.[12] Figures 6-5a and 6-5b show the surface of a human eye bank cornea immediately after a primary, parallel-faced anterior corneal flap was created. The comparative unit created a typical chattering of Bowman's layer and the superficial corneal stroma just as the original microkeratomes had done,[11] whereas the UniversalKeratome created a smooth resection. Figures 6-5a and 6-5b compare the scanning electron microscopic features immediately after the second (myopic power cut). The diameter of the comparative microkeratome power cut is smaller than that created with the UniversalKeratome for the same refractive error correction. Note the same chatter marks in the beginning of the secondary cut with the comparative unit (Figure 6-6, left), whereas there are no chatter

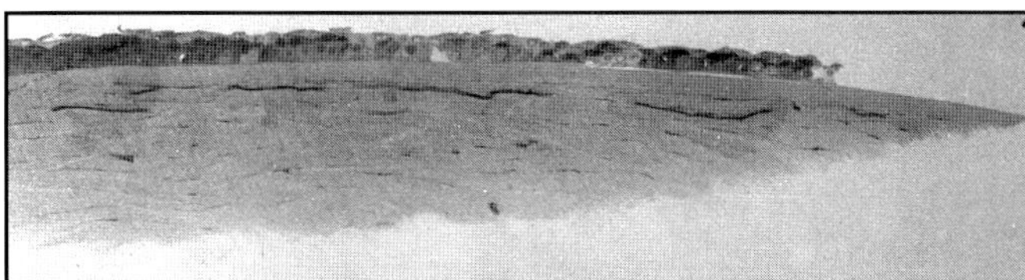

Figure 6-4a.
Light microscopic sectional views of a myopic power cut obtained in an eye bank eye with the Automated Corneal Shaper. Note the parallel faces of the Automated Corneal Shaper lenticle compared to the lenticular shape of the UniversalKeratome tissue. Figures 6-4a and 6-4b are at the same magnification (320x) and represent the amount of tissue resected to correct the same amount of myopia. Reprinted with permission from Binder P, Lambert R, Koepnick R, et al. A comparison of the Phoenix and Chiron microkeratomes for the correction of high myopia. *J Cataract Refract Surg.* 1996;22:1175-1188.

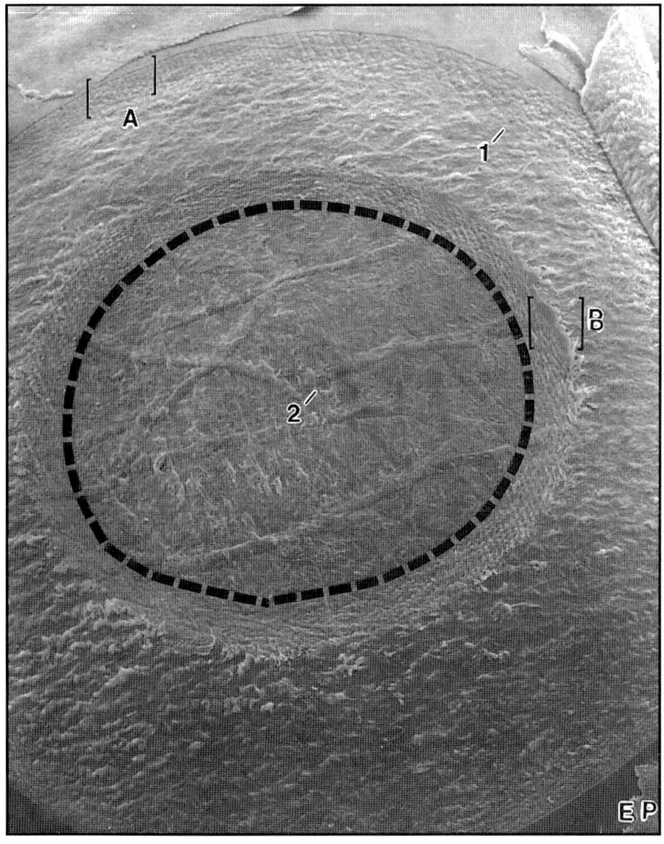

Figure 6-5a.
SEM view of the surface of an eye bank eye that has undergone automated lamellar keratoplasty with the UniversalKeratome. The diameter of the power cut is easily seen with the Automated Corneal Shaper, whereas the edge of the UniversalKeratome power cut cannot be detected at the SEM level. Note the irregular cut edge of Bowman's layer created by the Automated Corneal Shaper. 30x. 1′ = primary cut; 2′ = secondary cut. The area in brackets (b) on the left is the slope from the primary cut to the secondary cut. Reprinted with permission from Binder P, Lambert R, Koepnick R, et al. A comparison of the Phoenix and Chiron microkeratomes for the correction of high myopia. *J Cataract Refract Surg.* 1996;22:1175-1188.

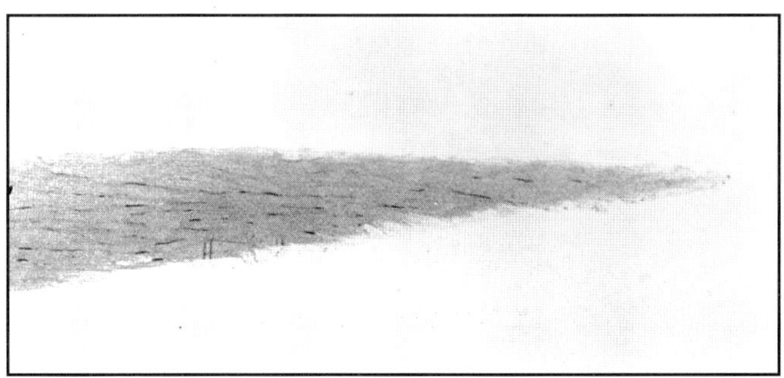

Figure 6-4b.
Light microscopic sectional views of a myopic power cut obtained in an eye bank eye with the Phoenix Keratek Inc UniversalKeratome. Note the parallel faces of the Automated Corneal Shaper lenticle compared to the lenticular shape of the UniversalKeratome tissue. Figures 6-4a and 6-4b are at the same magnification (320x) and represent the amount of tissue resected to correct the same amount of myopia. Reprinted with permission from Binder P, Lambert R, Koepnick R, et al. A comparison of the Phoenix and Chiron microkeratomes for the correction of high myopia. *J Cataract Refract Surg.* 1996;22:1175-1188.

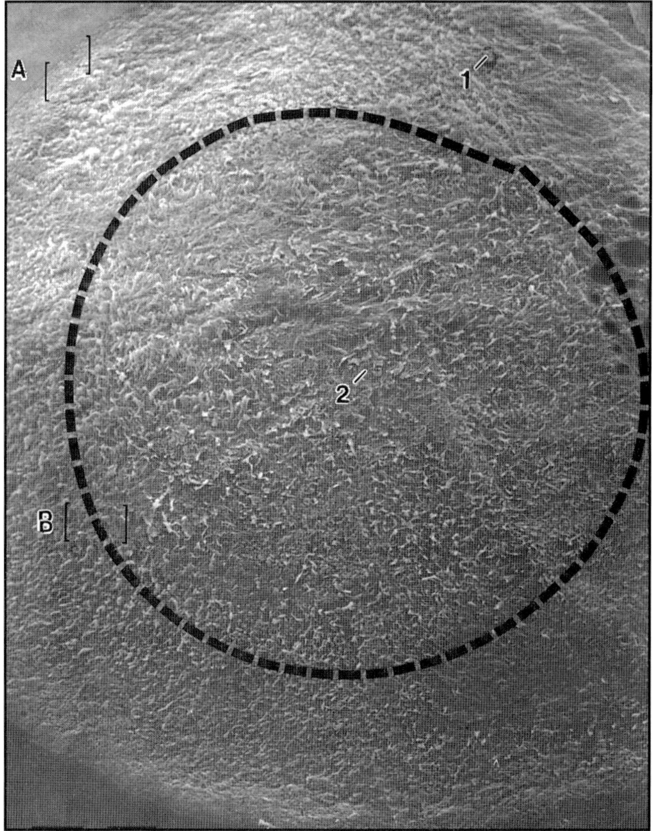

Figure 6-5b.
SEM view of the surface of an eye bank eye that has undergone lamellar lenticular keratoplasty with the UniversalKeratome. Reprinted with permission from Binder P, Lambert R, Koepnick R, et al. A comparison of the Phoenix and Chiron microkeratomes for the correction of high myopia. *J Cataract Refract Surg.* 1996;22:1175-1188.

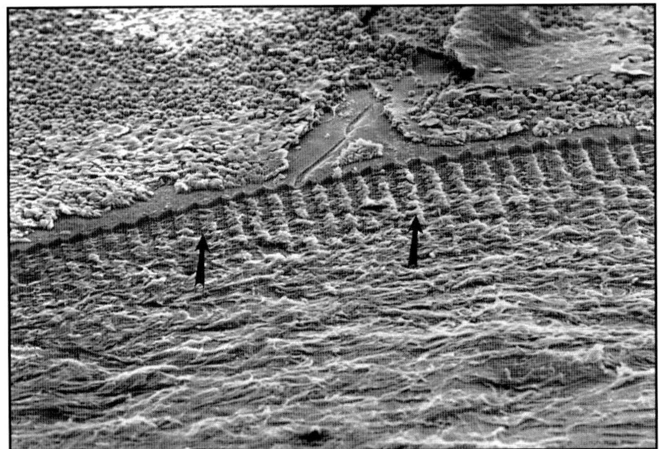

Figure 6-6.
High power SEM view of the edge of the power cut seen with the Automated Corneal Shaper (area marked in brackets as a in Figure 6-5, left). Note the chatter marks on the sloping edge of the power cut. Reprinted with permission from Binder P, Lambert R, Koepnick R, et al. A comparison of the Phoenix and Chiron microkeratomes for the correction of high myopia. *J Cataract Refract Surg.* 1996;22:1175-1188.

marks with the UniversalKeratome (Figure 6-6, right). Furthermore, the other unit creates a smaller final optical zone diameter (which explains postoperative visual complaints) since there is a taper from the beginning of the secondary cut to the final achieved diameter (arrows, left) which is always smaller than attempted. The surface of the optical zone was found to be smoother with the UniversalKeratome. These acute morphologic results demonstrate that the optical theory and design of the UniversalKeratome are correct and that the UniversalKeratome is capable of creating optically correct and extremely smooth resections.

CLINICAL RESULTS

The first sighted eyes were operated in October 1995. Subsequently, KMIS and LASIK procedures have been performed on eyes with spherical equivalent refractive errors between -6.87 and -25 D (Table 6-3). The ultrasonically determined cap thickness resections were variable; postoperative refractive errors for KMIS were undercorrected during the development of the predictive algorithms. The initial microkeratome designs had a traverse speed of 0.5 mm/sec; the slow traverse speed was thought to be the cause of edema of the corneal cap. Subsequent traverse speed modifications have used traverse speeds from 0.75 to 1.5 mm/sec. The LASIK results were dependent on laser algorithms that are currently undergoing modification.

Early metal blade designs combined with a wide lateral throw of the blade during the 14,000 cycles per second oscillation deposited metallic fragments into the interface. These particles did not interfere with vision. Modifications of blade design have included wider cutting surfaces that are "mirror-finished" to reduce the chances of interface metallic foreign bodies. Early designs of the PMMA optical cap combined with less than adequate blade sharpness created irregular cap edges; subsequent blade modifications and the reduction of the PMMA cap diameter from 9.0 to 8.5 mm has greatly reduced these complications. Visual and refractive results obtained in sighted eyes are listed in Table 6-3. Based on the laboratory tests and clinical results the Phoenix Keratek UniversalKeratome has been demonstrated to be easy to use and be capable of creating excellent clinical results.

COMPARISON OF CURRENTLY PERFORMED KMIS AND LASIK

The current KMIS procedure is entirely different from the currently performed LASIK procedure and, consequently, the two procedures cannot be compared. These two procedures differ in all respects except that a microkeratome is used in the first step of each procedure. Table 6-4 compares the differences between the current procedures. The excimer laser produces very smooth surfaces and predictable tissue excision, whereas current microkeratomes resect tissue volume and shapes that are dependent on IOP, blade quality, traverse speed, blade oscillation, and corneal deformation. Figures 6-7a and 6-7b compare the surface of an eye bank eye immediately following a standard LASIK procedure with the surface of an eye following a Phoenix UniversalKeratome power cut (KMIS) of the same diameter and attempted myopic correction. The surfaces are comparable. The predictability of tissue shape excision and potential differences in postoperative wound healing will determine if these two modalities produce equivalent visual and refractive results.

TABLE 6-3

First LASIK Cases Performed by Frank Lavery, MD, and Perry S. Binder, MD, Using the Phoenix Keratek Inc UniversalKeratome

Preop Sphere	Preop Astig	Diameter PMMA	Cap Thickness	Preop BSCVA	Preop UCVA	Follow-Up (mos.)	Postop UCVA	Postop Sphere	Postop Astig	Postop BSCVA
-9.50	2.25	8.5	133	20/25	<20/200	1	20/200	1.50	0.00	NR
-20.75	1.00	8.5	155	20/40	<20/200	1	20/125	-3.00	1.50	NR
-4.25	5.25	9.5	165	20/25	20/60	1	20/25	0.50	3.00	NR
-24.00	1.50	8.5	187	20/60	CF	1	20/200	-1.00	3.00	20/125
-12.50	1.25	8.5	133	20/30	<20/200	1	20/125	-1.00	5.00	20/30
-11.00	1.75	8.5	134	20/40	<20/200	1	20/125	-3.00	1.00	20/60
-10.00	1.00	8.5	87	20/15	<20/200	1	20/15	0.00	0.00	20/15
-9.00	0.75	8.5	169	20/20	<20/200	1	20/30	-0.75	0.75	20/30
-10.25	1.00	8.5	109	20/20	<20/200	1	20/80	2.00	0.00	20/30
-14.50	1.00	8.5	200	20/30	<20/200	1	20/60	-3.50	0.00	20/30
-26.25	0.75	8.5	103	20/100	CF	1	20/125	-4.00	1.00	20/100
-23.50	1.75	8.5	180	20/80	CF	1	CF	-8.75	2.00	20/100
-11.00	1.25	8.5	125	20/15	<20/200	1	20/15	-0.25	1.75	20/20
-12.00	0.75	8.5	103	20/30	<20/200	1	20/80	-2.00	3.00	20/60
-10.00	1.50	8.5	101	20/20	<20/200	1	20/125	1.00	1.00	20/20
-7.00	1.75	8.6	100	20/20	CF	3	20/70	-4.00	5.00	20/20
-11.00	2.25	8.6	130	20/20	CF	3	20/80	-1.75	2.25	20/30

NR=not reported, CF=count fingers.

SUMMARY

The Phoenix UniversalKeratome advances the field of microlamellar refractive surgery by minimizing human error while improving the optical quality of tissue resection, as well as predictability of tissue resection. Expected improvements in surgical nomograms and instrument advances make the future of lamellar refractive surgery bright.

References

1. Lyle W, Jin G. Initial results of automated lamellar keratoplasty for correction of myopia: one year follow-up. *J Cataract Refract Surg.* 1996;22:31-43.

2. Ibrahim O, Waring GI, Salah T, et al. Automated in situ keratomileusis for myopia. *J Refract Surg.* 1995;11(6):431-441.

3. Bosc J, Montard M, Delbosc B, et al. Non-freeze myopic keratomileusis: retrospective study of 27 consecutive operations. *J Fr Ophthalmol.* 1990;13:10-16.

4. Rozakis G, ed. *Refractive Lamellar Keratoplasty.* Thorofare, NJ: SLACK Inc; 1994.

5. Crews K, Mifflin M, Olson R. Complications of automated lamellar keratectomy. *Arch Ophthalmol.* 1994;12:1514-1515.

6. Ruiz L, Rowsey JJ. In situ keratomileusis. *Invest Ophthalmol Vis Sci.* 1988;29(suppl):392.

7. Polit F, Ibrahim O, El-Maghraby A, et al. Cryolathe keratomileusis for correction of myopia of 4.00 to 8.00 diopters. *Refract Corneal Surg.* 1993;9:259-267.

8. Pallikaris I, Papatzanaki M, Stathi E, et al. Laser in situ keratomileusis. *Lasers Surg Med.* 1990;10:463-468.

9. Brint S, Ostrick D, Fisher C, et al. Six-month results of the multicenter phase I study of excimer laser myopic keratomileusis. *J Cataract Refract Surg.* 1994;20:610-614.

10. Bas A, Onnis R. Excimer laser in situ keratomileusis for myopia. *J Refract Surg.* 1995;11(suppl):S229-S233.

11. Binder P, Akers P, Zavala E, et al. Refractive keratoplasty: microkeratome evaluation. *Arch Ophthalmol.* 1982;100:802-806.

12. Binder P, Lambert R, Koepnick R, et al. A comparison of the Phoenix

TABLE 6-4

Comparison of Current KMIS Procedures With Currently Performed LASIK and the Phoenix Keratek Inc UniversalKeratome*

	KMIS	LASIK	UniversalKeratome
Optical zone diameter (mm)	4.2 to 5.0	6.0	6.0
Excised tissue shape	Parallel	Lenticular	Lenticular
Tissue excision	Mechanical	Laser	Mechanical
Cap diameter (mm)	7.2 to 8.0	8.6 to 9.0	8.6 to 9.0
Cap thickness (μm)	160	130 to 160	130 to 160
Microkeratome passes	Two	One	Two
Optical surface quality	Rough	Smooth	Smooth

*Comparison based on clinical experience of the author, reported clinical data, and results of unpublished laboratory experiments.

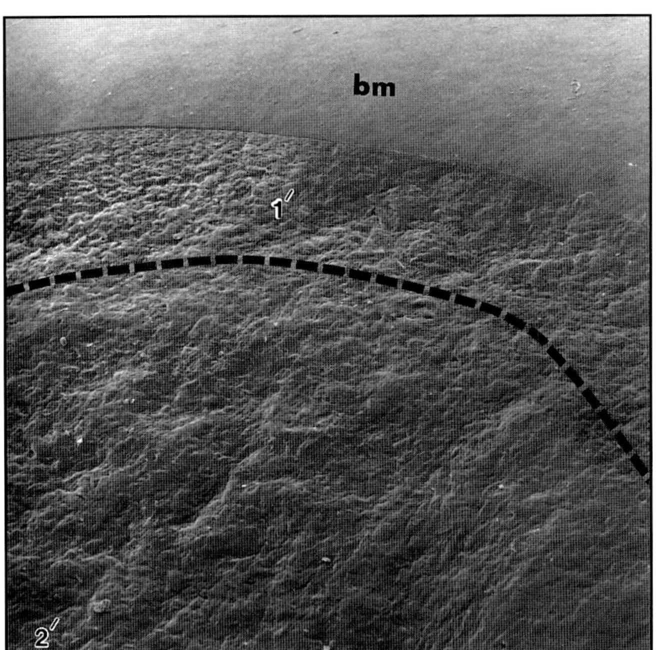

Figure 6-7a.
SEM comparison of the ocular surface of eye bank eyes immediately following a LASIK procedure performed with the UniversalKeratome and a current argon-flouride excimer laser (Figure 6-7a) (58x) with the surface of a KMIS performed using the UniversalKeratome (Figure 6-7b) (34x) for the same degree of myopia using the same 6.0-mm optical zone diameters. There is no difference in the surface smoothness with either procedure. Note the same smooth cut edge of Bowman's layer (bm) created with the UniversalKeratome in both figures. 1′ = primary cut; 2′ = secondary cut (LASIK, left; KMIS, right).

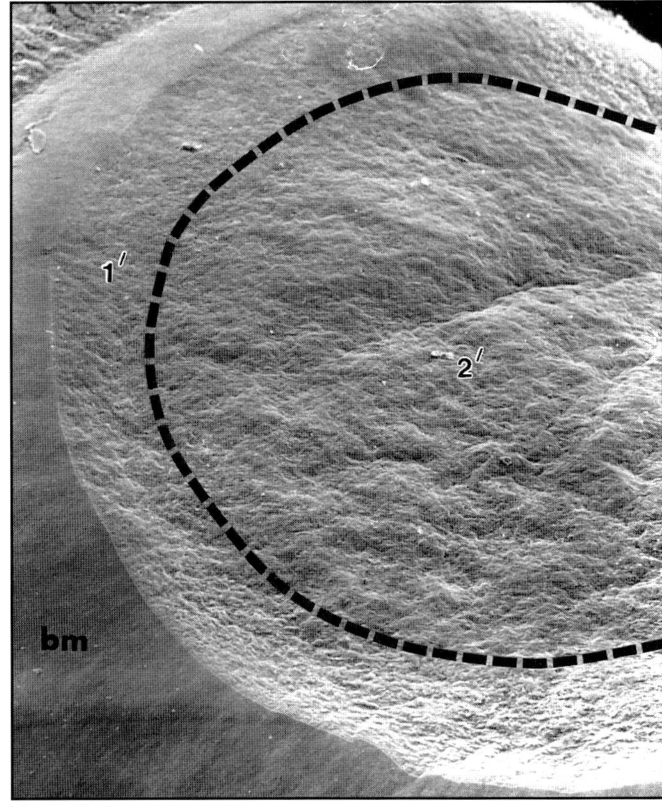

Figure 6-7b.
SEM comparison of the ocular surface of eye bank eyes immediately following a LASIK procedure performed with the UniversalKeratome and a current argon-flouride excimer laser (Figure 6-7a) (58x) with the surface of a KMIS performed using the UniversalKeratome (Figure 6-7b) (34x) for the same degree of myopia using the same 6.0-mm optical zone diameters.

and Chiron microkeratomes for the correction of high myopia. *J Cataract Refract Surg.* 1996;22:1175-1188.

13. Hoffman C, Rapuano C, Cohen E, et al. Displacement of corneal lenticle after automated lamellar keratoplasty. *Am J Ophthalmol.* 1994;118(1):110-111.

14. Arenas-Archila E, Sanchez-Thorin J, Naranjo-Uribe J, et al. Myopic keratomileusis in situ: a human preliminary report. *J Cataract Refract Surg.* 1991;17:424-435.

15. Price FJ. Keratomileusis. Contemporary refractive surgery. In: Thompson, Waring GO III, eds. *Ophthalmology Clinics of North America*. Philadelphia, Pa: WB Saunders Co; 1992:673-681.

16. Laroche L, Gauthier L, Thenot J, et al. Nonfreeze myopic keratomileusis for myopia in l58 eyes. *Refract Corneal Surg.* 1994;10:400-412.

17. Maldonado A, Nano H. In situ myopic keratomileusis results in 30 eyes at 15 months. *Refract Corneal Surg.* 1991;7:223-231.

18. Gomes M. Keratomileusis-in-situ using manual dissection of corneal flap for high myopia. *Refract Corneal Surg.* 1994;10(suppl):S255-S257.

19. Kohlhaas M, Draeger J, Lerch R-C, et al. Different techniques of lamellar refractive keratoplasties for the correction of myopia. *Eur J Implant Refract Surg.* 1995;7:70-76.

20. Leahey A, Burkholder T. Complications of automated lamellar keratektomy. *Arch Ophthalmol.* 1994;112:1514-1515.

21. Littlefield T, Binder P, Geggel H, et al. The Phoenix Keratek, Inc. UniversalKeratome®. *Biomedical Optics.* 1997;2:106-114.

Chapter 7

COMPARISON OF MICROKERATOMES

Richard W. Yee, MD, Mohammed N. Khan, MD,
Asma T. Khan, Alice Chuang, PhD,
Narayanan Ramesh, MBBS

Photorefractive keratectomy (PRK) was a major innovation in corrective eye surgery that came about due to the excimer laser. The powerful and accurate excimer laser is able to ablate minute amounts of corneal tissue, from the epithelium inward, without the use of a blade and can be adjusted for correction of various degrees of myopia. The results of PRK were for the most part successful,[1,2] except in cases of high myopia that displayed significant postoperative side effects.[3-5] Wound healing of the ablated epithelium and Bowman's layer is a postoperative concern, with corneal haze and regression being common findings. The regrowth of the epithelium and Bowman's layer after surgery was also a concern due to regeneration of varying thicknesses of individuals, making accurate correction of high myopia difficult.

The introduction of laser in situ keratomileusis (LASIK) alleviated some of these complications.[6,7] LASIK is an innovative procedure combining the use of excimer laser and keratomileusis in which a corneal flap of 130- to 160-µm thickness is created with a microkeratome to expose the stroma. The stroma is then ablated with excimer laser to correct for myopia. The use of a corneal flap aims to minimize damage to the anterior corneal layers. A further advantage of ablating through only the stroma as opposed to the combination of epithelium, Bowman's layer, and stroma is the formation of new connective tissue at the site of the wound with no unwanted epithelial edema.[8,9]

Additionally, LASIK provides early stabilization of postoperative refraction as compared with PRK by sparing Bowman's layer. Thus, with increasing use of LASIK

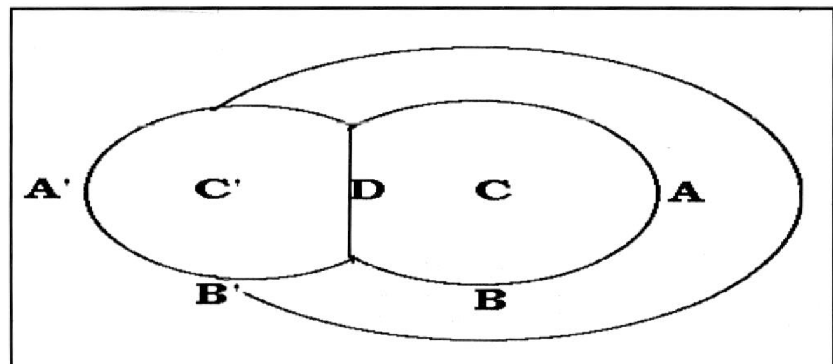

Figure 7-1.
Schematic of cornea shown with underside of resected flap and underlying stromal bed. A′=lateral flap edge, B′=bottom flap edge, C′=flap center, A=lateral stromal edge, B=bottom stromal edge, C=stromal bed center, and D=hinge.

and proliferation of microkeratome types, at least two questions arise regarding microkeratomes: which type of microkeratome to use and whether different microkeratomes cause different levels of damage to the epithelium and stroma during the creation of the corneal flap. Two microkeratomes, Chiron Automated Corneal Shaper (Chiron Vision Corp, Claremont, Calif) and SCMD (a manual microkeratome manufactured by SCMD of Fountain Hills, Ariz and distributed by Microtech), are representative of two classes currently in use. SCMD is turbine nitrogen gas-driven for higher cutting speed and contains a permanent head plate as a safety feature. Anecdotally, some ophthalmic surgeons prefer the control that the manual SCMD enables them to have. In contrast, other surgeons prefer the controlled speed of automated microkeratomes for more consistent cuts.

In our research we have used scanning electron microscopy (SEM) quantitative grading of damage by independently trained observers to compare the quality of cuts on porcine corneas made by Chiron and SCMD microkeratomes, with the idea that the smoothest and cleanest cuts may help reduce postoperative complications.

MATERIALS AND METHODS

Surgical Procedure

In the first experiment, six pairs of fresh pig eyes were prepared for cutting and creation of corneal flaps by two microkeratomes, the automated Chiron and the manual SCMD. For each pair of eyes, a coin was flipped to determine which microkeratome was to be used first, thus maintaining randomness. Each pig eye was placed and centered on a globe plexiholder, and the epithelium was carefully scraped off. A suction cup was placed on each eye, generating an IOP greater than 65 mmHg. A corneal thickness of 160 µm was cut at automated speed (Chiron) or a corneal thickness of 130 to 150 µm was cut across manually at normal, even-paced speed using a #1 vacuum ring and a stop ring of 8 mm (SCMD). The following rpm speeds were used: 7000 rpm for Chiron and 14,000 rpm for SCMD at a pressure of 42 psi.

After the flap was created and resected to expose the stromal bed, a few drops of 2% glutaraldehyde were placed on the stromal bed and the underside of the flap to preserve the flap in its open position. After 30 seconds, a few drops were again added. Then the eye was immediately placed in a labeled cup that was half-filled with 2% glutaraldehyde. Each blade (for both Chiron and SCMD) was used for only two eyes and then disposed of.

Electron Microscopy

Tissue processing for SEM was done in two batches.[10] Each sample was fixed in 3% glutaraldehyde for at least 24 hours and then washed for 5 minutes in malonic-sodium-phosphate buffer (pH 7.3 to 7.4). The buffer was removed and the tissue fixed in 2% osmium tetroxide for 1 hour at 4°C. Each sample was sequentially washed for 5 minutes in water, 5 minutes in 50% ethanol, 5 minutes in 70% ethanol, 15 minutes in 95% ethanol, and three times each for 15 minutes in 100% ethanol. Each sample was then treated with hexamethyldisilazane (HMDS) for 30 seconds to 1 minute and, after decanting HMDS, allowed to air dry for 1 hour. Each sample was mounted onto SEM stub and sputter coated. The underside of the flap and stromal bed of each cornea was then scanned using SEM at a magnification of 150x, with all seven designated positions on the corneal flap and stromal bed scanned separately (Figure 7-1).

Grading of Damage

After obtaining pictures of all seven positions for each cornea, pictures of each position for all 12 eyes were grouped together and shuffled, with the identity (which pair of eyes and which microkeratome used) being hidden. Graders received verbal and written instructions on specific grading criteria for each position correlated with sample pictures. Based on their visual assessment of damage in a particular position, graders then gave each

TABLE 7-1

Grading of Corneal Damage at Designated Positions on SEM After Chiron or SCMD Microkeratome Use on Paired Porcine Eyes

Position*	Chiron	(Mean SD)**	SCMD	(Mean SD)**	p Value***
Overall	3.042	(0.700)	2.083	(0.639)	<0.0001
A	3.08	(0.736)	2.25	(0.387)	0.05
A′	3.375	(0.607)	2.667	(0.645)	0.09
B	3.333	(0.665)	2.167	(0.465)	0.0006
B′	3.583	(0.683)	1.875	(0.518)	0.0002
C	2.958	(0.459)	1.75	(0.418)	0.0026
C′	2.625	(0.468)	2.167	(0.890)	0.399
D-hinge	2.667	(0.736)	2.042	(0.697)	0.266
D-stroma	2.708	(0.843)	1.75	(0.74)	0.181

*Refer to Figure 7-1 for descriptions of positions.
**Grading: 1=excellent, 2=good, 3=fair, 4=poor.
***p value obtained from one-way ANOVA with random effect model.

picture a score of 1 to 4 (1=excellent, 2=good, 3=fair, 4=poor).

STATISTICAL METHODS

Weighted kappa statistics measuring the agreement between graders were calculated. The average scores of each location of each eye obtained from four graders were computed for further analysis. A one-way ANOVA with random effect model was employed to compare the differences in mean score between Chiron and SCMD microkeratomes. A p-value less than 0.05 is considered statistically significant.

RESULTS

The kappa statistics indicate the intergrader agreement between graders one and two was 59% better than if graders' ratings were by chance. Similarly, the kappa statistics between graders one and three was 73%, between graders one and four was 68%, between graders two and three was 65%, between two and four was 48%, and between three and four was 65%. These indicate a moderate agreement among graders (>0.6 represents good reliability, 0.4 to 0.6 represents moderate reliability, and <0.4 represents poor reliability[11]).

Table 7-1 shows the mean and standard deviation of the overall mean score and the mean score of each location. Overall, SCMD had a significantly lower score than Chiron (mean difference = 0.96, $p<0.0001$). For each location, SCMD had a mean score lower than Chiron. Locations A, B, B′, and C showed statistically significant differences (see Table 7-1). Location A′ did not reach a statistically significant level ($p=0.09$), which may be due to the small sample size (six pairs). Locations C′, D at hinge, and D at stromal bed did not show a statistical difference between Chiron and SCMD.

DISCUSSION

Due to the increasing use of the LASIK procedure, we believe that the choice of a microkeratome is an important one. Chiron and SCMD microkeratomes were chosen to represent two major classes of microkeratomes, automated and manual, respectively. SEM was chosen to evaluate the quality of the cuts because of its powerful ability to display detailed surface topography of the corneal stroma, thus making visual recognition of corneal damage easier. When graders were trained, they were instructed to disregard any shrinking or artifactual matter due to tissue preparation. In order to maintain fairness, these aspects had no impact on their evaluation.

As was stated before, SCMD overall showed better scores. In addition, SCMD was shown to be statistically significant at locations A, B, B′, and C. In a side-by-side comparison of one pair of porcine eyes cut by the two microkeratomes as is shown in Figures 7-2a and 7-2b (position A′ for first pair of eyes), it is visually apparent that Chiron produced the worse cut with shredded flap edges. Generally, the Chiron cuts produced chatter marks, jagged edges, lines, and shards. Although SCMD may have produced such characteristics in some eyes, it did not do so to the extent that Chiron did judging from qualitative photographs (Figures 7-2a through 7-7b) and from quantitative grading assessments (see Table 7-1). Figures 7-2a through 7-7b further show the differences in the cuts made by both microkeratomes in various pairs of eyes. The presence of chatter marks, jagged edges, lines, and shards is taken to be an indicator of damage[12] of the epithelium and stroma with the assumption that more damage, as determined by SEM, results in more and longer postoperative complications. Such studies have yet to be undertaken, but this study provides evidence of greater visually apparent damage induced by Chiron than by SCMD.

The control that an ophthalmic surgeon has during a cut with a manual microkeratome may account for SCMD's better performance. With automation, a surgeon has essentially no control over the electrically controlled microkeratome, possibly causing more damage. However, other variables may have also contributed to SCMD's superior results, including higher rpm speed, quality of blade, and overall design of microkeratome. Further studies will need to be conducted in order to determine the exact reason(s) for less damage induced by SCMD.

References

1. McDonald MB, Frantz JM, Klyce S, et al. Central photorefractive keratectomy for myopia. The blind eye study. *Arch Ophthalmol.* 1990;108:799-808.
2. Seiler T, Wollensak J. Myopic photorefractive keratectomy with the excimer laser: one year follow up. *Ophthalmology.* 1991;98:1156-1163.
3. Seiler T, Jean V, Pham T, Derse M. Statistical analysis of myopic regression after excimer laser PRK. *Invest Ophthalmol Vis Sci.* 1991;32(suppl):S721.
4. Sher NA, Barak MN, Daya SM, et al. Photorefractive keratectomy (PRK) using 193 nm excimer laser in high myopia. *Invest Ophthalmol Vis Sci.* 1992;33(suppl):S762.
5. Tavola L, Garancini P, Carones F, Brancato R. Does any variable influence the regression after PRK? *Invest Ophthalmol Vis Sci.* 1992;33(suppl):763.
6. Kim H-M, Jung HR. Laser assisted in situ keratomileusis for high myopia. *Ophthalmic Surg Lasers.* 1996;27:S508-S511.
7. Marinho A, Pinto MC, Pinto R, Vaz F, Neves MC. LASIK for high myopia: one year experience. *Ophthalmic Surg Lasers.* 1996;27:S517-S520.
8. Pallikaris IG, Papatzanaki ME, Siganos DS, Tsilimbaris MK. A corneal flap technique for laser in situ keratomileusis. *Arch Ophthalmol.* 1991;109:1699-1702.
9. Tuft SJ, Zabel RW, Marshall J. Corneal repair following keratectomy: a comparison between conventional surgery and laser photoablation. *Invest Ophthalmol Vis Sci.* 1989;30:1769-1777.
10. Hyatt MA. *Principles and Techniques of Scanning Electron Microscopy.* New York, NY: Van Nostrand Reinhold and Co.
11. Altman DG. *Practical Statistics for Medical Research.* New York, NY: Chapman and Hall; 1995:403-409.
12. Hoffmann RF, Bechara SJ. An independent evaluation of second generation suction microkeratomes. *Refract Corneal Surg.* 1992;8:248-254.

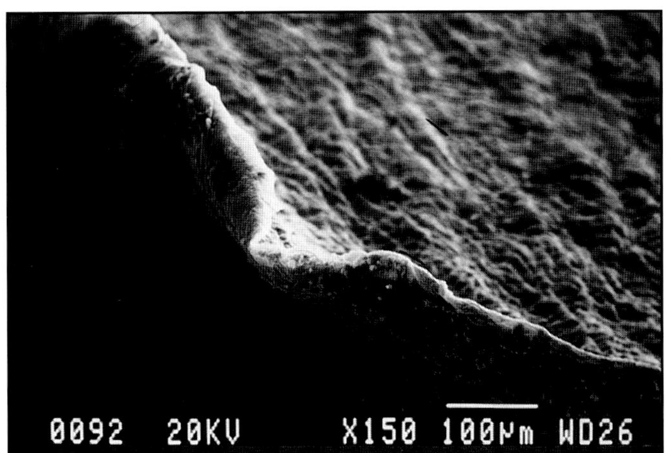

Figure 7-2a.
SEM of position A′ on paired porcine corneas (150x). Cut by SCMD. Note fairly smooth edge lined with small waves. No chatter marks are seen. (Bend in surface is artifactual due to drying during SEM tissue preparation.)

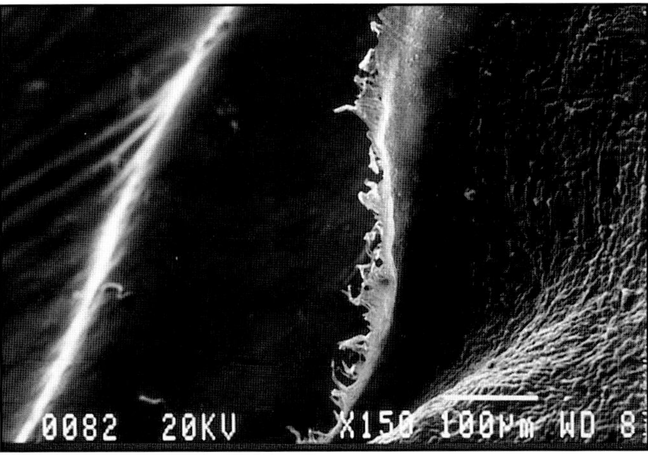

Figure 7-2b.
Cut by Chiron. In contrast, edge of flap is torn and shredded deeply. Few chatter lines are seen at the top edge of flap. No smooth surface is seen.

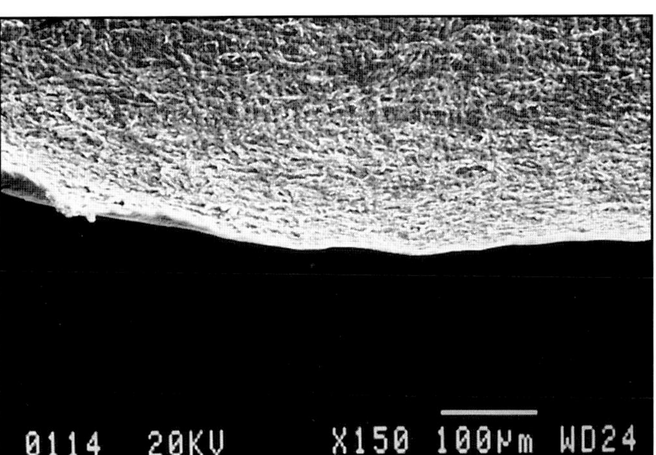

Figure 7-3a.
SEM of position B′ on paired porcine corneas (150x). Cut by SCMD. Right two thirds of flap is smoothly consistent, but left one third shows rough edge in the form of waves. No chatter marks are seen.

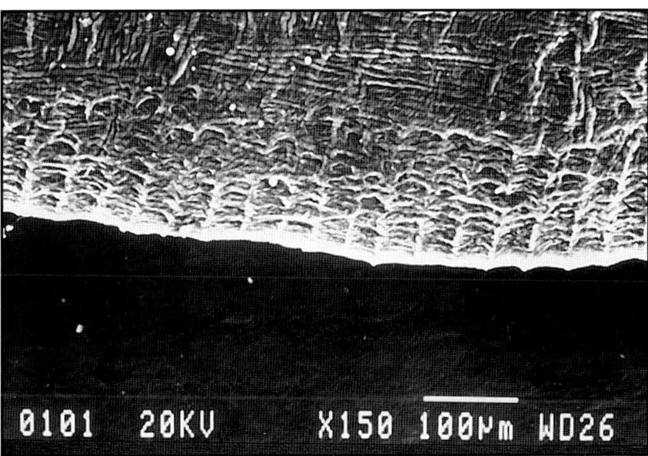

Figure 7-3b.
Cut by Chiron. Entire flap edge is smoothly consistent except for prominent chatter marks (length between 50 to 100 μm) which extend to flap edge.

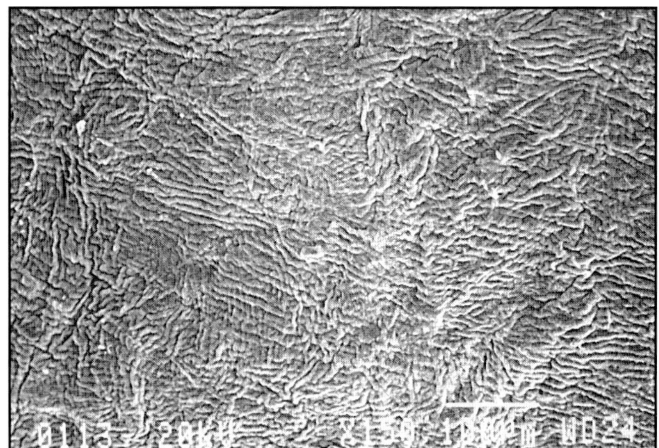

Figure 7-4a.
SEM of position C′ on paired porcine corneas (150x). Cut by SCMD. Surface is somewhat smooth and homogeneous except for bottom middle, where an indentation (>100 μm) and several small ridges are seen. White material can be seen strewn on the surface of this micrograph and the one in Figure 7-4b. This material was considered to be either artifactual or shards from another part of the cornea.

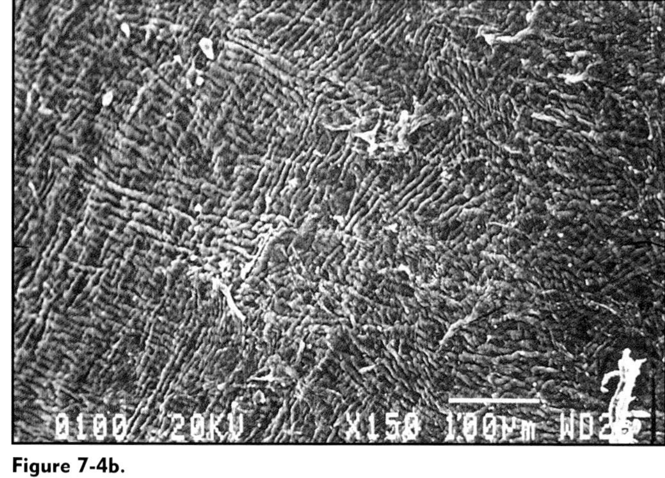

Figure 7-4b.
Cut by Chiron. Surface is fairly homogeneous and smooth (excluding artifacts and shards). No indentations or ridges are present except for several slight ridges (<100 μm) in the center.

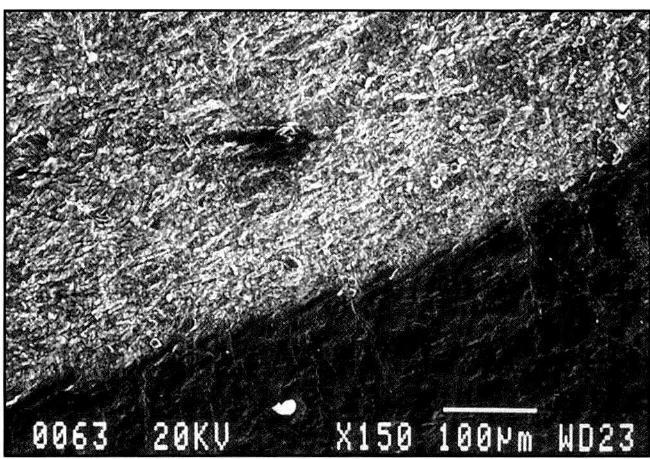

Figure 7-5a.
SEM of position A on paired porcine corneas (150x). Cut by SCMD. Edge is jagged with some cut marks and lines that extend beyond edge onto surface of cornea.

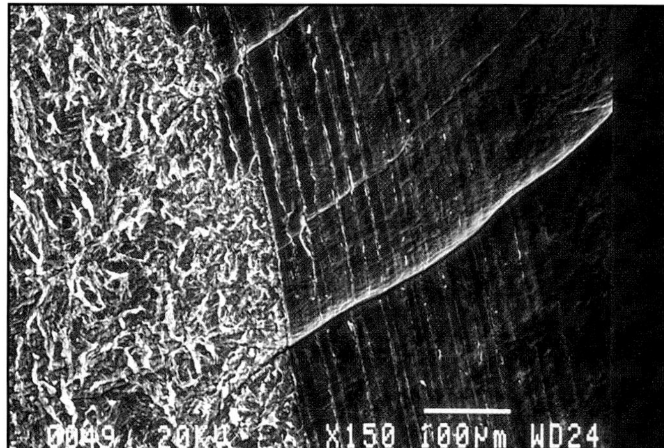

Figure 7-5b.
Cut by Chiron. Jagged edges are seen, but unlike the micrograph in Figure 7-5a, the cut marks are less frequent (only two are seen), but cut much deeper into stroma. The cut marks, or chatter, extend much further (>300 μm) beyond the edge onto the cornea than in Figure 7-5a (<50 μm).

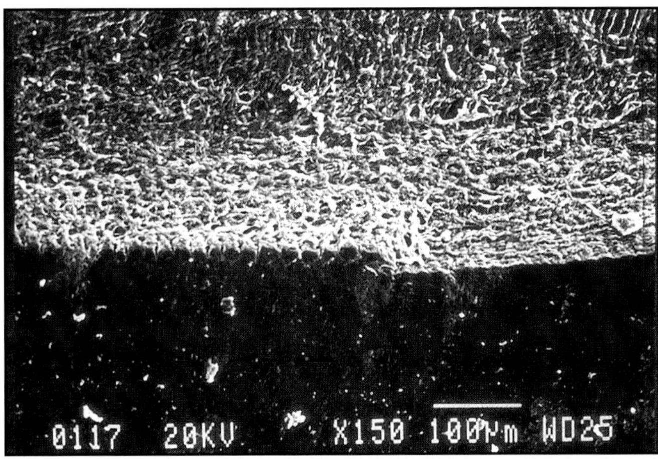

Figure 7-6a.
SEM of position B on paired porcine corneas (150x). Cut by SCMD. While the right one third has a smooth edge without chatter marks, an abrupt transition is made to the left two thirds where the stromal edge is broken by prominent small chatter marks which extend about 100 μm into the stroma.

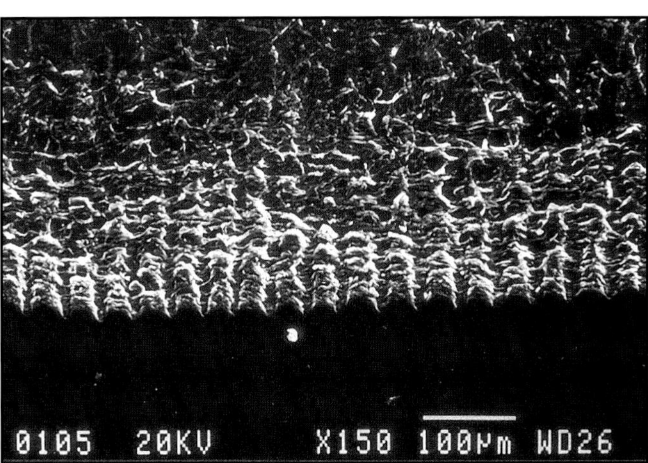

Figure 7-6b.
Cut by Chiron. Jagged edges produced by prominent large chatter marks (length between 100 to 150 μm) that are more widely spaced than those in Figure 7-6a.

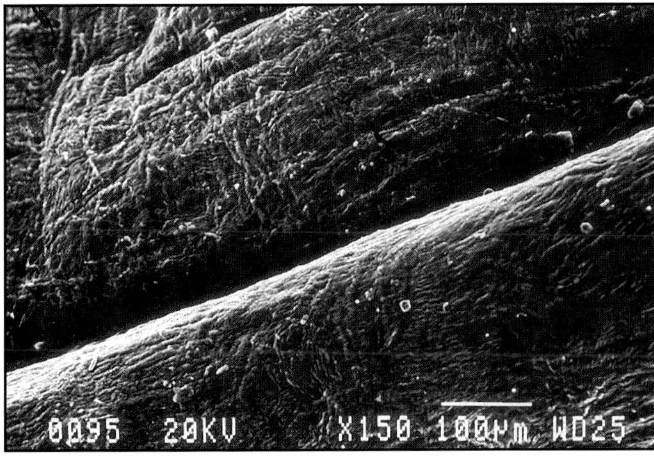

Figure 7-7a.
SEM of position D on paired corneas (150x). Cut by SCMD. Hinge area is fairly smooth and flowing. No jagged edges are seen. Adjacent stroma is homogeneous except for slight ridges on both sides of hinge.

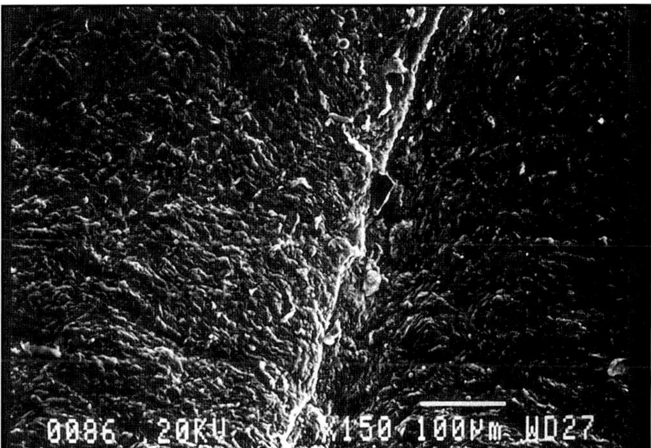

Figure 7-7b.
Cut by Chiron. Hinge area is not straight or consistent. Artifactual or misplaced shards can be seen. Adjacent stroma is not homogeneous and several ridges can be seen the length of the hinge.

Chapter 8

THE PICOSECOND LASER

Mark Speaker, MD, PhD, Vincenzo Marchi, MD,
Tibor Juhasz, PhD, Marc A. Goldberg, MD

INTRODUCTION

The current trend in laser refractive surgery favoring intrastromal surgical techniques is an outgrowth of perceived and demonstrated advantages over predecessor surface ablation techniques. A critical advantage of intrastromal surgery includes an avoidance of damage to corneal epithelium and Bowman's layer with associated reductions in undesirable outcomes such as pain, lengthy recovery times, stromal scarring or haze, and regression of effect.[1] An issue to be considered in developing intrastromal surgery techniques is how best to gain access to, as well as remove, stromal tissue without damaging surrounding corneal stroma. The picosecond laser is one of several promising technologies currently under development for intrastromal refractive surgery.

The picosecond laser, originally produced by Intelligent Surgical Laser (ISL) (San Diego, Calif), and now owned by Escalon Medical Corp (Skillman, NJ) was first described as a refractive tool in 1986.[2] It is a pulsed solid-state neodymium-yttrium lithium fluoride (Nd-YLF) laser for intrastromal photorefractive keratectomy (IPRK) which operates in the infrared at 1053 nm with a pulse duration of 20 picoseconds. The infrared pulses are not absorbed by normal corneal tissue so that corneal epithelium and Bowman's layer are undisturbed as the picosecond laser beam passes through them to the specified focal point in the stroma where optical breakdown occurs.[2-4] In addition, the ultrashort pulse width of the picosecond laser allows for tissue cutting or removal at threshold energies of approximately 10 μJ (compared to millijoule thresholds of nanosecond YAG lasers), limiting the effects of optical breakdown to approximately a 10-μm radius, so that collateral damage to Descemet's membrane and the endothelium does not occur.[2,5-8]

Optical breakdown at the focal point of the picosecond laser achieves a plasma mediated photodisruption of corneal tissue. The gas bubbles produced in the wake of the optical breakdown diffuse through remaining cornea and are undetectable within 30 to 60 minutes. The delivery system of the picosecond laser allows for a precise scanning ablation of a three-dimensional ablation zone.[9] Because of the 10 μm spot size of each pulse of the picosecond laser, thousands of pulses are necessary to achieve a sufficient amount of tissue removal for a desired refractive effect. In order to deliver the multiple pulses accurately and completely, the ISL laser utilizes a delivery system that centers and immobilizes the cornea for laser application. The cornea is stabilized by a cone containing a quartz applanating lens (coupling the cornea to the delivery system) and a limbal suction ring, ensuring immobilization as well as centration.

Layering of thousands of pulses within the stroma in intrastromal picosecond laser keratomileusis (IPRK) creates a potential space within the stroma. The resultant collapse of the overlying corneal tissue (ie, epithelium, Bowman's layer, and anterior stroma) can create a flattening of the corneal surface, and a desired hyperopic effect of greater than 10 D in rabbit and cat corneas.[9] Treatment with this technique produced little change in human corneas, however, possibly because of the presence of Bowman's layer.

Because the results of intrastromal ablation were inconsistent in human corneas, the laser was adapted to lamellar refractive techniques. Using a spiral pattern at a depth of 180 μm in the center, a lamellar cut can be made in less than 1 minute that produces a flap identical to that produced by microkeratomes. At this point in the technique, scattered stromal bridges are encountered which have to be divided by sweeping with a blunt instrument such as a spatula. The flap can then be elevated leaving as large or small a hinge as desired. Electron microscopy has demonstrated that the cut surface of the flap is comparable to that produced with a microkeratome (RR Krueger, MD, personal communication). The excimer laser can then be used to perform a central stromal ablation under the flap. This technique has been referred to as picosecond laser keratomileusis, or PELK.

The picosecond laser can also be used to outline a lenticle 100 μm in thickness and of varying diameters. The edges of the lenticle may then be connected to the surface with a lamellar cut allowing the lenticle to be extracted with forceps from the stroma. This procedure is called PLK and is effectively equivalent to an ALK performed without a microkeratome. In blind human eyes, corrections of over 20 D have been achieved using this technique. Through PLK, the scanning laser delivery system of the ISL laser can allow for the delineation of a variety of intrastromal lenticles with plus, minus, or toric power. The PLK procedure may therefore prove useful for the range of refractive errors, and as such, human studies on sighted eyes are currently being undertaken to evaluate the practical utility of the procedure.[9]

SURGICAL INDICATIONS

The preoperative evaluation and potential indications for IPRK are identical to those for surface ablation with the excimer laser. Low and moderate myopes are likely the best candidates for this procedure. PLK and PELK, however, as mentioned above, extend the potential indications for the picosecond laser to high myopia and hyperopia as well as astigmatism.

PLK SURGICAL TECHNIQUE

The ISL picosecond laser (model 4000, The Eye Laser) (Figures 8-1a and 8-1b) is the laser currently used to perform PLK. It operates at a wavelength 1053 nm with a pulse width of 40 picoseconds, with a frequency of 1 kHz and a 10 μm spot size. Preoperatively, patients receive topical tetracaine or Marcaine for anesthesia. As with most current forms of refractive surgery, this level of anesthesia is generally adequate. The cornea is then marked using a 6-mm optical zone marker with the entrance pupil for centration. After calibrating the laser with a vinyl test cornea, with particular attention to the z-axis (depth) calibration, the microscope laser delivery system is centered around the previously placed optical zone mark. The delivery system

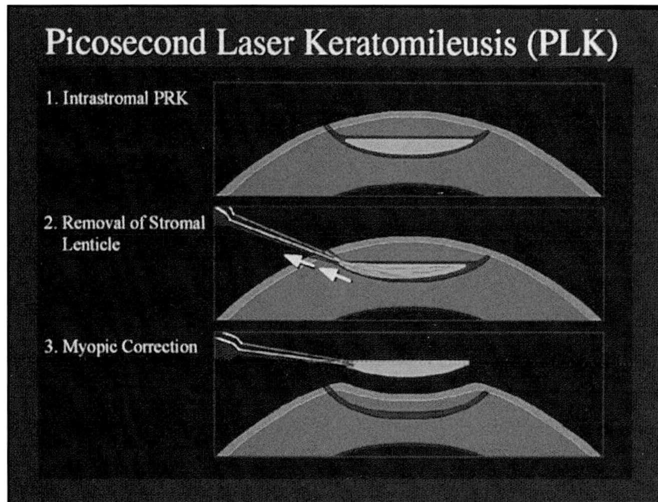

Figure 8-1a.
Schematic of PLK procedure.

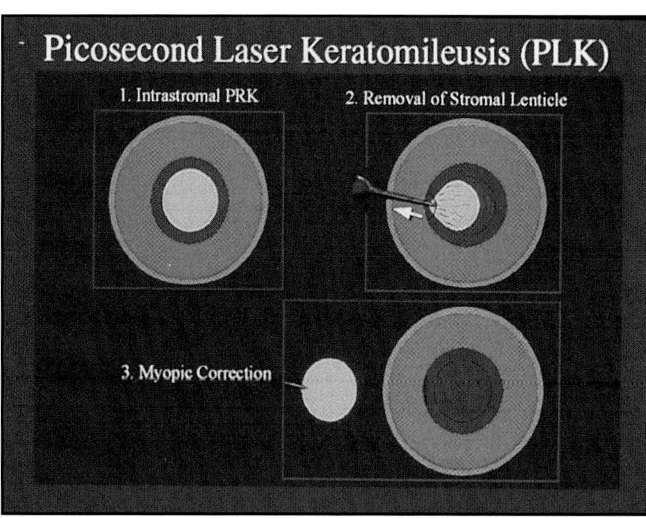

Figure 8-1b.
Schematic of PLK procedure.

consists of a cone containing a quartz applanating lens and stabilized by a limbal suction ring connected to vacuum. With suction applied and the applanated delivery hardware in place, a laser pattern consisting of two simple lamellar horizontal cuts at different depths, and an annular vertical cut connecting the two lamellar cuts is delivered. These three cuts delineate a 4-mm stromal lenticle. An additional ring-shaped horizontal cut around the lenticle extends access from the stromal lenticle to the corneal surface. Forceps are then used to grasp the lenticle through a shallow incision of 45° to 60° peripheral to the lenticle, and the lenticle is removed through this incision (Figure 8-2). A topical antibiotic drop is applied postoperatively.[9]

POSTOPERATIVE COURSE AND OUTCOME

Postoperatively in IPRK and PLK, patching or a bandage contact lens is generally not required. Postoperative antibiotic and steroid drops in a qid dosage may be discontinued after 1 to 2 weeks.

Picosecond laser surgery has been studied to date in both cat and human corneas (Figure 8-3).[7,9-11] IPRK can effect a hyperopic topographic change of about 12 D which remains stable up to 6 months post-surgically in cat corneas.[10,12] Although some stromal haze may develop within the first 4 post-surgical weeks in the cat corneas, this haze is markedly reduced or eliminated by 3 to 6 months.[10,12] Human and animal studies are also currently underway examining the safety and efficacy of PLK and PELK. The advantages of the picosecond laser compared with a microkeratome relate to superior safety, a flatter learning curve, greater flexibility in making lamellar incisions, and the necessity of raising the IOP during the procedure obviated. Disadvantages include the more complex technology and increased expense of a laser compared to a microkeratome.

The picosecond laser is still in early phases of development and study. Its efficacy and safety have been demonstrated in early animal and human investigations.[9-13] Long-term studies of both PLK and PELK will of course be necessary in the future to better evaluate safety, efficacy, and stability of the procedures, but it is clear that the picosecond laser shows great promise as an applicable intrastromal refractive surgery technology for the future.

References

1. Tuft SJ, Zabel RW, Marshall J. Corneal repair following keratectomy: a comparison between conventional surgery and laser photoablation. *Invest Ophthalmol Vis Sci.* 1989;30:1769-1777.

2. Troutman RC, Veronneau-Troutman S, Jacobiec FA, et al. A new laser for collagen wounding in corneal and strabismus surgery: a preliminary report. *Trans Am Ophthalmol Soc.* 1986;84:117-132.

3. Vogel A, Schweiger P, Freiser A, et al. Intraocular Nd:YAG laser surgery: light tissue interactions, damage range, and reduction of collateral effects. *IEEE J Quant Electron.* 1990;26:2240-2260.

4. Niemz MH, Hoppeler TP, Juhasz T et al. Intrastromal ablations for refractive corneal surgery using picosecond infrared laser pulses. *Lasers Light Ophthalmol.* 1993;5:145-152.

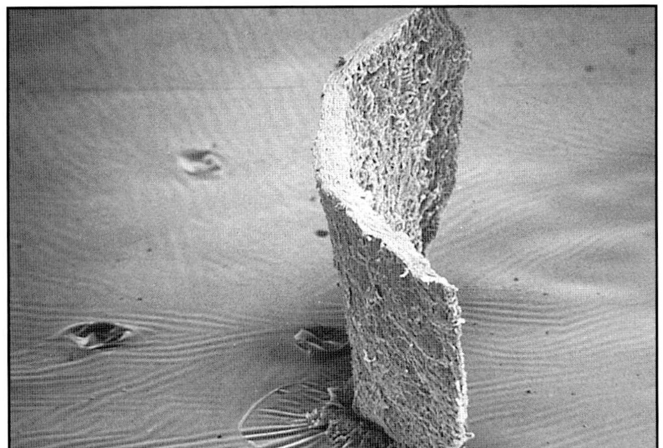

Figure 8-2.
SEM of stromal lenticle removed from PLK in blind human eye.

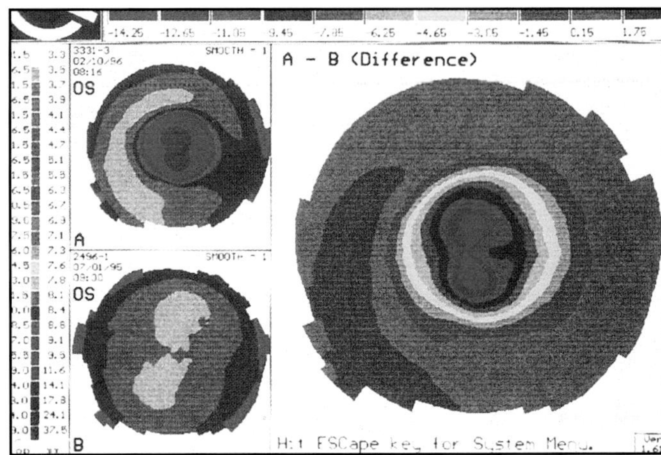

Figure 8-3.
Corneal topography of blind human eye 7 months after PLK (V Marchi).

5. Zysset B, Fujimoto G, Puliafito CA, et al. Picosecond optical breakdown: tissue effects and reduction of collateral damage. *Lasers Surg Med*. 1989;9:193-204.

6. Habib MS, Speaker MG, Juhasz T, et al. Acute effects of myopic intrastromal ablation of the cat cornea with the Nd:YLF picosecond laser. *Invest Ophthalmol Vis Sci*. 1994;35(suppl):2026.

7. Habib MS, Speaker MG, McCormick SA, et al. Wound healing following intrastromal photorefractive keratectomy (IPRK) with the Nd-YLF picosecond laser in the cat cornea. *J Refract Surg*. 1995;11:442-447.

8. Nissen M, Speaker MG, Davidian ME, et al. Acute effects of intrastromal ablation with the Nd:YLF picosecond laser on the endothelium of rabbit eyes. *Invest Ophthalmol Vis Sci*. 1993;34(suppl):1246.

9. Habib MG, Speaker MS, Goldberg, MA, Abramson JL. Intrastromal corneal laser surgery. In: Elander R, Rich L, Robin J, eds. *Textbook of Refractive Surgery*. Philadelphia, Pa: WB Saunders. In press.

10. Aquavella J, Hanuch O, Agrawal S, et al. Myopic intrastromal photorefractive lamellar keratectomy in the cat cornea. *Invest Ophthalmol Vis Sci*. 1996;37(suppl):S572.

11. Habib MS, Speaker MG, McCormick SA, et al. Fluorescence studies of corneal healing following intrastromal photorefractive keratectomy with the Nd-YLF picosecond laser. *Ophthalmic Surg and Laser Ther*. Submitted for publication.

12. Habib MS, Speaker MG, Kaiser R. Myopic intrastromal photorefractive keratectomy (IPRK) with the neodymium-yttrium lithium fluoride picosecond laser in the cat cornea. *Arch Ophthalmol*. 1995;113:499-505.

13. Speaker MG, Habib MS, Marchi V. Results of a safety study of myopic intrastromal photorefractive keratectomy (IPRK) with the Nd:YLF picosecond laser in blind human eyes. *Invest Ophthalmol Vis Sci*. 1995;36(suppl):S985.

Chapter 9

NONMECHANICAL MICROKERATOMES USING LASER AND WATERJET TECHNOLOGY

Ronald R. Krueger, MD, MSE, Barbara Parolini, MD,
Eugene I. Gordon, PhD, Tibor Juhasz, PhD

INTRODUCTION

LASIK, or laser in situ keratomileusis, performed under an anterior corneal flap is a new refractive procedure that is able to correct high amounts of myopia as well as other refractive disorders. The procedure may be regarded as an extension or modification of in situ keratomileusis[1] combined with the laser ablative properties of photorefractive keratectomy (PRK).[2] This procedure offers intrinsic advantages over that of excimer laser PRK in that Bowman's layer and the epithelium remain intact with increased stability and reduction of wound healing, postoperative pain, and visual recovery time. Although LASIK is in its infancy, several reports of the initial clinical outcome have been quite promising[3-8] and randomized clinical trials are underway in the United States and elsewhere assessing clinical outcome and predictability of the procedure.

Despite its inherent benefits, a major drawback with LASIK is the demanding nature of the surgery itself, which is due in part to the surgical skill required to operate and maintain an expensive, technically complex microkeratome used in making the initial anterior corneal flap. The most widely used microkeratome for LASIK is that of the Chiron Automated Corneal Shaper which is a modification of the Barraquer/Krumeich/Swinger (BKS) microkeratome used in keratomileusis.[9] The Chiron Automated Corneal Shaper features a 25° blade angle, steel blade oscillation at 8000 cycles per minute, a suction fixation ring that elevates the IOP to greater than

60, and an adjacent set of gears that advances the microkeratome at a predetermined speed and retracts it when flap cutting is completed. These multiple components and features of the Chiron Automated Corneal Shaper contribute to a higher incidence of intra- and postoperative complications associated with this form of laser refractive surgery. Microkeratome-related complications related to suction and increased IOP include vascular occlusion; subretinal neovascular hemorrhage; thin, thick, and irregular flaps; and intraoperative discomfort and anxiety.[10] The high-speed oscillating blades also may contribute to cutting chatter within the bed and along its edge, which may contribute to irregular astigmatism and epithelial ingrowth.[10] Finally, the adjacent gears can result in jamming of the unit by eyelashes or other obstructive elements, which would result in an irregular cut and need to abort the procedure. The additional risk of these complications is reported to increase the risk of significant complication after laser refractive surgery for low myopia from that of 0.5% in PRK to greater than 3% in LASIK.[11] Consequently, many advocate that LASIK be considered for correction of only higher levels of myopia where PRK complications increase because of wound healing.

Yet many are enthusiastic about LASIK and attempts have been made to introduce new microkeratomes that may improve the simplicity of performing the procedure and quality of lamellar cutting, and reduce the incidence of microkeratome-related complications. Among the newer mechanical microkeratomes, several offer automated advancement without using gears (Schwind, Phoenix UniversalKeratome, Draeger, and Refractive Technologies Flapmaker), while others offer only manual advancement (Eye Technology MLK, SCMD, and Moria). Modifications in the blade angle approach (range: 0° to 25°), the oscillating frequency of the steel blade (range: 8000 to 16,000) and the material of the blade (Schwind: sapphire blade, Mastel: diamond blade) have been attempted to improve flap cutting and reduce chatter and irregular astigmatism. Although a decrease in mid-peripheral chatter along the stromal bed has been observed in microkeratomes with a lower advancement drive:blade oscillation ratio (D:B ratio), peripheral edge irregularities and translamellar cutting along the flap can still be seen (RR Krueger, unpublished results). Improvements in the surgeon view of the procedure (Schwind, Phoenix UniversalKeratome, and Draeger) have also been made, and a rotating rather than oscillating blade has been introduced by Draeger. Although these improvements may not directly impact the complication rate, the absence of high suction and high-speed motorized blade oscillation seen in the Mastel microkeratome may offer some safety improvements. However, Mastel does introduce potential complications associated with a mechanical nonoscillating device (ie, tissue drag, etc.) that requires clinical correlation, which is unavailable.

Consequently, efforts have been made to consider an alternate method of lamellar sectioning that does not require the use of mechanical microkeratomes. Two such alternative technologies include that of the ISL neodymium:YLF (yttrium lithium fluoride) picosecond laser (Escalon Medical Corp, Skillman, NJ) and the HydroBlade Keratome (Medjet Inc, Edison, NJ). The former is a laser microkeratome that deposits laser pulse energy intrastromally to create a corneal flap without a mechanical blade or significant suction.[12] The latter is a water jet microkeratome that uses a thin, high pressure beam of water in place of a mechanical blade to cleave a lamellar flap without suction or tissue hydration.[13] The following sections will thoroughly consider each of these technologies and review their potential benefits over conventional mechanical microkeratome techniques.

THE ND:YLF PICOSECOND LASER

Ronald R. Krueger, MD, MSE, Tibor Juhasz, PhD

History and Mechanism

DEVELOPMENT IN OPHTHALMOLOGY

Since the early 1980s, photodisruption with the neodymium YAG laser has been successfully used in intraocular surgery.[14-16] Laser capsulotomy and iridotomy have become standard procedures in ophthalmology, utilizing ultrashort pulses of nanosecond duration by a method known as optical Q-switching.[17] Another more sophisticated method of optical pulsing is passive mode locking whereby a series of seven to 10 pulses each of picosecond duration is fired within a total envelope of 35 to 50 nsec (Figure 9-1). Although the individual mode lock pulse is 500 times shorter and of less energy than a Q-switch pulse, the sufficient precision and simplicity of Q-switching led to its widespread use in anterior segment surgery.[18,19]

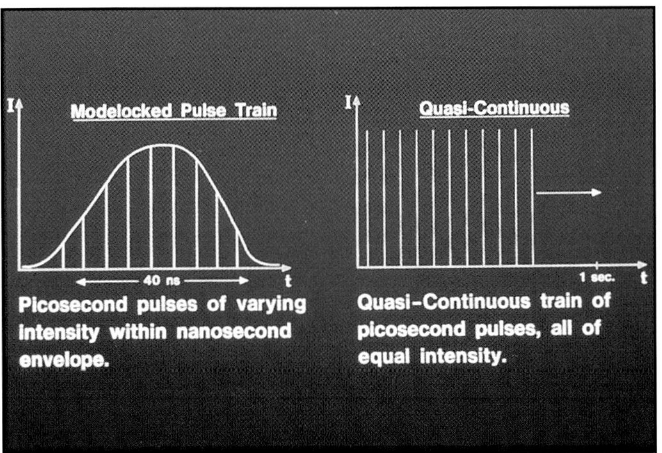

Figure 9-1.
Mode-locking and quasi-continuous.

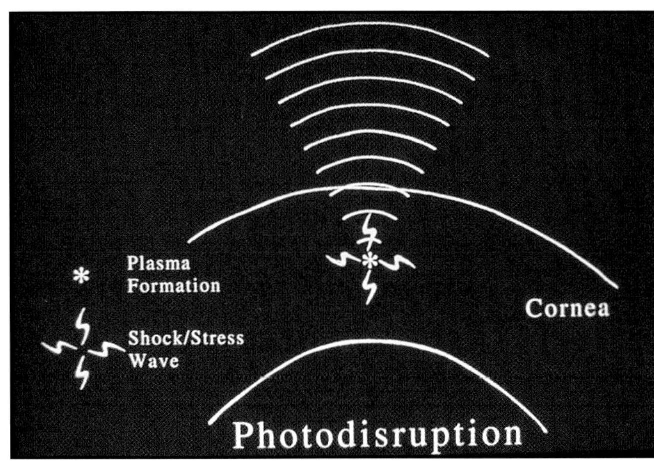

Figure 9-2.
Optical breakdown: mechanism of photodisruption which includes a plasma spark, shockwave, and cavitation bubble.

Recently, attention to picosecond pulsing has been renewed in ocular surgery because of its superior precision and energy confinement.[20,21] Using active rather than passive mode locking techniques, picosecond pulses of similar magnitude can be generated in a quasi-continuous fashion. This allows for a continuous succession of pulses that can be used for more sophisticated applications such as corneal surgery.

MECHANISM OF PHOTODISRUPTION

The mechanism of photodisruption occurs because of a phenomenon called optical breakdown, whereby laser light of high power density (~10^{10} to 10^{12} W/cm^2) ionizes tissue by stripping electrons from their atoms without absorption of light.[17] When optical breakdown is achieved, a localized plasma of high temperature and pressure is created which vaporizes the tissue, producing a shockwave and cavitation bubble (Figure 9-2). Beyond the plasma, the divergent laser energy as well as the shockwave are highly spatially dependent and both dissipate with a very short distance. Optical breakdown is most efficient and spatially confined when using a short pulse, a wide cone angle (angle of focus), and the fundamental mode of laser ablation.[17] Each of these requirements is achieved when using the picosecond Nd:YLF laser in clinical application.

NONCORNEAL OPHTHALMIC APPLICATIONS

Besides the picosecond laser's use in corneal surgery, which is the primary focus of this chapter, it has numerous other intraocular applications even beyond those of posterior capsulotomy, iridotomy, iridoplasty, and anterior vitreolysis which are recognized with the Q-switch Nd:YAG laser. The picosecond laser is capable of higher precision, high frequency pulse application which can be useful in anterior capsulotomy, Ab externo sclerectomy,[22] Ab interno sclerostomy,[23] lens fragmentation,[24] and posterior vitreolysis.[25] Clinical investigation using the Nd:YLF picosecond laser in these applications is currently underway, the details of which are not the scope of this chapter.

Laser Instrumentation

The laser system used for picosecond pulse generation is a commercially available neodymium-doped YLF ophthalmic picosecond laser (ISL model 4000, Escalon Medical Corp, Skillman, NJ) (Figure 9-3). It consists of a diode pumped Nd:YLF oscillator and Nd:YLF regenerative amplifier that generates optical pulses with a wavelength of 1053 nm, pulse duration of 30 picoseconds, pulse repetition rate of 1000 Hz, and maximum pulse energy of 1 mJ.

The delivery system for intrastromal pulse application utilizes a series of computer-controlled scanning X-Y-Z mirrors which direct the focused pulse energy through a mounted contact lens held in apposition with the target cornea (Figure 9-4). A ring suction device and plano-plano contact lens are used to ensure delivery of the most uniform and symmetric pattern of pulses, which can be evidenced by the cavitation bubbles within the cornea.[26] One of several different geometric patterns of pulse energy delivery can be selected and applied predictably at

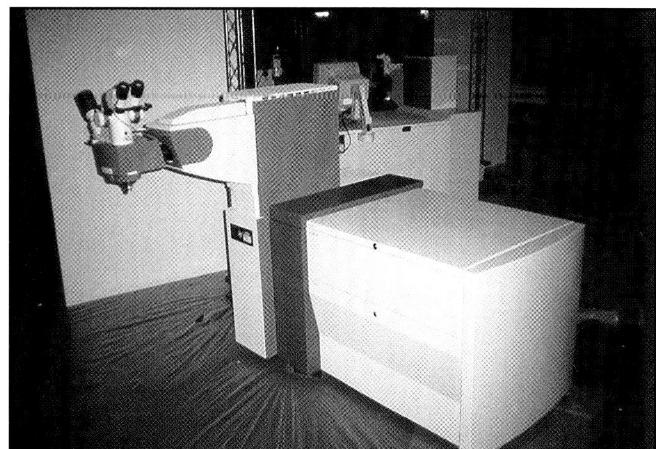

Figure 9-3.
The Nd:YLF ophthalmic picosecond laser system.

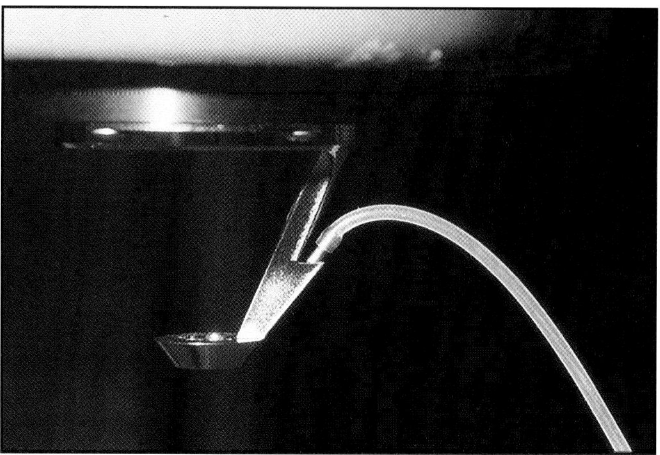

Figure 9-4.
Contact lens delivery system that flattens the cornea under suction to ensure the most uniform and predictable pattern of pulse delivery.

any corneal depth and Z-axis curvature pattern. A computer determines the three-dimensional treatment pattern and controls the position of the focused 10-μm diameter laser spot. For lamellar flap dissection, a parallel (plano) expanding spiral of pulses is applied at 160-μm depth followed by a series of more anterior pulses in a cylindrical pattern to externalize the flap.

Principles of Corneal Photodisruption

BIOPHYSICS AND THEORY

The essential principle behind picosecond intrastromal photodisruption is the separation and removal of a small amount of stromal collagen from within the cornea by focusing highly transmissive infrared laser light through a transparent tissue (the cornea). The theory and practical biophysics of this process, however, is more complicated and involves an understanding of the energy parameters and interaction involved.

When focusing picosecond laser pulses into corneal stromal tissue, the formation of a microplasma occurs as soon as a certain power density is reached. The expansion of this plasma generates a shockwave that disrupts and vaporizes a certain volume of tissue due to the localized high pressure gradient. The threshold for plasma formation and disruption in corneal stroma is on the order of joules per square centimeter,[21] and varies in proportion to the square root of the pulse duration.[27] Since the size of the laser pulse is focused to 10 μm in diameter, the threshold energy need be only 10 or 20 μJ for microplasma formation to occur. The amount of corneal tissue removed during the photodisruption process increases with increasing energy and is typically 7 to 10 μm in diameter,[28] although reports of as little as 0.1 μm have been cited.[27]

Immediately following shockwave formation, the plasma expansion results in the formation of a cavitation bubble which rapidly increases in size before collapsing to a steady state value within 0.1 ms.[28] The steady state size of the cavitation bubble is on the order of tens of microns in diameter (at near threshold energies) and is typically at least 20 μm during treatment. It persists in the cornea for at least 30 minutes before disappearing.[28] When multiple intrastromal pulses are sequentially placed in a spiral pattern, a whitish opacity is observed beneath the corneal surface as seen in Figure 9-5.

INITIAL TRIAL OF ISPRK

The initial concept for correcting refractive error with the Nd:YLF picosecond laser was that of intrastromal photorefractive keratectomy (ISPRK).[29] Early experimental animal studies appeared quite promising for this technique of intrastromal ablation, and these studies gave us a great deal of information regarding the safety of this technology. First of all, intrastromal picosecond pulses were found to demonstrate no detectable endothelial damage if limited to the anterior stromal (ie, more than 200 μm from the endothelium).[30] Second, there appeared to be no significant histological wound healing response in corneas treated with the laser.[31] Third, evidence of intrastromal tissue removal could be seen pachymetrically[29] and mass spectroscopy of cavities revealed carbon dioxide, carbon monoxide, and water vapor, suggesting a gaseous elimination of vaporized collagen.[32] Finally, topographic flattening of cat corneas have been shown after ISPRK, which strongly suggested its utility as a minimally invasive keratorefractive procedure.[29]

Based on this experimental research, a Phase I FDA feasibility study was conducted in the United States in 10 blind eyes to further demonstrate ISPRK's safety and efficacy. Although safe and painless, no significant refractive effect (cycloplegic refraction, pachymetry, and topography) could be demonstrated in these blind human eyes over a 1-year follow-up period (RR Krueger, unpublished results). An explanation for this lack of change in corneal curvature and thickness can be seen ultrastructurally and understood by reviewing the biophysical findings.[26]

As was mentioned above, the typical zone of disruption and tissue removal with the picosecond laser is between 7 to 10 µm, while the typical cavitation bubble size is greater than 25 µm.[28] Consequently, ISPRK is performed with a 20- to 25-µm spot separation in order to avoid collision with adjacent bubbles. The additive effect of the picosecond pulses placed in sequence is enough to separate lamellar layers, but actual tissue removal is restricted to a smaller area. This process of tissue removal can be further confounded if lamellar cavities are larger than the spot separation such that pulses are placed within cavities rather than within tissue.

ULTRASTRUCTURE OF ISPRK

Ultrastructural studies of ISPRK performed in freshly enucleated cadaver eyes demonstrate representative areas of both tissue loss and tissue separation.[26] Figure 9-6 illustrates the horizontal border of an interlamellar cavity with undisturbed stromal collagen fibrils adjacent to the surface. Figure 9-7 demonstrates tissue loss by the termination of fibrils, while Figure 9-8 demonstrates separation of collagen fibrils along a cavity's vertical (apical) border.

These findings suggest that picosecond intrastromal photodisruption results in both tissue loss and tissue separation, which makes it difficult to use as a purely intrastromal refractive surgical procedure. Initial clinical attempts to define an ISPRK nomogram failed, primarily due to the distortion of tissue from intrastromal cavities. Perhaps future work with femtosecond pulses can sufficiently reduce the size and lifetime of intrastromal cavities to allow for accurate pulse placement and predictable tissue reduction.

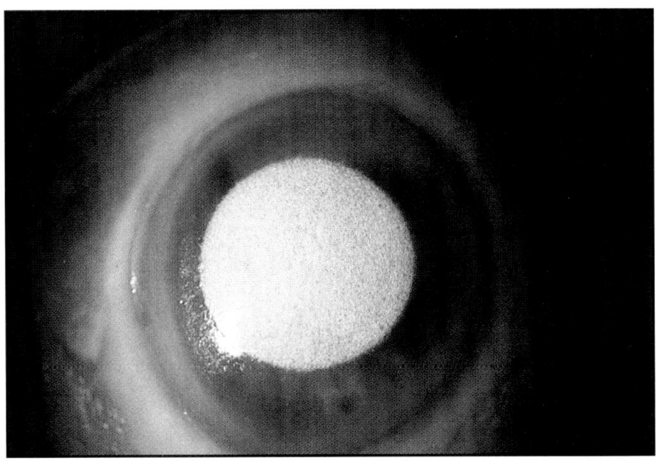

Figure 9-5.
A myriad of intrastromal bubbles after ISPRK in a cadaver eye leading to a whitish opacity beneath the corneal surface.

Picosecond Laser Microkeratome

INTRASTROMAL CUTTING TOOL

Since predictable tissue loss during picosecond intrastromal photodisruption is confounded by a broader area of tissue separation, the picosecond laser acts more as a precision intrastromal knife than as an intrastromal tissue vaporization tool. Consequently, it can be used to make precision cuts in the cornea intrastromally to be used in refractive and corneal surgery. Both lamellar and perpendicular incisions (Figure 9-9) are possible with the picosecond laser, so perhaps its greatest potential use is as a laser microkeratome.

Investigational studies of the picosecond laser in flap cutting for LASIK have been performed both histologically and in preliminary clinical trials. Histologically, smooth lamellar intrastromal dissections of 6 mm in diameter were generated 160 µm below the corneal surface in human cadaver eyes within 48 hours of enucleation. Picosecond Nd:YLF pulses of 40 or 60 µJ energy and 20-, 25-, or 30-µm spot separation were applied in an expanding spiral fashion. Deturgescence with 15% dextran was performed prior to the procedure to ensure a central corneal thickness of 580 to 620 µm. IOP was held constant by a height-adjusted fluid reservoir at greater than physiologic pressures of 30 to 40 mmHg to compensate for the applanation and suction of contact lens delivery system. The corneas were immersed in 1/2 Karnovsky's fixative and the next day washed, post fixed in 2% aqueous osmium tetroxide, dehydrated through

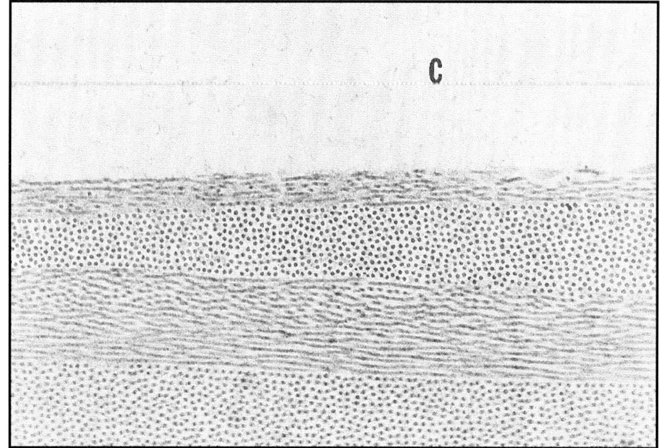

Figure 9-6.
Horizontal border of an interlamellar cavity (c) with undisturbed collagen fibrils adjacent to the surface.

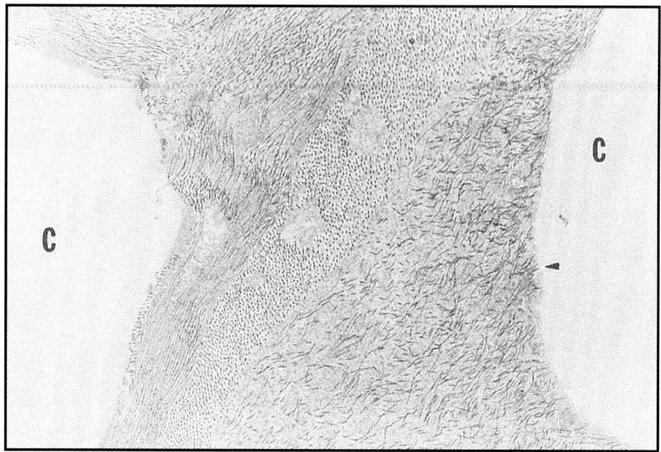

Figure 9-7.
Collagen tissue strand between cavities (c) demonstrating disruption of the collagen matrix and termination of fibrils along the right cavity border (arrowhead) (TEM: 25,000x).

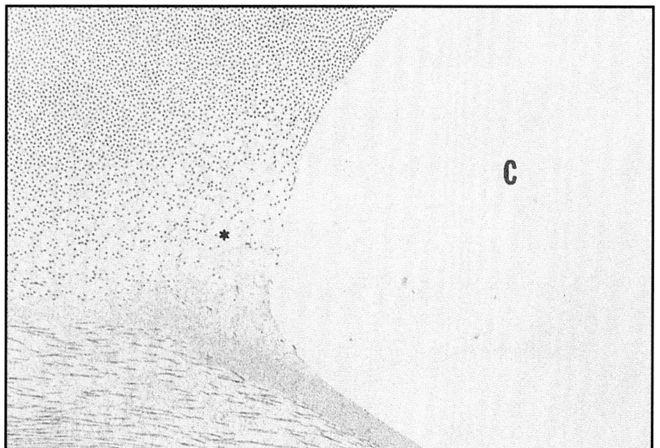

Figure 9-8.
Apical border of a horizontally elongate cavity (c) demonstrating both fibrillar separation (asterisk) (TEM: 50,000x).

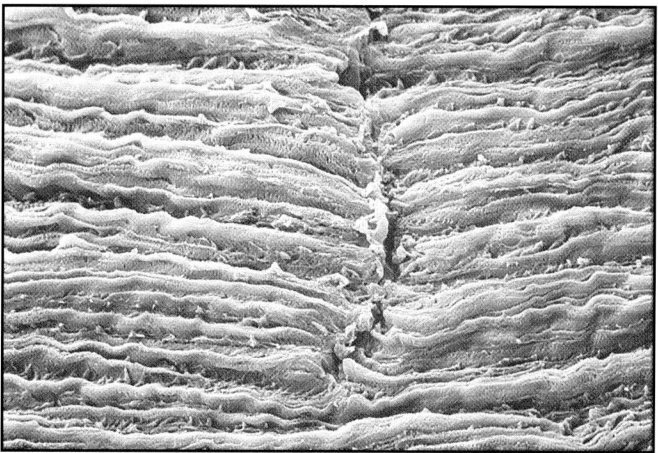

Figure 9-9.
Intrastromal RK-like incision produced by picosecond laser photodisruption in a plane perpendicular to the corneal surface. The overlying epithelium and underlying endothelium, although not shown, are undisturbed (SEM: 1500x).

graded ethanol, and critical point dried. After being coated with palladium, they were examined on a JEOL JSMT300 scanning electron microscope.[12]

The anterior corneal flaps created with smaller (20 µm) spot separation were much easier to detach from the stromal bed, regardless of the energy per pulse.[12] This finding was supported by scanning electron microscopy (SEM) images which show a fairly smooth stromal bed at 20 µm, and even 25-µm spot separation, with both energies, 40 and 60 µJ/pulse (Figure 9-10). The stromal bed appears rougher when generated with a spot separation of 30 µm, being the same at both energies tested. Higher magnification micrographs (Figure 9-11) reveal more lamellar protrusions on the stromal beds with larger separations, perhaps because of stromal tearing during separation. These results illustrate the relative smoothness of picosecond laser flap generation which is comparable to that of conventional microkeratomes. The ease of separation and greater relative smoothness of the 20-µm spot separation suggests its use for clinical application.

THE STEPS OF LASER FLAP GENERATION

The steps of the procedure for flap generation involve centration, applanation, lamellar pulse application, externalization, and flap dissection. The first two steps, centration and applanation, involve the use of a flat (plano)

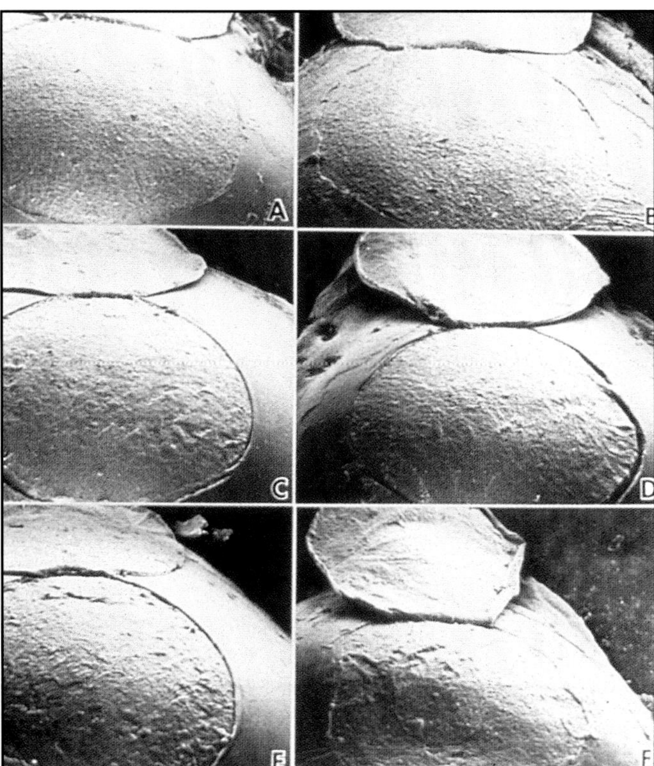

Figure 9-10.
Stromal bed and underside of flap generated by a spiral pattern of laser pulses of 40 μJ/p (a, c, e) or 60 μJ/p (b, d, f). The smoothest surfaces are achieved using a spot separation of 20 μm (a, b) with progressively less smoothness at 25 μm (c, d) and 30 μm (e, f) (SEM: 15x).

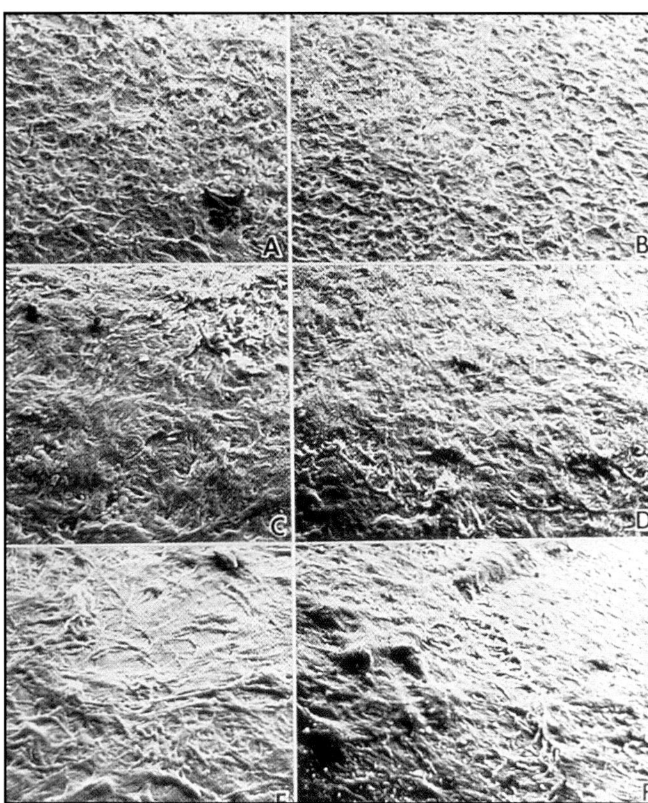

Figure 9-11.
High magnification micrograph of stromal bed from Figure 9-10 showing a more rough lamellar appearance to the 30-μm spot separation (e, f) than the 25 μm (c, d) or 20 μm (a, b) which is probably indicative of stromal tearing (SEM: 100x).

quartz contact lens mounted onto a metal coupling device that is coupled to the delivery arm of the laser. The patient is asked to lie in a supine position beneath the operating microscope. After the application of anesthetizing drops, the contact lens coupling device is aligned and applanated over the entrance pupil while the patient fixates on a coaxial illumination source in the microscope. Suction is applied to fix the globe to the device, and typical IOPs need not exceed those of ~40 mmHg (recorded during the histological analysis). The contact lens device is then coupled to the delivery arm to align the eye with the computer-controlled X-Y scanning optics of the laser. Although a sophisticated tracking system was initially implemented, difficulty in intrastromal Z-depth alignment and surface displacement due to cavitation bubbles made a contact lens applanation device necessary. The contact lens device allows precise depth placement of pulses intrastromally and prevents displacement of the anterior corneal surface due to cavitation.

The next two steps, lamellar pulse application and externalization, refer to two patterns of laser pulses programmed by the laser software for generating an anterior corneal flap. The first pattern is an expanding spiral with a spot separation of 20 or 25 μm at a depth ranging from 180 to 200 μm. The pulse energy varies from 20 to 40 μJ/pulse, and a maximum disc shaped incision of 6-mm diameter is achievable within the current laser hardware. The second pattern is a successive series of 6-mm circles along the disc's circumference in a cylindrical pattern with each successive circle being 10 μm closer to the cornea's anterior surface. A short cord of the circumference is left uncut creating a hinge. Externalization is complete when circumferential pulses are placed anterior enough to break through the epithelium so that the gas from cavitation can be seen collecting underneath the contact lens. Suction is then released and the contact lens applanation is positioned away from the eye.

The final step is dissection. The epithelium is penetrated with a blunt instrument directly across from the hinge

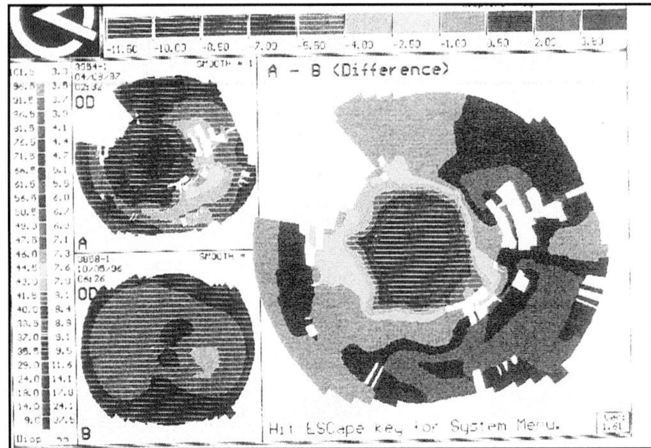

Figure 9-12.
Videokeratograph of a well-centered picosecond laser flap and -15 D excimer laser ablation. At 6 months postoperatively, 11.5 D of topographic flattening can be seen centrally.

and the flap is gently lifted from the stromal bed with minimal manipulation and blunt dissection. A 6-mm anterior corneal flap is created without the use of a mechanical microkeratome. Once the stromal bed is exposed, the patient is moved to the excimer laser to complete the keratomileusis.

EARLY CLINICAL RESULTS

Clinical application of this technology has been tested in partially sighted human eyes in Rome, Italy, by Professor Vincenzo Marchi. In a series of 14 eyes in 14 patients (age range: 34 to 78 years, visual acuity: 20/400), picosecond laser flap generation was performed followed by excimer laser ablation of the exposed stromal bed using a Lambda Physik excimer laser (Model LPX 200 MC, Goettingen, Germany).[33] A small, single zone ablation pattern, ranging from 3.5 to 4.5 mm in diameter was placed beneath the flap and eyes were enrolled in one of three treatment groups of -5.0, -10.0, and -15.0 D. Following excimer treatment, the flaps were replaced onto the reshaped bed, and postoperatively, combined antibiotic corticosteroid drops were instilled in the eye with a soft contact lens.

The results in the -5.0 D group demonstrated a smooth flap separation in three of the four participating patients. One of the four was removed from further study because of flap damage secondary to difficulty in dissecting the flap. The other three all experienced undercorrection secondary to marked myopic regression from the small excimer ablation zone.

In the -10.0 D group, four of the five patients experienced smooth flap separations, with minimal manual dissection. All four had well-centered or minimally decentered flaps, with overall undercorrection and regression of effect over 6 months. One of the five patients had a badly decentered flap, resulting in irregular astigmatism and removal from the study.

In the -15.0 D group, four of five patients had a well-centered or mildly decentered flap with a smooth flap separation. A topographic example of a well-centered flap and laser ablation is seen in Figure 9-12. Each patient was nearly fully corrected with only slight regression over the 6-month postoperative period. As in the -10.0 D group, one patient of five had a badly decentered flap and ablation which resulted in removal from the study (Figure 9-13).

Overall, marked regression was seen in nearly all patients, but with greater stability in the high, -15.0 D, group than the other two (Figure 9-14).[33] This significant regression has been shown to be associated with small ablation zone sizes,[34,35] and in our study appears to be more prevalent in the lower diopter corrections. The limitation of a 6-mm flap in the existing picosecond laser delivery system led to the tendency of a smaller ablation zone size and consequent undercorrection.

The complication of poor centration of the flap over the pupillary center in two eyes is due to the application of the applanation contact lens onto the cornea. As the lens is lightly pressed down on the epithelium, the cornea tends to slip under the mechanical pressure of the lens. This problem is accentuated further by the relatively small flap diameter. Larger flap diameters and a modified applanation approach are being investigated to eliminate this problem in the future.

The final complication encountered in one case involved difficulty in separating the flap from the underlying bed resulting in flap damage. The cause of this problem is not well understood, but may be due to excessive flap interface interconnections. No other patient experienced similar problems.

The remaining eyes, 79% (11/14), experienced no further complication with no case of epithelial ingrowth, flap wrinkling, significant haze, postoperative pain, or foreign body sensation. Figure 9-15 is a representative slit lamp photograph of a cornea 6 months after picosecond laser flap generation in excimer LASIK. One can see only trace interface haze and no evidence of flap irregularity or epithelial ingrowth.

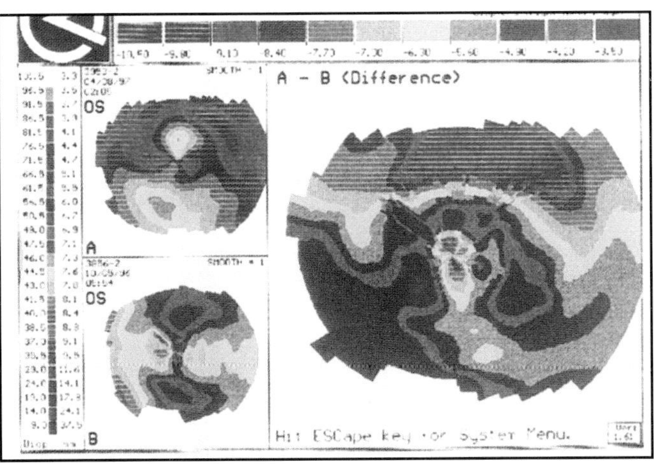

Figure 9-13.
Videokeratograph of a grossly decentered picosecond laser flap and -15.0 D excimer laser ablation. Variable topographic flattening and irregular astigmatism can be seen.

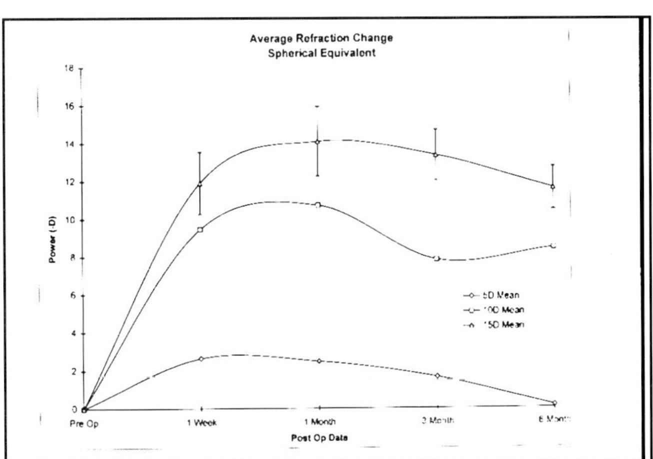

Figure 9-14.
Time plot of mean spherical equivalent refractive change for the -5.0, -10.0, and -15.0 D treatment groups. Although undercorrected, the mean and standard deviation value in the -15.0 D group is more stable than in the other two groups. Regression due to small optical zone size can be seen in each group.

ADVANTAGES OVER MECHANICAL MICROKERATOMES

The potential advantages of picosecond laser flap generation for LASIK is the utility of one technology, the laser, for both flap cutting and ablation. The present clinical example uses two different lasers, the picosecond Nd:YLF and excimer, but future applications may integrate the fifth harmonic of the 1053 nm Nd:YLF to produce a solid-state ultraviolet (UV) source (211 nm).[36] This would allow the picosecond Nd:YLF laser to be used for both flap generation and UV scanning spot ablation. Other advantages of this technology over that of mechanical microkeratomes include its precision and reproducibility in producing uniform thickness flaps, the relative smoothness of the flap interface, the lack of high IOP suction, and the lack of high-speed oscillating blades. The only disadvantages of the present technique are the 2 to 3 minutes required to apply the pulses and develop the flap, the small flap diameter and poor centration limited by present hardware, and the occasional difficult dissection which is as yet poorly understood. These disadvantages are minimal or can be overcome with further refinements in the technology.

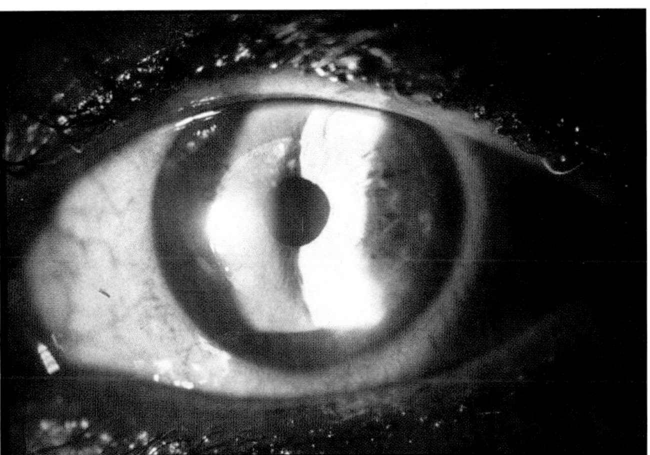

Figure 9-15.
Slit lamp photograph of a cornea 6 months after picosecond laser flap cutting in excimer LASIK. There is no flap irregularity or epithelial ingrowth, and only trace interface haze.

Picosecond Laser Keratomileusis

CONCEPT AND STEPS OF PLK

An alternate refractive application of the Nd:YLF picosecond laser is that of picosecond laser keratomileusis (PLK). The procedure involves the application of two layers of pulses, the first being a deep, concave, lenticular-shaped pattern and the second being an anterior lamellar flap pattern which intersects with the first pattern in the periphery. The steps of procedure, like in flap generation, include centration and applanation, but are then followed by lenticular pulse application before continuing with lamellar pulse application and externalization. Dissection is then carried out for the flap and the lenticular interface to peel back and retract the flap before peeling back and removing the disc-shaped lenticle. The pattern of picosecond laser

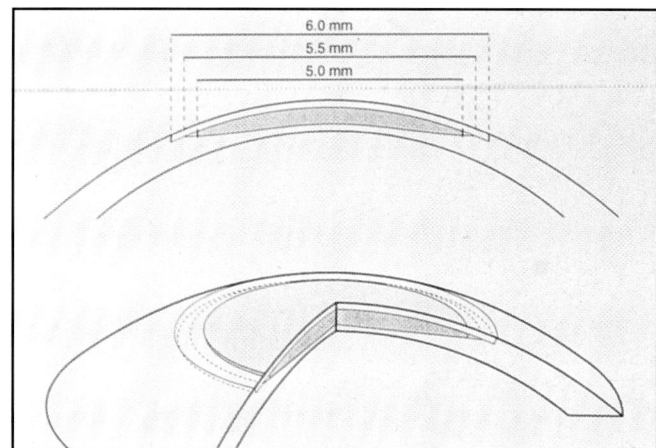

Figure 9-16.
Pattern of PLK. The shaded area represents the intrastromal lenticle delineated by a 5.5-mm posterior dissection and 6.0-mm anterior corneal flap.

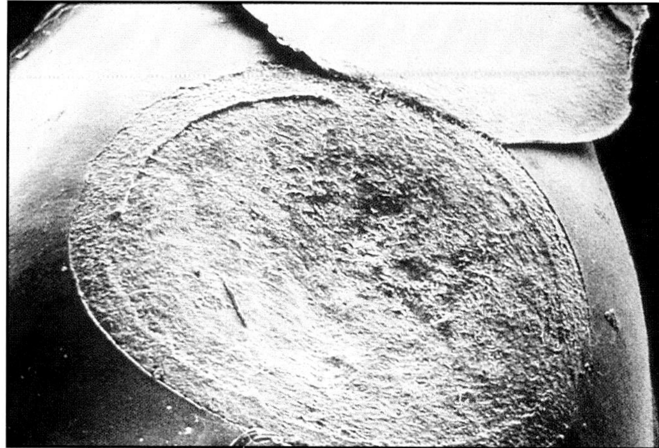

Figure 9-17.
SEM of the stromal bed following PLK. The central concave surface represents the region where the lens-shaped lenticle was removed beneath a 6-mm diameter flap (SEM: 15x).

pulse application is shown in Figure 9-16 as an artist's rendition. Here the intrastromal lenticle is delineated by a 5.5-mm diameter posterior dissection which is followed by a 5.0-mm diameter circular disc-shaped dissection and subsequent externalization to create a 6-mm diameter flap.[12] Because our chosen pattern allows the flap to be larger than the lenticle we are able to form a hinge. The technique is similar in concept to that of ALK.

SEM of the stromal bed following PLK is shown in Figure 9-17. Here one can see a 6-mm folded back flap with a 5-mm diameter circular dissection concentric to the outer edge of the exposed stromal bed. The central concave surface represents the region where the lens-shaped lenticle was removed. During the photodisruption process, the posterior concave layer of pulses is first applied in an expanding spiral pattern, which is then converted to a constricting spiral pattern to define the central portion of the anterior flap. This ensures adequate tissue separation near the point where the lenticle's anterior and posterior surfaces meet so that the lenticle is sufficiently detached from the surrounding tissue to be easily removed once the flap is raised.

EARLY CLINICAL RESULTS

The PLK procedure has been performed in clinical trials in a series of partially sighted eyes by Professor Marchi in Rome, Italy. In one example of bilateral PLK, a severely myopic patient with a refraction of -22.0 D (20/200) OD and -21.5 D (20/200) OS had the procedure performed in both eyes within 6 months of each other.[37] The central depth of the posterior concave layer was 320 µm with a uniform anterior flap of 200 µm in each eye. A 120-µm lenticle of 3.2-mm diameter was carefully dissected free and removed after lifting the flap. The flap was then repositioned with good postoperative healing in each case.

Postoperatively at 7 months, the first treated (left) eye had a refraction of -0.75 D (20/70) and corneal topography demonstrated a well-centered central zone of 21 D of flattening (Figure 9-18a). The subsequently treated (right) eye at 2 months postoperative had a refraction of -2.0 D (20/70), and corneal topography showed 22.5 D of flattening centrally (Figure 9-18b). The change in corneal thickness by pachymetry was 121 µm in the left and 122 µm in the right, which is consistent with the programmed lenticle thickness of 120 µm. Overall, the outcome of these two eyes in a single patient with PLK demonstrated good reproducibility in the treatment of high myopia.

Future Developments of Intrastromal Laser Surgery

SMALLER LASER AND LARGER FLAP

The current ISL Model 4000 picosecond laser is a flash-lamp-pumped Nd:YLF laser which uses one resonating cavity as an oscillator and another as a regenerative amplifier. The dimensions of the system are 50 x 79 x 53 inches with a separate power supply (29 x 29 x 50 inches) and delivery system (27 x 27 x 31 inches). The current delivery system uses optics that limit the treatment zone

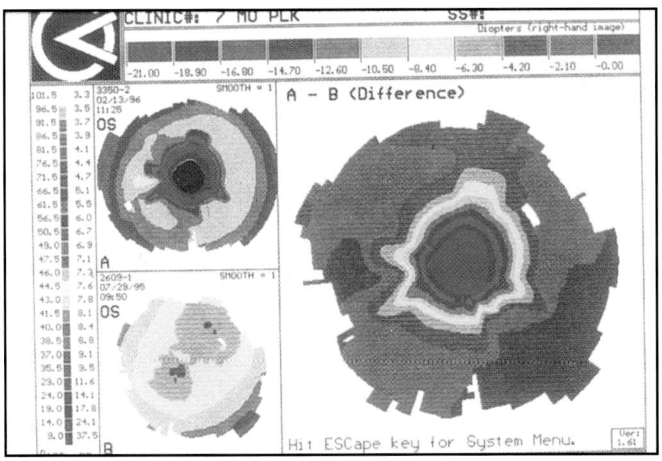

Figure 9-18a.
Videokeratography of a patient treated with PLK, removing a 120-μm intrastromal lenticle of 3.2-mm diameter beneath a 200-μm, 6-mm flap. Left eye at 7 months postoperative.

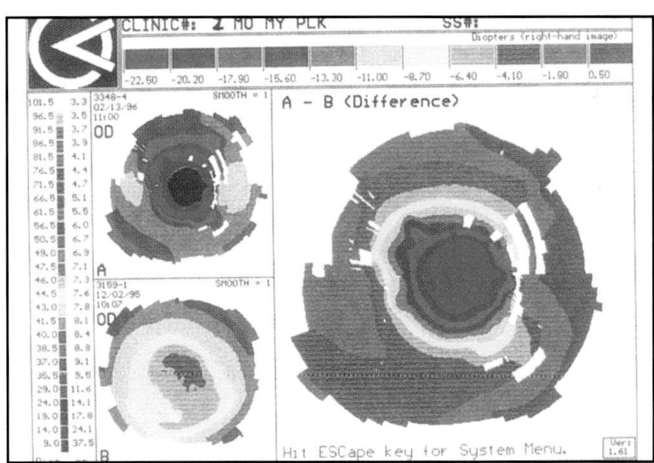

Figure 9-18b.
Right eye at 2 months postoperative.

diameter to 6 mm, which is currently too small for LASIK.

At the time of this writing, a new prototype laser system is operational that is much smaller in size and capable of forming a large diameter flap. The new system is an all-in-one laser, which means it uses the same resonating cavity as both an oscillator and regenerative amplifier and only a single Nd:YLF crystal pumped by a diode laser (Figure 9-19).[38] The dimensions of the system are consequently quite smaller (24 x 11 x 6 inches) and it can be easily transported and requires no special power requirements. A small power supply (13 x 13 x 4 inches) and cooler (12 x 12 x 18 inches) is also required in addition to a same-sized delivery system. A series of wider field, wider diameter lenses is incorporated in the delivery system to increase the treatment zone diameter to 10 mm. The new system will likely not be sold by Escalon Medical Corp, but by a new, yet unnamed company.

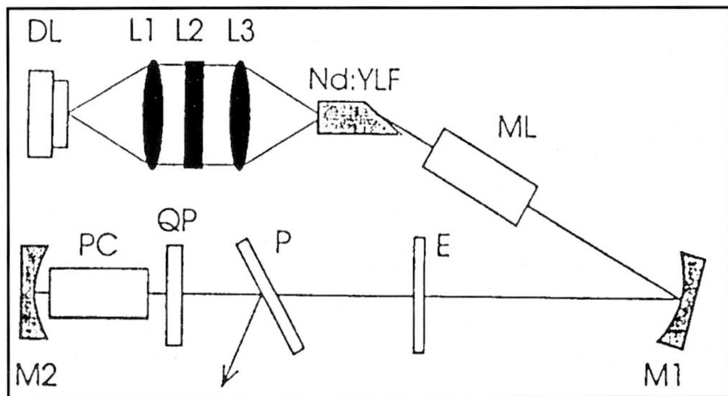

Figure 9-19.
Schematic diagram of the all-in-one laser, which simplifies and reduces the size of the Nd:YLF picosecond laser.

PICOSECOND LASER ULTRAVIOLET PHOTOABLATION

One of the listed advantages of the picosecond laser microkeratome is that the same laser could be frequency shifted to the fifth harmonic of the 1053-nm wavelength to produce a solid-state UV source of 211 nm.[36] This can be done by passing the picosecond laser light through three (type I) BBO crystals to generate the second, fourth, and fifth harmonics from the laser output. The harmonics can then be separated by a prism to isolate the fifth harmonic wavelength at 211 nm for photoablation (Figure 9-20).[36] The 211-nm wavelength has been shown to have a strong absorbance, similar to 193 nm,[39] and when using the picosecond pulse, the zone of collateral damage or pseudomembrane is again similar to that of 193 nm. Commercial, solid-state ultraviolet laser sources are already available through Novatec Laser Systems Inc (Carlsbad, Calif) and LaserSight Technologies Inc (Orlando, Fla), but neither of these use a picosecond laser source. The novel approach of using a picosecond laser as both an ultraviolet source for photoablation and infrared source for flap cutting makes for an attractive consolidation of technology for use in refractive surgery.

FEMTOSECOND LASER PHOTODISRUPTION

Finally, one of the most exciting and revolutionary refinements of the picosecond laser technology is shortening the laser pulse by nearly 200 times to the femtosecond range. Femtosecond laser photodisruption is

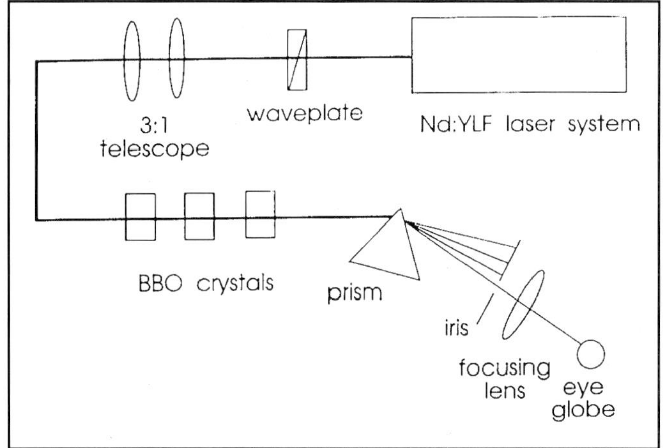

Figure 9-20.
Schematic diagram of a frequency shifted Nd:YLF picosecond laser to produce UV (211 nm) picosecond laser light. The fifth harmonic is generated by passing the laser light through three BBO crystals, and a prism is used to separate and filter out the other harmonics.

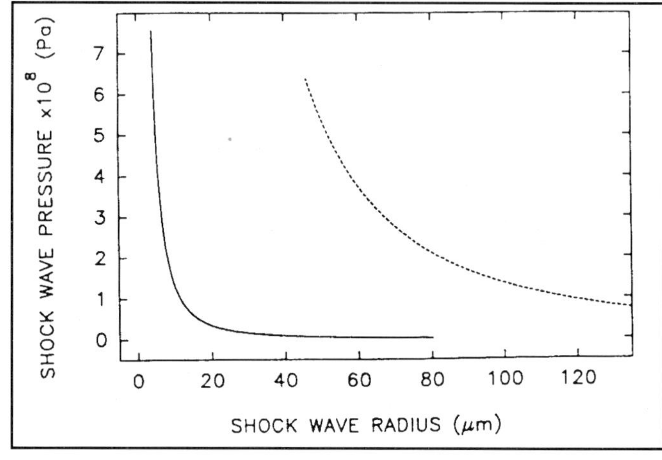

Figure 9-21.
Graph of shockwave pressure as a function of shockwave radius for femtosecond (left) and picosecond (right) photodisruption. The shockwave reduces to a soundwave within 20 μm and 200 μm, respectively.

the state-of-the-art of ultrashort pulse laser technology, and this bears significance in corneal surgery by reducing the size and duration of the shockwave and cavitation bubble, and by reducing the amount of energy necessary for photodisruption. Shockwaves with the femtosecond laser pulse decay to a soundwave within 20 μm and 10 nsec, whereas it takes 200 μm and 100 nsec for the picosecond laser shockwave to decay (Figure 9-21).[40] This increases the safety of the corneal endothelium by increasing the allowable depth of intrastromal photodisruption to less than 200 μm from the endothelial surface, which is necessary for the picosecond laser.[30]

Cavitation bubble size and duration is also reduced with the femtosecond laser. At 10 times the threshold fluence, the maximum bubble radius in the cornea with the femtosecond laser is 23 μm (seen within 650 nsec),[40] whereas with the picosecond laser it is ~125 μm (seen within ~5 μsec).[28] After 1 ms (the time of the next successive pulse), the bubble radius decays to 7 μm and 40 μm, respectively.[40] Although fluences that are less than 10 times the threshold have smaller cavitation bubbles, one can see where the femtosecond laser would have less problems in adjusting the spot separation (to avoid placing pulses within cavities) than the picosecond laser. Full disappearance of the femtosecond bubbles in corneal tissue occurs within 15 to 30 seconds, contrary to 15 to 30 minutes with picosecond laser-induced bubbles.[40]

Finally, less threshold energy is required for photodisruption with the femtosecond laser and this is in proportion to the square root of pulse duration.[27,40] Since the 150 fsec pulse is 200 times shorter than the 30 psec pulse, it requires 14 times less energy to achieve optical breakdown and plasma formation. The cavitation bubble size at laser fluences close to threshold is directly proportional to the laser energy, suggesting that cavitation bubble sizes are reduced even further (~14 times) at near threshold fluences.

The net effect of femtosecond laser photodisruption in flap cutting for LASIK can be shown histologically and directly compared with that of a mechanical microkeratome. Figures 9-22a and 9-22b demonstrate the SEM of lamellar surfaces cut with the femtosecond laser at 2 μJ/pulse and 10-μm spot separation (see Figure 9-22a) in comparison with a Chiron microkeratome flap cut (see Figure 9-22b) under the same magnification. The Chiron Automated Corneal Shaper produces edge chatter and torn lamellar tissue fragments along the surface, whereas the femtosecond laser produces a smooth surface with minimal undulation. In addition, the separation of lamellar flaps with the femtosecond laser requires no significant dissection as they are simply lifted from the underlying bed without intervening attachments. Further research with this laser is expected to refine and simplify the lamellar flap cutting process in LASIK and provide a more attractive way of cutting and separating corneal lamellar tissue intrastromally.

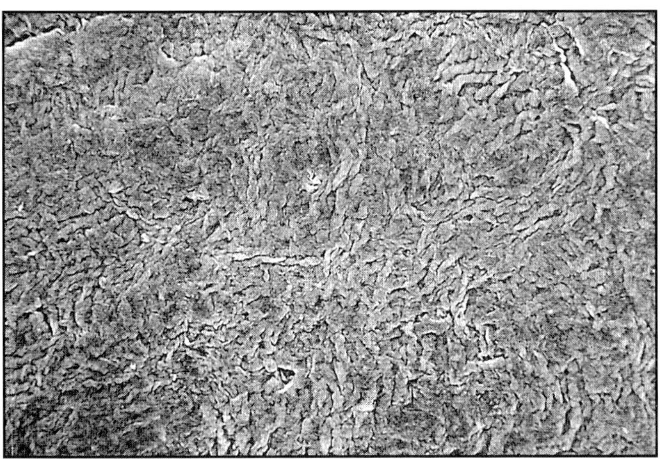

Figure 9-22a.
SEM of a lamellar surface cut by a femtosecond laser at 2 μJ/pulse and 10-μm spot separation.

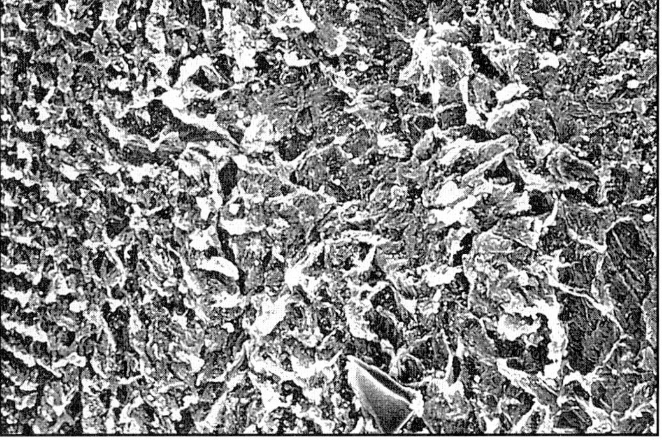

Figure 9-22b.
SEM of a lamellar surface cut by a Chiron Automated Corneal Shaper microkeratome. Edge chatter and stromal tearing is apparent with the Chiron Automated Corneal Shaper and is absent in the femtosecond laser surface (SEM: 200x).

THE HYDROBLADE KERATOME

Barbara Parolini, MD, Eugene I. Gordon, PhD

History of the Waterjet Technology

The use of the waterjet for cutting soft material and tissue is not a new concept. Anecdotally, it was first used by the Babylonians for cleaning, and has been used in mining for cutting stone for more than 100 years. It is used now extensively for cleaning surfaces and food preparation. The concept of using a high-pressure waterjet for industrial cutting of soft material was introduced by Dr. Norman C. Franz of the Department of Wood Science at the University of Michigan in the mid-1960s. He began research on controlling jets of water for cutting a variety of wood products and soft non-metallic materials. Research in the mid-1970s pointed toward the use of higher pressures and in the 1980s included abrasives to cut metals, utilizing waterjet pressures up to a practical limit of 80,000 psi.[41]

How the Waterjet Works in Surgical Applications

TISSUE SEPARATION MECHANISMS

Cutting of soft, relatively rigid material by a waterjet is accomplished by fatiguing and breaking structural bonds by a process that is complex and not totally understood. In understanding cutting of tissue, the classic text by Eisner is fundamental to much of what is described here.[42] Eisner describes cutting, cleaving, and erosion as the fundamental mechanisms of tissue separation. The sectility of the tissue is essential to the choice. In the case of low sectility material, *cutting* with a blade of rigid material is desirable since as the sharp edge of the blade stretches and fatigues the tissue, bonds are broken and the tissue separates under the blade edge. Moving blades enhance the tissue separation since the fatigue is increased. However, in the case of mechanical microkeratomes, cutting with metal and sapphire blades is necessarily damaging since there is a tearing and shredding component associated with blade friction. The damage associated with blade cutting is exceptionally high in the cornea and is undesirable. Moreover, the blade forces on the tissue are high which compress or stretch the tissue and compromise the accuracy of the cut.

Since the cornea is highly sectile in a direction roughly parallel to the lamellar interface, the collagen bonds between lamellae are weak. Tissue that is highly sectile favors *cleaving* as the separation mechanism, which limits tissue damage. In a cleaving mode, only the bonds between lamellae are broken, preserving the basic integrity of the lamellae and the keratocytes. This reduces light scatter and haze and minimizes trauma. Hence, it follows that lamellar surgery is best done in a cleaving mode. The waterjet can operate in a cleaving mode, and is therefore an ideal tool for lamellar surgery.[42] In particular, a waterjet that is scanned along a lamellar plane perpendicular to the direction of the water flow operates in a cleaving mode only if the tissue is not under compression.[13] When the tissue is under compression it results in loss of tissue and erosion which should be avoided in lamellar surgery. Hence, whenever the corneal tissue is to be cleaved by a waterjet, it must be under slight tension in a direction perpendicular to the anterior surface. In contrast, when tissue is to be removed, such as in epithelial removal, erosion is appropriate and the tissue should be under compression.[13] Careful attention must be given to the method of applanation, which depends on the objective of the surgery.

Another characteristic of the waterjet is its ability to cut, cleave, or erode certain tissue when the water speed is above a threshold value, but not when it is below. The threshold value depends on the tissue and it is different for each tissue in a heterogeneous structure. The water speed may be set above the threshold value for cutting the tissue of interest but below the threshold value for damage to adjacent material. Hence, the waterjet is capable of anisotropic tissue separation or removal when the beam speed is chosen properly. In the case of the epithelial removal, it is possible to totally erode away the epithelium in a prescribed area without loss or damage to Bowman's layer.

It might be instructive to think of the waterjet as if it were a thin, circular, cylindrical wedge like a needle. It exerts radial outward forces on tissue by the collision of water molecules moving at the surface of the beam. The slight inward deflection of the water molecules toward the inner part of the beam produces a reactive outward force on the tissue. By virtue of the extremely high speed of the water, the available forces are much greater than can be applied by a solid needle of the same diameter. Solid material blades have a limit on the acceleration they can sustain. An oscillating blade in a microkeratome moves at a maximum speed of a few meters per second (m/sec). The waterjet, in the microkeratome application, moves at a speed of about 450 m/sec. In other words, the waterjet may be thought of as a rapidly moving, unidirectional needle of enormous rigidity.

MICROKERATOME DESIGN

The results described here were obtained on a laboratory microkeratome utilizing computer-controlled, X-Y linear position drives with 1 µm placement accuracy, a filtering system for the sterilized water with 0.1 µm pores, and water pressure capability up to 20,000 psi. The beam forming orifice is a ruby jewel with a specially shaped aperture (36-µm diameter) and a shaped nozzle. The resulting beam diameter is typically about 0.9 times the orifice diameter, about 33 µm. Other orifice diameters ranging from 10 µm to 100 µm are used depending on the application.

BEAM CHARACTERISTICS

The waterjet microkeratome (the HydroBlade) is implemented by using a circular, parallel beam of sterile, highly filtered water (other fluids are possible) moving at supersonic speed. The speed of the beam depends on the stagnation pressure (ie, the hydrostatic water pressure before the beam gains speed) and passes through the orifice. For an appropriately constructed orifice, the emerging homogeneous beam (Figure 9-23) looks like a fine monofilament ("fish line") near the orifice. The fish line region of the beam is capable of sustaining radial oscillations, but the amplitude in an appropriately formed beam is too low to be visible. As the perimeter of the beam interacts with the surrounding air or other medium, the homogeneity of the beam is gradually compromised, and micron-sized droplets form. Once the beam loses its homogeneity, it slows down and breaks into a fine mist beyond the fish line region (the incoherent region). The length of the fish line region depends on the orifice shape and diameter, the nozzle design, and the stagnation pressure. The achieved fish line lengths are typically more than adequate, and the loss in speed is negligible in the homogeneous region.

For lamellar surgery, the beam parameters are not especially critical. Typical settings include a stagnation pressure, which is 20,000 pounds per square inch (psi) or 1360 atmospheres, and a beam diameter of 33 µm. This produces a fish line length of about 10 cm. The measured water flow rate in the beam is about 367 µL/sec. The force exerted by the beam when it is stopped is 20 gram wt. The maximum beam speed can be calculated from the stagnation pressure using Bernoulli's equation and empirical fudge factors to give 460 m/sec. The speed at the surface of the beam is lower due to friction. The average beam speed is established by two experimental measurements:

1. Using the measured water flow rate and the momentum change per unit time, the beam force average speed can be calculated to be about 462 m/sec.

2. From the beam diameter (@33 μm) and the flow rate, we calculate the average speed to be about 430 m/sec.

Since the beam area is not known accurately, to at least the degree of difference between the two measurements, we take 450 m/sec as the appropriate value within a few percent. From the flow rate and the average speed, we calculate that the beam carries a continuous kinetic power of about 35 watts (95 j/mL). The measured temperature rise of the spent beam in a crude calorimeter is in the region of 10°C.

The globe is kept at normal IOP, which increases by no more than 15% during the cut (as measured by a needle tonometer). The beam is mechanically scanned in a direction perpendicular to its length, defining a cutting plane. The emerging beam beyond the cutting region is only slightly changed with some scattering, since only the surface of the beam is in contact with the tissue. During a cleave, the exiting beam force, as measured on a force transducer, is reduced by only 1.5 gram wt. (~7%) for the longest cleave dimension, 8 mm. Some of the water is scattered, and not stopped, and simply does not fall on the transducer. This beam force reduction equals the force on the tissue.

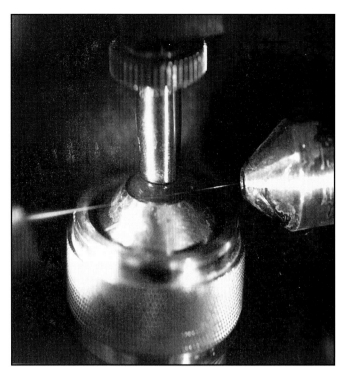

Figure 9-23.
Beam of the HydroBlade Keratome. The emerging homogeneous beam near the orifice looks like a fine monofilament ("fish line"). An enucleated eye is held in an eye-chuck; only the cornea is protruding.

The cleave, within the plane across 8 mm of cornea at a scan speed of 10 mm/sec, takes 0.8 sec (compared to 2 sec for a microkeratome blade cut), and requires no more than 294 μL of sterile water. By measurement of the flap thickness and the residual corneal thickness, one cannot say that absolutely no tissue is lost since the measurement error is a few microns. However, by electron microscopic observation of the cleaved surfaces, one can say with certainty that no tissue is lost during the cleave and that it appears as a perfect blunt dissection. The short time for the cleave and the negligible force on the cornea during the process (a maximum of 1 to 2 gram wt. compared to tens of gram wt. for a conventional scalpel cut) ensures the precision of the cut. Even an unsupported cornea at normal IOP does not visibly move or compress when it is cut by a waterjet. In this case, the waterjet can shave off layers as thin as a few microns.

Beam contact with the tissue along its path is for only about 18 μsec and the water moves only parallel to the surface of the cut tissue, and not into the tissue, hence there is no hydration. Absence of hydration is verified by the complete absence of aeration in the tissue, which would be expected if there was hydration, since the water in the beam contains air in a concentration well above the normal concentration at atmospheric pressure. When hydration is produced intentionally, as by directing the beam into the tissue, there is substantial aeration. This is further confirmed by transmission electron microscope observation of the cross section after a blunt dissection (Figure 9-24).

There is minimal heating of the tissue. The maximal temperature rise of the water when it is stopped and transfers no heat to its surroundings is 23°C. If energy is transferred to tissue during collisions, the overall temperature rise must be less. We think a skin of liquid about 1-μm thick is stopped and transfers energy to the surrounding tissue with a similar heat capacity but much thicker. The contact time is 3.3 milliseconds at most. Accordingly, the temperature rise must be much less than 23°C and this rise lasts for only a few milliseconds.

There are no shockwaves generated by the waterjet, although a low background acoustic spectrum might be detected based on waterjet studies on hard materials.[43]

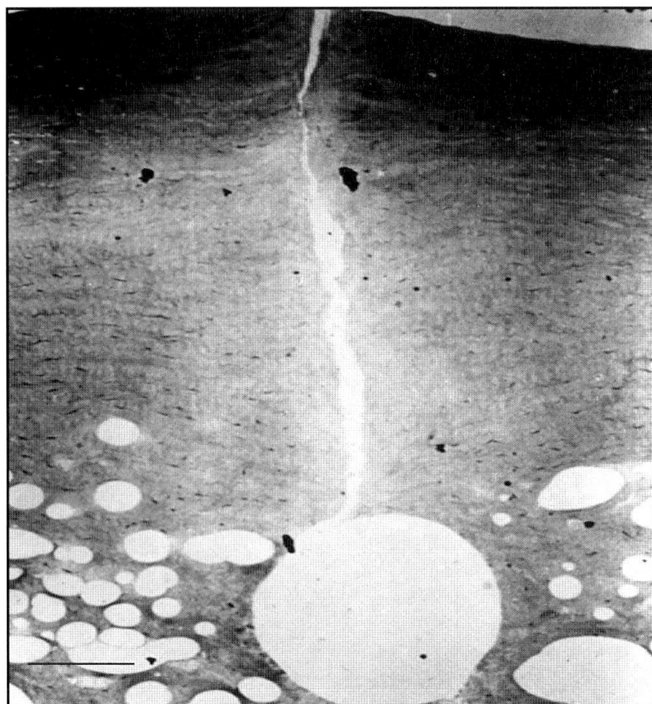

Figure 9-24.
TEM of a cross-section of a cornea after a blunt dissection performed with a waterjet, intentionally directed into the tissue to produce hydration. Hydration is revealed by aeration (TEM: 1500x).

The fact is that there are no known physical or chemical mechanisms other than the mechanical force of 1 g that might impact the safety of the procedure or the condition of the tissue. As noted, the magnitude of the mechanical force is substantially lower than that associated with mechanical blade cuts.

The Waterjet as a Microkeratome

LAMELLAR CLEAVING

The physical explanation for how the HydroBlade cleaves is fairly complex but a simple way to understand the physics is to consider that water molecules or micron-sized droplets at the boundary of the beam collide with tissue as the beam begins to come into contact with the cornea. This boundary water is deflected and changes its transverse momentum from virtually zero to some finite value directed inward into the beam. The equivalent outward reactive force on the tissue from the beam behaves much like a dull circular wedge of enormous rigidity. It cleaves along the easiest path, sacrificing beam energy, and scattering as it goes. The stagnation pressure and the beam velocity are large enough to cleave completely through the tissue for the chosen scan speed, which is typically 10 mm/sec. The emerging beam shows relatively little degradation.

When necessary, the waterjet beam is perfectly capable of cutting a shaped lenticle across lamellae similar to a blade. However, cutting across lamellae and breaking all the fibrils within takes substantially more energy than an interlamellar cleave in which only a few fibrils need to be cut. Therefore, the chosen scan rate is lower when producing a shaped lenticle in which lamellae must be cut.

The nature and shape of the incised tissue is defined by the shape of the anterior surface of the cornea during the planar waterjet cut. The anterior shape during the cut is established by a suction template, since incision by a waterjet without erosion requires that the tissue not be under significant compression. A suction template deforms the tissue by pulling it toward and into the template rather than by compression applanating the tissue. A flat suction template spaced a predetermined distance away from the plane of the cut produces a parallel, lamellar flap. A perimetric hinge of predetermined width may be produced by blocking the jet near the end of the scan so that it does not cut all the way from side to side. A slightly concave template allows removal of a plano convex lenticle of predetermined refraction. Lenticles with positive, negative, or astigmatic refraction may be removed. The position of the hinge on the perimeter can be chosen wherever desired by establishing the scan direction.

The design features of the actual template (Figure 9-25) are complex and include a micro-roughened surface that grips the anterior corneal surface and ensures the stability of the cornea during the cleave. This minimizes corneal oscillations, and ensures accuracy in achieving the desired thickness of the lenticle and position of the cleaved boundary region. In producing a flap, the template design consists of a circular cylindrical trephine as the boundary within which is the circular template. A small circular gap between the perimetric boundary of the template and the inner wall of the trephine provides space for vacuum suction which converts the template surface into a vacuum chuck. The trephine is used to create a well-defined, shallow gutter region surrounding a central corneal plateau with vertical walls. The jet therefore enters the lamellar structure without the need to cut through lamellar layers.

EXPERIMENTAL AND ULTRASTRUCTURAL ANALYSIS

Paired cadaver eyes from the same donor, 48 hours after enucleation, were mounted in preparation for flap cutting. A flap was created in one eye, using a Chiron Automated Corneal Shaper microkeratome. The Medjet waterjet microkeratome was used to produce an 9-mm diameter, 150-µm thick flap in the other eye. Samples were immediately fixed in Karnovsky's solution (2.5% glutaraldehyde and 2% paraformaldehyde). After 48 hours of fixation, the corneas were bisected through the treated area. One half was processed for SEM and the other half for transmission electron microscopy (TEM). The corneas were post fixed in 1% osmium tetroxide, washed, and dehydrated using graded alcohol concentrations.

SEM: With a critical-point drying apparatus, the alcohol was exchanged with CO_2. The dried samples were then mounted and coated with a 20-nm layer of gold. Documentary photomicrographs were obtained with an AMRAY 1200 B scanning electron microscope.

Parallel cleaving with a HydroBlade to generate a corneal flap produces a new stromal (lamellar) surface such as would be expected with ideal blunt dissection. Figure 9-26a shows a removed cadaver eye flap which is 8 mm in diameter and about 150 µm thick. The outer surface and the cleaved underside surface are essentially indistinguishable. The associated surface of the stromal bed is seen in Figure 9-26b without a tear film.

The mechanical microkeratome (Figure 9-27a) pulls and rips tissue while the HydroBlade (Figure 9-27b) cuts only the few collagen fibrils linking vertically adjacent lamellae. Figure 9-28a illustrates that the keratocytes are not removed in the process of HydroBlade cleaving. They are removed in microkeratome blade cuts as seen in Figure 9-28b and in PRK ablated surfaces. In TEM and SEM studies of the cornea cross section after resection, there is absolutely no evidence of subsurface change (EI Gordon, unpublished data).

Resection of non-parallel lenticles (cutting through the lamellae) takes more energy from the beam. The trajectory of the cut is along the interlamellar boundary and then quickly across the lamella and then along the boundary again. The transit across the lamellae requires cutting many more fibrils than in an interlamellar cleave (Figures 9-29a and 9-29b). The locus of the across-the-lamella transit is generally a narrow circular ring, and it was anticipated that this would be the site of haze in the post-surgical live cornea because the fibril spacing is increased at the position of the cut. Elimination of optical back-scattering haze depends critically on maintaining the normal spacing of fibrils. In contrast, no haze was expected in the interlamellar cut region. Experimental observation in rabbits, in fact, confirm our expectation that low level haze occurs only where the cut is across the lamella. It does not occur along the cleaved interlamellar boundary. Thus, a low level haze in Dutch Belted rabbits can be seen in the form of a bull's-eye pattern (Figure 9-30) which generally dissipates in less than 15 weeks.

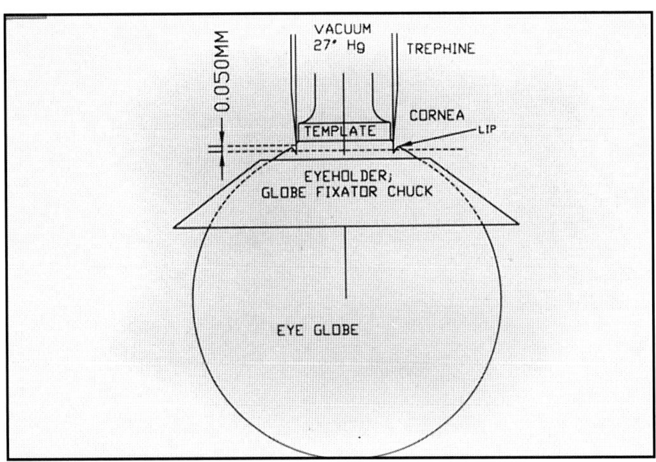

Figure 9-25.
Schematic representation of the template. The template design consists of a circular cylindrical trephine as the boundary within which is the circular template. A small circular gap between the template and the inner wall of the trephine provides a vacuum suction ring which converts the template surface into a vacuum chuck.

ADVANTAGES OVER MECHANICAL MICROKERATOMES

The HydroBlade Keratome is much less damaging to the cornea than oscillating blades in common use and potentially much safer. The HydroBlade is intended for use in lamellar surgery, particularly for "damage free" removal of pathologic tissue in lamellar keratoplasty and for producing parallel hinged flaps in LASIK.

The difference in the mechanism of lamellar cleaving with the HydroBlade Keratome in comparison to that of the mechanical microkeratome is ideal blunt dissection while the latter is gross sharp cutting. Confirmation by high magnification SEM comparisons between conventional blade microkeratomes and the

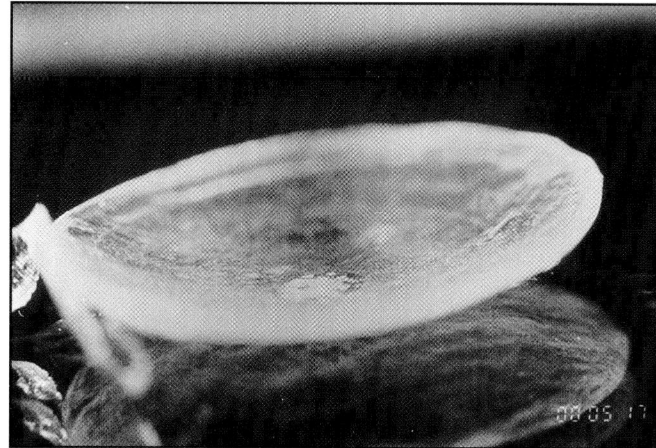

Figure 9-26a.
Flap removed from cadaver cornea. The diameter is 8 mm and the thickness is 150 μm.

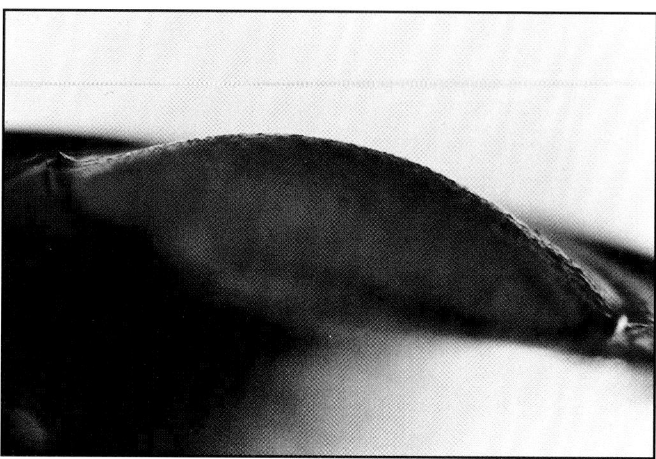

Figure 9-26b.
Stromal surface of the same eye after flap removal.

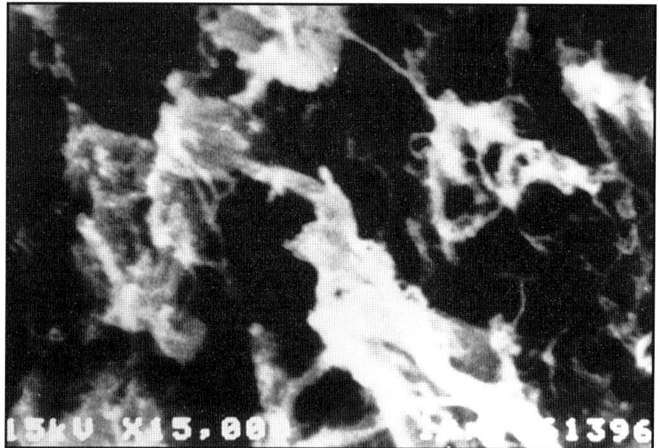

Figure 9-27a.
Cadaver corneal surface after creating a flap with a Chiron Automated Corneal Shaper keratome. The mechanical keratome pulls and rips tissue (the white areas are the ends of cut lamellae) (SEM: 15,000x).

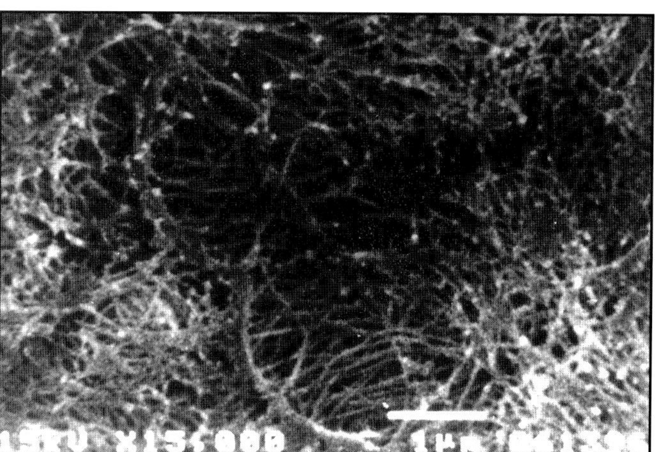

Figure 9-27b.
Cadaver corneal surface after creating a flap with the HydroBlade. Only the collagen fibrils linking vertically adjacent lamellae are cut (the white spots are the bulbous ends of cut interconnecting fibrils) (SEM: 15,000x).

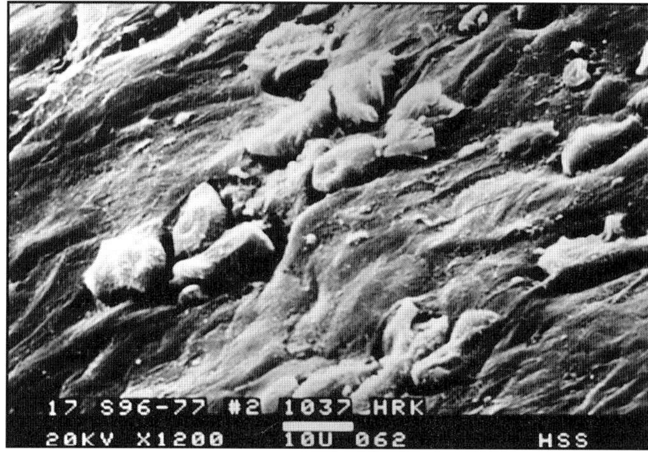

Figure 9-28a.
Cadaver corneal surface after creating a flap with the HydroBlade. The keratocytes are not removed (SEM: 1200x).

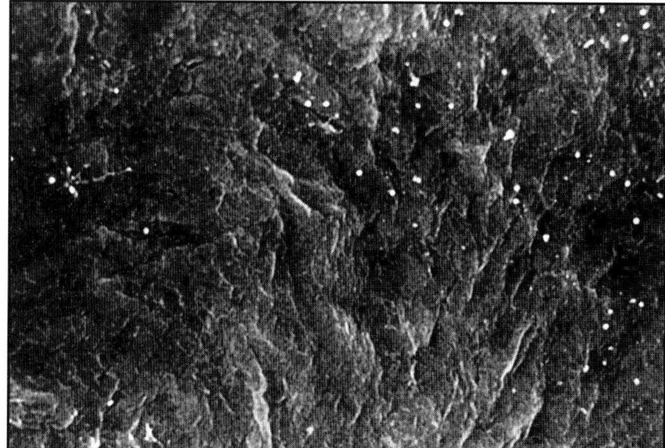

Figure 9-28b.
Cadaver corneal surface after creating a flap with the Chiron Automated Corneal Shaper keratome. The keratocytes are removed (SEM: 1000x).

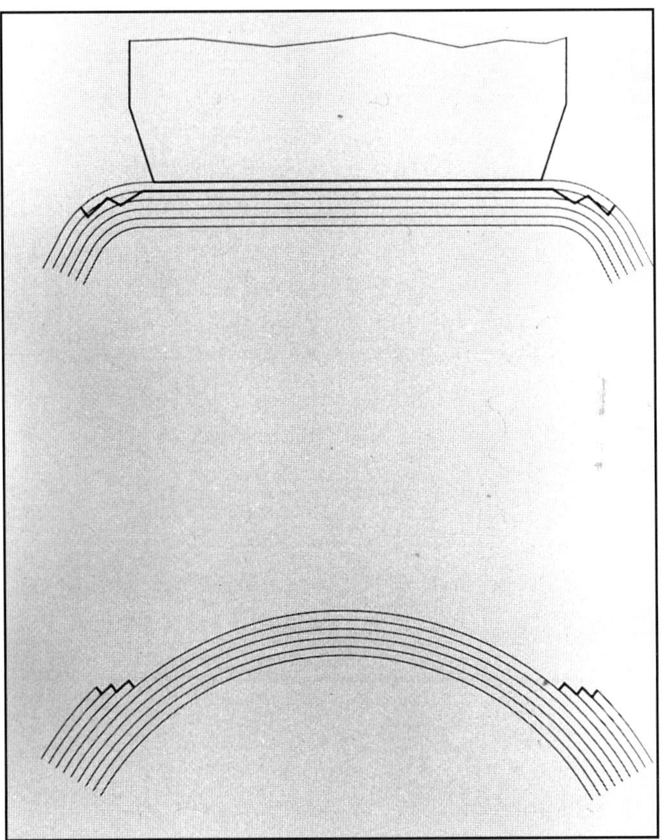

Figure 9-29a.
Schematic representation of interlamellar cutting.

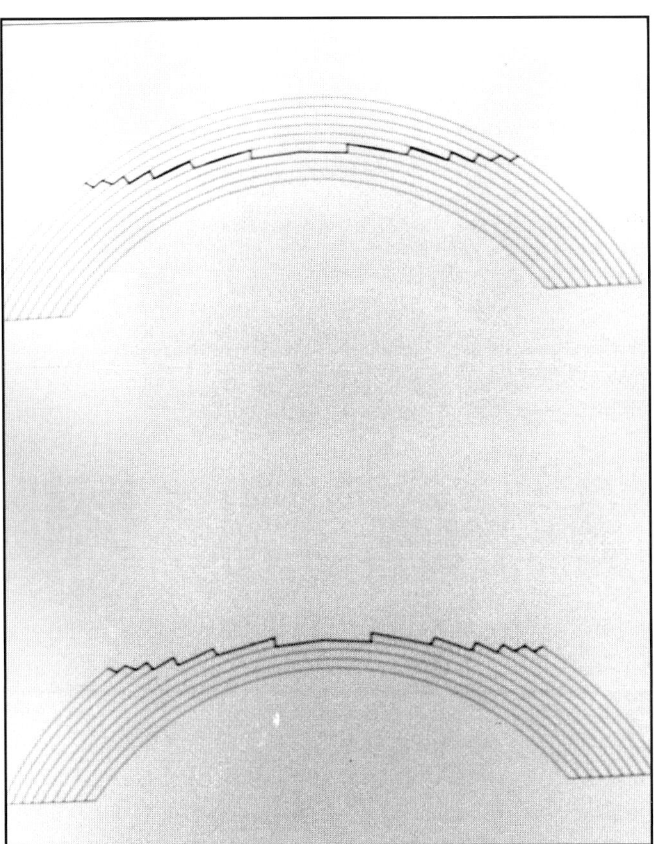

Figure 9-29b.
Schematic representation of across lamellae cutting.

HydroBlade Keratome demonstrate the marked difference in surface quality. One cannot imagine a less damaging separation of lamellae to produce a lamellar flap than that seen with the HydroBlade Keratome. Similarly, lenticular shaping is expected to produce surfaces and lenticles that can be defined within microns to produce accurate refractive changes. We anticipate that the keratocytes that remain on the surface with HydroBlade Keratome cuts and the lack of damage to the fibrils and lamellae should result in less trauma and more stable and quicker healing, especially for hinged flaps such as used in LASIK. We anticipate less epithelial ingrowth, irregular astigmatism, haze, regression, and flap- or suction-related complications.

It is expected that the increased safety, ease of use, and low cost of the HydroBlade Keratome will lead to greater acceptance and lower costs for the associated procedures, bringing this technology within reach of many more individuals.

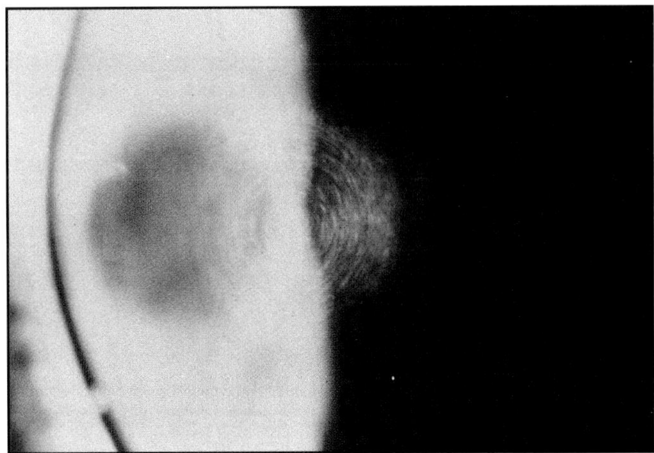

Figure 9-30.
Slit lamp photo of a rabbit cornea that is cut with the HydroBlade. Low level haze occurs only where the cut is across the lamella. It does not occur along the cleaved interlamellar boundary. The haze is observed in the form of a bull's-eye pattern and it was generally low level.

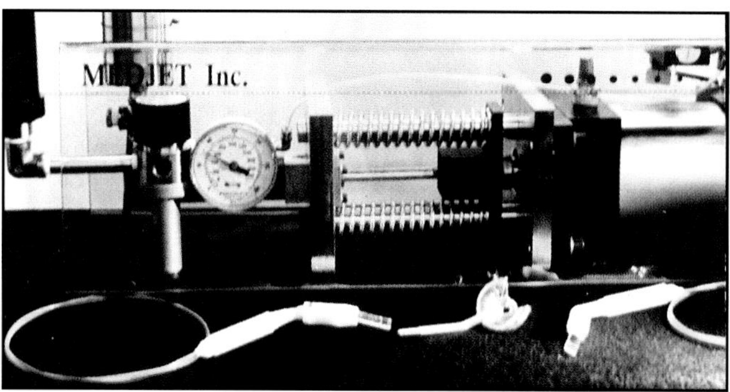

Figure 9-31.
HydroBrush keratome and Eye Mask.

The Waterjet in Epithelial Debridement

EPITHELIAL EROSION

The waterjet can operate in a cleaving mode, only if the tissue is not under compression. When the tissue is under compression, then it separates tissue by *erosion*. Hence, whenever a layer of corneal tissue is to be removed, such as in epithelial removal, erosion is appropriate and the tissue should be under compression. Simple applanation is adequate. It is also necessary when removing a layer such as the epithelium that the underlying layer have a higher water speed or sectility threshold for erosion. In this way, by controlling the water speed and the flow rate, the entire layer may be removed without any damage to the underlying layer. Accuracy in positioning the beam, thickness of the beam, etc, simply are not issues for concern.

APPARATUS

The design of the apparatus (Figure 9-31) is based on a discovery at Medjet that when a circular waterjet beam impinges at a small angle (eg, 15°) on a smooth, flat surface, a surface waterjet sheet is formed. The waterjet sheet exhibits complex propagation modes. However, the basic mode may be thought of as a gradually widening, thin sheet of rapidly moving water. The speed of the water along the surface decreases rapidly through friction because of the large surface area in contact with the plate. The speed of the water in the sheet and the flow rate are determined by the distance from the point of impact, the initial speed determined by the stagnation pressure, and the fixed size and shape of the orifice. Turning the waterjet on and then off at a fixed time later establishes a flow quantity. Under an appropriate set of parameters of water speed and quantity, the water sheet produced by the HydroBrush Keratome will remove epithelium with no damage to the underlying layer.

At the threshold for damage to the underlying layer, water (actually sterile saline solution) will begin to hydrate the tissue. Hydration is readily discerned since the water in the jet contains air in a concentration well above the maximum amount that is normally dissolved at atmospheric pressure. Thus, when the water comes to rest in the tissue, it effervesces and aeration of the tissue can be observed. Hence, aeration is observed at the threshold for damage. Under operating conditions, the quantity of water needed to fully remove the epithelium is about one quarter the amount needed to observe aeration.

The sterile saline solution used in the Medjet HydroBrush Keratome is provided in a 15 mL, thin-walled, flexible, sterile bottle. The bottle is attached to the working head through a small diameter, flexible, high pressure plastic tube (burst strength of 15,000 psi). A working fluid provides hydrostatic pressure at 5700 psi to the bottle. The saline solution within the flexible bottle assumes the same stagnation pressure and it flows out of the bottle, through the tube to the 100-μm diameter orifice, and initiates the waterjet beam. The waterjet beam impinges on the underside of a Lexan applanating plate which is where the removal occurs. The flow rate is about 2 mL/sec and the procedure is complete in about 6 seconds. The flow lasts for an absolute maximum of 8 seconds; the exposure time for the beginning of aeration is about 30 seconds, several times the operation time, so the procedure is totally safe.

The region of epithelial removal is defined by an Eye Mask. The Eye Mask is actually a hand-held globe fixation device with a prescribed circular opening, 6 mm or more in diameter. The opening is centered and placed over the area to be cleared of epithelium. The selected corneal area protrudes slightly through the Eye Mask. The underside of the applanating plate is lightly touched like a wand to the corneal apex with a force of about 1 gram wt. and the flow is initiated by a foot pedal. To ensure complete removal of the epithelium in the circular area, the applanating plate is moved a few millimeters to each side once during the procedure. The spent saline solution is collected in a mask of absorbent material around the eye.

For either the HydroBlade or the HydroBrush

Keratome, the high pressure working fluid to pressurize the sterile saline solution in the bottle is provided by an extremely simple, single stroke intensifier. A 12- to 16-g, liquid CO_2 cartridge, such as used in an air rifle, provides the working pressure to drive the intensifier. Although the equilibrium vapor pressure of the CO_2 gas is about 850 psi at room temperature, an equalizer limits the available pressure to a value of 220 psi. This is applied to a piston within a gas cylinder, rated to 250 psi. The gas piston, working against a light spring, drives another piston within a hydraulic cylinder. This hydraulic piston has a much smaller diameter which produces the high hydrostatic pressure driving the jet. The foot pedal controls a valve in the flow path, initiating the waterjet. Once the gas piston reaches a stop, the working pressure drops quickly. After the procedure, the CO_2 cartridge is removed, the residual working pressure is released, and the spring pushes the gas piston back to its starting position. The process is ready to be repeated. No electrical power is used.

EXPERIMENTAL AND ULTRASTRUCTURAL ANALYSIS

Extensive histological studies have been performed in rabbits and human cadaver eyes. The corneal surface, after epithelial removal performed with the HydroBrush, is compared to the corneal surface after epithelial removal performed with a surgical blade (#64 Beaver Mini-Blade) and analyzed with light microscopy (LM), SEM, and TEM. The same tissue processing is performed as outlined in the analysis of lamellar cleaving for SEM. Further analysis of LM and TEM are as follows:

LM: The samples were embedded in Spurr low viscosity embedding medium; 1-μm sections were cut and stained with toluidine blue. Documentary photomicrographs were obtained using an Olympus BX60 microscope.

TEM: The samples were embedded in Spurr low viscosity embedding medium; ultra-thin sections were cut and stained with uranyl acetate and lead citrate. Documentary photomicrographs were obtained using a Philips 300 TEM microscope. The same results can be observed in human and rabbit eyes.

Epithelial removal performed with the HydroBrush will be referred to as Hydro-Epithelial Keratectomy, or HEK. The results presented here have been performed in rabbits, but similar outcomes have been observed in human cadaver eyes. The HydroBrush exposes a smooth and clean surface (Figure 9-32a). Epithelial removal with a blade produces an irregular surface with a large amount of cellular debris at the base of the debridement zone (Figure 9-32b). The debris represents particles larger than 2 μm, filaments, and individual cells or clusters of cells. The HydroBrush produced sharp edges (Figure 9-33a). The edges are not always well defined after epithelial removal with the blade, and cells with irregular shape are present on the corneal surface (Figure 9-33b).

At TEM (Figures 9-34a through 9-34d) it can be noticed that not only is the basal lamina present, but also the basal epithelial cell membrane with the hemidesmosomes. The surface exposed by the blade is variable, and either cellular debris with patches of basal lamina or bare stroma can be observed.

ADVANTAGES OVER CONVENTIONAL TECHNIQUES

Blade scraping leaves the surface in a different condition compared to HEK. When the removal is obtained by manual scraping, the region of greatest sensitivity to shear stress lies between the lamina densa and the lamina lucida of the basal lamina.[44] This finding was reconfirmed by our studies; histology showed that, after blade removal, patches of lamina densa of the basal lamina are present, even if not uniformly. The blade exposes a surface on which debris and cells, isolated or in clusters, can still be found, even if the appearance of the wound using the operating microscope immediately after the procedure is similar to that of the wound obtained after HEK. Histologically, the surface after HEK always appears as even, smooth, and regular. The HydroBrush is so gentle that it leaves intact not only the basal lamina but even the basal cell membrane with the hemidesmosomes.

The basal lamina forms the scaffold for the organization of the epithelium, and it is the boundary that separates the epithelium from the stroma. It is an extracellular secretory product of the basal epithelial cells. The absence of basal lamina can result in the ingrowth of epithelial cells into the stroma[45] and stromal hydration.

The thickness of the basal cell membrane is less than 0.5 μm,[46] and therefore we do not expect that its presence could in any way affect the excimer laser ablation. On the other hand, it can possibly positively affect the rate of wound healing, providing a natural surface for the

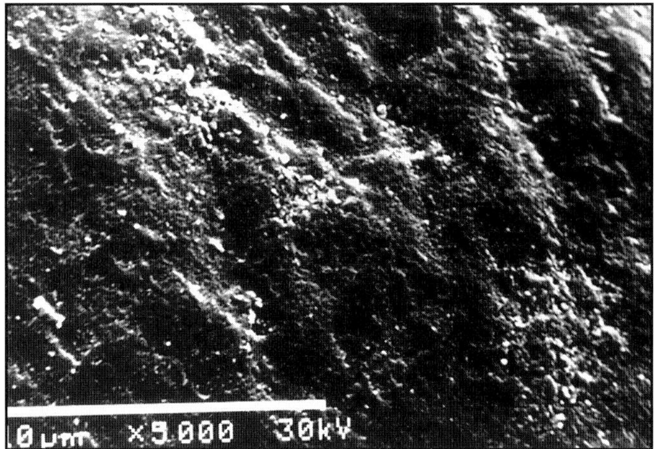

Figure 9-32a.
Surface of the rabbit cornea after epithelial removal with the HydroBrush which exposes a smooth, clean surface (SEM: 5000x).

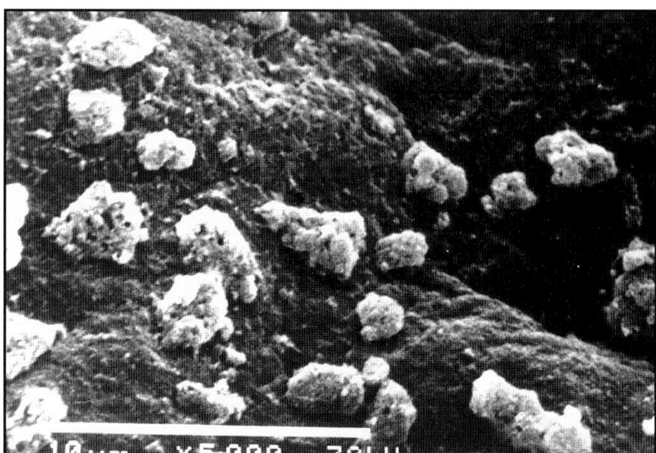

Figure 9-32b.
Rabbit cornea. Epithelial removal with a blade produces an irregular surface. A large amount of cellular debris is observed at the base of the debridement zone as particles larger than 2 μm, as filaments, and as individual cells or clusters of cells (SEM: 5000x).

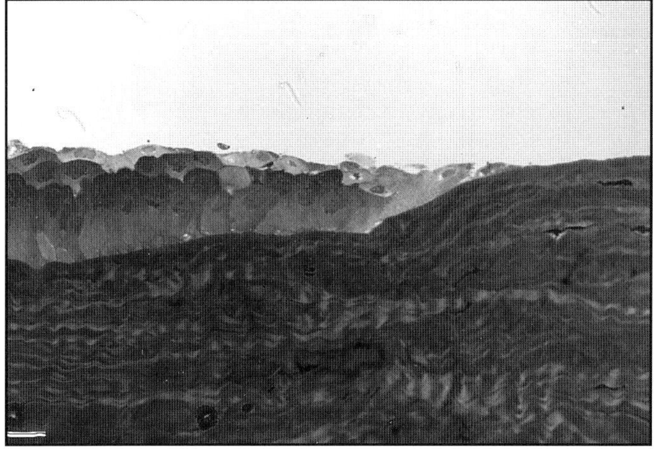

Figure 9-33a.
Rabbit cornea. Sharp epithelial border produced by the HydroBrush (LM: 125x, Mag bar = 80 μm).

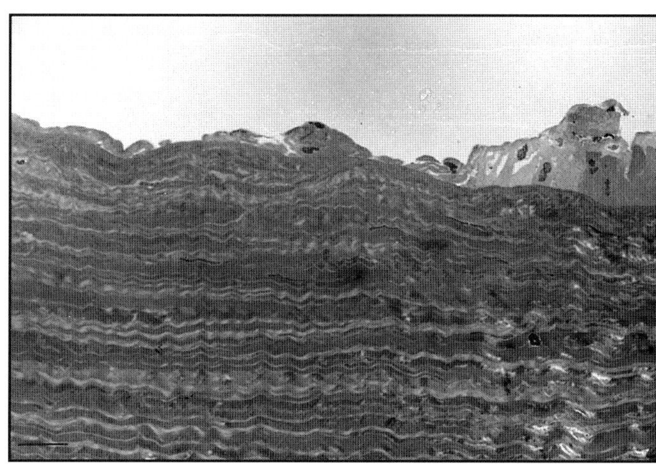

Figure 9-33b.
Rabbit cornea. The edges are not always well defined after epithelial removal with the blade and cells with irregular shape are present on the corneal surface (LM: 125x, Mag bar = 80 μm).

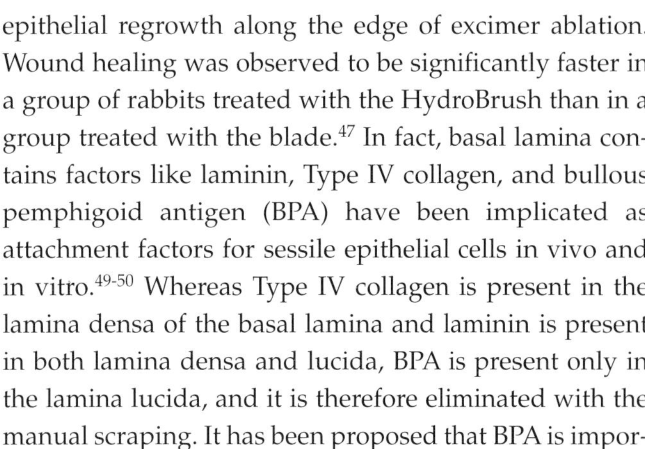

epithelial regrowth along the edge of excimer ablation. Wound healing was observed to be significantly faster in a group of rabbits treated with the HydroBrush than in a group treated with the blade.[47] In fact, basal lamina contains factors like laminin, Type IV collagen, and bullous pemphigoid antigen (BPA) have been implicated as attachment factors for sessile epithelial cells in vivo and in vitro.[49-50] Whereas Type IV collagen is present in the lamina densa of the basal lamina and laminin is present in both lamina densa and lucida, BPA is present only in the lamina lucida, and it is therefore eliminated with the manual scraping. It has been proposed that BPA is important in cell attachment because antibodies to BPA cause detachment of epidermal cells in vitro, and detachment occurs in vivo in patients with these antibodies.[51]

For PRK, a smooth and clean surface is extremely important to avoid risks of uneven photoablation with the laser. The debris affects the smoothness of the photoablated zone since the debris is not readily ablated and acts as a mask.[52] With PRK the basal lamina is eliminated by the ablation, but we speculate that the presence of both the basal lamina and the basal cell membrane at the boundary of the ablated zone could facilitate the start of the epithelial regrowth.

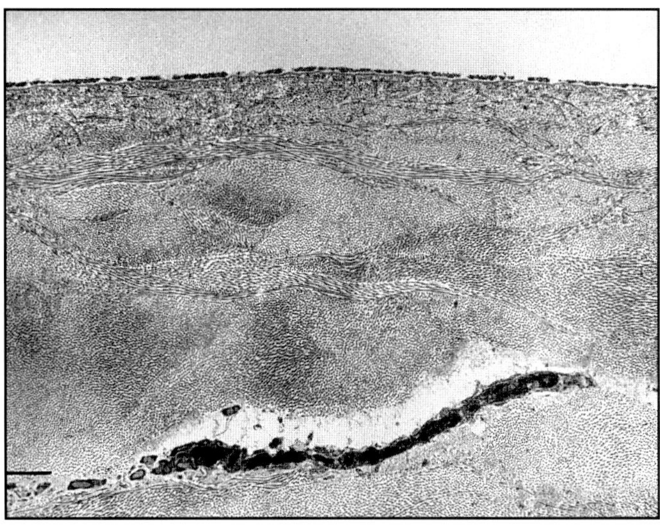

Figure 9-34a.
Rabbit cornea. Epithelial removal with the HydroBrush. The surface is even and extremely clean (TEM: 7600x).

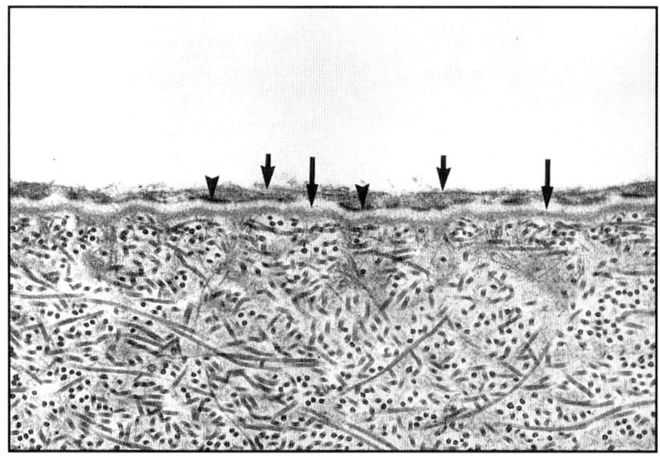

Figure 9-34b.
Rabbit cornea. Epithelial removal with the HydroBrush. The basal lamina (long arrows) and the basal epithelial cell membrane (short arrows) with the hemidesmosomes (arrowheads) are intact (TEM: 27,000x).

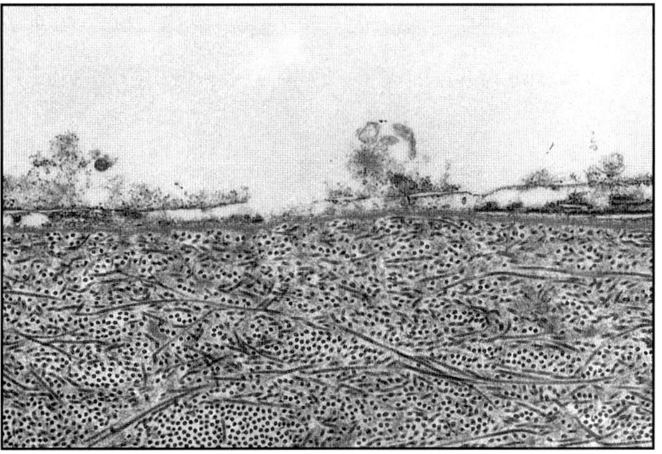

Figure 9-34c.
Rabbit cornea. Epithelial removal with the blade. The surface is variable. Cellular debris with patches of basal lamina can be observed (TEM: 23,000x).

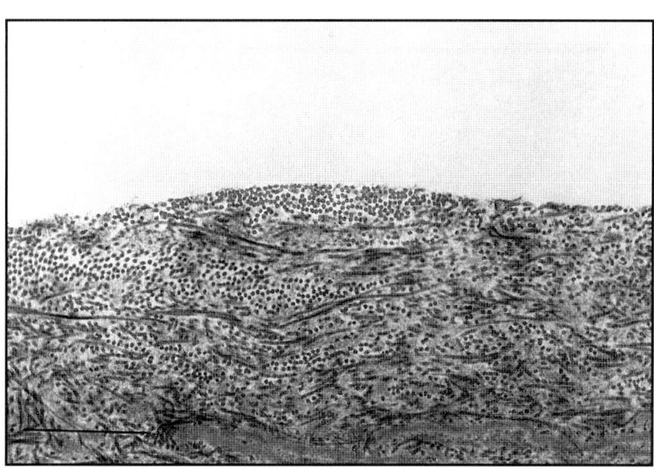

Figure 9-34d.
Rabbit cornea. Epithelial removal with the blade. The surface is variable. Bare stroma can be observed (TEM: 23,000x).

The boundary of the epithelial removal zone, in the case of HEK, is much better defined with little or no cell damage in contrast to the blade, which leaves a poorly defined boundary with significant cell damage. It is known that cell damage and tissue destruction activate host defense mechanisms, including soluble plasma factors (complement and clotting cascades) and immune competent cellular components (neutrophils, monocytes, macrophages, and endothelial cells).[53,54] The result may be that HEK promotes a faster start of the healing process, less tissue hydration, and less cellular and cytokine damage to the underlying stroma. If this is so, then the rate of healing of the epithelium after PRK may be faster with less stromal inflammation, swelling, and keratocyte death.

The shape of the wound is regularly round after HEK, as determined by the shape of the internal opening of the Eye Mask. It is difficult to maintain a circular shape by manually scraping the epithelium even if a round tip mini-blade is used, as in this study. It has been shown that a round epithelial erosion heals faster than a complex lesion.[55]

The HydroBrush does not hydrate the cornea, as proved by the absence of aeration within the cornea following the procedure and by pachymetry. We have demonstrated that aeration would occur if the tissue were hydrated by the waterjet (EI Gordon, unpublished data).

The use of a brush of water provides an easy-to-use, more precise, and faster method to remove the corneal epithelium. It avoids the risk of leaving debris and damaging the underlying stroma, and there is no initial stromal hydration change. The uncontrolled swelling at the initiation of PRK is minimized.

Future Developments of Waterjet Technology

As already mentioned, the waterjet is capable of cutting, like a blade, across lamellae as in producing lenticles, the shape of which is defined by the shape of a suction template. A flat suction template produces a parallel, lamellar flap. A hinge of predetermined width may be produced by blocking the jet during the scan so that it does not cut all the way from side to side. A slightly concave template allows removal of a plano convex lenticle of predetermined refraction. Lenticles with positive, negative, or astigmatic refraction and a combination of hinged flaps and lenticle cutting may be obtained.

The small diameter, minimal shearing forces, differential cutting ability, and the ability to make trajectory cuts under precision control have already borne fruit in bloodless liver sectioning, cosmetic surgery, and orthopedic surgery, and almost certainly will play a role in cancer treatment and many other areas that currently require too much precision for blade techniques. The requirements for corneal surgery are very high and the waterjet has already shown its unique attributes in overcoming the skills challenge.

The bridge to the surgery of the 21st century crosses the waterjet.

The authors of "The HydroBlade Keratome" would like to thank the Medjet staff, Parid Turdju, Peretz Feder, Ekram Kahn, Herbert Waggener, Joseph Calderone Jr, MD, Marco Zarbin, MD, David Dillman, MD, Robin Beran, MD, William Constad, Mark Abelson, MD, George O. Waring III, MD, Lee Nordan, MD, and Ronald R. Krueger, MD, MSE.

References

1. Ruiz LA, Rowsey JJ. In situ keratomileusis. *Invest Ophthalmol Vis Sci.* 1988;29:392.
2. Marshall J, Trokel S, Rothery S, Krueger RR. Photoablative reprofiling of the cornea using an excimer laser: photorefractive keratectomy. *Lasers Ophthalmol.* 1986;1:21-48.
3. Pallikaris IG, Paptzanaki ME, Stathi EZ, Frenschock O, Georgiadis A. Laser in situ keratomileusis. *Lasers Surg Med.* 1990;10:463-468.
4. Buratto L, Ferrari M, Rama P. Excimer laser intrastromal surgery. *Am J Ophthalmol.* 1992;113:291-295.
5. Salah T, Waring GO, El Maghraby A, Moadel K, Grimm S. Excimer laser in situ keratomileusis under a corneal flap for myopia to 2 to 20 diopters. *Am J Ophthalmol.* 1996;121:143-155.
6. Pallikaris IG, Siganos DS. Excimer laser in situ keratomileusis (LASIK) versus photorefractive keratectomy for the correction of high myopia. *J Refract Corneal Surg.* 1994;10:499-510.
7. Guell JL, Muller A. Laser in situ keratomileusis (LASIK) for myopia from -7 to -18 diopters. *J Refract Surg.* 1996;12:222-228.
8. Knorz MC, Liermann A, Seiberth V, Steiner H, Wiesinger B. Laser in situ keratomileusis to correct myopia of -6.00 to -29.00 diopters. *J Refract Surg.* 1996;12:575-584.
9. Swinger CA, Barraquer JI. Keratophakia and keratomileusis: clinical results. *Ophthalmology.* 1981;88:709-715.
10. Pallikaris I, Siganos D. LASIK complications management. In: Talamo JH, Krueger RR, eds. *The Excimer Manual: A Clinician's Guide to Excimer Laser Surgery.* Boston, Mass: Little, Brown and Co; 1997:329-338.
11. Seiler T. Barraquer lecture: can LASIK replace PRK? *Ophthalmology.* 1996;103(9A):103.
12. Ito M, Quantock AJ, Malhan S, Schanzlin DJ, Krueger RR. Picosecond laser in situ keratomileusis with a 1053-nm Nd:YLF laser. *J Refract Surg.* 1996;12:721-728.
13. Gordon E, Parolini B, Abelson M. The HydroBlade™ Keratome principles and microscopic confirmation of surface quality. *J Refract Surg.* In review.
14. Aron Rosa D, Aron JJ, Griesemann J, Thyzel R. Use of the neodymium YAG laser to open the posterior capsule after lens implant surgery: a preliminary report. *J Am Intraocul Implant Soc.* 1980;6:352-354.
15. Fankhauser F, Roussel P, Steffen J, Van der Zypen E, Chererkova A. Clinical studies on the efficacy of high power laser irradiation upon some structures of the anterior segment of the eye. *Int Ophthalmol.* 1981;3:129-139.
16. Steinert RF, Puliafito CA. *The Nd:YAG Laser in Ophthalmology.* Philadelphia, Pa: WB Saunders; 1985.
17. Academy of Ophthalmology Committee on Ophthalmic Procedure Assessment. Nd:YAG photodisruption. *Ophthalmology.* 1993;100:1736-1742.
18. Lin CP. Laser tissue interactions: basic principles. *Ophthalmol Clin North Am.* 1993;6(3):381-391.
19. Steinert RF, Puliafito CA, Trokel SL. Plasma formation and shielding by three ophthalmic neodymium-YAG lasers. *Am J Ophthalmol.* 1983;96:427-434.
20. Zysset B, Fujimoto JG, Puliafito CA, Birngruber R, Deutsch TF. Picosecond optical breakdown: tissue effects and reduction of collateral damage. *Lasers Surg Med.* 1989;9:193.
21. Niemz MH, Klanenik EG, Bille JF. Plasma-mediated ablation of corneal tissue at 1053 nm using a Nd:YLF Oscillator/Regenerative Amplifier Laser. *Lasers Surg Med.* 1991;11:426-431.

22. Cooper HM, Schuman JS, Puliafito CA, et al. Picosecond neodymium: yttrium lithium fluoride laser sclerectomy. *Am J Ophthalmol.* 1993;115:221-224.

23. Gross RL, Feldman RM, Orengo-Nania S, Font RL. Nd:YLF laser sclerostomy in rabbits. *Invest Ophthalmol Vis Sci.* 1993;34(4):736.

24. Gwon A, Fankhauser F III, Puliafito C, Gruber L, Berns M. Focal laser photophacoablation of normal and cataractous lenses in rabbits: preliminary report. *J Cataract Refract Surg.* 1995;21:282-286.

25. Cohen BZ, Wald KJ, Toyama K. Neodymium:YLF picosecond laser segmentation for retinal traction associated with proliferative diabetic retinopathy. *Am J Ophthalmol.* 1997;123:515-523.

26. Krueger RR, Quantock AJ, Juhasz T, Ito M, Assil K, Schanzlin DJ. Ultrastructure of picosecond laser intrastromal photodisruption. *J Refract Surg.* 1996;12:607-612.

27. Stern D, Schoenlein RW, Puliafito CA, Dobi ET, Birngruber R, Fujimoto JG. Corneal ablation by nanosecond, picosecond and femtosecond lasers at 532 and 625 nm. *Arch Ophthalmol.* 1989;107:587-592.

28. Juhasz T, Hu XH, Turi L, Bor Z. Dynamics of shockwaves and cavitation bubbles generated by picosecond laser pulses in corneal tissue and water. *Lasers Surg Med.* 1994;15:91-98.

29. Habib MS, Speaker MG, Kaiser R, Juhasz T. Myopic intrastromal photorefractive keratectomy with the neodymium-yttrium lithium fluoride picosecond laser in the cat cornea. *Arch Ophthalmol.* 1995;113:499-505.

30. Habib MS, Speaker MG, McCormick SA, Kaiser R. Acute effects of intrastromal ablation on the corneal endothelium of the cat with the Nd:YLF laser. *Invest Ophthalmol Vis Sci.* 1994;35(suppl):2026.

31. Habib MS, Speaker MG, McCormick SA, Kaiser R. Wound healing following intrastromal photorefractive keratectomy with the Nd:YLF picosecond laser in the cat. *J Refract Surg.* 1995;11:442-447.

32. Habib MS, Speaker MG, Schnatter WF. Mass spectroscopy analysis of the byproducts of intrastromal photorefractive keratectomy. *Ophthalmic Surg Lasers.* 1995;28:481-483.

33. Marchi V, Krueger R, Gualano A, Juhasz I, Suarez C. Clinical analysis of the Nd:YLF picosecond laser as a nonmechanical microkeratomes. *Arch Ophthalmol.* In review.

34. O'Brart DPS, Gartry DS, Lohmann CP, Kerr Muir MG, Marshall J. Excimer laser photorefractive keratectomy (PRK) for myopia: comparison of 4.00 mm and 5.0 mm ablation zones. *Refract Corneal Surg.* 1994;10:87-94.

35. O'Brart DPS, Corbett MC, Lohmann CP, Kerr Muir MG, Marshall J. The effects of ablation diameter on the outcome of excimer laser photorefractive keratectomy: a prospective, randomized double-blind study. *Arch Ophthalmol.* 1995;113:439-443.

36. Hu XH, Juhasz T. Study of corneal ablation with picosecond laser pulses at 211 nm and 263 nm. *Lasers Surg Med.* 1996;18:373-380.

37. Krueger R, Juhasz T, Marchi V. The picosecond laser as a nonmechanical microkeratome for LASIK and picosecond lamellar keratoplasty (PLK). *J Refract Surg.* In press.

38. Turi L, Juhasz T. Diode-pumped all-in-one-laser. *Optics Letters.* 1995;20:1541-1545.

39. Puliafito CA, Steinert RF, Deutsch TF, Hillenkamp F, Dehm EJ, Adler CM. Excimer laser ablation of the cornea and lens: experimental studies. *Ophthalmology.* 1985;92:741-748.

40. Juhasz T, Kastis GA, Suarez C, Bor Z, Bron WE. Time-resolved observations of shockwaves and cavitation bubbles generated by femtosecond laser pulses in corneal tissue and water. *Lasers Surg Med.* 1996;19:23-31.

41. Richard K. Miller. *Waterjet Cutting: Technology and Industrial Applications.* Lilburn, Ga: The Fairmont Press, Inc; 1991.

42. Eisner G. *Eye Surgery, An Introduction to Operative Technique.* Berlin, Germany: Springer-Verlag; 1990:64.

43. Li HI, Geskin ES, Gordon EI. Investigation of the pure waterjet-workpiece interaction. V International Waterjet Conference. Saint Andrew, Scotland, 1993.

44. Fujikawa LS, Foster CS, Gipson IK. Basement membrane components in healing rabbit corneal wound: immunofluorescence and ultrastructural studies. *J Cell Biol.* 1984;98:129-138.

45. Segawa K. Electron microscopic studies on the human corneal epithelium: dendritic cells. *Arch Ophthalmol* 1964;72:650-655.

46. Jakus MA. Further observations on the fine structure of the cornea. *Invest Ophthalmol Vis Sci.* 1962;1:202-225.

47. Parolini B, Turdiu P, Abelson M, Zarbin M, Gordon E. Hydroepithelial keratectomy performed with the HyrdoBrush™. *J Refract Surg.* In review.

48. Terranova VP, Rohraback DH, Martin GR. Role of laminin in the attachment of PAM 212 (epithelia) cells to basement membrane col lage. *Cell.* 1980;22:719-726.

49. Hintner H, Fritsch PO, Foidart JM, Stingl G, Schuler G, Katz SI. Expression of basement membrane zone antigens at the dermo-epibolic junction in organ cultures of human skin. *J Invest Dermatol.* 1980;74:200-204.

50. Hay ED. Collagen and embryonic development . In: Hat E, ed. *Cell Biology of the Extracellular Matrix.* New York, NY: Plenum Press; 1981:379-410.

51. Gammon WR, Merrit CC, Lewis SM, Sams WM, Carlo JR, Wheeler CE. An in vitro model of immune complex mediated basement membrane zone separation caused by pemphigoid antibodies leukocytes and complement. *J Invest Dermatol.* 1982;78:285-290.

52. Hersh PS, Carr JD. Excimer laser photorefractive keratectomy. *Ophthalmic Practice.* 1995;13:9-14.

53. Guirao X, Lowry SF. Biologic control of injury and inflammation: much more than too little or too late. *World J Surg.* 1996;20:437-446.

54. Clark RAF. Wound repair. *Curr Opinion Cell Biol.* 1989;1:1000-1008.

55. Arbour JD, Brunette I, Boisjoly HM, Shi ZH, Dumas J, Guertin MC. Should we patch corneal erosions? *Arch Ophthalmol.* 1997;115:313-317.

Chapter 10

MICROKERATOMES

John F. Doane, MD, Stephen G. Slade, MD, FACS,
Stephen A. Updegraff, MD

With the introduction of laser in situ keratomileusis (LASIK), there has been tremendous interest on the part of surgeons and industry to bring forth a microkeratome that offers the highest quality, predictability, repeatability, and ease of use. In theory, a microkeratome designed for LASIK should give the surgeon access to the corneal stroma to apply laser energy to remove corneal tissue to effect a refractive change. This being said, there are many variations on a theme. In fact, laser technology has taken this idea one step further to completely do away with microkeratomes by creating a corneal flap with the use of intrastromal lasers. Necessity being the mother of invention, one is led to believe with the tremendous activity in the microkeratome industry that a better product can be designed. This chapter will describe the early history of microkeratome development, discuss goals of microkeratome design and evaluation, and list technical attributes of individual devices.

HISTORY

Corneal lamellar refractive keratoplasty has its roots in the work of Professor Jose Ignacio Barraquer beginning in 1949 in Bogota, Colombia.[1-5] Dr. Barraquer developed myopic keratomileusis which used two instruments he designed, a manually driven microkeratome (Figure 10-1) and the cryolathe (Figure 10-2), to reshape the cornea and alter its refractive power. Dr. Barraquer's technique involved resecting a 300-µm lamel-

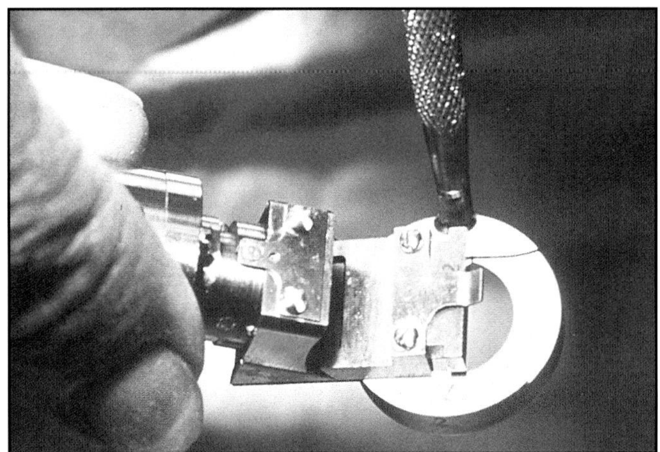

Figure 10-1.
Original Barraquer manual microkeratome on suction ring.

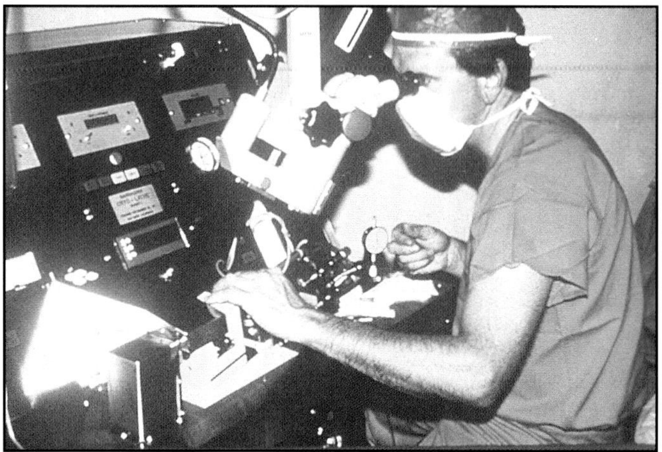

Figure 10-2.
Cryolathe used in freeze myopic keratomileusis.

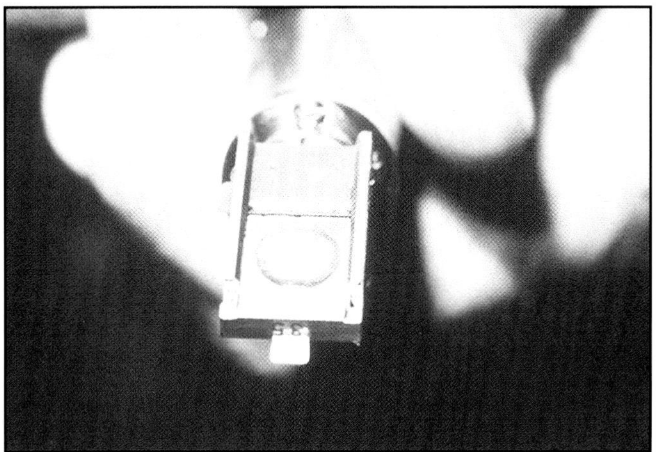

Figure 10-3.
Disc of lamellar corneal tissue displayed on Barraquer microkeratome.

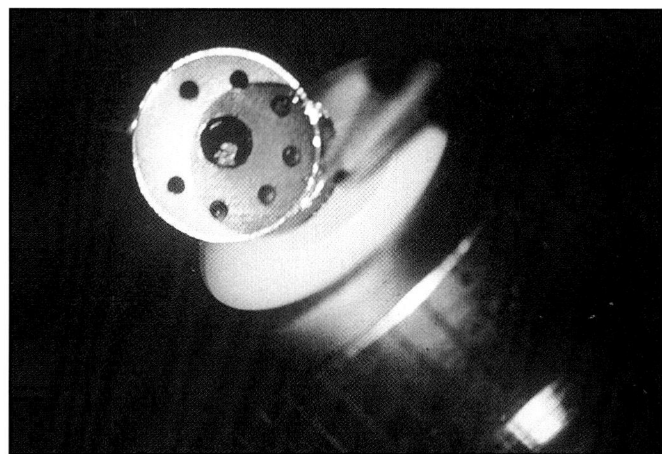

Figure 10-4.
Chiton green stained corneal disc being transferred on corneal spatula.

lar disc of corneal tissue (Figure 10-3), staining it with Chiton green dye for easier handling (Figure 10-4), placing it on the cryolathe freezing block and sculpting or reshaping the stromal surface with dictates entered into the computer (Figures 10-5 and 10-6), and then suturing it back into position (Figure 10-7). This technique did not prove to be applicable to a large number of surgeons in general due to the difficulty in mastering the manual keratome and the complexity of the cryolathe.[6,7]

In an attempt to avoid the side effects of tissue processing seen with the cryolathe, the Barraquer-Krumeich-Swinger (BKS) non-freezing system was developed. In this technique, after a keratectomy was performed to obtain a corneal disc of tissue, the corneal cap was inverted (epithelial side down) over a formed suction dye (Figure 10-8). Once in place, a second pass of the keratome was made to remove tissue centrally for myopia corrections and peripherally for hyperopia corrections[8] (Figures 10-9 and 10-10). This technique did not gain widespread acceptance, owing to the complexity of the system as well as the inaccurate results of a manual keratectomy by the majority of surgeons attempting the procedure, but it did lead researchers to investigate the damage present in corneal tissue after freezing and to demonstrate the clinical advantage of rapid healing when corneal tissue is not heavily processed.[9-12]

This being realized, we again turn our attention to Bogota, Colombia, to witness the next advance in microkeratome development. Drs. Barraquer and Luis Antonio Ruiz felt the next direction to explore was keratomileusis in situ. This technique involved two passes of the microkeratome over the eye, the first to remove a planar cap of tissue and the second to perform the refractive cut which was

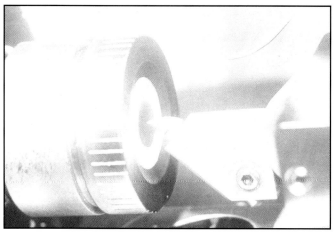

Figure 10-5.
Corneal disc on cryolathe cutting block before shaping.

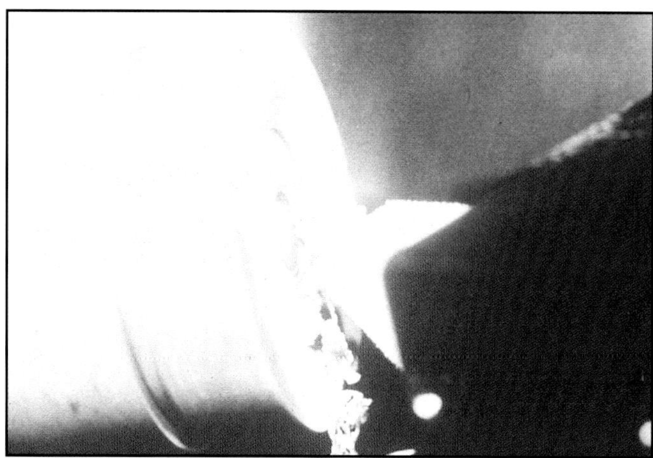

Figure 10-6.
Corneal disc being reshaped on cryolathe.

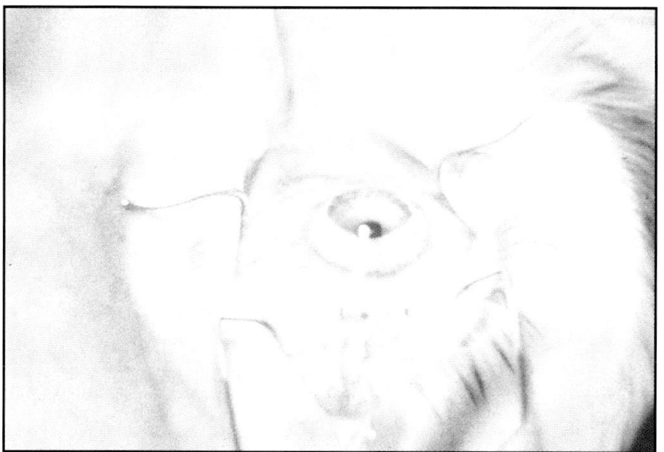

Figure 10-7.
Disc reposited to corneal bed in preparation for suturing.

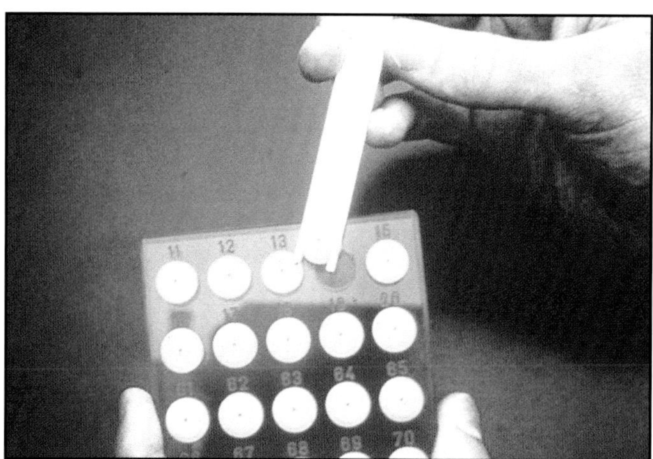

Figure 10-8.
Barraquer-Krumeich-Swinger non-freeze system custom dyes.

based upon the planned correction. Importantly, there was no processing of tissue so these unwanted effects could be avoided. Initially, they used a manual microkeratome as did other surgeons. The results with the early manual microkeratomes resulted in a wide range of correction. Typically, uncorrected vision did improve, but best corrected vision often decreased due to irregular astigmatism.[13,14] The next challenge was to develop a microkeratome that would be accurate, consistent, and provide acceptable safety. The Ruiz-Steinway, Draeger, and first-generation Micro Precision keratomes were all developed to improve accuracy, reproducibility, smoothness of the keratectomy, ease of use, and reliability. The keratome developed by Dr. Ruiz has gained the largest usage worldwide. This device is an automated geared microkeratome that is passed over a geared suction ring track (Figure 10-11). The automation of the passage of the keratome allows for a consistent velocity of passage and a uniform thickness to the keratectomy. The suction ring used with this device for keratomileusis in situ (ALK) has three interlocking pieces (Figures 10-11 and 10-12) that allow for intraoperative adjustment, which is unlike prior systems that utilized several different suction rings with varying shoulder heights to achieve different diameter keratectomies. With the advent of LASIK, microkeratome manufacturers now only have to provide one or relatively few suction rings since only one pass of the keratome is required.

THE MICROKERATOMES

The following section briefly describes the attributes of various microkeratomes used historically, currently in widespread clinical use, or under investigation or design.

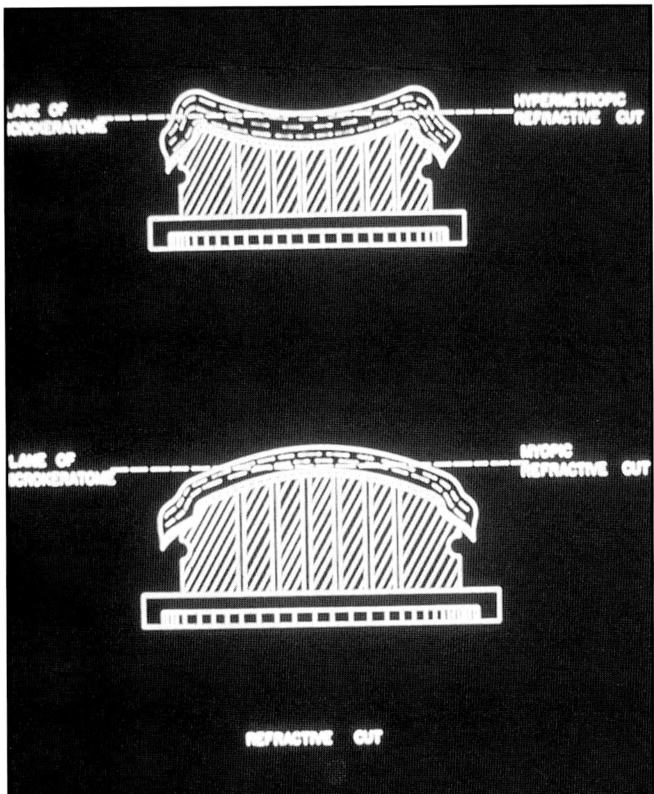

Figure 10-9.
Animated depiction of corneal disc on dye for hyperopic correction (top) [note anticipated peripheral removal of tissue] and corneal disc on dye for myopic correction (bottom) [note anticipated central removal of tissue].

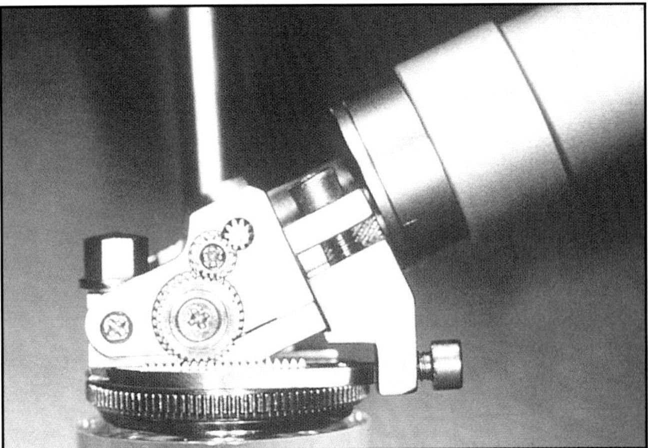

Figure 10-11.
Ruiz designed Chiron Automated Corneal Shaper which includes microkeratome with stopper in place on the three-piece suction ring used for ALK. Note gear advancement mechanism and impingement of stopper screw onto the lateral side of the suction ring.

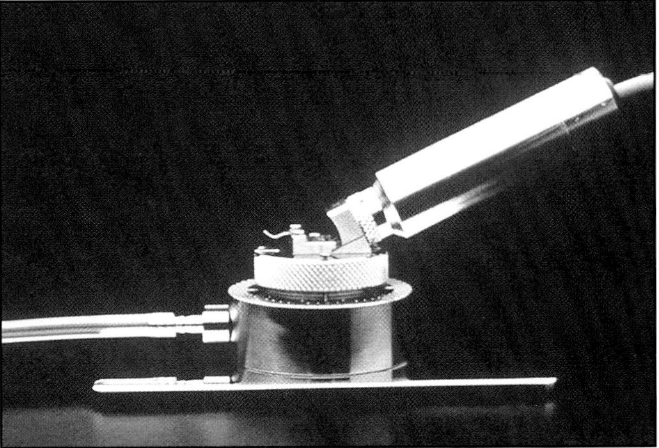

Figure 10-10.
Barraquer-Krumeich-Swinger microkeratome on suction dye platform.

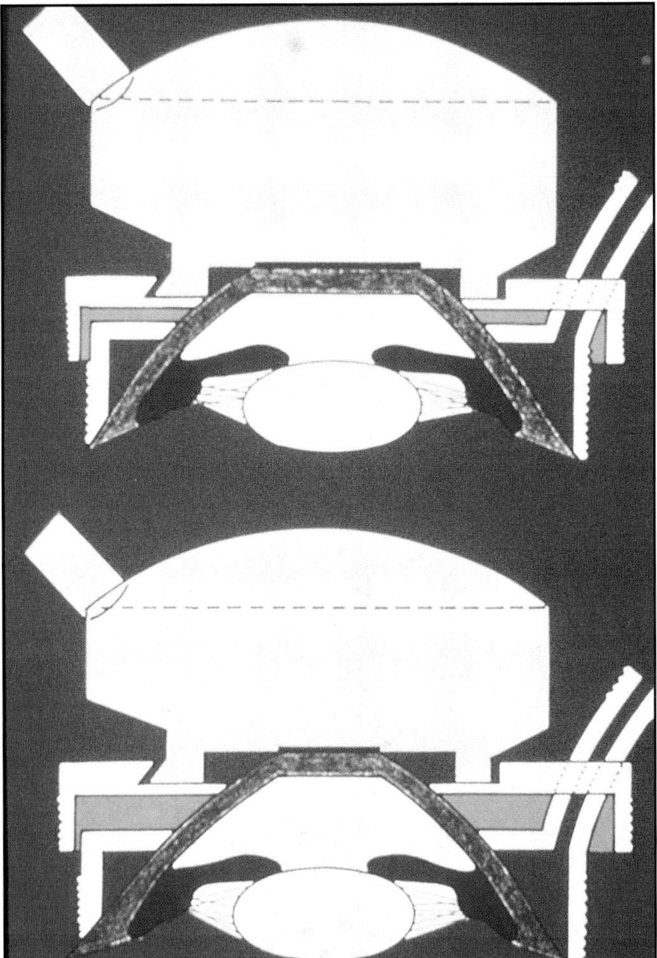

Figure 10-12.
Animated picture of three-piece suction ring collapsed (top) allowing for the largest possible diameter keratectomy and parallel plates separated with smaller diameter keratectomy achieved.

TABLE 10-1

MICROKERATOMES

Device Name	Manufacturer
Barraquer Original	
Barraquer 1996 Model	
Barraquer-Krumeich-Swinger	Eye Tech-M.Y. A. AG
Draeger Lamellating Rotokeratome	Storz Inc
Ruiz Automated Corneal Shaper	Chiron Vision Corp
TurboKeratome (SCMD)	Visionaerie Inc
Lamellar Keratoplasty System	Plancon Instruments/Moria
Micro Precision	Eye Technology Inc
UniversalKeratome	Phoenix Keratek Inc
Flapmaker	Refractive Technologies Inc
Schwind Microkeratom	Herbert Schwind Gmbh & Co
Visijet Hydrokeratome	Surgijet
Medjet	
Guimarães Microkeratome	
Mastel Diamond Lamellar Keratome	Mastel Precision Surgical Instruments Inc
Lasers*	

*At the time of this publication several laser manufacturers have developed or are in the process of developing techniques to create a flap of tissue under which a layer of stroma has been removed, in effect performing LASIK without a microkeratome.

There are undoubtedly several more under development that have not been publicly divulged at this time. Table 10-1 lists all microkeratomes known to us and Table 10-2 categorically lists attributes of five of the most highly touted in clinical practice at this time. Table 10-2 in no way implies superiority or lack thereof of the microkeratomes that are mentioned or not discussed. Notably, to date there has been no direct side-by-side comparative evaluation of the different microkeratomes reporting clinical data.

Original Barraquer Microkeratome

The original Barraquer microkeratome consisted of a microkeratome head with steel blade that was passed manually over the cornea (see Figures 10-1 and 10-3). This system utilized multiple suction rings of varying shoulder heights to achieve desired keratectomy diameters. IOP was checked with the Barraquer tonometer. A new microkeratome is under development by Drs. Barraquer and Carriazo in Bogota, Colombia.

Barraquer-Krumeich-Swinger Microkeratome

This device requires a manual pass of the keratome to achieve a lamellar cap of tissue. This is subsequently placed epithelium side down over a custom suction dye and the refractive cut is completed (see Figures 10-8 through 10-10). The system is sterilizable.

Draeger Lamellating Rotokeratome

This device was discontinued by Storz Inc, St. Louis, Mo. This microkeratome as described for LASIK consists of a microkeratome with a single thickness applanation (depth) plate or head and only one size suction ring. The metal blade rotates at 500 revolutions per minute and has a blade

TABLE 10-2

MICROKERATOME COMPARATIVE DATA

	ACS	UK	Microkeratom	Micro Precision	Turbo Keratome
Blade translation	Automatic	Automatic	Automatic	Manual	Manual
Translation speed*	2.3	9	<7	Surgeon control	Surgeon control
Blade material	Metal	Metal	Sapphire	Metal	Metal
Reusable blade	Single use	Single use	Reusable	Single use	Single use
Blade angle	25°	0°		9°	25°
Blade edge	Bi-faceted	Uni-faceted		Bi-faceted	Bi-faceted
Blade drive	Electric motor	Electric motor		Pneumatic	Pneumatic
Blade speed OPM	8000	14,000		20,000	15,000
Blade direction	Sideways	Oscillatory		Sideways	Sideways
Thickness setting	Individual plates	Disp. lenses		Adjustable	Fixed head
Diameter setting	Adjustable ring	Disp. lenses		Mult. rings	Mult. rings
Diameter verification	Appl. lenses	Disp. lenses		Appl. lenses	Appl. lenses
Pressure increase	Suction pump	Suction pump	Suction pump	Suction pump	Suction pump
Pressure verification	Tonometer	Not possible	Manometer	Tonometer	Tonometer
Sterilizable	Yes	No	Yes	Yes	Yes
Single unit	No	Yes	Yes	No	No
Surgeon view of surgery	No	Yes	Yes	No	No

*Translation speed in seconds for forward pass, blade speed in oscillations per minute.
ACS=Chiron Vision Corp Automated Corneal Shaper, UK=Phoenix Keratek Inc UniversalKeratome, Microkeratom=Herbert Schwind GmbH & Co Schwind Microkeratom, Micro Precision=Eye Technology Inc Microlamellar Keratome, TurboKeratome=Visionaerie Inc SCMD, Disp. lenses=custom disposable lenses, Mult. rings=multiple suction rings, Appl. lenses=applanation lenses, Tonometer=Barraquer style tonometer.

angle approach of 0°. It is powered by an electrical power source and is used as a single unit. It does allow the surgeon to directly view the surgical field as the case occurs. The device is automatically advanced. The system is sterilizable.

Ruiz Automated Corneal Shaper

The Ruiz-designed microkeratome is manufactured by Hansa of Miami, Fla, and distributed by Chiron Vision Corp (Claremont, Calif) as either a LASIK-only unit or a combined ALK/LASIK unit. The combined unit can have either a single suction ring for LASIK or adjustable height ring for ALK (see Figures 10-11 and 10-12) whereas the LASIK unit has only a single-size suction ring. The microkeratome heads can be fit with a variable number of depth plates depending on the thickness of keratectomy desired. Both units are designed with stops (see Figure 10-11) to allow for the creation of a hinge in the flap. The keratome heads in both units are powered by an electrical motor with the metal blade moving sideways at 8000 oscillations per minute. The blade has an angulation of 25°. The unit consists of two pieces: the microkeratome with motor and the suction ring with handle. The surgeon does not have a direct view of the leading edge of the blade as the surgery is performed but can see the flap come into the receptacle on the top side of the microkeratome. The microkeratome is advanced by activation of an electrical motor over a geared track on the suction ring allowing for consistent velocity passage (Figures

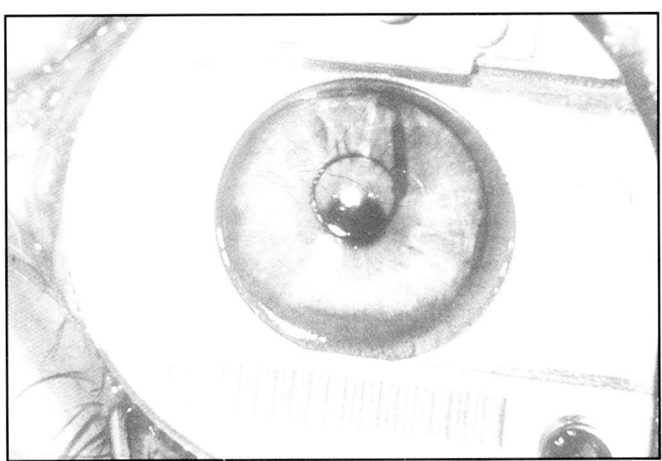

Figure 10-13.
Automated Corneal Shaper three-piece suction ring over ink-marked cornea. Note geared track on suction ring that accepts gearing on microkeratome body for automated advancement of the keratome.

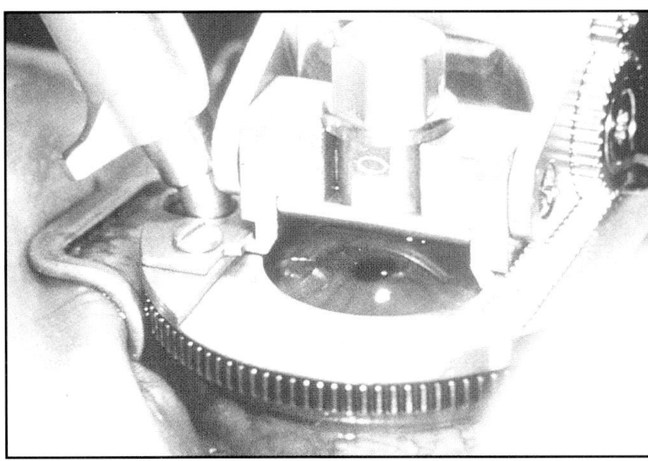

Figure 10-14.
Automated Corneal Shaper microkeratome head advancing over suction ring, which has been applied to the corneal surface.

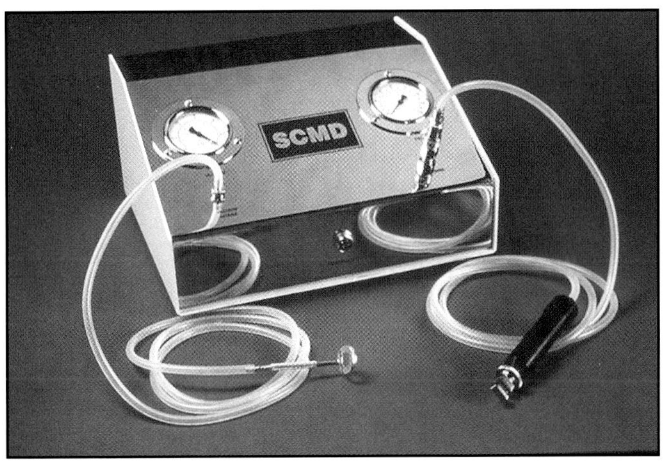

Figure 10-15.
TurboKeratome by Visionaerie Inc includes microkeratome, suction ring, and module.

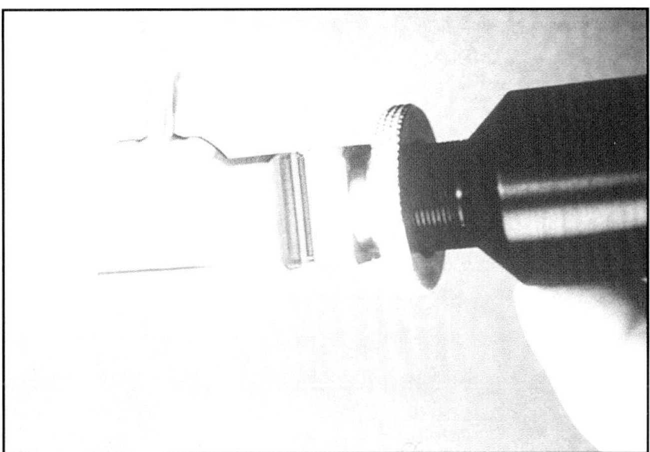

Figure 10-16.
TurboKeratome microkeratome head being inserted into the suction ring.

10-13 and 10-14). The system is sterilizable.

TurboKeratome (SCMD)

The TurboKeratome is distributed by Visionaerie Inc of Wilmington, Del (Figure 10-15). This microkeratome as sold for LASIK comes with a fixed keratome head (no depth plate) that achieves a 150-µm flap thickness. It comes with multiple suction rings to achieve varying diameter keratectomy flaps and four stop rings that give varying hinge dimensions. The bi-faceted metal blade has an angulation of 25° with side-to-side movement and oscillates 15,000 times per minute. The blade drive is powered by a nitrogen gas turbine operating at 60 pounds per square inch and achieves six times greater torque than electrical motors per the manufacturer. The microkeratome is manually advanced by the surgeon (Figure 10-16). The system is sterilizable.

Lamellar Keratoplasty System

This device is made by Plancon Instruments of Antony, France, and is distributed by Moria of France. The Plancon microkeratome has removable depth plates from 50 to 200 µm in 5-µm increments. It utilizes a bi-faceted metal blade that oscillates at 14,000 cycles per minute via nitrogen gas turbine. The unit comes with multiple suction rings depending on the diameter keratectomy desired. The ker-

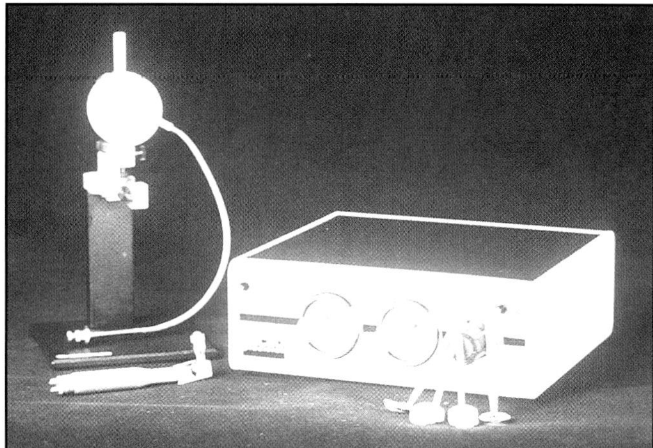

Figure 10-17.
Micro Precision's Microlamellar Keratome system.

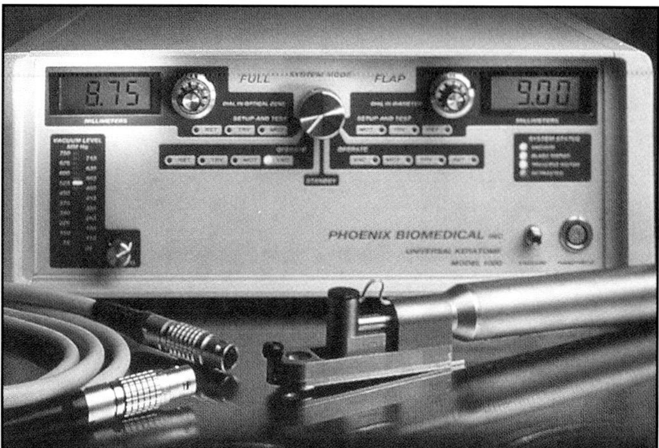

Figure 10-18.
Phoenix Keratek Inc's UniversalKeratome.

atome is advanced manually across the cornea by the surgeon who does not have a direct view of the operating field. The system is sterilizable.

Micro Precision Microlamellar Keratomileusis System

This device is distributed by Eye Technology Inc of St. Paul, Minn (Figure 10-17). The system features a patented adjustable plate which allows for a range of lamellar resections from 0 to 466 μm in 1-μm increments. A micrometer handle is attached to the adjustable plate and provides for calibration and verification of desired thickness. This unit also comes with multiple suction rings which allow for varying diameter flaps, but does have an adjustable ring under development. The suction rings and microkeratome head have dual dove-tail rail systems, which the manufacturer states cause less jumping and chatter marks in the stroma leading to a smoother keratectomy bed surface. The unit includes a "stop pin" system which helps create a hinged flap. The metal blade is bifaceted and angulated at 9°. The blade drive has sideways movement with 20,000 oscillations per minute. The blade drive is powered by a pneumatic turbine which the manufacturer states has six times the torque of electric motors. The microkeratome is manually advanced by the surgeon. The systems is sterilizable.

UniversalKeratome

The unit is manufactured and distributed by Phoenix Keratek Inc of Scottsdale, Ariz (Figure 10-18). This microkeratome comes as a single unit with no handled suction rings (Figure 10-19). This system is unique in that it has customized polymethylmethacrylate optical inserts (Figure 10-20) that can be used to achieve a planar disc of tissue with subsequent ablation with an excimer laser with the LASIK technique or lenticular inserts that can be used for a lenticular resection of tissue in the keratomileusis in situ technique. The metal blade is unifaceted and oscillates at 14,000 cycles per minute and has a 0° angulation. The device can be calibrated to create a hinge in the flap. The surgeon has direct view of the surgical field through the optical inserts but is unable to check the IOP immediately before the passage of the blade. This device is automatically advanced with an electrical motor drive. The microkeratome cannot be sterilized, but the blade and optical inserts can be autoclaved or chemically sterilized.

Flapmaker Disposable Microkeratome

This device (Refractive Technologies Inc, Cleveland, Ohio) is completely disposable and requires no assembly. It is sterilizable and requires no cleaning or maintenance. The unit is gearless. It is driven by flexible shafts that reportedly provide uniform motion of the microkeratome with blade oscillation at 12,500 cycles per minute. The unit is made of clear acrylic and enables the surgeon to directly visualize the case. The Flapmaker is purchased with a fixed preset resection depth with a variety of choices available to the surgeon. The surgeon is able to control flap diameter and can adjust for hinge creation.

Schwind Microkeratom

This device is made by Herbert Schwind Gmbh & Co of Germany. This comes as a single microkeratome unit

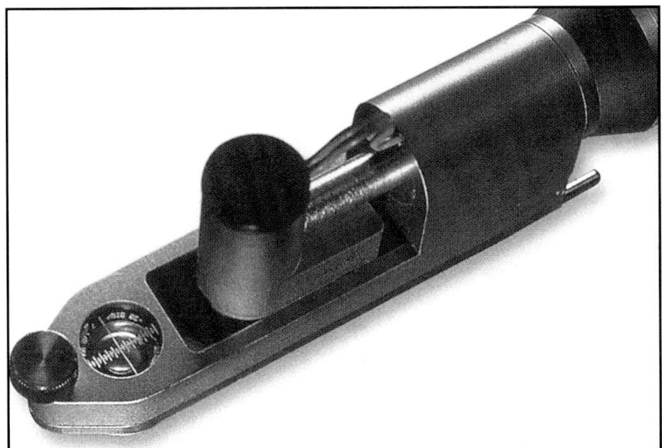

Figure 10-19.
UniversalKeratome is a single-piece unit. Note optical insert with calibrated surface.

(Figure 10-21) with accompanying power pack and foot controls. This device has an electrical motor system with drive cables that connect to the microkeratome head for advance and return of the cutting blade. The vacuum system consists of two suction rings. One is for stabilizing the peripheral cornea and the other is for stabilizing the lamella during the incision. This system is unique in that it has a sapphire blade that can be reused reportedly with long life expectancy. The blade cuts to a fixed 150-µm depth with an oscillation rate of 1350 cycles per minute and the surgeon has a direct view. The system can be sterilized.

Clear Corneal Molder Microkeratome

Dr. Ricardo Guimarães of Belo Horizonte, Brazil, has developed this device for use in LASIK.

Mastel Diamond Lamellar Keratome

This instrument has been designed by Mastel Precision Surgical Instruments Inc of Rapid City, SD. The system features diamond blades, clear viewing applanation, and manual operation. The flap created has a hinge parallel to the eyebrow.

Water Scalpels

Two high pressure water incising instruments are currently under design and development. Surgijet is developing the Visijet Hydrokeratome. This instrument uses a water beam size of 36 to 50 µm operating at 6 to 12,000 psi. The manufacturer reports good lamellar incisions with no collateral damage. Since the procedure only lasts 2 seconds when incising the cornea, the manufacturer speculates that significant stromal hydration will be unlikely. Possible treatments include myopia, hyperopia, and astigmatism with either direct reshaping of the surface or flap creation with removal of stromal tissue. In the last application, the Hydrokeratome would perform functions of both the microkeratome and an excimer laser. The second water scalpel under development is the Medjet high water pressure microkeratome. It is being designed and tested with the assistance of Dr. David Dillman of Danville, Pa.

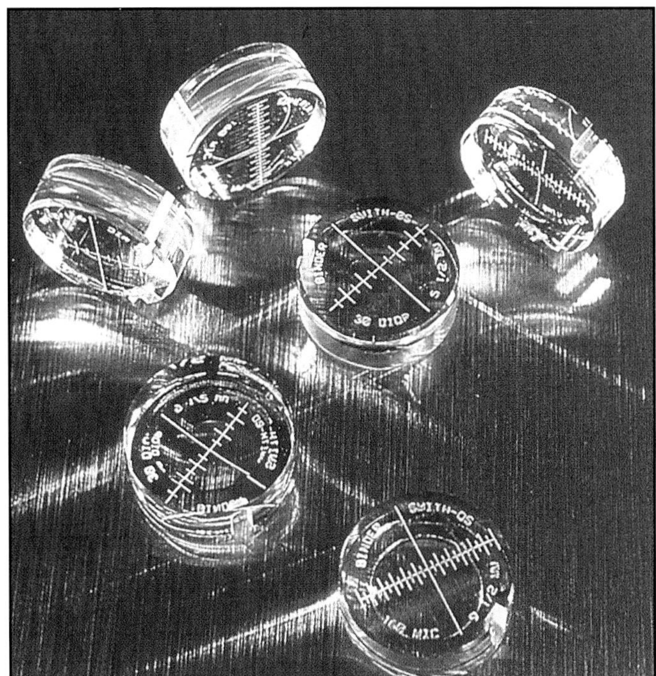

Figure 10-20.
UniversalKeratome PMMA optical inserts.

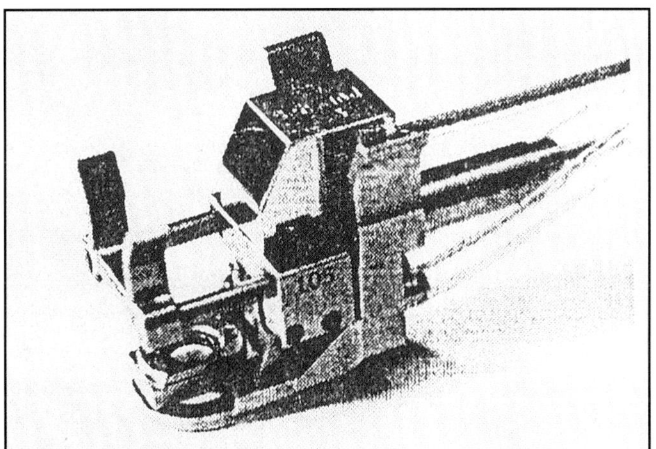

Figure 10-21.
Schwind Microkeratom is a single unit with double suction ring.

Laser Keratomes

Several lasers capable of intrastromal ablation through

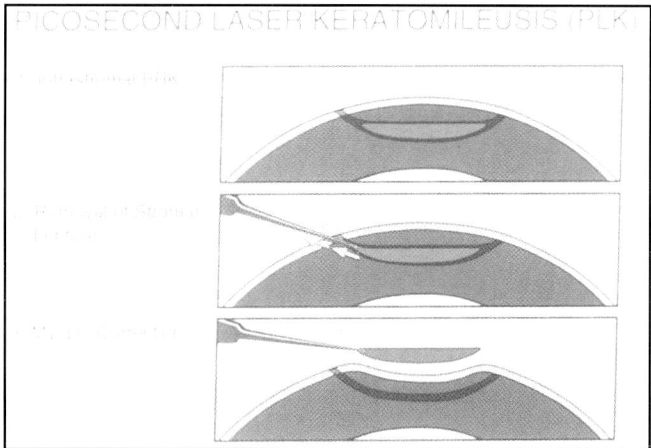

Figure 10-22.
Side view of intrastromal laser application to create a corneal flap and also create a lenticular piece of corneal stromal tissue that can be removed with forceps. This system would negate the use of a classical microkeratome.

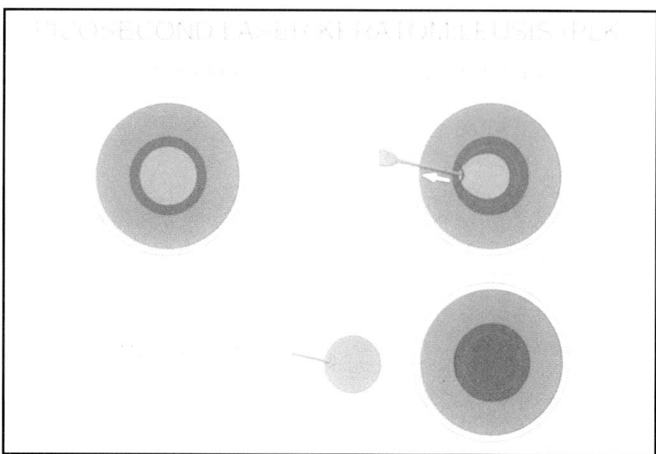

Figure 10-23.
Top view of intrastromal laser application to create a corneal flap and also create a lenticular piece of corneal stromal tissue that can be removed with forceps. This system would negate the use of a classical microkeratome.

an intact corneal surface are currently being tested to create a corneal flap. These lasers will simultaneously remove corneal stromal tissue to effect a refractive change (Figures 10-22 and 10-23).

MICROKERATOME SELECTION

Historically, microkeratomes for corneal refractive surgery have been difficult instruments to master. Regardless of what device a surgeon elects to use, they must come to master all aspects of its design, limitations, cleaning, maintenance, operation, and potential side effects. There are several salient features that can be discussed to champion one microkeratome over another including:

- Visibility of the cornea during the creation of the keratectomy.
- Automated systems that control the rate of the pass of the microkeratome.
- Blade angulation and its impact on adherence of the keratectomy and secondary epithelial ingrowth.
- Blade oscillation rate.
- Blade oscillation rate to keratome advancement rate.
- Torque delivered to the cutting blade.
- Suction to create a lamellar corneal flap and ability to check the IOP intraoperatively.
- Case after case dependability, repeatability, and durability.

With all the above said, creation of a flap of corneal tissue for LASIK is still surgery and conveys a certain amount of risk. Is there a perfect system? Not yet, and possibly never. The most important decision to make in the selection of a microkeratome is education on the part of the surgeon and his or her staff. To this end the safest and most reliable application of microkeratome technology for patient care will be achieved.

REFERENCES

1. Barraquer JI. Oueratoplastia refractiva. *Estudios Inform Oftal Inst Barraquer.* 1949;10:2-21.
2. Barraquer JI. Keratomileusis. *Int Surg.* 1967;48:103-117.
3. Barraquer JI. Results of myopic keratomileusis. *J Refract Surg.* 1987;3:98-101.
4. Barraquer JI. Method for cutting lamellar grafts in frozen corneas: new orientations for refractive surgery. *Arch Soc Am Ophthalmol.* 1958;1:237.
5. Bores L. Lamellar refractive surgery. In: Bores L, ed. *Refractive Eye Surgery.* Boston, Mass: Blackwell Scientific Publications; 1993:324-391.
6. Slade SG, Updegraff SA. Advances in lamellar refractive surgery. *Int Ophth Clinics.* 1994:147-162.
7. Nordan LT, Maxwell WA. Keratomileusis. In: Schwab IR, ed. *Refractive Keratoplasty.* New York, NY: Churchill Livingstone; 1987:41-68.
8. Swinger CA, Krumeich J, Cassiday D. Planar lamellar refractive keratoplasty. *J Refract Surg.* 1986;2:17-24.
9. Binder PS. What we have learned about corneal wound healing from refractive surgery (Barraquer Lecture). *Refract Corneal Surg.* 1989;5:98-120.
10. Binder PS, Zavala EY, Baumgartner SD, et al. Combined morphologi-

cal effects of cryolathing and lyophilization on epikeratoplasty lenticles. *Arch Ophthalmol.* 1986;104:671-679.

11. Zavala EY, Krumeich J, Binder PS. Laboratory evaluation of freeze vs nonfreeze lamellar refractive keratoplasty. *Arch Ophthalmol.* 1987;105:1125-1128.

12. Buratto L, Ferrari M. Retrospective comparison of freeze and nonfreeze myopic epikeratophakia. *Refract Corneal Surg.* 1989;5:94-97.

13. Arenas-Archila E, Sanchez-Thorin JC, et al. Myopic keratomileusis in-situ: a preliminary report. *J Cataract Refract Surg.* 1991;17:424-435.

Flapmaker Disposable Microkeratome

ALEXANDER DYBBS, PHD

The Flapmaker (Refractive Technologies Inc, Cleveland, Ohio) microkeratome is an automatic, completely assembled, disposable microkeratome as shown in Figure 1. It is made of a hard, clear, polycarbonate plastic and is single use.

It is based upon the principle of the carpenter's plane as developed by Barraquer. The blade, made from surgical stainless steel, oscillates at 12,500 rpm and is controlled by a unique patented flexible cable that is electronically driven. The blade extends a fixed distance from a clear fixed plate and is at a 26° angle to the plate. Resection depths of 130 or 160 µm are available. The microkeratome is mounted in a suction plate and is driven across the cornea at 6.8 mm/sec by a patented flexible cable that is electronically controlled.

The Flapmaker comes completely assembled with a blade inserted for either 130- or 160-µm resection depth. No assembly is needed. Three connections are made: the suction tube, the blade oscillation flexible cable, and the flexible drive cable. The flaps made with this microkeratome are 10.5 mm in diameter and are thus suitable for both myopia and hyperopia. The microkeratome has several unique features.

- It is clear, thus the surgeon can observe the flap as it is being made.
- Its blade only oscillates in the forward motion, thus avoiding any possibility of recutting the stromal bed or the flap.
- It has no gears to jam or be stopped by eyelashes.
- It has an adjustable electronic stop for the hinge position, which prevents free caps from being made.
- It has a preset resection depth, thus eliminating the possibility of cutting through the globe.

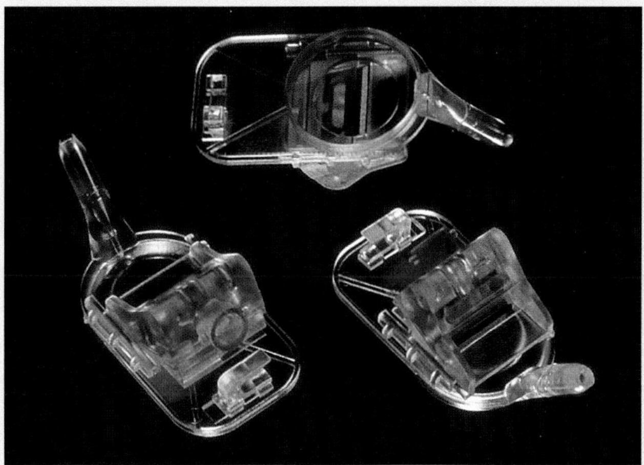

Figure 1.
The Flapmaker Disposable Microkeratome.

SECTION 4

PROCEDURE

Chapter 11

PREOPERATIVE EVALUATION

Dimitrios S. Siganos, MD, Ioannis G. Pallikaris, MD

HISTORY

Checking Stability of Refraction

LASIK and PRK are refractive procedures performed usually in patients who are 18 years or older. This is the age at which refraction is considered to have stabilized. We ask the patients for their earlier refractive status, the spectacle or contact lens power they are using, and any previous spectacle prescription. The patient is asked about frequency of changing spectacles or contact lenses. If a discrepancy is found between the patient's previous refractive status and the one he or she presents, then thorough checking of clarity or condition of the optical media is a must. One should be aware of the possibility of keratoconus, cataract in progression, or corneal warpage syndrome.

Contact Lens Wearers

Soft contact lens wearers are advised to stop wearing their contact lenses at least 3 weeks prior to preoperative evaluation and surgery. The contact lens flattens the cornea and an examination conducted immediately after contact lens removal might underestimate myopia. Furthermore, soft contact lenses are responsible for the corneal warpage syndrome. In such a case, evaluation of that eye is better performed after asking the patient not to wear his or her contact lenses for at least 3 months. The same applies for hard contact lens wearers, who in either case should not be evaluated unless they have omitted their contact lens use for 3 to 4 months. We have seen topographies of hard contact lens wearers giving the impression of keratoconus even 2 months after they had discontinued their contact lens use. The topographies of these same eyes were absolutely normal when a 4-month period had lapsed.

Diabetes

Although we have treated about a dozen diabetic patients with PRK or LASIK, none of them developed any complications related to refractive surgery. The epithelial healing was as fast as with the non-diabetic population, and no complications of any kind were encountered. However, the problems that persons with diabetics, especially the poorly controlled or the insulin dependent, may face are that:

- Refraction is usually not stable, as the crystalline lens absorbs more water due to increased glucose in the surrounding aqueous humor, rendering the eye more myopic. In a person who has diabetes who has undergone a refractive procedure for the correction of myopia, this transient increase in myopia might be considered as regression or undercorrection.
- Persons with diabetes develop cataracts earlier than non-diabetics. This could be attributed to excimer laser surgery as well. In the initial PRK Summit Technology data submitted to the FDA, a small percentage had developed cataract. Whether cataract was the result of excimer laser exposure or the steroids used following PRK was not identified.

These two situations, as well as possible complications related to their disease such as defective or slow wound healing, higher susceptibility to infection, etc, must be clearly explained to persons with diabetes who are candidates for PRK, and should be stated in the informed consent form.

EXAMINATION

Uncorrected Visual Acuity

This is a measurement that should, ideally, be taken in all cases. Although it sounds needless, especially in high myopes, uncorrected visual acuity, particularly for near, is important. This is because of patient expectations and the possibility of the eye ending up hyperope. In such a case, the patient could think that he or she had deteriorated as the individual was able to read before surgery, something that he or she is unable to do after LASIK. This especially applies in patients where presbyopia has intervened. A 50-year-old patient who previously had -4.0 D of myopia and is now perfectly corrected (ie, emmetrope), unless fully informed prior to surgery, would consider that the refractive surgery abolished his or her reading vision, which was previously without spectacles. Many patients who have jobs requiring the constant use of near vision should be well informed prior to surgery about the possibility of the early hyperopic shift or that of overcorrection and the consequences. These patients should avoid having both eyes operated at the same sitting.

Best Corrected Visual Acuity—Manifest Refraction

Contrary to what most studies indicate, or perceive as a success of a refractive surgical procedure, we believe that, along with contrast sensitivity, this is *the* most important factor to evaluate. Postoperative unaided visual acuity is a measure of efficacy and predictability; however, safety of a refractive surgical procedure such as LASIK is best corrected visual acuity. We now consider anecdotal the phrase "gain of best corrected visual acuity." It is true that, owing to the high minification of the retinal image of high myope, there may be a loss of best spectacle corrected visual acuity. However, best corrected visual acuity or contrast sensitivity testing in moderate and high myopia should always be determined using a soft or, preferably, hard contact lens, having a spherical equivalent as close as possible to that of the patient's refraction. Overrefraction should never be more than ± 2.5 D. Ideally, the optometric department of any refractive surgery center should have all powers of contact lenses so that all patients could be properly evaluated. We always use contact lens determination of best corrected visual acuity in myopia over 6.5 D and hyperopia over 4 D. Irrespective of the patient's refractive error, best corrected visual acuity should be tested in any condition where the patient's best corrected visual acuity with spectacles is lower than 20/20. A suboptimal best corrected visual acuity (ie, less than 20/200) could be an indication of a subclinical keratoconus, a corneal warpage syndrome, irregular astigmatism, etc, all of which are contraindications, whether temporary or absolute, to having refractive surgery performed on such eyes.

Slit Lamp Examination

Evaluation of the anterior segment on slit lamp examination is mandatory to rule out various diseases or pathology. The lids are checked for any disease or blepharitis that should ideally be treated prior to LASIK surgery. The cornea is examined for clarity, scars, and presence of dystrophies or degenerations, especially keratoconus. However, subclinical keratoconus might be missed unless a corneal topography is obtained. Many surgeons consider keratoconus as not being an absolute contraindication for LASIK or PRK. Actually, we have performed LASIK or PRK in more than 20 such patients and only in a very small percentage were the results unpredictable. There are few reports in the literature on this subject that coincide with our results. The stability of refraction and a preoperative central corneal thickness of 500 µm or more are important factors in performing LASIK on a keratoconus patient. The patient should also understand that the results may end up suboptimal, that keratoconus may deteriorate, and that a corneal transplantation may become necessary following LASIK.

Corneal neovascularization as a result of contact lens wear should also be recognized. In LASIK, the suction produced by the microkeratome suction ring usually ruptures these vessels and conjunctival hemorrhage may result. This is usually not a serious complication, but it might decrease visibility during surgery and the conjunctival hemorrhage may produce anxiety, especially in female patients during the first 20 postoperative days (ie, the usual period needed for absorption).

The anterior chamber is checked for evidence of active iritis and a very thorough examination of the crystalline lens is conducted under full mydriasis. A 50-year-old patient with -11.0 D and nuclear sclerosis or other evidence of peripheral lens opacities would benefit more from a clear lens extraction than from a LASIK procedure.

The Pupil

Measuring the size of the pupil in dim illumination is important to avoid glare problems postoperatively. LASIK is a procedure that is mostly used to correct moderate and high degrees of myopia. It is well known that the thickness of corneal tissue to be removed for a certain amount of myopia is directly proportional to the ablation zone diameter. Since in LASIK large corrections are attempted, ideally small zones are utilized in order to avoid getting too deep in the cornea. This is true and useful as long as a transition zone or a multipass technique is used. Otherwise, prismatic effects of the reshaped corneal optics are liable to induce glare and halo phenomena more commonly than PRK. If the dim-light pupil diameter is more than 5 mm, such phenomena are to be expected and are more pronounced the greater the attempted correction.

Schirmer Test

This test is performed in order to avoid treating cases with xerophthalmia, something that may delay healing. This is more important in photorefractive keratectomy (PRK) than in laser in situ keratomileusis (LASIK). However, some of the preservatives in drugs used following LASIK may accentuate xerophthalmia symptoms.

Cycloplegic Refraction

We use one drop of phenylephrine 5% and one drop of Cyclopentolate 1%, the latter to be repeated 5 minutes later, and we determine cycloplegic refraction about 30 to 40 minutes after instillation. Cycloplegic refraction in moderate and high myopes, and more noticeably in hyperopes, should be also performed by using contact lenses, for the reasons mentioned earlier.

Although hyperopes tend to be the group presenting high amounts of spasm of accommodation, we have seen myopes with differences between manifest and cycloplegic refraction of more than 2 D.

What to do in such a case? When the cycloplegic refraction is lower than the manifest, we ask the patient to come back at a later date to recheck his or her manifest refraction. The spasm might be caused by overcorrection of his or her spectacles or contact lenses. A slow fogging technique may be all that is required. However, if the difference between manifest and cycloplegic refraction still persists, we then use the cycloplegic refraction—always corrected to the corneal plane—as the attempted correction, especially if the patient is in his or her late 20s or older.

The patient's history and preoperative examinations will determine whether or not the patient should be subjected to refractive surgery. Primarily, the patient must be well informed regarding alternative refractive surgical procedures, so that our decision on which procedure is appropriate for the patient meets his or her expectations. In our decision-making process, we must take well into consideration the patient's age and occupation.

One problem we frequently come across is that younger patients seek refractive surgery before their myopia is considered stable or before the age of 18 years due to occupational needs. In this case, it must be explained that they will probably need to undergo a second refractive operation in the years to come. The patients must be aware of the legislation regarding the job they want to obtain, because it differs among countries. Very often, a young person obtains an uncorrected visual acuity of 20/20 so as to meet the entry demands for a military academy, but a minor scar at the corneal periphery or on epithelial ingrowth could be disastrous. On the whole, it is preferable to subject a young patient with low myopia to PRK for the correction of his or her refractive error, with our goal being overcorrection, instead of undergoing LASIK. Young patients who plan to proceed with academic studies should be informed that their myopia might increase in the next 5 to 10 years. On the other hand, patients over 40 years of age are eligible for clear lens extraction if their myopia is over -14 D. The combination of having a clear lens extraction performed on one eye and LASIK performed on the other is a fine solution for high myopes. Patients with myopia over -16 D should consider undergoing a phakic IOL of anterior chamber or ICL. Patients over 45 years of age should be thoroughly examined for cataract development because there could be a need for a future (in 10 to 20 years) cataract operation. Thus, these patients must be informed that they can undergo one operation and achieve two goals at one time (myopia correction and a cataract extraction).

The preoperative examination helps us decide the kind of refractive surgery to be performed. At the analysis of each of the preoperative examinations done, I will explain how these can lead us to determine a certain surgery.

The patients who are contact lens wearers must discontinue wearing lenses at least 3 weeks prior to the examination date, especially if they are half hard. If the manifest refraction results are stable (within 0.5 D) and the corneal topographic map does not show signs of any corneal abnormality, then we can proceed with the operation. Patients with subclinical keratoconus shown on the corneal topographic map or with abnormal effect due to contact lens wear should discontinue wearing their lenses for 2 or 3 months. The inclusion and exclusion criteria remain the same.

Fundus Examination

A thorough retinal examination under good mydriasis is a must prior to LASIK surgery. Almost all candidates are moderate to high myopes, and we have encountered numerous peripheral retinal degenerations, holes, tears, breaks, and macular pathology. Since we had one case that developed retinal detachment following LASIK, we prefer to treat peripheral pathology with the argon laser prior to LASIK. For macular pathology, we use photodocumentation, and fluorescein angiography is performed when needed. The most important aspect is for the patient to understand that correction of his or her refractive error is only optical and not anatomical, and that, as a myopic eye, he or she will always be more liable to retinal detachment than the natural emmetrope.

DECISION MAKING

One or Two Eyes?

In any case, if any complication occurs during surgery of the first eye, the idea of treating both eyes in the same sitting should be avoided. There are both advantages and disadvantages in performing simultaneous LASIK. The advantage for the patient is that he or she gets over his or her bilateral error of refraction at the same time and that the postoperative follow-up time and visits are shortened to those required had only one eye been treated. Another advantage is that the patient does not have to experience aniseikonia, or actually having monocular vision for a period of time by using spectacles if he or she is contact lens intolerant, or that the patient does not have to wear a contact lens in the fellow eye until he or she decides to have that operated on as well.

Among the disadvantages is the inability to check immediately for a postoperatively recognized complication such as a bilaterally decentered ablation zone. Another disadvantage is that any residual error, whether over- or undercorrection that has occurred in one eye, could not be accounted for in the operation of the fellow eye.

Which Eye to Operate First?

Usually the non-dominant eye is selected, unless otherwise requested by the patient. The non-dominant eye is the one having the lowest best corrected visual acuity and highest astigmatism and refractive error.

What Is the Intended Correction?

Most patients ask for a plano refraction. However, many myopes at the age of declining accommodation may benefit from an intended undercorrection, as it will allow them for some time to read without the need for spectacles (see also Uncorrected Visual Acuity). Many of the myopes of this age either remove their spectacles to read, or have deliberately undercorrected spectacles so as not to need two pairs or bifocal or multifocal spectacles. Many of them have also never recognized their reading problem.

CONCERNS

Ptosis

Patients should be warned about the possibility of experiencing slight ptosis after the operation. This is attributed to the use of steroids, although the mechanism is not clear. Although we do not use steroids for a long period following LASIK, about 4% of our patients complain of postoperative drooping of their eyelid. This is usually temporary, although some patients believe it never recovered. Although we are not aware of such a policy being adopted by any refractive surgery center, a way to compare, as well as for medicolegal purposes, would be that of taking photos of the patient as is done in strabismus and plastic surgery centers. After all, refractive surgery is considered by some authorities as a cosmetic surgery.

Clinical Parameters Assessed in the Preoperative Evaluation (Uncorrected and Best Corrected Visual Acuity)

Due to the fact that LASIK is a relatively new technique, these data are often used in presentations, analyses, publications, and in protocols, so it is best to use standardized examination procedures for visual acuity evaluation. For example, Americans use the ETORS chart whereas Europeans use the decimal scale. It is wise to optimize the conditions for the patient's examinations used for the evaluation of the visual acuity. It is of great importance that the patients are assessed under the same conditions prior to and after the surgery, so as to have a clearer indication as to whether there has been an improvement of the visual acuity or some visual loss. For the visual acuity evaluation of patients with high myopia, it is best to use contact lenses, preferably hard, for these contact lenses simulate vision obtained after the refractive operation. Furthermore, these contact lenses minimize any optical effects that are apparent with wearing glasses and provide us with more information regarding the function of the macula. Prior to astigmatic correction, many refractions must be obtained either on the same or different days. There is an intense problem when the correction applies to low myopias with relatively low astigmatisms. Changes on the axes' power if the astigmatism is higher than -3 D must be taken under consideration and a consensus value should be obtained. For patients with myopia over -14 D and low astigmatism of up to -1 D, a thorough assessment of the astigmatism is of little importance. The reason is that, with the correction of high myopia, a large tissue segment is removed and the amount of potentially included astigmatism is quite high. In these cases, the patient must be informed of the need for a second "refinement" operation for the correction of the remaining astigmatism and/or myopia.

Chapter 12

THE PROCEDURE

Ioannis G. Pallikaris, MD, Dimitrios S. Siganos, MD,
Thekla G. Papadaki, MD

Laser in situ keratomileusis (LASIK) is a procedure that can be performed in an outpatient operating suite; however, always under sterile conditions.

EQUIPMENT

The equipment used can be divided into two groups. The first group contains the material that is ready prior to surgery and will be used, and the second group comprises instruments that may be used (ie, they should be ready there but not opened unless needed). The room should include an air ionizer for best maintenance and operation of the excimer laser machine

Material that is opened:

- Material for skin cleansing and draping (gauze, steri-drape, Betadine solution)
- Medication
- Anesthetic eye drops, such as proparacaine
- Combined antibiotic-steroid eye drops, such as diclofenac sodium eye drops
- Cyclopentolate eye drops
- Mask, cap, and sterile powderless gloves
- The microkeratome set
- A wire Barraquer lid speculum
- LASIK marker, to be painted with gentian violet

- A Barraquer applanation tonometer
- BSS in syringes of 10 mL
- Corneal paper shields or other flap protector
- Beaver knife
- Air cannulas (25 and 31 gauge)
- Collibri forceps
- Pallikaris LASIK cannula or any irrigation-aspiration cannula
- Cellulose microsponges
- Aquarium air pump
- Laser device
- Ultrasonic corneal pachymeter

Material ready in case of need:

- Pierse forceps
- Grasping forceps
- Scissors
- Curved tying forceps
- Needle holders
- 10/0 nylon sutures
- Bandage soft contact lenses

PERSONNEL REQUIRED

An experienced physician requires no assistance for the actual performing of the procedure. At least one well-trained medical assistant is required to prepare the patient, provide the surgeon with the proper instrumentation, and test and maintain the microkeratome in good working condition. A technician or engineer must be also available to calibrate the excimer laser and provide maintenance.

PATIENT PREPARATION

The procedure should be explained to the patient to facilitate cooperation and help alleviate anxiety. The patient should be told that he or she might experience some discomfort (a feeling of pressure) at the first stages and a blurring of his or her vision as the operation proceeds. He or she should become familiar with the noise of the microkeratome and that of the excimer laser, and should be advised to hold as still as possible during the operation.

PATIENT POSITIONING

Topical anesthetic is applied to the operating eye, one drop 5 minutes apart for a total of three drops. The patient is given a cap to wear and lies on the operating table so that he or she is aligned with the laser beam.

Betadine solution is used to prepare the eyelids and a fenestrated sterile, plastic, adhesive drape is placed so that eyelashes are removed from the operating field.

PROCEDURE

The technician calibrates the laser according to the manufacturer's instructions.

Both the surgeon and assistant wear sterile gloves and assemble the microkeratome. The surgeon must doublecheck the instrument at the beginning of every case by him- or herself. A new blade should be used for every case. The surgeon performs several tests to ensure proper movement of the gears, proper sliding of the blade without binding, proper suction of the ring, and proper advancement of the microkeratome through the dove-tail of the suction ring.

The patient's refractive data are inserted in the computer. Data are preferably doublechecked by the assistant and the technician.

An important tip here is the following: At least 3 D of the attempted correction should be given in a zone of 7 mm or larger. According to Munnerlyn's algorithm for a given correction, the larger the zone, the deeper the ablation, and vice versa. In very high myopia, it is wise to use a small zone in order to ablate the minimum amount of tissue. However, if the actual ablation zone is 5 mm, the topographic zone tends to be smaller. Given that the patient might have a pupil that is greater than 4.5 mm at rest, this could create substantial optical problems, such as glare and halos, that are more intense the greater the attempted correction. Also, in very deep ablations, the transition zone between ablated and non-ablated cornea could possibly induce, beside spherical aberrations, prismatic effects that may not affect visual acuity as an amount, but may do so quality wise. Correcting at least 3 D at a large ablation zone provides for a smoother transition zone and less potential optical aberrations.

The surgeon removes his or her gloves and washes his or her hands using an ordinary scrub (Betadine). The surgeon then puts on sterile powderless gloves. Usual sterile gloves may be used if powderless gloves are unavailable, but care should be taken to remove excessive powder by washing off with sterile saline prior to the operation, since it is possible for powder to be trapped under the corneal flap and cause interface opacities.

The lid speculum is inserted, taking care to include the eyelashes so that they are out of the operative field. One more drop of topical anesthetic is instilled. **The patient's head positioning is of extreme importance.** The cornea should be at the center of the palpebral fissure. The surgeon should explain to the patient that he or she must keep his or her head steady and move only according to the surgeon's instructions. The patient is asked to fixate on the operating microscope's light and the cornea is marked (see also Chapter 14, *Assisting Instrumentation*). Marking ensures better repositioning of the flap at the end of the procedure.

The exact procedure for creating the corneal flap varies depending on which microkeratome is used. The procedure with the Chiron Vision Corp Automated Corneal Shaper is going to be described here since it is the most widely used. Information regarding the operation of other types of microkeratomes is given in Chapter 10.

The corneal surface is profusely irrigated using BSS for about 20 to 30 seconds while the suction tube removes the excess water. Good irrigation is essential to remove debris, etc. The corneal surface is then wiped off with a cellulose microsponge. The suction ring is inserted. Before activation of the suction ring, the ring is placed slightly eccentric to the nasal side of the cornea, by about 1 mm. This maneuver allows for better centration of the treatment area, while it protects the hinge of the flap from accidental ablation. In case the base of the flap is intended to be in any other position (eg, superiorly), then the suction ring is placed eccentric by 1 mm toward the intended base of the flap. Suction is activated by the assistant.

In enophthalmic eyes or in eyes having a small palpebral fissure, it is sometimes difficult to place the suction ring of the microkeratome. It is difficult, but not impossible. Some surgeons would go for a lateral canthotomy; however, in a very large series of eyes, we have never resorted to this procedure. By mobilizing the patient's head, positioning of the suction ring seems to be always possible. Even if the suction ring does not properly rest during its positioning, it does so when suction is turned on. In any case, most microkeratome manufacturing companies are currently reducing the suction ring diameter to comfortably fit in all eyes. In hyperopic small eyes the smaller suction ring is used.

Applanation tonometry is performed while the corneal surface is dry to ensure IOP has reached the minimum of 65 mmHg. The surgeon checks for the last time that the 160-μm thickness plate is inserted and that the stop screw of the Hansa stopper is properly adjusted.

The surface of the globe and the head of the microkeratome are moistened with BSS. The keratome's head is inserted into the dove-tail of the ring and advanced manually until the gears of the corneal shaper are firmly engaged to the gear track of the suction ring. The surgeon holds the suction handle with one hand and supports the motor cord with the other hand. The footswitch is depressed in the forward position. The microkeratome advances mechanically and stops as the shaper hits the stop. The footswitch is then depressed in the reverse position. The suction is switched off and the ring and head are removed from the eye.

During forward movement of the keratome, one should always look for the flap being created, and during the reverse movement that the flap returns back to the cornea. This is a first indication that one gets a flap and not a cap. Prompt attention at this point is extremely useful, especially in the case that a cap has been produced. Then the surgeon knows where the cap might be found.

Before lifting the flap, it is profusely irrigated once more to remove cells and debris, while the aspiration tube removes the excess water. The border of the flap is gently grasped at the temporal site with Pierse forceps, taking care not to injure the epithelium, and the flap is gently reflected nasally (Figure 12-1). Alternatively, the flap can be lifted by inserting the tip of a dry air cannula underneath the hinge. The cannula is then moved in a wave-like motion from the temporal to the nasal side (Figure 12-2). A Merocel microsponge is used to carefully remove excessive moisture from the edges of the hinge and the flap border prior to the ablation (Figure 12-3). The stromal surface of the flap is then covered by the flap protector (Figure 12-4).

Ultrasonic pachymetry of the stromal bed is performed and the thickness of the flap is calculated. This step is very important especially in high myopic correc-

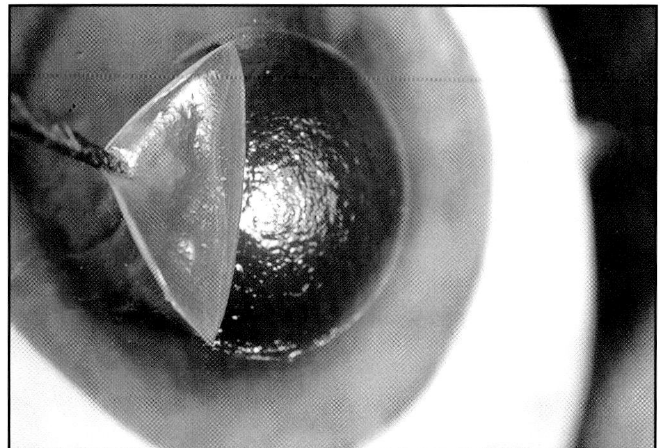

Figure 12-1.
The border of the flap is gently grasped at the temporal site with Pierse forceps, taking care not to injure the epithelium, and then the flap is gently reflected nasally.

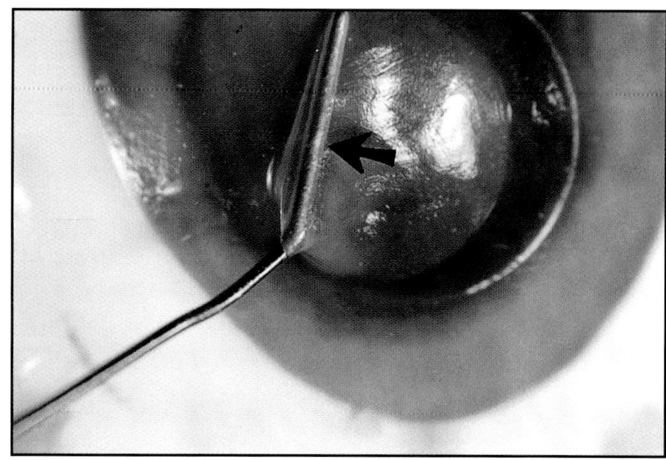

Figure 12-2.
Alternatively, the flap can be lifted by inserting the tip of a dry air cannula underneath the hinge. The cannula is then moved in a wave-like motion from the temporal to the nasal side.

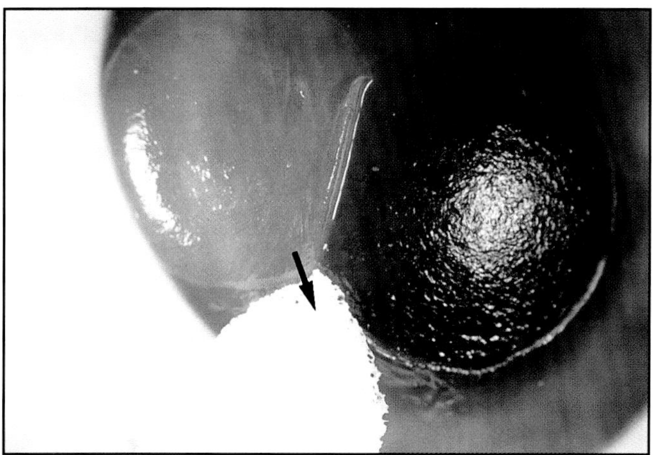

Figure 12-3.
A Merocel microsponge is used to carefully remove excessive moisture from the edges of the hinge and the flap border prior to the ablation.

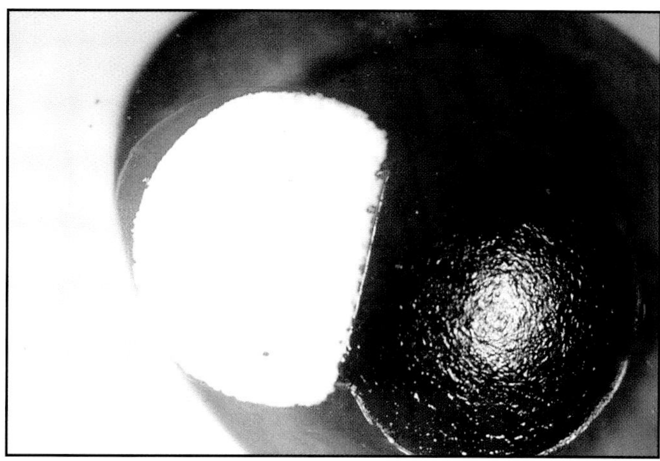

Figure 12-4.
The stromal surface of the flap is covered by the flap protector.

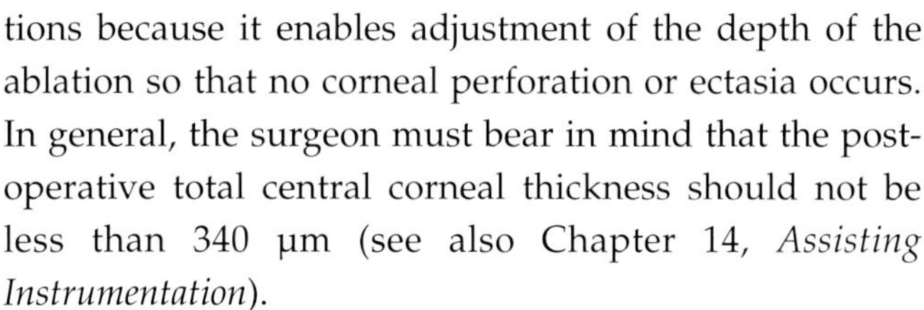

tions because it enables adjustment of the depth of the ablation so that no corneal perforation or ectasia occurs. In general, the surgeon must bear in mind that the postoperative total central corneal thickness should not be less than 340 μm (see also Chapter 14, *Assisting Instrumentation*).

Most microkeratomes are set or preset to produce a 150- to 160-μm flap. However, and from our experience, flap thickness was almost never 160 μm. Flap thickness ranged from 90 to 190 μm. What could be the importance of this? Actually, there is no magic number for the flap thickness. The flap should not be very thick, in order not to go deep in the stroma for ablation, and not so thin that it could not be easily handled. Anyhow, if the flap is thicker than 170 μm, there is a strong possibility that the edge at the base would "protrude," creating irregular astigmatism. On the other hand, when the flap is thinner than 120 μm, there is a tendency for the flap to create wrinkles.

Another important issue here in dealing with flap thickness is uniformity of refractive results. Two eyes having the same refractive error and exactly the same pattern of attempted correction/ablation would end up having a different outcome if there was a difference in flap thickness between the two eyes. This is because different levels of cornea stroma have different ablation rates. This is one of the reasons there is not yet a standard algorithm for LASIK.

Centration

If a needle is used to mark the center prior to ablation, then the cornea should be wet in order to be able to get a reflection. If the mark is not visible, then the area is passed with a Merocel sponge and the mark appears clearly. One should always mark lightly, as there is a danger of perforating the cornea. The Pallikaris centration device is specially designed so that it is always aligned with the original centration.

In case of astigmatism, we prefer centration on the optical axis and not the pupil center. Another tip is that if there is a capability of choosing the position of the base of the flap, then it is preferable to align the hinge of the flap so that it is parallel to the steeper axis. The reason is that more ablation will be effected there and more space is needed in that direction.

Laser Ablation

If the excimer laser utilizes a mask (such as the Aesculap-Meditec MEL 60), then the proper mask is placed on the eye, and suction is activated by the surgeon. In lasers not utilizing a mask or not having an incorporated tracking system, the globe may be fixed by the surgeon so that the whinny beams are focused on the corneal bed and centered over the pupil. Grasping by the forceps might induce some discomfort to the patient. To alleviate this, two pieces of a Merocel sponge soaked in 0.75% bupivacaine (Marcaine) may be applied after the creation of the flap (but before lifting it) for about 1 minute at the superior and inferior limbal conjunctiva where the forceps will touch. A Thornton ring can also be used to stabilize the eye.

The assistant goes through the patient's data once and doublechecks with the technician to ensure that the proper attempted correction is given. The surgeon activates the laser with the foot pedal and ablation is given. When ablation is complete, the surgeon switches the suction off and removes the mask from the eye.

If the ablated surface appears to be irregular, one could try to make it smooth. This can be done in the following way. A wet (with artificial tears) Merocel is passed over the ablated surface. Then a 9-µm PlanoScan phototherapeutic keratectomy (PTK) ablation is usually sufficient to make the surface regular.

Repositioning of the flap is the next step which can be performed using two techniques (Table 12-1):

TABLE 12-1

Comparison of Dry and Wet Techniques

Dry Technique	Wet Technique
Advantages:	
Faster visual rehabilitation (hours)	Lower incidence of flap folds or wrinkles
Lower incidence of epithelial islands or debris	
Disadvantages:	
Higher incidence of flap folds or wrinkles	Slower visual rehabilitation due to edema (24 to 72 hours)
Higher incidence of epithelial islands or debris	

1. The dry technique—A small suction tube with moderate suction or the Pallikaris LASIK suction tube is moved over the area of the bed to remove epithelial cells or debris that could be included in the interface. No irrigation of the corneal bed or the stromal surface of the flap is performed. The corneal surface is then thoroughly irrigated with BSS using an irrigation-aspiration cannula, so that debris and excessive epithelial cells are removed (Figure 12-5).
2. The wet technique—The ablated bed and the stromal surface of the flap are irrigated thoroughly (flushed) with BSS using an irrigation-aspiration cannula. A wet Merocel microsponge is used to remove excessive moisture, and this manipulation is repeated several times until cells and debris are totally removed from the surface of the globe. The Merocel movement can be aided by pressing it with an air cannula (Figure 12-6). The movement is repeated twice, once nasally and once temporally, starting from the base of the flap. The flap is then repositioned using an air cannula as described in the dry technique.

Two microsponges are used to gently manipulate the cornea so that the marks on the flap are properly aligned with the corresponding marks on the peripheral corneal ring.

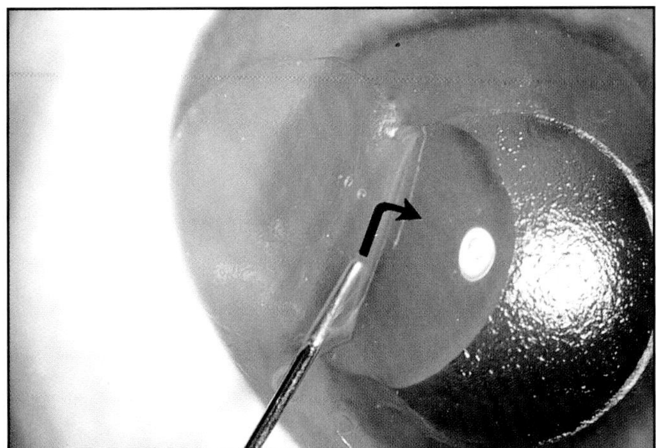

Figure 12-5.
The dry technique—One or two drops of BSS are placed on the corneal bed at the hinge of the flap. An air cannula is inserted beneath the epithelial surface of the flap. The cannula is moved slowly temporally (arrow), parallel to the corneal surface, and the fluid on the bed allows the flap to settle gently in its primary position.

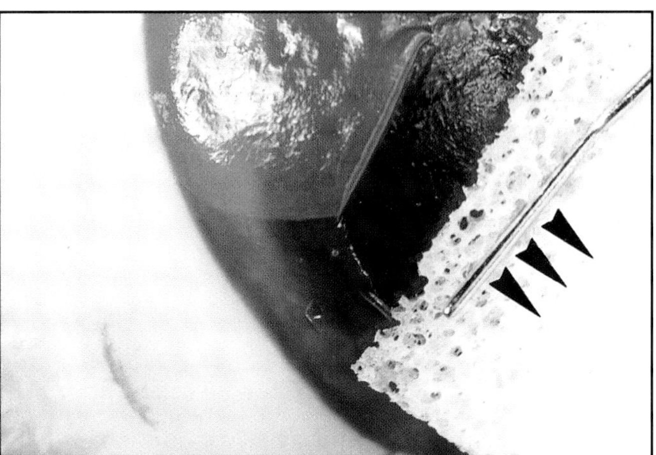

Figure 12-6.
The wet technique—A wet Merocel microsponge is used to remove excessive moisture, and this manipulation is repeated several times until cells and debris are totally removed from the surface of the globe. The Merocel movement can be aided by pressing it with an air cannula (arrows).

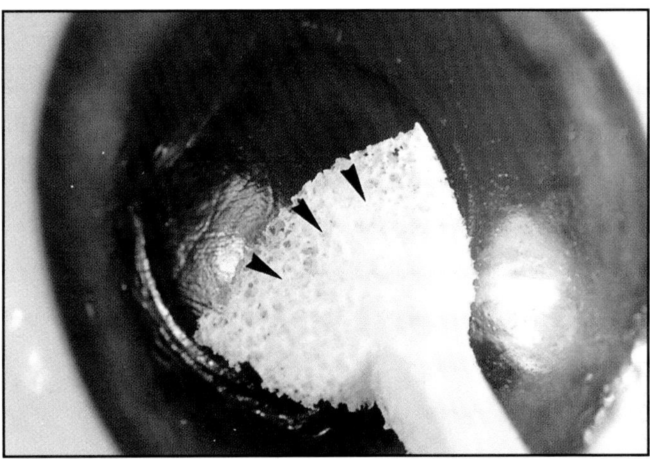

Figure 12-7.
A Merocel sponge just wet in its periphery is used to lightly press the center of the cornea for a few seconds.

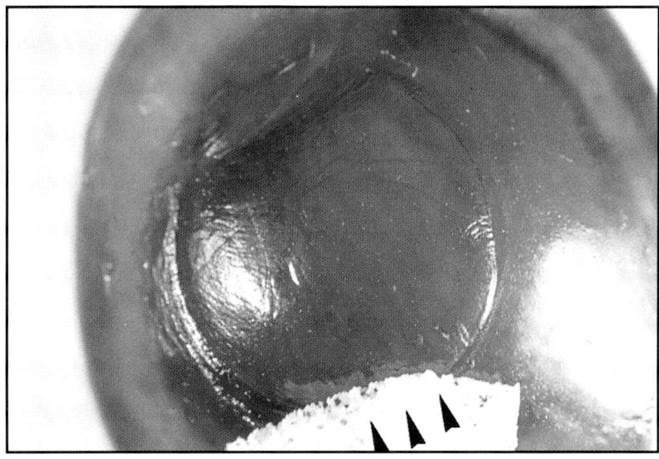

Figure 12-8.
A dry spear (arrows) is used to remove excessive moisture from the borders of the aligned flap, aiding its seal to the bed.

As soon as the flap is repositioned, the surface of the cornea is dried using air through an aquarium air pump, or, alternatively, by leaving the eye open in atmospheric air for 5 minutes. Dehydration of the corneal surface allows the flap to adhere easily on the bed. Adequate adherence of the flap is detected by depressing the peripheral cornea with the tip of a cellulose microsponge. The formation of radiating lines that extend to the flap ("striae sign") indicates that the flap is adherent to the bed.

A Merocel sponge just wet in its periphery is used to lightly press the center of the cornea for a few seconds (Figure 12-7). Following that, a light "massage" is applied to the cornea with the wet sponge in the direction of the diclofenac sodium; one drop of a combined antibiotic-steroid solution (eg, tobramycin-dexamethasone) and of cyclopentolate 1% eye drops are instilled. We usually do not apply any contact lens. However, it is the surgeon's decision whether or not to apply a bandage soft contact lens. A bandage soft contact lens is usually applied only in cases where there is an epithelial defect. Eye patching is rarely used, while sutures are reserved for the rarest cases of a total cup, when drying of the corneal surface proves insufficient to keep the disc in place (Figure 12-8).

PATIENT FOLLOW-UP

At the end of the procedure, the patient is given oral and written instructions regarding the early postoperative care and is helped to the recovery room. The most important instruction is not to rub his or her operated eye. Thirty to 60 minutes later, the surgeon reevaluates the patient under the operating microscope or at a slit lamp to ensure that the flap is properly in place.

If the flap is misaligned or by any means irregularly positioned, it should be lifted back and repositioned. Repositioning, however, increases the risk for epithelial cell accumulation at the stromal-flap interface. The patient is reexamined on the following day to ensure complete healing of the surgical trauma.

RELATED READING

Automated Corneal Shaper™. Operator's manual. Rev 1.4. Chiron Vision Corp; March 1994.

Pallikaris IG, Papatzanaki ME, Siganos DS, Tsilimbaris MK. A corneal flap technique for laser in situ keratomileusis. *Arch Ophthalmol*. 1991;109(12):1699-1702.

Pallikaris IG, Papatzanaki ME, Siganos DS, Tsilimbaris MK. Tecnica de colajo corneal para la queratomileusis in situ mediante laser. Estudios en Humanos. *Arch Ophthalmol* (Esp ed.). 1992;3(3):127-130.

Pallikaris IG, Siganos DS. Excimer laser in situ keratomileusis and photorefractive keratectomy for correction of high myopia. *Refract Corneal Surg*. 1994;10(5):498-510.

Pallikaris IG, Siganos DS. Laser in situ keratomileusis to treat myopia: early experience. *J Cataract Refract Surg*. 1997;23(1):39-49.

Chapter 13

POSTOPERATIVE MANAGEMENT

Dimitrios S. Siganos, MD, Ioannis G. Pallikaris, MD

Although laser in situ keratomileusis (LASIK) is a more complicated procedure than photorefractive keratectomy (PRK), its advantages outweigh its difficulties—both for the patient, who can see earlier, does not feel any pain, and does not have the possibility of developing a "surprise" regression, and for the surgeon, who once sure of his or her procedure, has ensured the patient of a comfortable postoperative period, during which the findings are recorded.

WHAT TO CHECK FOR?

Immediately after the LASIK operation, there is corneal edema that subsides in the next postoperative days. Immediately postoperatively, the ablation zone appears irregular and eccentric due to the unevenly distributed edema (Figure 13-1). The next postoperative day, the ablated area is more centered and most of the edema at the flap edge has subsided (Figure 13-2).

Usually the flap has adhered well and the margins are hardly seen. If the wet technique is used, the flap is sometimes edematous. In these cases, edema tends to be more at the margins and the base of the flap. The latter, owing to its "stretch" during surgery, tends to recover last. The surgeon should inspect for folds in the flap. Where the flap has been well aligned, the folds caused by edema will disappear in almost all cases. If there is a slight doubt about the alignment of the flap, then the patient should be

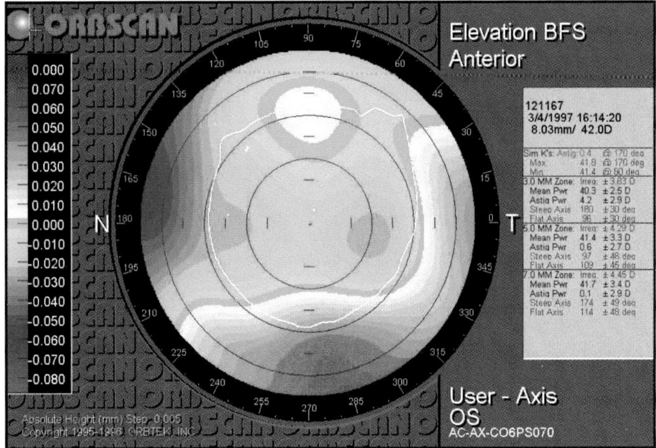

Figure 13-1.
Thirty minutes postoperatively.

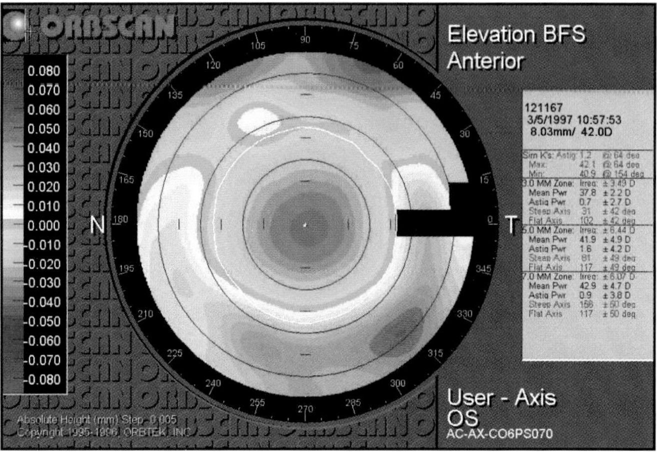

Figure 13-2.
One day postoperatively.

brought back to the laser room to have the flap everted, the interface washed, and the flap repositioned. A lot of BSS and certainly the wet technique are used. The next day, the flap is very easily lifted and the water used in the wet technique allows the flap to take its position. This will obviate the need for later, more difficult surgery caused by increased adhesiveness of the flap and will reduce the time the eye may not be seeing due to an irregular astigmatism caused by the misaligned flap.

Sometimes the flap gives a faulty impression of being misaligned or rotated. This happens when the postoperative edema is not uniformly distributed. It might be more in one part of the margin or at one end of the base. Corneal topography in this case may also show a misleading decentration as part of the ablated zone appears elevated. The way to differentiate it is by the absence of folds, in the event that the flap is properly aligned and the alignment marks that sometimes persist through the second day coincide. In such a case nothing is done. Topography is not very meaningful the first week for the reason mentioned above—not uniform corneal edema. Therefore, it is better performed at 1 week or later.

Fluorescein testing should always be done. A small epithelial defect is treated by either a bandage soft contact lens or by pressure patching of the eye. No matter how small the defect, it should be treated as a serious matter. Its presence might mean local edema of that area, hence imperfect adherence of the flap, hence an invitation for epithelial cells to also grow under the flap. A quick refraction is performed recording the unaided visual acuity and visual acuity using the pinhole.

MEDICATION

We usually prescribe combined drops of dexamethasone and antibiotic for 10 days. We used to prescribe the drops for 1 month in a tapered dose, starting four times a day and ending the fourth week once a day as we do in PRK cases.

However, steroids here would help during the first days to decrease flap edema. They have no role in preventing regression, a matter that is also controversial in PRK. However, in LASIK, the regression is in no way similar to that of PRK. If it happens, it does so not abruptly but very gradually over the postoperative course, and seems to be percentile, depending on the amount of the intended correction (ie, the more the attempted correction, the more the regression), but mostly in absolute numbers. The regression seen is in the order of 10% to 20% and the process tends to be completed by 2 years postoperatively. We have followed eyes for more than 7 years and 85% of the regression effect occurs during the first year.

We have conducted a study (unpublished data) using two different laser systems. Both stability and regression were different. We have also compared our initial results with our most recent ones and found a difference. From both studies it can be deduced that the quality and/or the pattern of ablation may play a serious role in the regression issue. Now, even in PRK, we see much less haze and/or regression compared to the first-generation lasers.

Chapter 14

ASSISTING INSTRUMENTATION

Ioannis G. Pallikaris, MD, Thekla G. Papadaki, MD

Apart from the microkeratome and the laser device, a variety of surgical instruments and ancillary equipment is needed in order to achieve a successful laser in situ keratomileusis (LASIK) procedure (Figure 14-1). Furthermore, retreatments and LASIK complications surgery would not be possible without the development of special instrumentation.

LASIK assisting instrumentation:

- A wire Barraquer lid speculum
- Markers
- Flap stabilizer
- An irrigation-aspiration cannula
- Scissors and corneal paper shields
- Needle holders
- Collibri, Pierse, and curved tying forceps
- Air cannulas
- Barraquer applanation tonometer
- Applanator lenses
- Cellulose microsponges

Instrumentation for retreatment procedures:

- Beaver knife
- Rotating brush
- The Vinciguerra recentering system

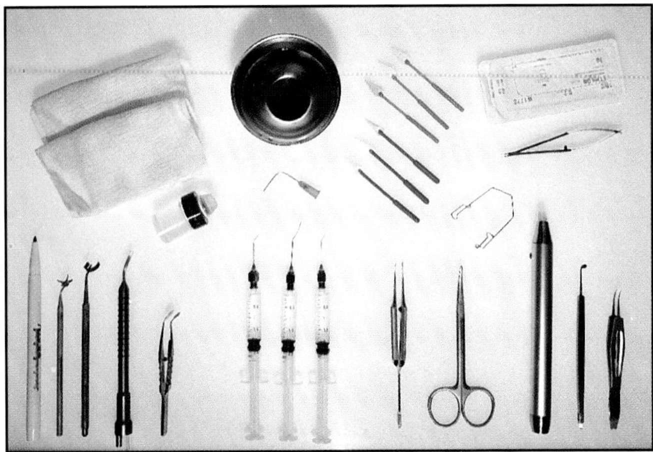

Figure 14-1.
The LASIK instrument tray.

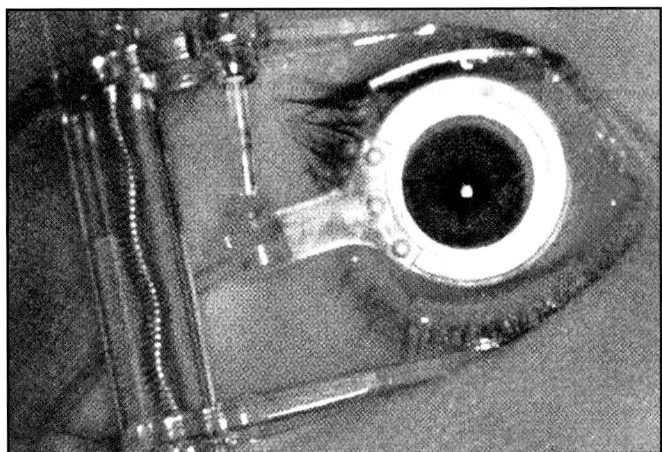

Figure 14-2
The eye fixation speculum consists of a vacuum fixation ring attached to the speculum, a 3-cc spring loaded syringe, and a self-locking speculum.

Ancillary equipment:

- Aquarium air pump
- Ultrasonic corneal pachymeter
- Air purifier with ionizer
- Computerized corneal topography

LID SPECULUM

A wire Barraquer lid speculum is preferred over a solid-blade one when performing LASIK. It provides maximum exposure of the eye and does not interfere with placement of the suction ring and route of microkeratome head when performing the cut. In very deeply set (enophthalmic) eyes, the surgeon may face difficulty in achieving sufficient suction with the speculum on. A possible solution to this problem is to omit the speculum during flap resection and to replace it prior to flap lifting.

The disposable eye fixation speculum (eyeFix Inc) is a new instrument designed for immobilizing and aligning the eye (Figure 14-2). It consists of:

- A luminescent vacuum fixation ring which is attached to the speculum. The design allows for the vacuum ring to be moved in and out of the surgical field.
- Attached 3-cc spring-loaded syringe which supplies vacuum to the ring.
- Self-locking speculum.

The eye fixation speculum can be used not only in LASIK, but also in any non-intraocular procedure requiring a securely fixed eye (Figure 14-3).

MARKERS

Marking is the first step and probably one of the most important in LASIK. It enables better centration of the suction ring and ensures proper repositioning of the hinged flap at the end of the procedure. It is also crucial in cases of total cap, because it allows for better cap alignment and prevents accidental positioning of the cap with the epithelial side down. To serve the purposes mentioned, marking in LASIK should include at least three points on the corneal surface:

- The center of the pupil.
- Two points at the periphery of the cornea positioned in such a way so that they could assist proper repositioning of a free cap.

Several markers have been proposed and new markers have been developed for use in LASIK. The marker I prefer is the Duckworth & Kent marker designed especially for LASIK (Figure 14-4). It is an arcuate marker, 10 mm in diameter, which bears two stems:

1. One 5-mm long, radially extending from the periphery to the center of the arc.
2. A 3-mm eccentric one, situated on the rim of the arc at right angles to the radial stem (Figure 14-5).

Another marker that could also be useful in LASIK is the four-blade, radial incision marker (Figure 14-6). It also bears a central ring with a crosshair that facilitates alignment with the visual axis. It is of particular use if the Phoenix Keratek Inc or the Schwind microkeratome is used, as it helps the surgeon achieve good centration by

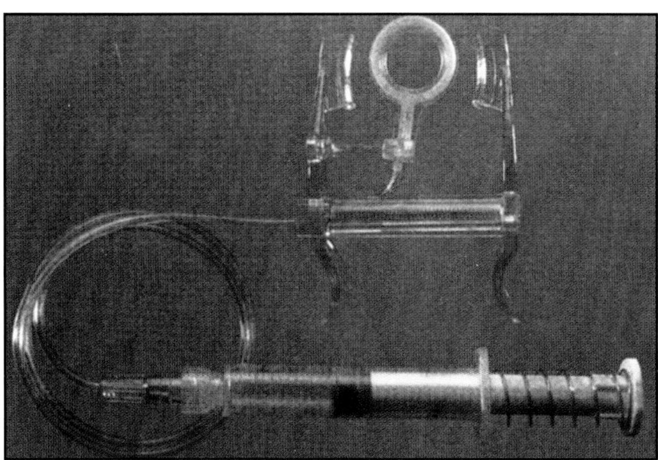

Figure 14-3.
The eye fixation speculum.

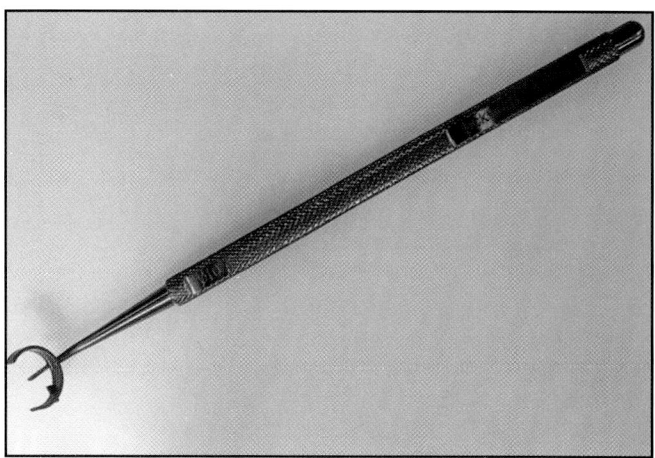

Figure 14-4.
The LASIK marker.

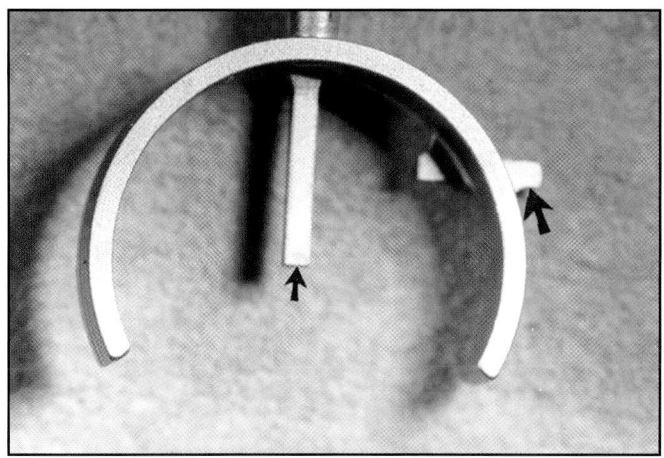

Figure 14-5.
Magnification of the front tip of the LASIK marker. It is a 10-mm arcuate marker which bears two stems: one 5-mm long stem, radially extending from the periphery to the center of the arc and a second 3-mm eccentric stem, situated on the rim of the arc at right angles to the radial stem.

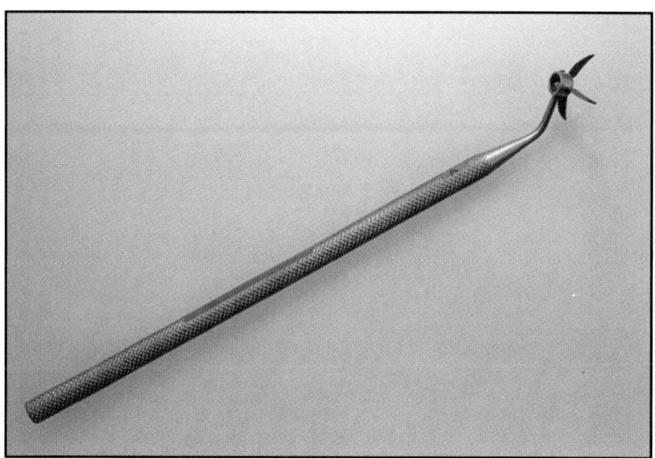

Figure 14-6.
The four blade, radial incision marker.

aligning the markings with the crosshair of the polymethylmethacrylate (PMMA) optical insert (see also Chapter 10, *Microkeratomes*).

FLAP STABILIZER

This is a special pair of forceps I designed, manufactured by Duckworth & Kent (Figure 14-7). It bears a tip curved at a 45° angle to the handle. The tip consists of a solid plate (10 mm) shaped like a hinged flap and a 6-mm ring. When the instrument is closed, the ring is smoothly apposed to the plate (Figure 14-8). Thus, the forceps is capable of securely holding the flap, while inflicting minimal or no injury to the resected corneal tissue. The flap stabilizer is used to immobilize the flap during retreatment procedures, where epithelial cell accumulation, debris, or other exogenous material has to be scraped out of the stromal side of the flap (Figure 14-9).

IRRIGATION-ASPIRATION CANNULA

It is a special cannula that I designed (Duckworth & Kent). The front tip of the cannula is slightly curved and consists of an aspiration tube with a sharp cutting rim. This tube incorporates a smaller, deeper set irrigation tube (Figure 14-10a). The latter bears a blunt rim of an inner

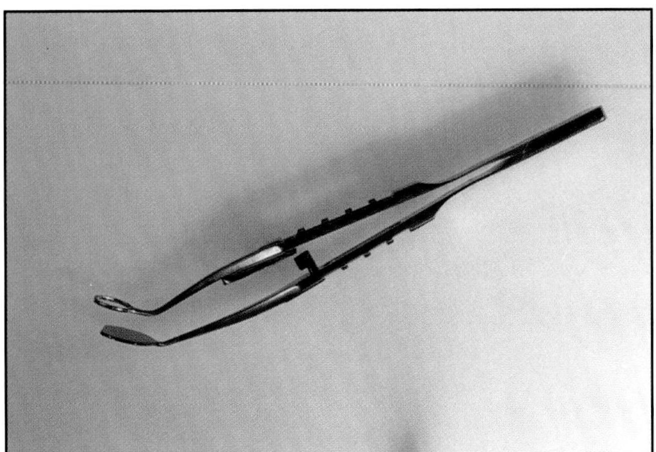

Figure 14-7.
The flap stabilizer.

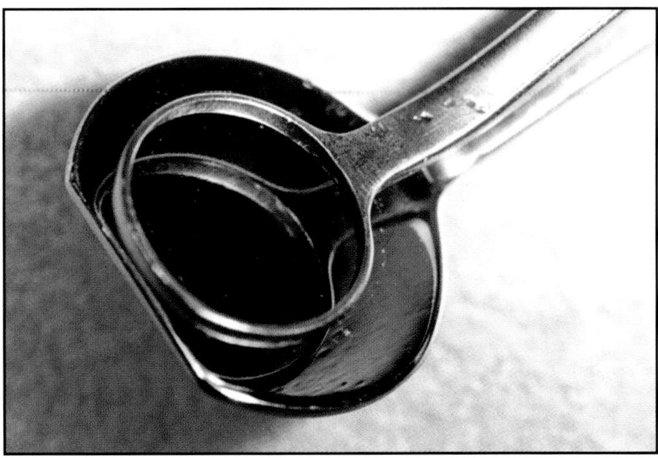

Figure 14-8.
The tip of the flap stabilizer. It consists of a solid plate, 10 mm in diameter, shaped like a hinged flap, and a 6 mm ring. When the instrument is closed the ring is smoothly apposed to the plate.

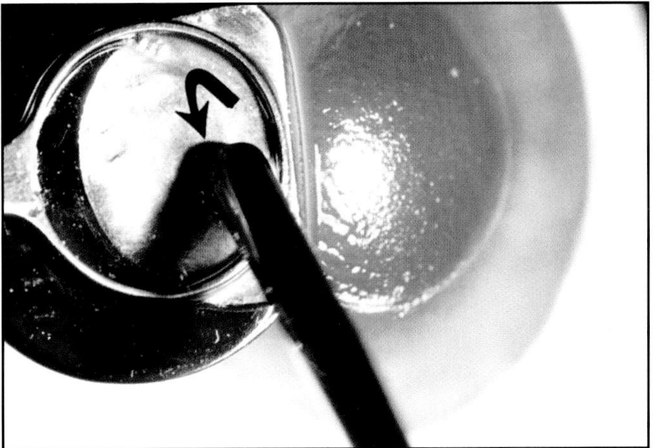

Figure 14-9.
The flap stabilizer is used to immobilize the flap when exogenous material has to be scraped out of its stromal side.

diameter that is slightly larger than the one third of the respective diameter of the irrigation tube. Thus, the irrigation rate never exceeds the aspiration rate when both tubes are used. The tip of the cannula can be used bare or covered with a silicone sheath.

The back tip bears two sites for connection with the irrigation and the aspiration unit, respectively (Figure 14-10b). The suction tubing is connected to the instrument through a port, while the tubing connecting the cannula to the BSS infusion device is flush against a tube, situated next to this port.

In LASIK, the cannula has the following applications.

1. Uncovered front tip (Figure 14-10c):
   - Scrapes and aspirates debris from the stromal bed using the wet technique (see also Chapter 12, *The Procedure*).
   - Scrapes, irrigates, and aspirates epithelial or other material deposits from the stromal side of the flap or the bed during reoperations (Figure 14-10d).
2. Silicone sheathed front tip (Figure 14-10e):
   - Aspirates debris from the conjunctival fornices during irrigation of the corneal surface.

SCISSORS AND CORNEAL PAPER SHIELDS

Scissors are used to cut a corneal paper shield or other similar material in the shape of a hinged flap. Thus, a mask is created, which is used to cover and protect the hinge and the stromal side of the flap from being accidentally ablated by the laser beam (see also Chapter 12, *The Procedure*).

Furthermore, scissors can be used to cut out material such as silicone or plastic in different shapes in order to create ablation masks. The latter can be used in the treatment of eccentric ablations ("smart masks" are under patent) (see Chapter 24, *LASIK Complications and Their Management*).

NEEDLE HOLDERS

LASIK is a sutureless technique. Nevertheless, the beginning surgeon must have a microsurgical needle hold-

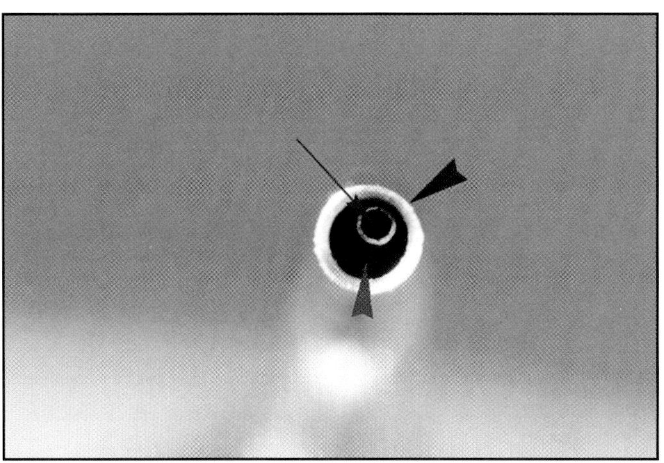

Figure 14-10a.
The front tip of the cannula is slightly curved and consists of an aspiration tube (red arrow) with a sharp cutting rim (arrowhead). This tube incorporates a smaller, deeper set aspiration tube (arrow).

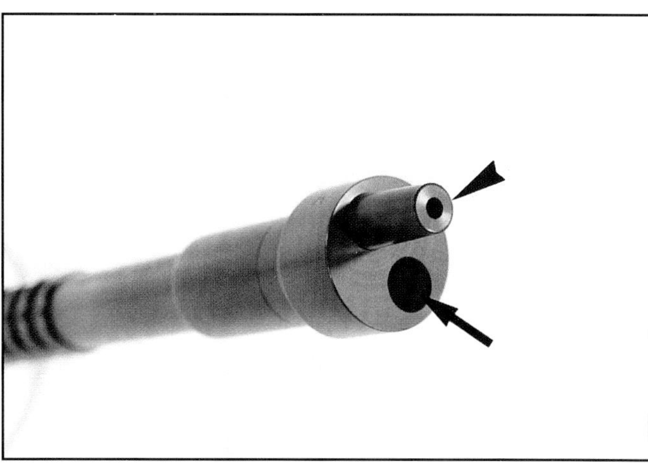

Figure 14-10b.
The back tip bears a port for connection with the suction tubing (arrow) and a tube for connection with the BSS infusion device (arrowhead).

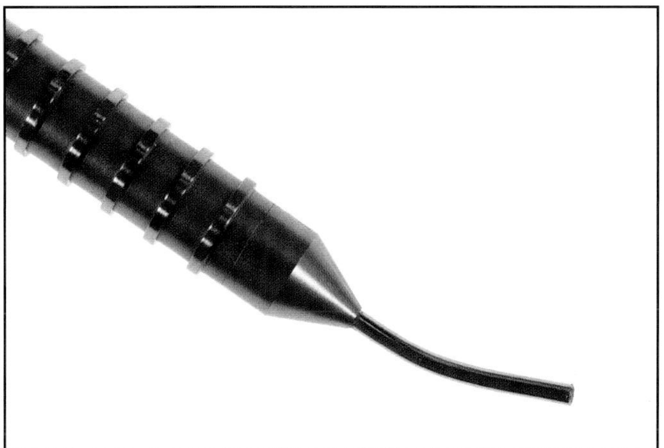

Figure 14-10c.
With the front tip uncovered.

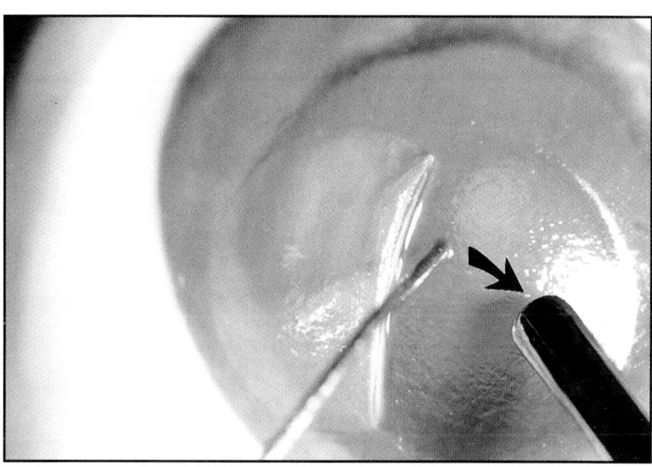

Figure 14-10d.
The irrigation-aspiration cannula scrapes, irrigates, and aspirates epithelial or other material deposits from the stromal side of the flap or the bed during reoperations.

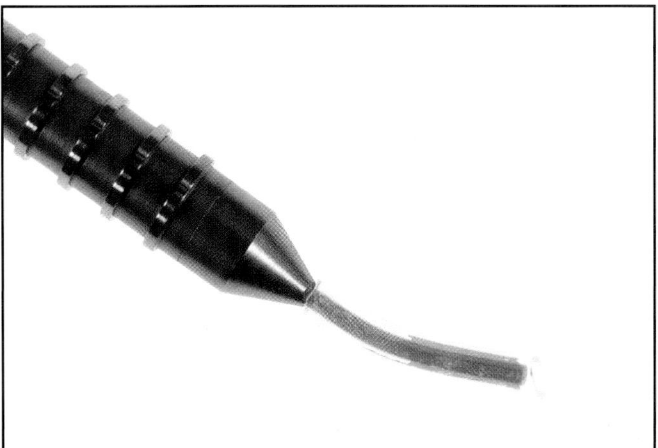

Figure 14-10e.
With the front tip covered with a silicone sheath.

er and 10/0 nylon sutures available for complicated cases, or cases ending up with a total cap where the resected corneal tissue could not sufficiently adhere by dry air.

COLLIBRI, PIERSE, AND CURVED TYING FORCEPS

Collibri, Pierse (Figure 14-11), curved tying forceps, or other comparable instrument is used for reflecting and repositioning the hinged flap as well as the corneal cap in cases of total resection.

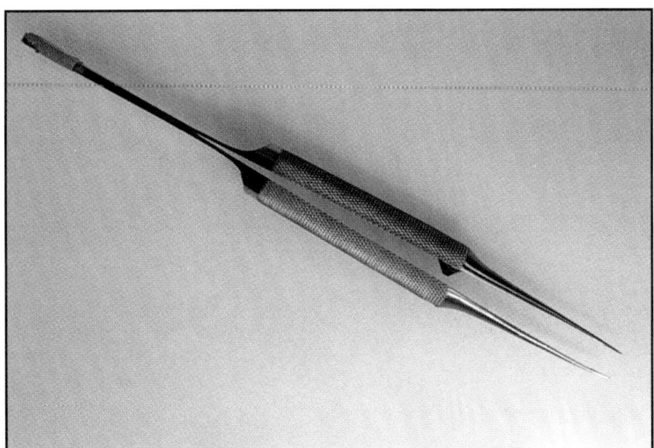

Figure 14-11.
Pierse forceps.

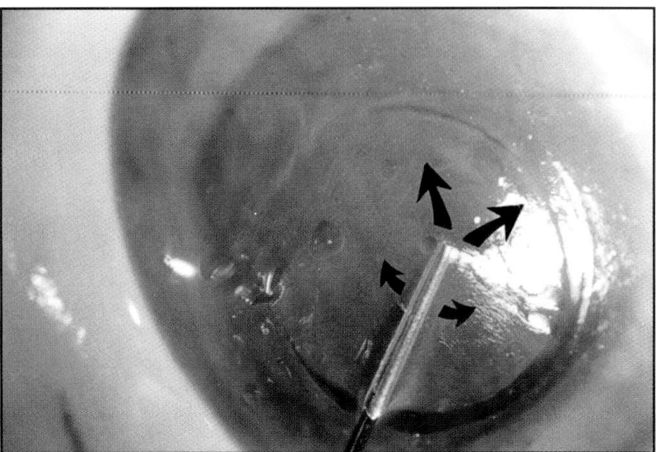

Figure 14-12.
Flap repositioning. The tip of an air cannula is inserted underneath the flap. The cannula is then moved outward, while the interface is thoroughly irrigated with BSS.

AIR CANNULAS

Air cannulas are used in:

- Reflecting and repositioning of the hinged flap (see also Chapter 12, *The Procedure*).
- Irrigating the corneal or stromal surface.
- Pressing a wet microsponge firmly against the cornea during cleansing of the stromal bed and the stromal side of the flap. The latter manipulation is repeated several times, until all visible debris has been swept out of the interface (see also Chapter 12, *The Procedure*).
- In cases where the flap is irregularly repositioned by the first attempt, proper alignment can be achieved by the following maneuver: the tip of an air cannula is inserted underneath the flap. The cannula is then moved outward, while the interface is thoroughly irrigated with BSS (Figure 14-12). In this way, any air bubbles or debris are removed from the interface, and the flap is repositioned without even being lifted.

BARRAQUER APPLANATION TONOMETER

The Barraquer applanation tonometer (Figure 14-13a) consists of a convex dome with an inscribed applanation ring on its flat, lower surface (Figure 14-13b). The diameter of the ring indicates a 65 mmHg pressure. The dome is suspended by a plastic ring vertically and perpendicularly over the center of the pupil. Given the weight of the dome, the tonometer applanates an area of varying diameter on the corneal surface, according to the IOP of the eye. The lower the IOP, the larger the diameter of the applanated area (Table 14-1).

Applanation tonometry prior to flap resection is a very critical step of the LASIK procedure. Unless IOP is confirmed to be at least 60 to 65 mmHg, the surgeon should not proceed to performing the cut. An IOP lower than 60 mmHg could result in an increased risk of complications such as thin, irregular, and even perforated flaps.

APPLANATOR LENSES

Applanator lenses measure the diameter of the exposed cornea and provide a reference for the hinge position. Therefore, they are used to estimate the diameter of the flap to be created. Each lens is made of PMMA and bears an inscribed ring and a metal handle (Figure 14-14). The ring diameter varies with different lenses and indicates the diameter of the flap to be created. Four different sizes are available: 7.75, 8.25, 8.75, and 9.25 mm. The lens of choice is fitted between the dove-tail of the suction ring with its handle at 90° from the suction handle (Figure 14-15). By comparing the size of the applanated area to that of the ring, one can judge the anticipated flap diameter.

In ordinary cases, it is at the surgeon's discretion to

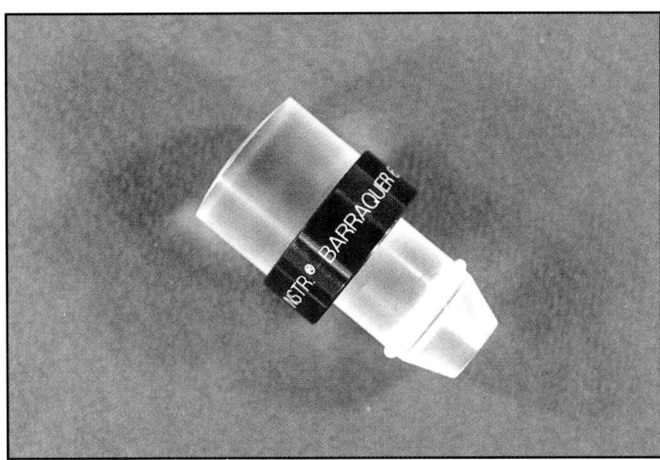

Figure 14-13a.
The Barraquer applanation tonometer consists of a convex dome with an inscribed applanation ring on its flat, lower surface.

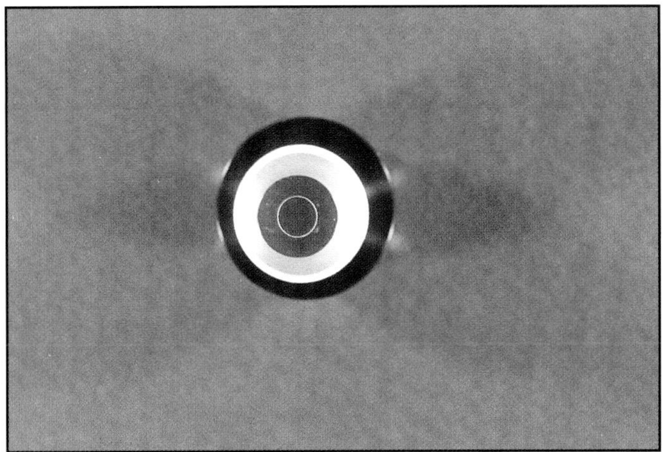

Figure 14-13b.
The Barraquer applanation tonometer. Surgeon view.

omit this step or not. Nevertheless, in cases of very small or flat corneas (<41 D), estimating the flap diameter allows for better adjustment of the position of the hinge, so that the risk of ending up with a total cap is markedly diminished.

However, modern microkeratome devices (Schwind, Phoenix Keratek Inc, Guimarães, and the Flapmaker) are designed in such a way so that they eliminate the need for applanator lenses. They incorporate transparent applanation plates and are designed to perform flaps of standardized thickness and diameter.

CELLULOSE MICROSPONGES

Merocel surgical spears are preferred over other brands because they seem to leave few or no remnants (ie, cotton threads) behind.

TABLE 14-1

Size of Applanation Area

Size of Applanated Area (Compared to the Diameter of the Inscribed Ring)	IOP	Manipulation
Equal to	65 mmHg	Borderline pressure. Sweep the cornea and repeat measurement.
Smaller than	>65 mmHg	Adequate pressure. Proceed to the cut.
Larger than	<65 mmHg	Do not cut. Reposition suction ring and wipe corneal surface. Repeat measurement.

Cellulose microsponges have many uses in LASIK:

- Soaked in proparacaine, cellulose microsponges are used to anesthetize the forniceal conjunctiva prior to the procedure. This way the patient's discomfort from the speculum-induced lid traction is minimized.
- Dry or soaked in BSS, they are used to clean the fornices from any mucous or other debris prior to the microkeratome cut.
- A dry spear is used to wipe excessive moisture from the corneal surface in order to achieve sufficient suction and obtain correct applanation tonometry readings.
- After reflecting the hinged flap aside, the tip of a dry spear is inserted under the hinge to absorb excessive moisture prior to ablation (see also Chapter 12, *The Procedure*).
- A spear soaked in BSS is used to keep the flap moist after ablation. The flap is thus more easily handled and the epithelium is protected from scraping.
- In the wet technique, a spear is used to wipe the stromal bed (see also Chapter 12, *The Procedure*).
- Following flap repositioning, a spear soaked in BSS just at its tip is used to "iron" the flap on the

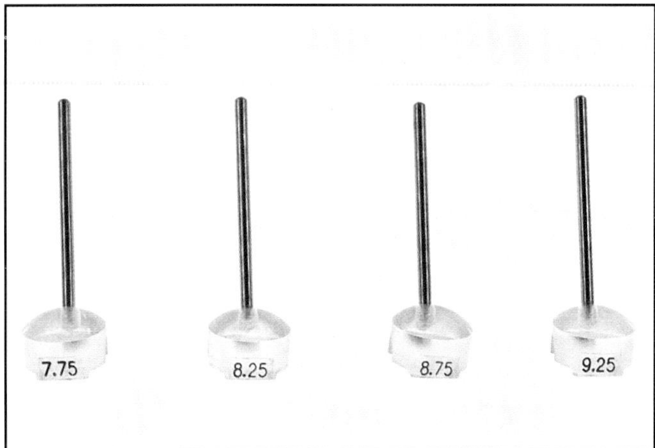

Figure 14-14.
Applanator lenses are used to estimate the diameter of the flap to be created. Each lens bears an inscribed ring and a metal handle. The diameter of the ring varies between different lenses and indicates the diameter of the flap to be created. Four different sizes are available: 7.75, 8.25, 8.75, and 9.25 mm.

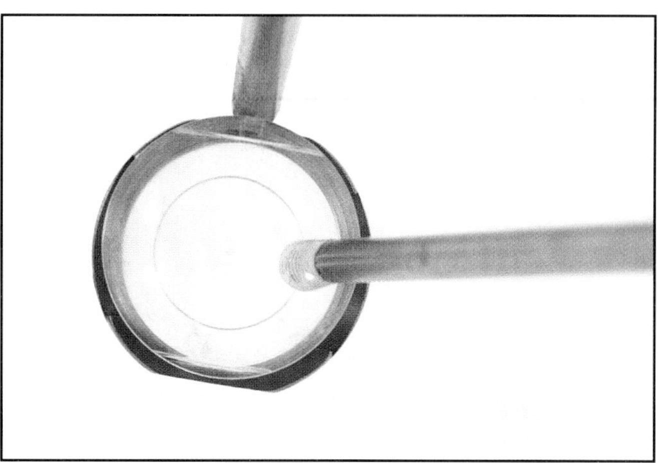

Figure 14-15.
The applanator lens of choice is fitted between the dove-tail of the suction ring with its handle at 90° from the suction handle. By comparing the size of the applanated area to that of the ring, one can judge the anticipated diameter of the flap.

bed. "Ironing" consists of wiping the flap in a nasal to temporal direction several times (hinge-away hinge direction) until the flap is properly aligned and no striae are visible under the operating microscope (see also Chapter 12, *The Procedure*).

- Spears cut out in different shapes can be used to protect the hinge and the stromal side of the flap from accidental ablation during the smoothing procedure. They can also serve as ablation masks during retreatment procedures ("smart masks" are under patent) (see Chapter 24, *LASIK Complications and Their Management*).
- Finally, a dry spear is used to remove excessive moisture from the borders of the aligned flap, thus adhering it to the bed.

BEAVER KNIFE

A Beaver #64 or a Hockey knife (Figure 14-16) is very useful in LASIK reoperations in two different surgical steps:

1. Detaching the flap from the stromal bed. Epithelium from a small area at the flap border is scraped away. At this site, the blade enters the interface and gradually dissects the flap from the stromal bed. The flap is then lifted with Pierse forceps or a comparable instrument.
2. Scraping out epithelial cells or other remnants that cause irregular astigmatism, or interfere with the visual axis from the interface.

THE ROTATING BRUSH

The rotating brush (Pal-Brush) (Figure 14-17) is very effective in the fast removal of the corneal epithelium prior to PRK. It is battery-powered and consists of a pen-like handle and disposable (brush material) brushes of 7 to 9 mm in diameter. The tip of the brush is placed on the cornea and is held perpendicular to the corneal surface. By pressing the motor button with the index finger, the brush rotates. In LASIK, the rotating brush is used in retreatment procedures, where cleansing of the stromal bed from epithelial ingrowth is required. The brush should be used with caution in cases of PRK over LASIK, even after the first postoperative year. There is always the risk that the flap will detach and twist by the rotating brush during deepithelialization.

THE VINCIGUERRA RECENTERING SYSTEM

Development of this system, used in treating decentered ablation zones, was based on the idea that recen-

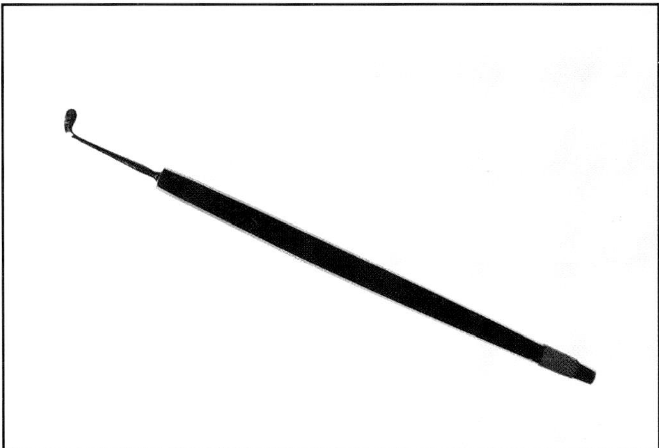

Figure 14-16.
Hockey knife.

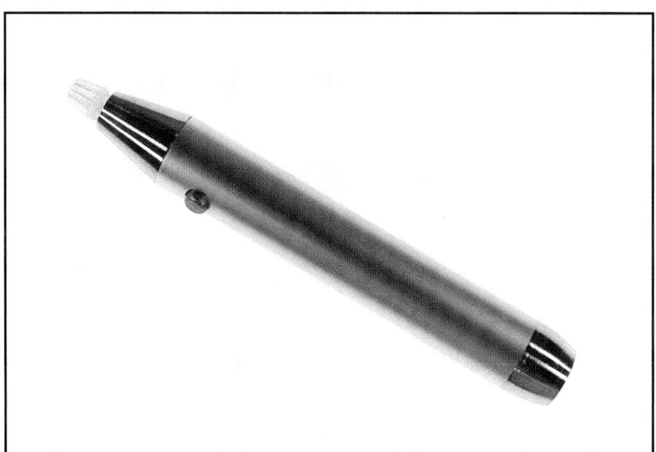

Figure 14-17.
Rotating brush.

tering of a decentered ablation zone requires ablation of a new larger and deeper zone that incorporates the decentered area. Attempted correction of reablation should be equal to that given during the initial procedure.

The Vinciguerra recentering system consists of (Figure 14-18):

- A suction mask bearing block positions situated at 45°, 90°, 135°, 180°, 225°, and 270°.
- A centering cross hair.
- Seven diaphragms.

The procedure is completed in three steps:

1. The mask is centered on the visual axis using the cross hair. The arm of the cross hair is aligned with the decentration axis (the imaginary line between the visual axis and the center of the decentered zone, which is estimated by corneal topography). The cross hair is then removed and the first diaphragm inserted in the same block position. The diaphragm is thus mathematically centered.
2. Subsequent ablations are performed with each of the seven diaphragms.
3. PTK is performed under intraoperative topographic monitoring to provide smoothness of the newly ablated area.

A special algorithm is used to calculate the number of microns to be ablated in each of the seven steps, so that the procedure will not change the intended refraction of the initial procedure. Detailed analysis of the algorithm is beyond the purpose of this chapter, and can be found elsewhere.

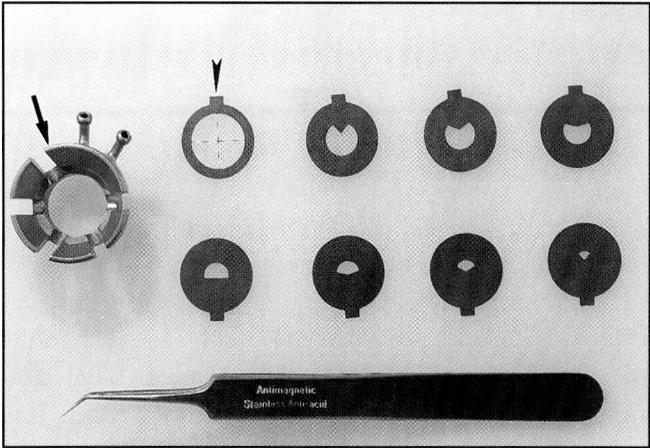

Figure 14-18.
The Vinciguerra recentering system. It consists of a suction mask that bears block positions situated at 45°, 90°, 135°, 180°, 225°, and 270° (arrow); a centering crosshair (arrowhead); and seven diaphragms.

AQUARIUM AIR PUMP

The aquarium air pump is a device that provides compressed air at an adjustable rate (low-medium-high). A rate of 1 to 2 L/minute (medium) is used at the end of the procedure to enhance flap adhesion. Air is directed to the corneal surface through a bent 21-gauge needle (Figure 14-19). The flap ranging dries prior to the central area.

Dehydration of the corneal surface allows the flap to adhere easily to the bed.

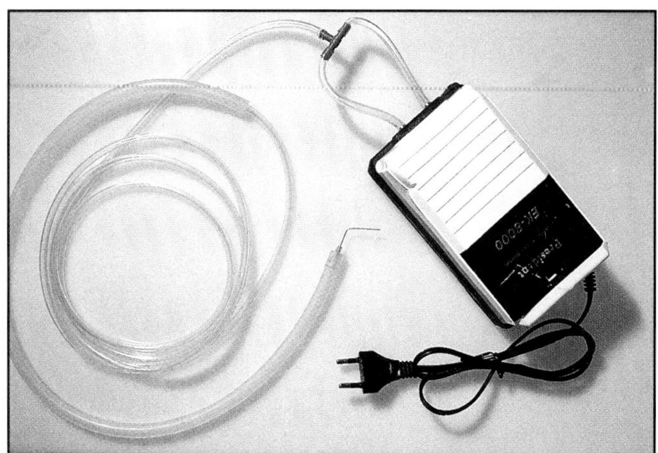

Figure 14-19.
The aquarium air pump.

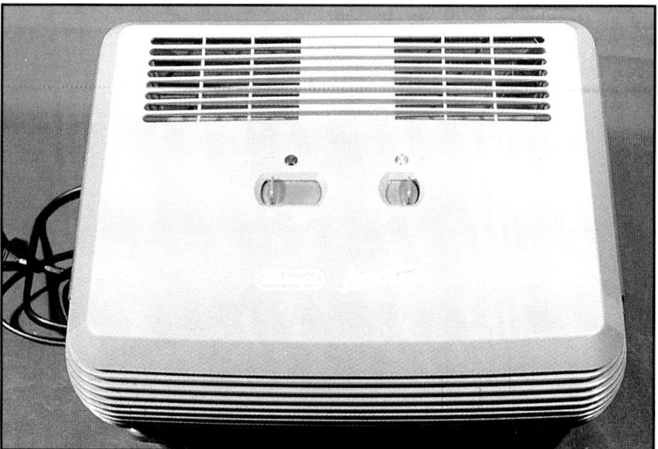

Figure 14-20.
The air purifier with ionizer.

ULTRASONIC CORNEAL PACHYMETER

The pachymeter we currently use is the Corneo-Gage Plus 2. The device is battery-powered and uses a probe with a 50 MHz transducer. It features multiple examination modes and therefore permits the user to select from RK, ALK, and laser keratectomy. The last is also used in LASIK. By properly placing the probe vertically to the patient's cornea, highly accurate, averaged (1000) measurements are obtained. Measurements are continuously taken and stored by the device in memory (ability to store data from 99 locations). Stored measurements can be reviewed and printed.

In LASIK, ultrasonic pachymetry is performed pre- and intraoperatively. Preoperative pachymetry allows for better surgical planning (ie, intended flap thickness and ablation depth). At this point, it is very important to note that a total corneal pachymetry of less than 450 μm is considered a borderline for LASIK, especially if a myopic correction of more than 8 D is intended. Intraoperative pachymetry of the stromal bed is of extreme importance, especially in high myopic corrections, as it enables adjustment of the ablation depth so that no corneal perforation or ectasia occurs. In general, the surgeon must have in mind that the postoperative total central corneal thickness should not be less than 340 μm. Provided that corneal pachymetry was obtained preoperatively, stromal bed pachymetry allows for precise calculation of flap thickness (by subtraction). The latter should especially be considered in case of retreatment procedures when the flap is already thinner. In general, when planning a reoperation, one must bear in mind that if the thickness of the primary flap is less than 100 μm, it is better not to attempt to detach it but to perform a second cut.

AIR PURIFIER WITH IONIZER

The air purifier (Figure 14-20) filters domestic air. This procedure is completed in three steps:

1. A fan motor draws the dirty air through the main grill to a prefilter. At this step the larger airborne particles (ie, lint, dust, and pollen) are removed.
2. The partially filtered air is then drawn through a HEPA (high efficiency particulate air) filter. This filter removes particles as small as 0.1 μm, even bacteria.
3. The air then passes through an activated carbon filter which removes odors. Purified air is returned to the room through the top-mounted grill.

The device also features an independently controlled ionizer. The latter, when switched on, releases a cloud of negative ions into the outgoing filtered air. These enhance further air filtration and help create a better balance of ions in the room and therefore reduce static electricity created by televisions and computer screens.

In LASIK, the air purifier is used to create an environment free of particles in the surgery room. It may also aid in keeping the excimer laser optics free of dust.

Chapter 15

HOW TO SHORTEN THE LEARNING CURVE

Alice Handzel, MD

INTRODUCTION

Dr. Jose Barraquer—the name is synonymous with the development of the innovative idea of keratomileusis.[1,2] The name laser in situ keratomileusis (LASIK) was conceived by Dr. Ioannis Pallikaris,[3,4] who was the first to perform this procedure on human eyes in 1989. Dr. Carmen Barraquer, who has performed a great number of LASIK surgeries, achieved perfection in it. These experienced LASIK pioneers paved the way for this excellent surgical procedure. As LASIK becomes more popular, numerous surgeons are either performing it already or planning to learn it and offer it to their patients. LASIK is considered a difficult procedure requiring meticulous training and high surgical skill. The notion of the learning curve is frequently used in association with LASIK, meaning that the LASIK novice is faced with a procedure that is completely different from what a "conventional" eye surgeon is used to and that the number of complications is high in the beginning.

How can we define a LASIK learning curve in the medical jargon? Usually it means the time after which the surgeon feels comfortable with a procedure (subjective), the complication rate decreases (objective), and the remaining complications are not dependent on the skill of the surgeon any longer. Gimbel[5] defines an "early learning process" which is quite adequate. The learning process is neverending. We should be open to feedback and strive for perfection.

In my opinion, LASIK is the best refractive procedure performed on the cornea we have as yet.

It is fascinating that in this refractive treatment we may respect the Bowman's layer, the importance of which we have always been taught. All the well-known benefits of the healing process in LASIK confirm the stabilizing effect of this tissue and we are satisfied to preserve it. The potential to reduce the complication rate is ascribed to saving Bowman's layer as well. The peripheral fine scar does not disturb our patients because it is of no functional significance.

After having seen the LASIK surgery, I was very enthusiastic about it, but felt uneasy about having to use the microkeratome. When learning to handle the microkeratome on pig eyes, it was a strange feeling just to hold on to a machine moving over the cornea and cutting it. As there is no direct contact to the tissue being cut, I had an impression of not being able to influence the performance of the machine. The uniqueness of working with the microkeratome stems from the fact that, once started, it is either a success or a failure and that there is very little a surgeon can do when the microkeratome blade is being advanced over the cornea. It was apparent that the success of the procedure greatly depended on a large number of details which all had to be correct before the cut of the cornea was initiated.

Wishing to minimize the stress of the learning curve, I tried to prepare myself as much as possible. For this reason I visited a number of surgeons performing this procedure before I started, and I participated in different training courses held by Drs. Slade, Casebeer, and Knorz.

Still impressed, I wanted to watch the "real" patients in a routine environment pre-, intra-, and postoperatively to see whether the healing and the recovery of vision were indeed as rapid as the surgeons claimed.

First I attended an automated lamellar keratoplasty (ALK) performed by Dr. Wiegand (Germany) in order to see the handling of the microkeratome. After that I visited Dr. Fouad Tayfour (Canada), met with Dr. Carmen Barraquer (Colombia), and visited Drs. Ioannis Pallikaris (Greece) and Klaus Ditzen (Germany). I also discussed the procedure with Dr. Carmen Barraquer as I met with her a second time after her video presentation.

In this chapter I will present the techniques of some very experienced LASIK surgeons, their improvements of the method, as well as modifications that I did to the procedure during and in an advanced stage of my learning curve; alterations which, according to my experiences, rendered the LASIK treatment easier and more comfortable during the first procedures and later on will be mentioned.

Every surgeon needs to work out his or her own technique, so I do not claim to show what is "good" or the "ultimate and only way," but just to present some different variations of LASIK surgery, so each surgeon can choose his or her own optimized technique. I hope this will help the beginners to shorten the early learning curve and to avoid the complications.

PREOPERATIVE TRAINING

Obviously, the individual learning curve depends on the individual experience. However, with respect to the LASIK learning curve, we can classify surgeons into three groups:

1. Surgeons who never performed ALK or photorefractive keratectomy (PRK) have to learn how to handle the microkeratome and the laser.
2. Ophthalmologists who have experience in PRK need to learn how to handle the microkeratome. This group will also have to accept that laser ablation in LASIK requires nomograms that are different from those they know from their PRK treatments. Both above mentioned groups have to learn the flap manipulation.
3. Surgeons who have already been performing ALK are in a better position, since they will have to learn the laser part only, which is easier than the microkeratome and flap handling.

It is very important to see live procedures done by experienced surgeons. There are not only the operations, but the different nomograms, manipulations, pre- and postoperative treatment, different instruments, cleaning and care of them, and experience, experience, experience!

I sought advice from three immensely experienced surgeons: Drs. Carmen Barraquer, Ioannis Pallikaris, and Fouad Tayfour.

The first live LASIK procedure I observed was performed in the Windsor Laser Eye Institute by Dr. Fouad Tayfour. He used the Summit excimer laser, Dr. Barraquer used the VisX 20/20, and Dr. Pallikaris used the Aesculap-Meditec. All the surgeons I met used the Chiron Automated Corneal Shaper.

It is very important to see surgeries done with differ-

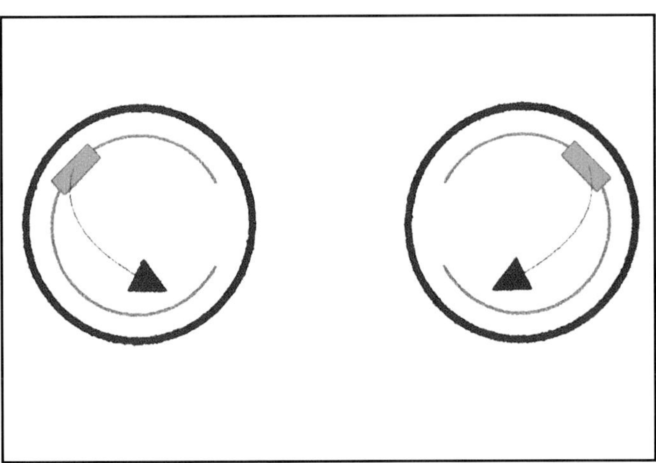

Figure 15-1.
Technique for lifting the flap using a forceps.

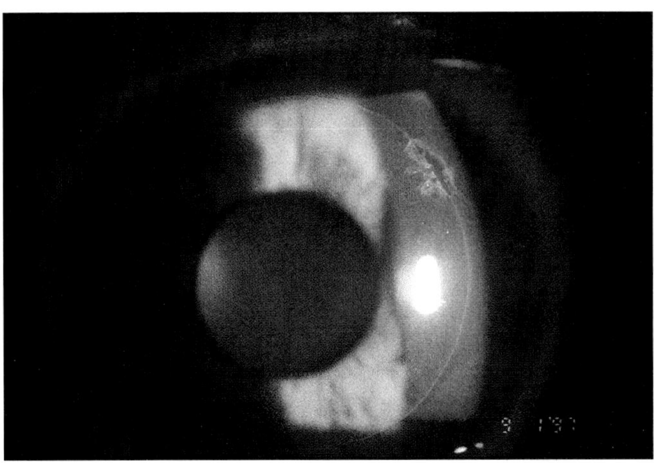

Figure 15-2.
Slit lamp photomicroscopy 2 hours after flap lifting and retreatment.

ent lasers under routine operating conditions. It helps to choose a laser one feels most comfortable with.

At that time, it was not possible to treat astigmatism with the Summit laser, and I believed that manipulations with the masks of the Aesculap-Meditec laser caused an additional danger of flap complications. Thus, I opted for the VisX 20/20 laser.

I met with Dr. Barraquer to obtain instructions about treatment, nomograms, and precautions specific for this laser and the Chiron microkeratome.

After having started my first operations, I saw her again to watch the procedure performed by her and to discuss details of and improvements in the operation technique. It was very important for me to meet her twice because we used the same laser and because the short-term feedback helped me perfect the procedure.

I took the opportunity to visit Dr. Pallikaris and see more LASIK procedures performed by him. We discussed incidence and management of complications and retreatments. These aspects were also discussed with Drs. Barraquer and Tayfour.

I saw Dr. Tayfour again to learn his technique of lifting the flap for removing pieces of epithelium and/or particles and retreatment of undercorrected eyes. He showed me his very elegant and safe method for reopening the flap.

The first step is done under the slit-lamp microscope after administering topical anesthesia and inserting an eye speculum. A Hockey knife is used to scratch a small epithelium area over a short section of the microkeratome cut from the original procedure at 1:00 or 11:00 (Figure 15-1), depending on the eye being retreated. Subsequently, the edge of the flap is slightly lifted with a Castroviejo forceps, only along a section of approximately 3-mm length and 2-mm width (Figures 15-2 through 15-4). The patient is then immediately placed under the laser microscope, without removing the speculum. The flap is opened by using the forceps to pull it continuously and very gently toward the hinge. This procedure seems to be safer than using a blunt spatula. No epithelium nor debris is introduced into the stromal interface. With this procedure I was able to reopen the flap for retreatment up to 9 months after the original surgery.

Before the first surgery on sighted eyes, the procedure was performed on approximately 300 pig eyes. In this phase, the creation of flap was intensively studied. An authorized technician from Chiron taught the operating room staff how to disassemble and assemble the microkeratome as well as how to clean and maintain it. The personnel and surgeon were instructed on which precautions needed to be taken. The checklist was created and discussed. Then the performing of flaps with and without a subsequent laser ablation were intensively rehearsed. The cooperation of the surgeon and staff was exercised. The entire procedure was repeatedly simulated.

This is a very important part of shortening the learning curve. It is strongly recommended that all surgeons starting LASIK do it until it becomes a boring, routine procedure. Apart from the straightforward, simple procedures, free caps should be deliberately created and repositioned. It is of utmost importance to learn and master

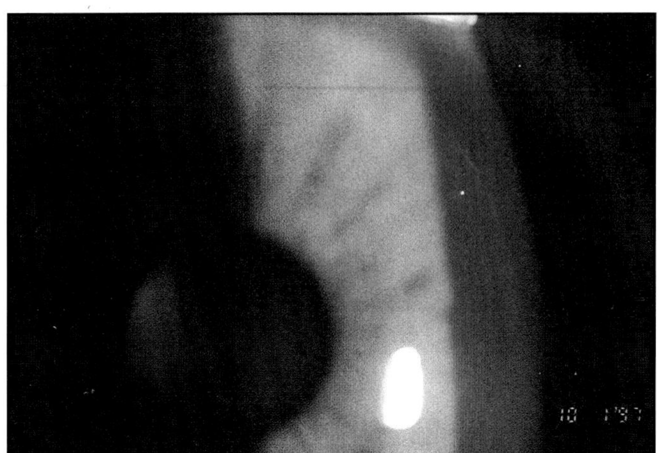

Figure 15-3.
Slit lamp photomicroscopy 1 day after flap lifting and retreatment.

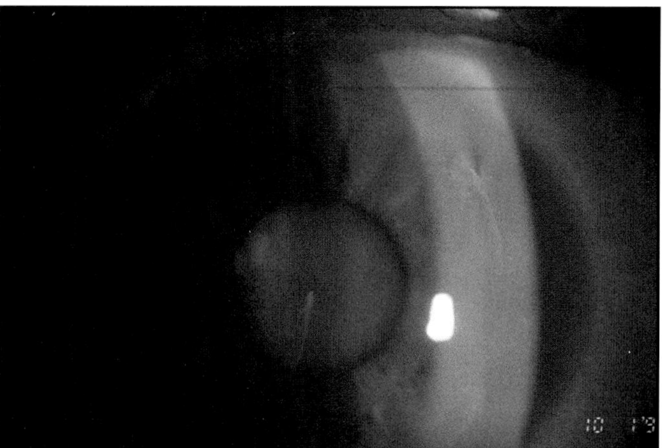

Figure 15-4.
Slit lamp photomicroscopy 1 day after flap lifting and retreatment.

the careful way of removing the cap from the microkeratome. Furthermore, it is essential to be able from the beginning to manage the complications and to do retreatment.

I was fortunate to have the support of Dr. Tayfour, who came to assist me on my first operating day. Later, I discussed with Drs. Tayfour and Barraquer the follow-up of all cases during my initial operations.

As Dr. J. Charles Casebeer pointed out,[6] every surgeon planning to use a microkeratome should participate in basic training courses followed by a mini-fellowship given by experienced surgeons. It is essential that an experienced surgeon supervises and supports the novice during at least the first operating day. Improperly handled, a microkeratome can severely damage an eye. Apart from this we should contribute as much as possible to maintaining high quality standards for this procedure. Therefore, only properly trained and skilled surgeons should be permitted to perform this procedure on sighted human eyes.

THE DETAILS

I would like to describe the LASIK procedure step by step, as well as other surgeons' and my own experience.

The Laser

The choice of the laser is not an easy task. There is very little objective information and new machines are entering the market at a very fast rate. Most large spot lasers do not seem to be capable of generating free programmable customized ablation patterns which could treat irregularities of the cornea in an easy and effective manner. Consequently, they are more likely to become outdated than the free scanning beam devices. On the other hand, the only excimer lasers that are currently approved by the FDA are large spot machines. The laser choice may thus be influenced not only by technological or economic factors, but also by the state regulations. I have been working with a large spot excimer laser and the results in treatment of myopia or myopic astigmatism are very good.

An important criterion for choosing the laser, especially for the LASIK procedure, is the total ablation depth for reasonable optical zone diameters. Most lasers offer a transition zone between the optical zone and not ablated part of the cornea, which is claimed to reduce halo effects and regression. Transition zones are more important for PRK than for LASIK. In LASIK, regression is not a significant factor.

For LASIK, the transition zone should be optional and its size should be arbitrarily programmable so that the total ablation diameter will not exceed the flap size. It is advantageous if the presence of a transition zone does not cause an increase in the total ablation depth, which should only depend on the size of the optical zone and on the amount of correction. This is a very important property for lasers to be used for LASIK.

Since this procedure is also used to treat high refractive errors, the ablation depth is a major concern. Therefore, it is very important to be able to combine different ablation diameters by directly applying or by simulating a multizone ablation in a single pass or in a multipass procedure. This allows the surgeon to achieve a sufficient optical zone diameter within a safe ablation depth limit. A minimum optical zone of 5-mm diameter is desirable, but sometimes when treating very high myopia a smaller zone (eg, 4.5 mm) has to be chosen. Knorz[7] suggests that the maximum ablation should not be deeper than 160 to 180 µm. I also do not exceed 160 µm of total ablation depth for high myopic errors. Especially in young patients, the possibility of retreatment should not be precluded; a margin for treatment that may become necessary in the future should be left to them. On the other hand, patients feel more comfortable with bigger optical zones, so that there is a trade-off between the ablation zone diameter and ablation depth when very high myopia is treated.

The lasers differ also in the support for the correct alignment of the ablation center. Some of them are equipped with different eyetracking devices.

It is obvious that the surgeon has to feel comfortable with the laser in order to obtain good results, but the predictability of the results is the crucial criterion.

Most LASIK surgeons apply their own modifications to the nomograms provided by laser manufacturers. These nomograms are based on their experience and analysis of the results. Therefore, a person starting on LASIK surgery should seek consultation from a colleague who is using the same laser, especially when high refractive errors are to be treated. Even then, one should adopt the advice with caution, as it is not certain that his or her nomograms will deliver the same result under different environments and combined with a possibly different surgical technique and different timing of the operation. Air humidity is also a factor that can influence the laser ablation. Although it is preferable to achieve the intended correction within a single treatment, the primary goal is not to overcorrect the patient. Undercorrection can be dealt with very easily, so it is not a real complication, but myopes, especially and not surprisingly presbyopic ones, are very sensitive against overcorrection.

Dr. Fouad Tayfour (personal communication) suggests that in cases of myopia of more than -10 D, the nomograms provided by the manufacturers should be adjusted. The part exceeding 10 D should be undercorrected by up to 60% on the corneal level depending on the laser in use. Example: a patient with a refraction of -16.0 D should receive a treatment of -10.0 D + (-6.0 D / 3) = -12.0 D on the corneal level. Dr. Carmen Barraquer applies a different adjustment formula (with a special factor) since she uses a different laser.

With the feedback from an increasing number of treatments, the surgeon can develop his or her own modifications to the nomograms and become less dependent on consultation with colleagues.

Preparation for the Operation—Cover the Eye?

There are various ways of preparing the eye for surgery. After disinfecting the eyelids, some surgeons use fenestrated adhesive plastic drape to keep the eyelashes folded back over the lids. Other surgeons advocate cutting of the eyelashes. Some do not like the drape because they fear that it can get into the way of the microkeratome, which would lead to flap complications. Many feel comfortable without the adhesive drape. If there are eyelashes that could interfere with the passage of the microkeratome, ask the assistant to fold them back with a Merocel surgical spear. Each way has its pros and cons. It is very important and common to all of them that the surgeon has to learn to assess if anything could interfere with the passage of the microkeratome and how to remove any potential obstacles.

As mentioned before, each surgeon has to find a method that he or she considers safe and comfortable.

The Eye Speculum

A variety of specula are used to separate the eyelids. Here again the decision is based on what is comfortable, or least uncomfortable, for the surgeon and the patient. The bigger specula may fold back the eyelids or eyelashes better, but they are more likely to get in the way of the microkeratome and some of the solid ones may even render impossible the placement of the suction ring. Specula that have parts that go deep into the conjunctiva cause patient discomfort and pain which lead to patient uneasiness during the surgery. I like the spring-loaded wire speculum Barraquer style which I use for my normal cases. It takes the least space. In difficult cases or when a patient tends to squeeze the lids I use a speculum (Geuder) with lockable wire bows which have an adjustable height and distance between the eyelids (Figure 15-5).

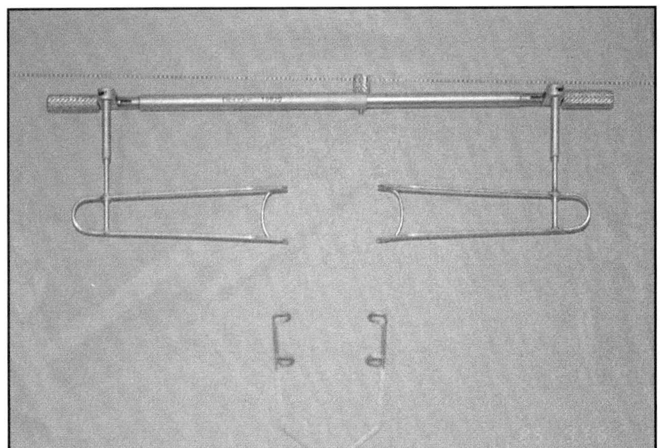

Figure 15-5.
Geuder eye speculum with lockable wire bows and Barraquer speculum.

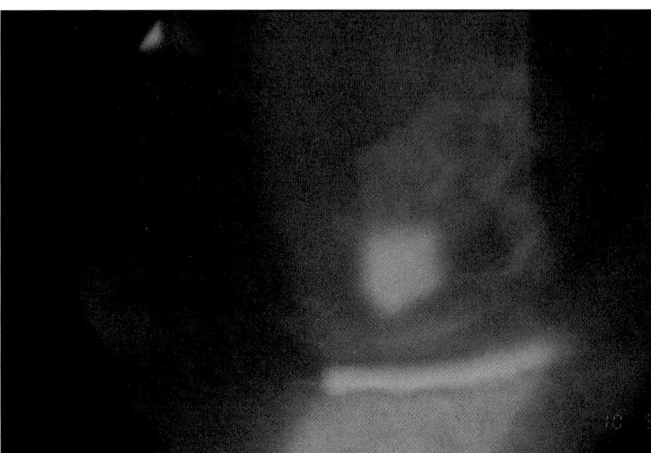

Figure 15-6.
Slit lamp photomicroscopy of a postoperative corneal erosion.

Anesthesia

Topical anesthesia is commonly used for LASIK. I apply anesthetic drops twice, approximately 1 minute apart, immediately before surgery. Excessive topical anesthesia can make the cornea prone to an erosion induced by the microkeratome cut. After 1 year of successfully administering the topical anesthesia twice, we started applying it three or more times in sensitive patients. We had two cases of corneal erosion (Figure 15-6), which healed without complications but eliminated the postoperative painlessness of LASIK. We returned to administering the topical anesthesia twice.

Marker

The marker has two purposes. It provides the reference for the placement of the suction ring and for the flap alignment after its reposition. Furthermore, it should allow an easy alignment, if a free cap is created instead of a hinged flap. Therefore, its marks should allow an alignment of a cap only in its original position with the epithelial side up. This is the reason why many markers (eg, RK markers) are not well-suited for LASIK. It is very helpful to have a marker allowing an easy and comfortable centration. Some ophthalmologists create their own markers. Drs. Chayet and Mendez were not satisfied with the markers that came with the laser and created their own marker supporting the reposition of a free cap. Many markers have the centration cross halfway down the depth of the marker ring. Even under the microscope it is difficult to see the cross for the centration. It disturbed me from the beginning, so I found another marker (Domilens, Figures 15-7 and 15-8) with the cross on the upper side, which is visible and thus helps in the centration process.

The Use of the Microkeratome

The flap resection and manipulation are the primary sources of complications specifically ascribed to LASIK. Therefore, it is self-evident that great care must be given to handling of the microkeratome. It should be thoroughly inspected before every use. The surgeon should check that the thickness plate is properly placed and that the stopper is firmly fixed in the intended position. Then the microkeratome should be placed on the dove-tail of the suction ring, advanced to the stop, and moved back by pressing appropriately the footswitch. The surgeon has to ascertain that the microkeratome moves smoothly over its entire track.

Most surgeons use the 160-μm plate, but the 130-μm plate is also used by some. Complications induced by insufficient flap thickness are more frequent with the 130-μm plate. A flap created with the 160-μm plate is more stable. Chiron supplies an adjustable suction ring, which allows a variation of the resection diameter, and a non-adjustable one with a fixed resection diameter of approximately 8.5 mm. With the adjustable ring, a flap of less than 8.5-mm diameter is obtained because there is an additional ring creating a distance between the suction ring and the patient's cornea. The adjustable ring is advantageous for lamellar keratoplasty and it is neces-

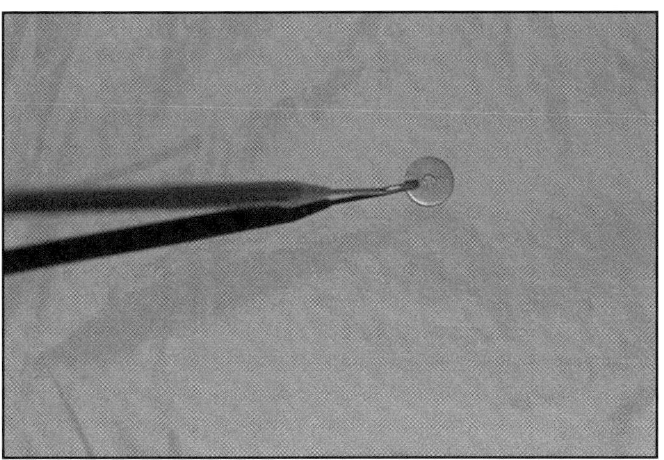

Figure 15-7.
Domilens marker.

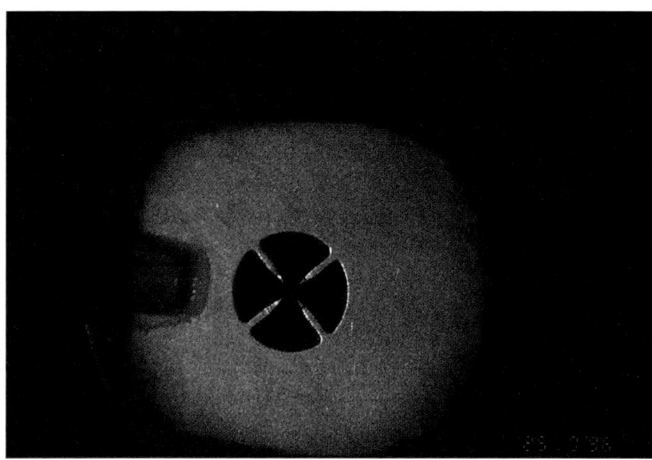

Figure 15-8.
Domilens marker.

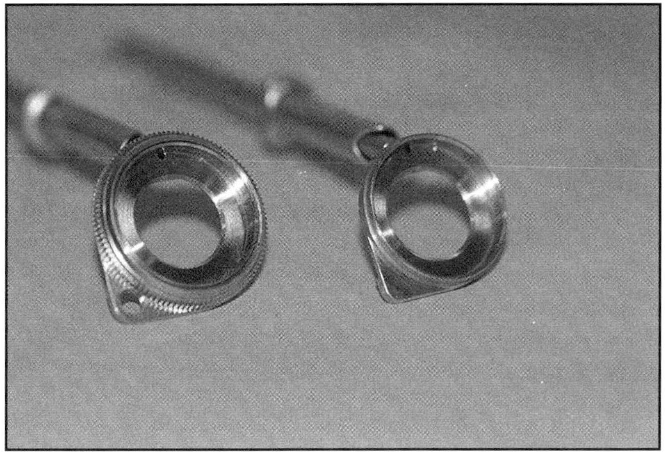

Figure 15-9.
Adjustable and non-adjustable suction ring for Chiron microkeratome.

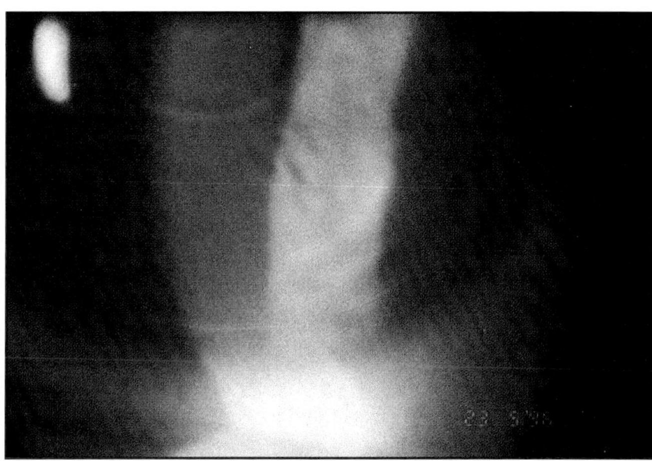

Figure 15-10.
Slit lamp photomicroscopy of a flap created with a non-adjustable ring 2 hours after surgery. (Note the peripheral cut. The still-present keratitis superficialis and the rest of the marker stamp are also visible.)

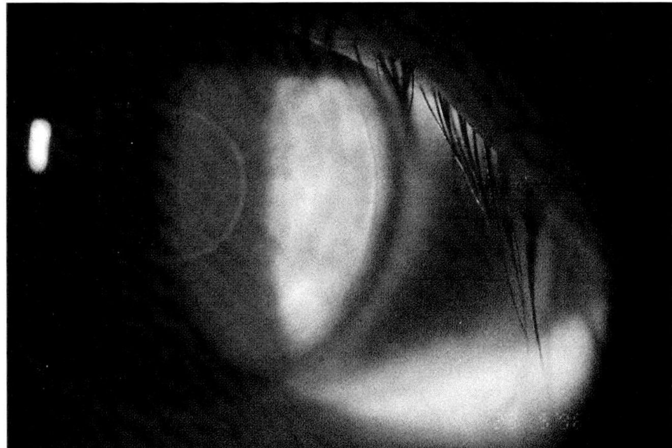

Figure 15-11.
Slit lamp photomicroscopy of a flap created with a non-adjustable ring 2 hours after surgery. (Note the peripheral cut. The still-present keratitis superficialis and the rest of the marker stamp are also visible.)

sary for ALK. For LASIK, however, I prefer the non-adjustable ring because it allows the creation of a flap of approximately 9.0-mm diameter (Figure 15-9), which is enabled by a more direct and more effective suction. I prefer bigger flaps because the fine scar is more peripheral. Additionally, a big flap is a prerequisite for treatment of hyperopia. The flaps created with a non-adjustable ring seem not only bigger but also thicker (Figures 15-10 and 15-11), more stable, and easier to manipulate. They are also less likely to develop wrinkles. Good flap quality also results in an easier and more comfortable retreatment.

The track of the microkeratome has to be inspected very thoroughly before activating the footswitch. Any potential obstacles should be removed. The eyelashes should be kept clear of the microkeratome's track and the eyelids should be separated in such a way the they do not prematurely stop the advancement of the microkeratome. If necessary, an assistant can help by folding back the eyelashes or gently pulling the eyelids, especially if they are so thick that they hang over the speculum.

Some surgeons decenter the suction ring nasally by 0.5 to 1.0 mm to obtain a correspondingly displaced flap. In some cases of a short flap, the laser treatment is still possible due to the nasal displacement.

Applanation

The cornea should be dry so that the rings engraved in the measuring instruments are seen clearly and the liquid on the corneal surface does not lead to a wrong pressure (too low) and resection diameter (too big) measurement. A Barraquer applanation tonometer is used to check the IOP. The flap diameter is then confirmed by an applanating lens. Some surgeons consider the diameter check superfluous when working with the non-adjustable ring and some worry that additional manipulations may lead to suction loss. Dr. Carmen Barraquer's opinion is that it is a second security check for the cut diameter and cut quality. Even after performing these tests, great care should be taken to ascertaining a stable adhesion of the suction ring to the cornea. This can be done by pulling the ring very gently.

There are different approaches to applanation. Checking IOP is considered essential by all surgeons, but some surgeons prefer to check the pressure by palpation instead of or in addition to using the Barraquer applanation tonometer. Some surgeons believe it to be sufficient only to check the IOP. I have been performing both checks.

The diameter check is very important because it shows the expected size of the flap. The stopper of the microkeratome has to set in such a way that a short flap hinge is created. For treatment of hyperopia, a very short hinge should be created. The stopper needs to be adjusted for this purpose.

Thus, for a given hinge size, the stopper adjustment depends on the flap diameter. If the flap diameter changes, the stopper needs to be readjusted. Inadequate stopper position may lead to a free cap or to a short flap.

Both applanation checks should always be performed. Every security measure recommended by LASIK experts should be followed in the learning curve.

AFTER THE CUT

Laser Ablation

The laser ablation is simple, provided that the laser has been programmed correctly. The correct centration is crucial for the result of the surgery. The surgeons use different techniques and sometimes additional instruments in order to obtain a proper centration. Some lasers are equipped with an eyetracker, which makes the laser beam follow the eye movements and helps to avoid a decentration. An eyetracker is not indispensable for myopic or combined myopic and astigmatic corrections. Myopic patients can fixate on the fixation light of the laser very well. An eyetracker is very helpful for the correction of hyperopia or hyperopic astigmatism. Some LASIK surgeons keep the suction ring on the eye, especially when treating hyperopia, in order to achieve its satisfactory immobilization.

Care should be taken not to allow the cornea to get too dry because the laser might ablate more tissue than under regular conditions. We also observed that patients whose cornea was very dry had more problems with the fixation of the red laser light.

On the other hand, the laser will ablate less than the programmed amount of tissue if the cornea is too wet.

Irrigation

There are many different ways of irrigating the intrastromal bed and the stromal side of the flap after laser ablation. Some surgeons perform a generous irrigation with open flap with or without brushing the stromal bed and the everted flap. I also applied this technique during my first two LASIK sessions. This technique bears a risk of transporting particles from the conjunctiva as well as pieces of epithelium into the intrastromal bed and of their remaining there. We experienced one bad case of epithelial ingrowth (Figure 15-12) working with this technique.

After observing an irrigation performed by Dr. Carmen Barraquer, I adopted her technique and had no cases of epithelial ingrowth ever since.

The flap is folded back immediately after laser ablation and the stromal bed is then irrigated under protection of the flap. Now I use this technique and I am highly pleased with the results. In retreated cases I occasionally find a small amount of peripheral epithelium pieces which are easily removed.

Another technique is extensive irrigation with the open flap, cleaning of the cornea and of the flap with a fine brush while a simultaneous suction removes the surplus liquid. Irrigation with an open flap and without suction is not recommended.

In case of a bilateral surgery, after the first cut, the slit of the microkeratome should be flushed vigorously from the upper side and the blade should be gently brushed in the cutting direction. This also reduces the risk of inducing an intrastromal epithelial ingrowth.

Drying the Edge of the Flap

There are different techniques for drying the edge of the flap to ensure sufficient flap adherence. Some surgeons use a stream of oxygen for drying the flap after its reposition. We use a Merocel sponge. We repeatedly and very gently touch the cornea along the flap edge with the sponge in order to draw BSS from the edge of the flap. We do it for approximately 2 minutes. After this the flap adherence is checked by depressing the peripheral cornea and ascertaining that peripheral folds extend into the flap. Other surgeons prefer to wait for 5 minutes after drying the flap edge.

We had one case of flap dislocation before the slit lamp check. The flap was repositioned very easily after thoroughly cleaning the stromal side of the flap and the interface with a wet Merocel sponge and after irrigation of the interface in the previously described manner. The flap was very well adapted, with no intrastromal particles or debris; only Descemet's folds were seen which disappeared later. Since then, the postoperative treatment (eye drops) is administered after the second slit lamp examination, 2 hours after the surgery, in order not to interfere with drying of the flap

POSTOPERATIVE CARE—BANDAGE CONTACT LENSES?

Many surgeons cover the eye with a bandage contact lens after surgery to protect the cut. We refrain from doing so because we heard about complications with contact lenses that caused a displacement of or tearing off the flap which led to problems in distinguishing the so-created cap from the contact lens. Other surgeons patch the eye for 2 hours after the procedure and then perform a slit lamp examination. Yet another group does not use contact lenses or patches and examines the eye at the slit lamp 30 minutes or 2 hours postoperatively. The patient is given protective eye shields for the first 24 hours postoperatively and at night for up to 3 weeks after the operation, depending on how confident he or she is that the eyes will not be rubbed during the night. I adopted the approach of the latter group. By doing this the chance of a corneal trauma is minimized and reveals good results.

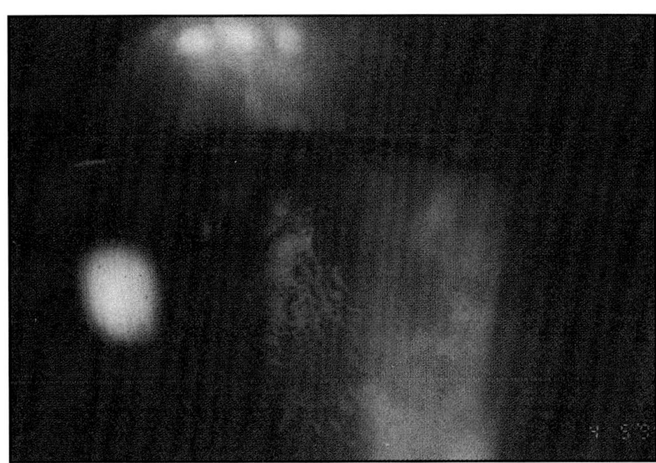

Figure 15-12.
Slit lamp photomicroscopy of an epithelial ingrowth.

Around the Procedure

During my various trips to see live surgeries, I also paid attention to the use of different instruments and other auxiliary devices, as well as to their cleaning and maintenance.

It was important for me to see how the microkeratome is cleaned and what additional instruments and other materials (eg, sponges) are used. In this section I would like to mention the things that I saw before starting to do the procedure, which later turned out advantageous.

Lint-free sponges are self-evident. Compared to learning the handling of the microkeratome and the excimer laser, this may be a minor issue, so it is usually not mentioned. I would like to stress that these sponges are very important. Particles of sponges that are used for cataract surgery do not look good in the intrastromal bed and they are very uncomfortable for the patient.

The cleaning of the microkeratome in our laser center consists of the following steps: rinsing in a Palmolive solution, cleaning with water, and then cleaning with alcohol and sterilization. We ceased using an ultrasound device for cleaning the head of the microkeratome. This step seems to release metal particles that can later be seen in the intrastromal bed. They are tiny and do not encumber the patient, but it always irritates the surgeon to see them under the slit lamp microscope. We saw fewer and smaller metal particles since we stopped using the ultrasound device.

The disposable microkeratome blades can be sterilized, but I prefer to use a new blade for each patient, for fear that the edge of the blade could be damaged by additional manipulations in the sterilizing process. In every case the edge has to be examined under the microscope before inserting it into the microkeratome. Gimbel[5] also inspects the blades under the microscope to make sure that there are no defects and no surface debris which is certainly to be recommended.

The air ionizator that was recommended to me by Dr. Carmen Barraquer proved very useful. It is also used in the watch and microchip industries to keep the air free of dust and particles. It is placed on the laser, above the patient's head. It is an additional security measure helping to avoid intrastromal debris and to improve the quality of the LASIK surgery.

BILATERAL SURGERY

There are also different opinions with respect to bilateral surgery. The main surgery risk and the complications causes are associated with the use of the microkeratome, whereas complications in the healing process are very rare. Therefore, many surgeons do surgery on both eyes in one session. Others prefer to wait until the healing of the first eye is completed before treating the second eye. Unilateral surgery is recommended in the learning curve. Usually I do bilateral surgery, unless the patient wants to wait for vision to recover in the first eye before undergoing surgery of the second eye. After unilateral surgery, patients with high refractive errors may experience severe problems (eg, headache, nausea, vertigo) caused by aniseikonia.[8] However, one should never try to talk a patient into having bilateral surgery. Patients should be informed about possible discomfort after unilateral surgery but the decision should be left to them.

If complications occur in the surgery of the first eye, the second eye procedure should be postponed, even if the complications are considered minor. This lets us stay on the safe side.

CONCLUSION

Every surgeon planning to learn LASIK can shorten the learning curve considerably and thereby avoid some complications and be better prepared for managing complications if they occur. In my opinion, the following points are essential:

- Participation in basic training courses.
- Visiting different experienced surgeons and watching their techniques as well as handling of different lasers.
- Different nomogram modifications that are used for different lasers will be noticed. It is important to learn about the modifications to the nomograms that are applied by experienced colleagues. The formula used for high myopia should be explained in great detail by the surgeon using it to the novice who plans to use the same laser. The same applies to other possible peculiarities (eg, centration) of the laser to be used. This helps in reducing the decentration, overcorrection, and retreatment rate.
- A LASIK novice should also carefully evaluate the organizational and medical issues related to the procedure. This is helpful to choose the most suitable solution for the medical and organizational aspects of pre- and postoperative care. One should also learn which instruments are used in the procedure and how they are maintained and cleaned. Special care is to be given to cleaning, assembling, and checking the microkeratome. Additional auxiliary devices, such as special filters for air condition or air ionizators, should be used to minimize the occurrence of dust particles and debris under the flap.
- Before starting, intensive training on a great number of pig eyes until LASIK becomes a routine procedure is strongly recommended. Surgery rehearsals with the entire team and an authorized technician should be performed repeatedly.
- Learn as much as possible about avoiding complications and handling them in case they occur.
- An experienced colleague should assist the novice LASIK surgeon at least during the first operating session.
- In the beginning, consultation from and supervision by experienced surgeons should be sought.

References

1. Barraquer JI. Queratomileusis para le correccion de la miopia. *Arch Soc Am Oftal Optom*. 1964;5:27-48.

2. Barraquer JI. Keratomileusis for myopia and aphakia. *Ophthalmology*. 1981;88:701-708.

3. Pallikaris IG, Papatzanaki ME, Stathi EZ, Frenschock O, Georgiadis A. Laser in situ keratomileusis. *Lasers in Surgery and Medicine*. 1990;10:463-468.

4. Pallikaris IG, Siganos DS. Excimer laser in situ keratomileusis and photorefractive keratectomy for correction of high myopia. *J Refract Corneal Surg*. 1994;10:498-510.

5. Gimbel HV, Basti S, Kaye GB, Ferensowicz M. Experience during the learning curve of laser in situ keratomileusis. *J Cataract Refract Surg*. 1996;5:542-550.

6. Casebeer JC. The introduction of new procedures and technology: a different view (editorial). *J Refract Surg*. 1996;3:331-334.

7. Knorz MC, Liermannn A, Seiberth V, Steiner H, Wiesinger B. Laser in situ keratomileusis to correct myopia of -6.00 to -29.00 diopters. *J Refract Surg*. 1996;5:575-584.

8. Enoch JM. Refractive aniseikonia: a source of binocular vision stress and asthenopia (letter to the editor). *J Refract Surg*. 1996;5:565-566.

SECTION 5

LASIK RESULTS AND COMPARISON WITH OTHER CORNEAL REFRACTIVE PROCEDURES

Chapter 16

THE PLANOSCAN-LASIK TECHNIQUE

Maria-Clara Arbelaez, MD

THE CORRECTION OF MYOPIA AND HYPEROPIA

Myopia

In the past years, excimer laser photorefractive keratectomy (PRK) has shown considerable results after treating myopic eyes up to -6 D. Compared to earlier methods, like myopic keratomileusis by freezing,[1] this technique caused less or no corneal haze due to less thermal and mechanical stress to the cornea. Several modifications reduced the thermal or mechanical exposure on the cornea by a significant amount, but all of them showed a poor refractive predictability or had other disadvantages for the patient. In 1983, the idea of using an argon-fluoride excimer laser with a wavelength of 193 nm (ultraviolet) was proposed. At this wavelength, the photon energy is so high that the covalent electronic connections of the molecules of the cornea are suddenly cracked and the produced gaseous fractions move away immediately.

With this new method, a significantly higher predictability of the correction was achieved. However, applying the treatment on the surface of the cornea causes regions with relatively large local slope and curvature differences, which could be the reason for an overactivation of the epithelium growth and the keratocytes in the stroma. Both are responsible for regression and haze.

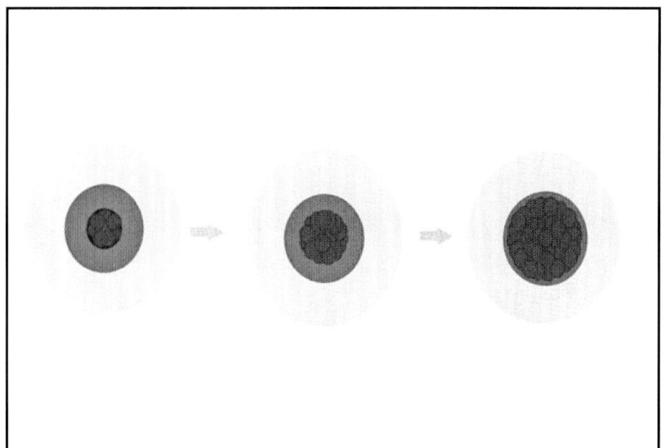

Figure 16-1.
In the PlanoScan algorithm, a laser beam with a fixed diameter of 2 mm is scanning in an irregular computer-controlled pattern over the cornea.

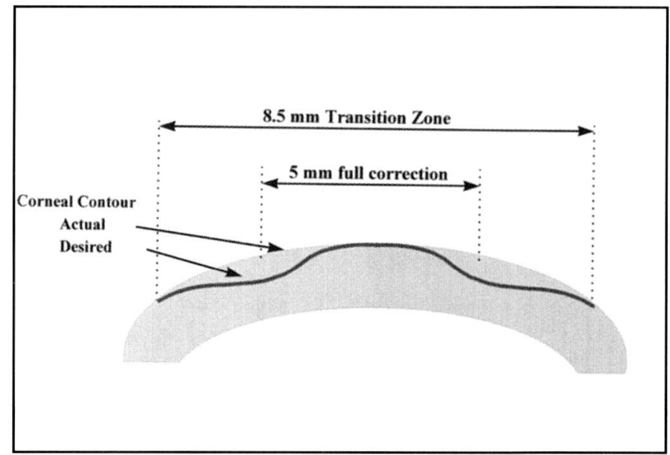

Figure 16-2.
Ablation profile of the cornea from a hyperopic treatment. The maximum of ablation is located not in the center region but in the outer part. To match the slope of treated and untreated surfaces as smooth as possible, a wide transition zone is established.

The next step of modifying this procedure has been laser in situ keratomileusis (LASIK). This procedure gives the possibility of applying the excimer treatment in the stromal bed and so avoiding an activation of the wound healing process on the surface. Thus, the possibility of regression can be reduced to a minimum, which remains due to the hyperactive wound healing capabilities of individual patients.

One of the general problems of treating mild myopia by PRK seems to be the creation of so-called central islands. This phenomenon is caused by the desired large corrected zones and the related large beam diameters (5.0 mm or more) of the excimer lasers and is one of the most prominent reasons for losing one or more lines in visual acuity.

To face the problem mentioned above, a new scanning algorithm, PlanoScan, was used. This method uses a laser beam with a fixed diameter of 2.0 mm, which scans over the surface of the cornea or over the stromal bed (Figure 16-1).

Using PlanoScan, the surgeon is able to create the same ablation profile (compared to a large area ablation) on the surface without the production of central islands.

Hyperopia

Up to now there have only been a few treatment methods for hyperopia. The technique of lamellar keratotomy, which has been used in 10% of eyes, showed a poor predictability. In several cases even irregular astigmatisms were induced. The usage of corneal inlets with lenticles for myopic patients seems to be a more simple technique with higher predictability, but the accurate centration of the lenticle seems to be a critical item. Treatments of hyperopia and hyperopic astigmatism with holmium YAG lasers show a large regression tendency and a significant fraction of patients even reach the original refractions.[2]

Also with the excimer laser PRK treatment of hyperopia, a high rate of regression has been observed up to now. This effect, which appears mainly above +4 D, is caused by the overactivation of the reepithelialization process. The amount of regression seems to be proportional to the absolute value of the correction and supports the theory that the higher the curvature change of the cornea, the more effective the reepithelialization will be. Due to the relatively complex curvature change of the corneal surface by a hyperopic treatment, this effect also arises in the case of reasonable zone sizes. The described situation is shown in Figure 16-2.

The deepening of the center part of the cornea is achieved by an ablation profile, in which the maximum ablation is located in the peripheral region. A large transition zone follows to reach the original curvature of the corneal surface at the outer boundary of the treatment area. As an example, a PRK treatment of +4 D with a corrected optical zone of 5 mm requires a total treatment zone of 9.0 mm in diameter. This large region has to be ablated due to the already explained slope transition of

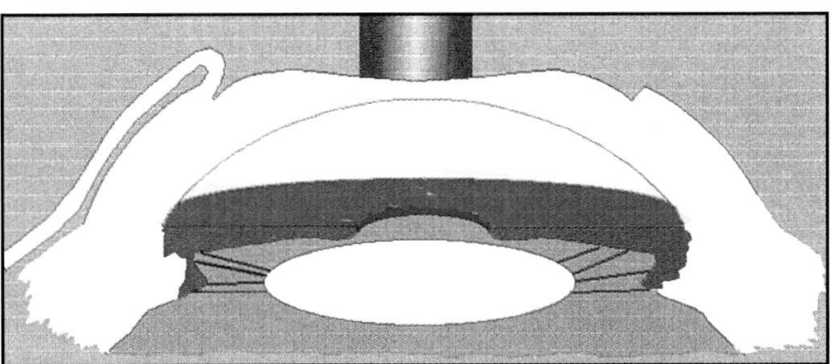

Figure 16-3.
With a microkeratome, a 160-μm thick surface parallel cut is done on the cornea. After putting the flap to the side, the excimer beam is applied to the stromal bed.

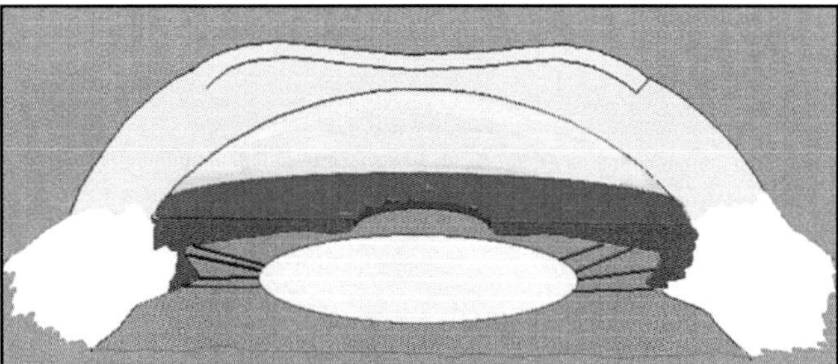

Figure 16-4.
After the laser treatment, the flap is repositioned to its original position. After 2 minutes, the flap is stable enough to remove the lid speculum.

the treated to the untreated cornea. It seems that the regression rate increases with the slope difference of these two regions.

Thus, the idea arose to apply this procedure in the stromal bed. A large advantage of this modification is also the missing defect of Bowman's membrane due to the epithelium abrasion and a correlated faster regain of the best corrected visual acuity. In addition to this, the wound healing is suppressed to a minimum and the patient feels no pain.

Therefore, LASIK combined with PlanoScan is a very effective method to correct hyperopic eyes.

THE TREATMENT PROCEDURE

The method of LASIK has shown a huge expansion during the past few years. The LASIK technique has two main advantages. Besides the very low regression tendency of the resulting refraction, an almost painless postoperative phase for the patient is also observed. In addition, the patients show a very fast recovery of visual acuity during a period of only 2 to 3 days. These effects result from the fact that the epithelium and Bowman's interface are untouched.

A typical LASIK treatment on a patient is initiated by a 160-µm thick lamellar cut on the cornea by an automatically driven microkeratome (Figure 16-3). The produced flap is connected to the surface of the cornea by a hinge. Putting this flap to the side allows an excimer laser treatment in the corneal bed. Finally, the flap will be positioned back to its original position (Figure 16-4). In certain cases (eg, with thin corneas), the thickness of the flap can be reduced to 130 µm or increased to 180 µm. Thus, a minimum of about 250 µm of the cornea can be saved, which is necessary to avoid ectasia.

This technique enables the surgeon to treat myopia even higher than -6 D without the significant regression tendency which can be seen in typical PRK cases.

There are two main issues in which the PlanoScan algorithm differs from the known full area ablation procedures. First, the diameter of the excimer laser beam is no longer variable but fixed to 2.0 mm, and second, the beam scans over the surface of the cornea. Clinical results show no central islands, which have been obviously produced by beams with diameters larger than 5 mm. Additionally, the thermal and mechanical stress of the cornea can be reduced to a minimum, because the scanning procedure is optimized in such a way that the position of each excimer pulse is as far away as possible from the previous one.

The PlanoScan algorithm is performed with a shot frequency of 25 Hz instead of 50 Hz. Thus, a typical treatment of a myopic eye with -6 D takes approximately 60 seconds. This value depends also on the size of the zone that has to be treated. The final configuration of the treatment parameters is a compromise between zone size and ablation depth.

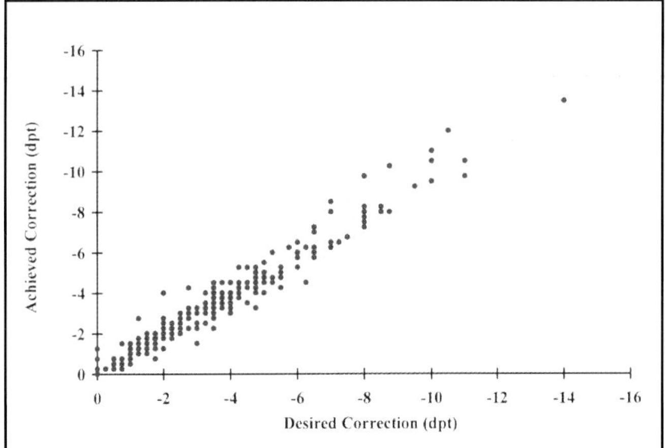

Figure 16-5.
Comparison of desired and achieved refractive spherical correction of 1-week postoperative examination.

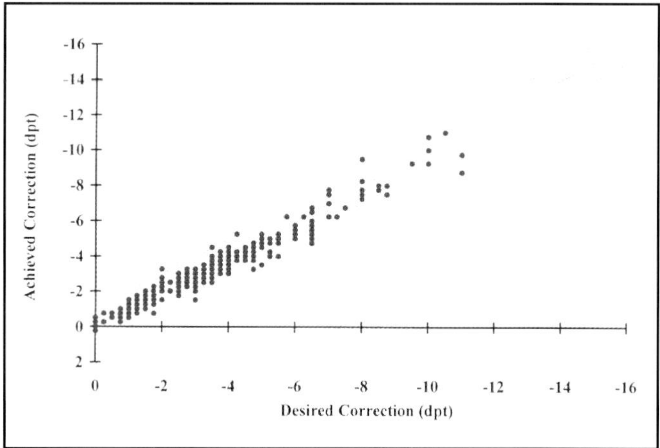

Figure 16-6.
Comparison of desired and achieved refractive spherical correction of 1-month postoperative examination.

THE RESULTS

Myopia

This section contains a study of 318 myopic eyes that have been treated by the PlanoScan-LASIK method on a Keracor 117 from Chiron Vision Corp (Technolas), using an excimer laser beam with a fixed diameter, which scans over the cornea. This procedure has been combined with the LASIK method. Follow-up data up to 6 months are presented and different aspects such as time stability and quality of vision are discussed.

The whole volume of patients was split into two groups with different preoperative spherical refractions (mild myopia: 0 to -6 D, high myopia: over -6 D).

For refraction corrections up to -6 D, 269 patients were treated with the PlanoScan method by a Keracor 116, upgraded to a Keracor-117 CT. To get complete information on the time behavior, the follow-up data from 1 week (postoperative) up to 6 months have been included in the analysis.

A direct verification for the predictability of the treatment method can be given by the calculated standard deviation of the achieved refraction for a given set of patients.

The comparison of those values from different follow-up times indicates the development of the refractions. Nevertheless, there is a strong influence of the patient numbers on the different calculated values, which shows a direct need of some statistical analysis concerning the individual confidence intervals for the mathematically calculated values.

In addition to the calculated standard deviation, a confidence interval for this value is determined. Two basic factors determine the boundaries of this interval. The first is the confidence level itself, which determines the probability (α) of making a mistake in the estimation of the standard deviation from a finite sample of data points. The second factor is the number of examinations that are included in the analysis. It is obvious that the larger this number is, the more accurate the standard deviation can be estimated. In the following analysis, a confidence level of 90% ($1-\alpha= 0.9$) has been used to specify the statistical error in the standard deviation. The only assumption that has been made in this case is a gaussian distribution of independent data points.

The direct comparison of desired and achieved corrections shows a very good correspondence in the values. The scattergrams in Figures 16-5 through 16-8 show the data volume that has been used for this analysis for the different follow-up times of 1, 4, 12, and 24 weeks.

As previously mentioned, the standard deviation of the difference between achieved and desired spherical refraction has been used as a measure for the efficiency of the treatment method.

The analysis of this data gives a 90% confidence interval of 0.42 D to 0.49 D for the standard deviation of 0.45 D for 1-month follow-up and an interval of 0.32 D to 0.44 D for the corresponding value of 0.37 D in the 6-month data for the group of patients with mild myopic treatments (Figure 16-9). For refraction corrections higher

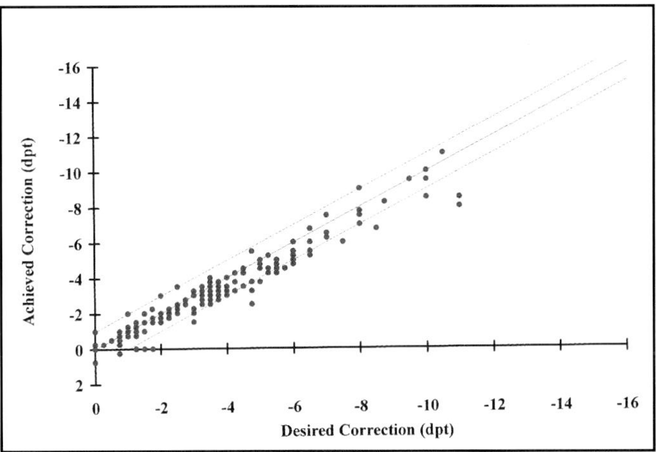

Figure 16-7.
Comparison of desired and achieved refractive spherical correction of 3-month postoperative examination.

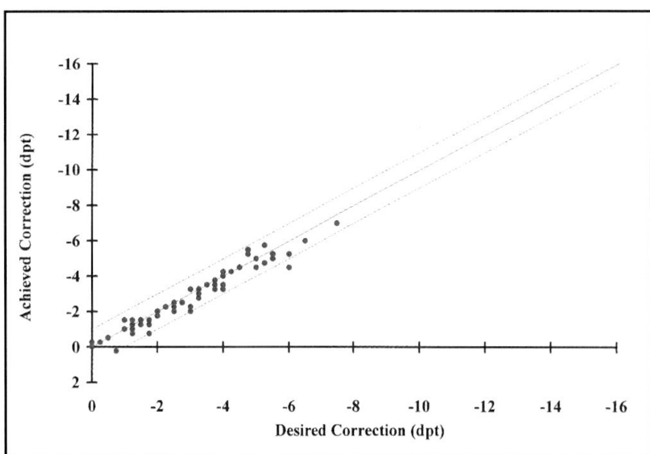

Figure 16-8.
Comparison of desired and achieved refractive spherical correction of 6-month postoperative examination.

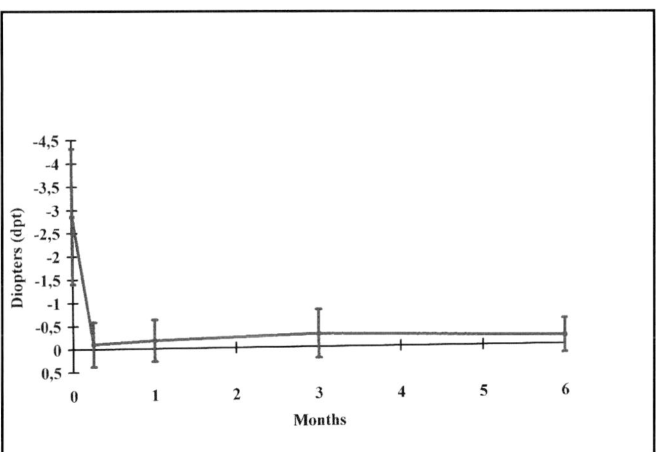

Figure 16-9.
Time development of the mean spherical refraction and standard deviation for corrections less than -6 D.

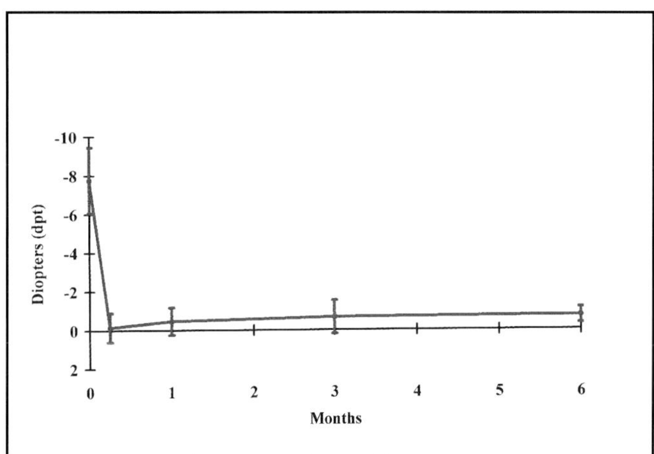

Figure 16-10.
Time development of the mean spherical refraction and standard deviation for corrections greater than -6 D.

than -6 D, the 1-month data show a standard deviation of 0.71 D with a 90% confidence interval of 0.60 D to 0.87 D and the corresponding 6-month data are 0.40 D with a range of 0.27 D to 0.84 D (Figure 16-10). The extremely large 90% confidence interval for the 6-month data is a direct result of the small number of six patients for this follow-up time.

In the case of treating the astigmatism, a similar analysis was made and the follow-up data indicate a very stable resulting refraction up to high cylinders. Figures 16-11 through 16-14 demonstrate follow-up data for 1, 3, and 6 months.

Two hundred seventy-seven patients had an astigmatic correction, and for the follow-up analysis of 1, 3, and 6 months, 222, 169, and 35 patients have been examined.

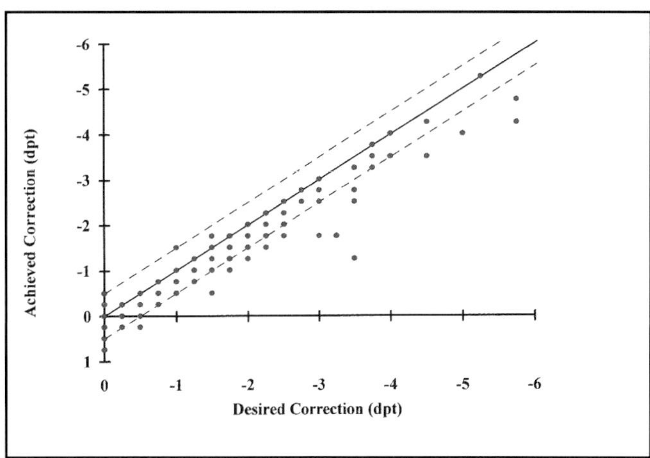

Figure 16-11.
Comparison of desired and achieved refractive cylindrical correction of 1-month postoperative examination.

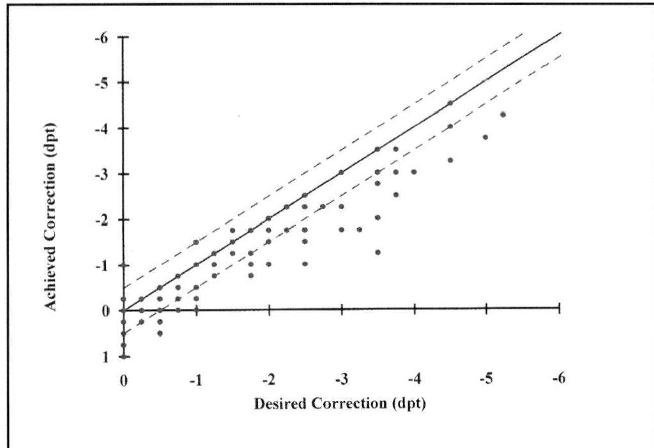

Figure 16-12.
Comparison of desired and achieved refractive cylindrical correction of 3-month postoperative examination.

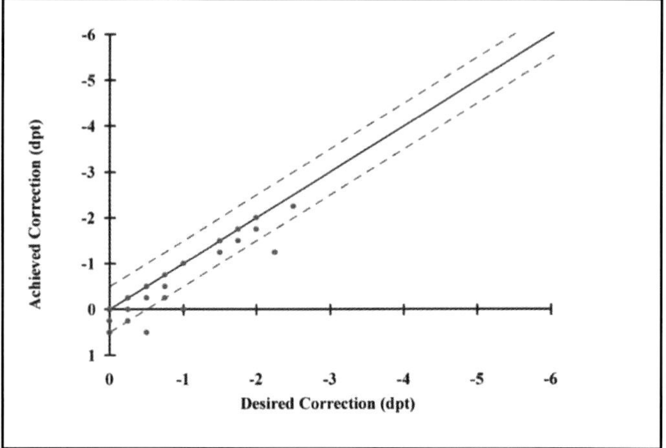

Figure 16-13.
Comparison of desired and achieved refractive cylindrical correction of 6-month postoperative examination.

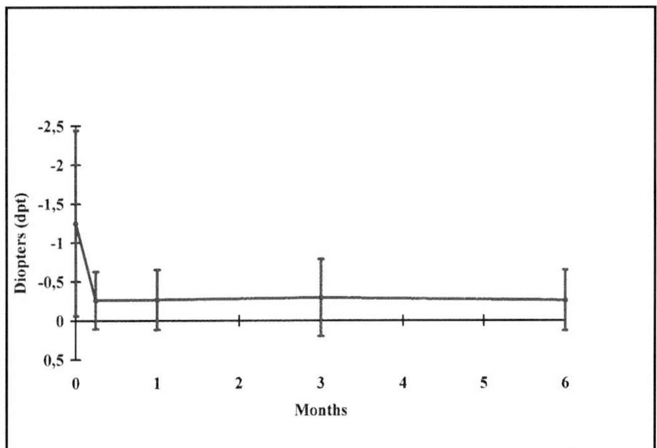

Figure 16-14.
Time development of the mean cylindrical refraction and standard deviation.

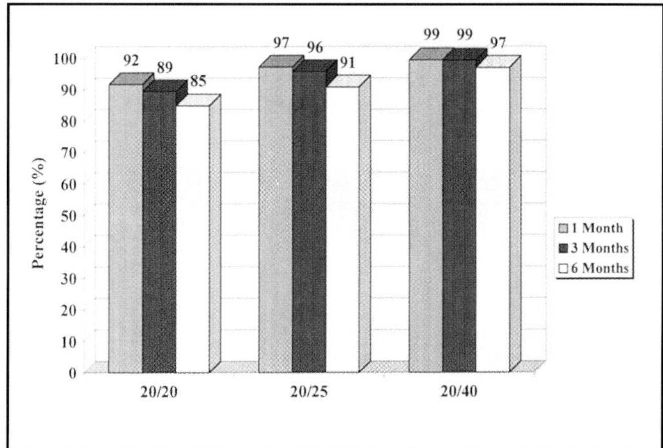

Figure 16-15.
Distribution of the best corrected visual acuity for treatments with a spherical correction less than -6 D.

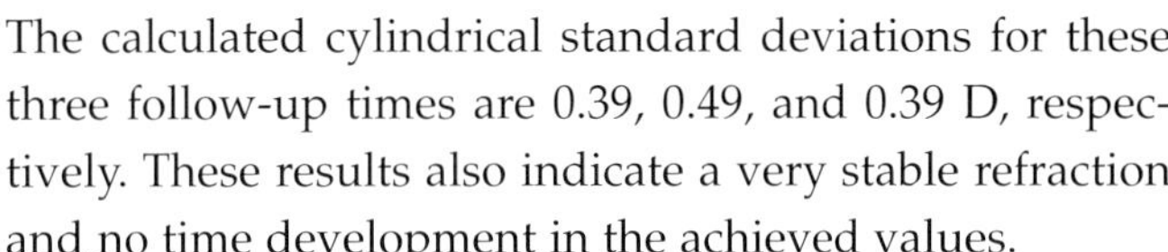

The calculated cylindrical standard deviations for these three follow-up times are 0.39, 0.49, and 0.39 D, respectively. These results also indicate a very stable refraction and no time development in the achieved values.

An important part of the analysis concerns the change of the vision of the patients, because this fact has a direct impact on the happiness of the treated person. Thus, the analysis of these parameters is of special importance.

The best corrected visual acuity after 6 months is 20/25 or better for 91% of the patients with mild myopia. Eighty-five percent of the patients even reach a best corrected visual acuity of 20/20. This time dependence of the visual acuity for mild myopia is shown in Figure 16-15. The numbers over the bars indicate the percentage of patients with the given best corrected visual acuity. The corresponding data for myopic treatments with more than -6 D is presented in Figure 16-16.

In the case of mild myopic treatments, 79% of the patients do not show a change in vision after 6 months, while 9% of them lose one line (Figure 16-17). For higher refractions, 58% of all patients have no change in the best corrected visual acuity after 3 months (Figure 16-18). This clearly shows the efficiency of the PlanoScan-LASIK technique.

The comparison of the best corrected visual acuity for different times shows that a large fraction of the patients with mild myopia (97%) reaches a vision level of 20/25 or better already 1 month after the surgery. For high myopic treatments, a corresponding percentage of 87% reaches a vision of 20/25 after 1 month. This very fast recovering

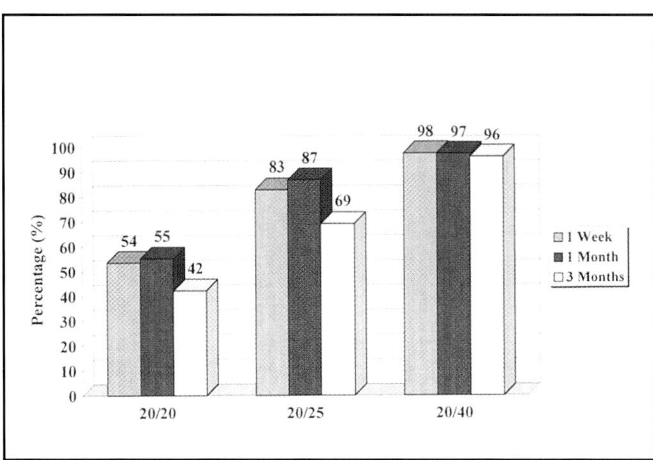

Figure 16-16.
Distribution of the best corrected visual acuity for treatments with a spherical correction greater than -6 D.

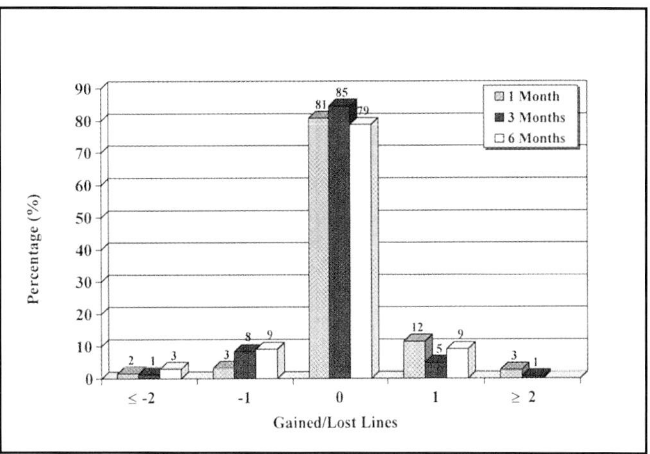

Figure 16-17.
Gained and lost lines in best corrected visual acuity for treatments with a spherical correction less than -6 D.

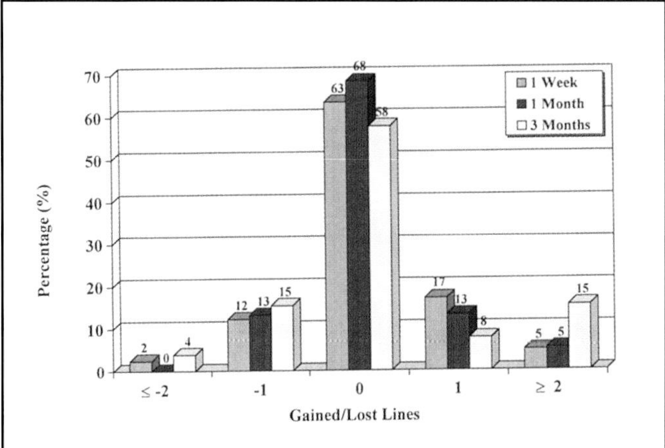

Figure 16-18.
Gained and lost lines in best corrected visual acuity for treatments with a spherical correction greater than -6 D.

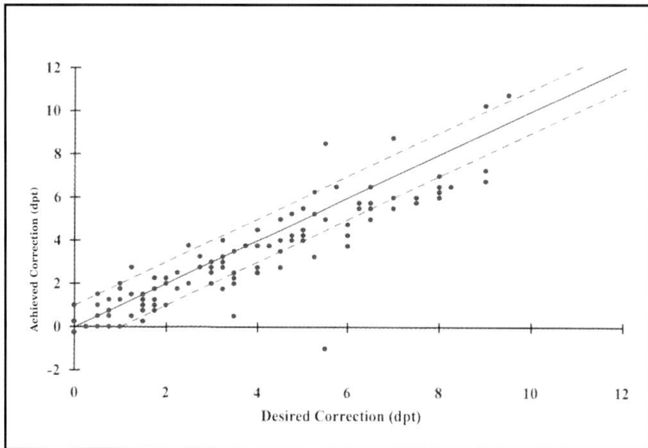

Figure 16-19.
Comparison of desired and achieved refractive spherical correction of 1-month postoperative examination.

tendency seems to be a direct result of the scanning algorithm, which allows a treatment with a reduced stress level for the cornea.

The calculated values of the standard deviation for spherical and astigmatic corrections show with a typical value of 0.37 D and 0.39 D, respectively, a high predictability in the achievable result. A time analysis of these values gives a very stable refraction with a 90% confidence interval.

In addition to these points, the fact of applying a LASIK treatment reduces the active cell growth region from the whole surface of the cornea to the edges of the cut. Thus, there is no significant influence of the epithelium growth on the resulting refraction. The only fact that has to be recognized is the possibility of epithelium ingrowth, what could happen in the case of some epithelium cells under the flap or a not completely closed edge of the cut. Both cases can be checked out and are in principle under control. Due to the LASIK technique, the Bowman's membrane is untouched and the cutting edge is only a small fraction of the whole interface.

Hyperopia

A total of 128 patients with a hyperopic correction range between 0 and +10 D have been treated and the existing follow-up data up to 6 months have been analyzed. The patients have been divided into two groups by their refractions: 0 to +4 D and +4 to +10 D. Figures 16-19 through 16-21 show the scattergrams of desired and achieved spherical refractions. The preoperative spheri-

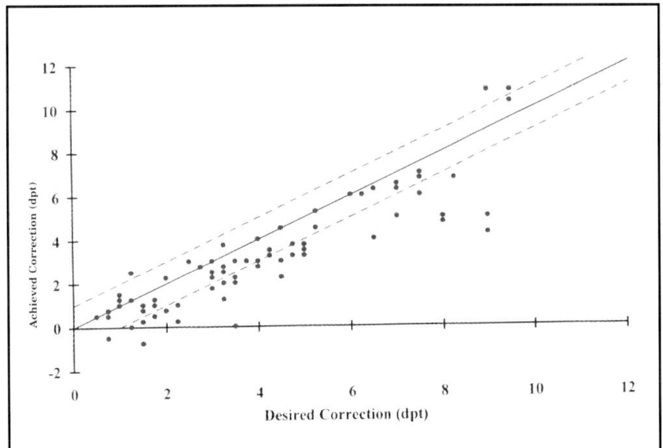

Figure 16-20.
Comparison of desired and achieved refractive spherical correction of 3-month postoperative examination.

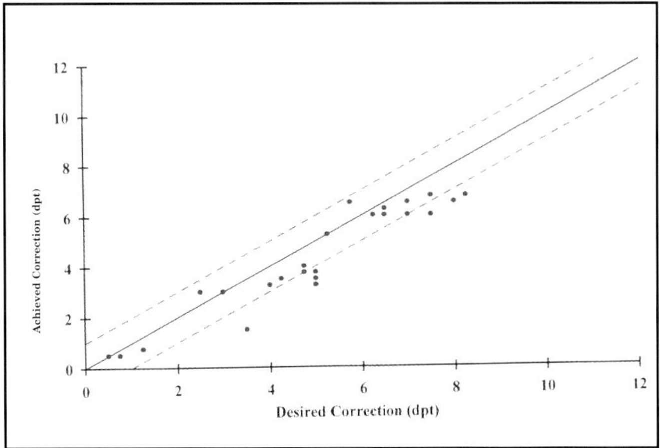

Figure 16-21.
Comparison of desired and achieved refractive spherical correction of 6-month postoperative examination.

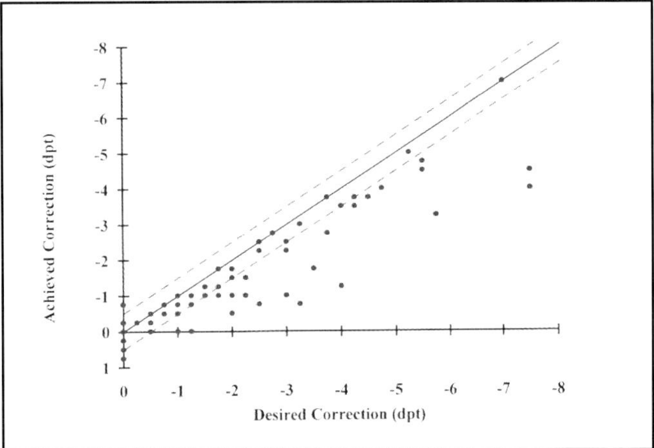

Figure 16-22.
Comparison of desired and achieved myopic cylindrical correction in combination with hyperopic treatments of 1-month postoperative examination.

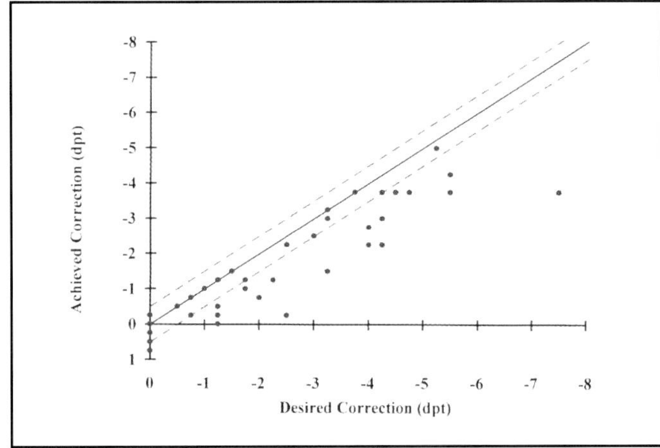

Figure 16-23.
Comparison of desired and achieved myopic cylindrical correction in combination with hyperopic treatments of 3-month postoperative examination.

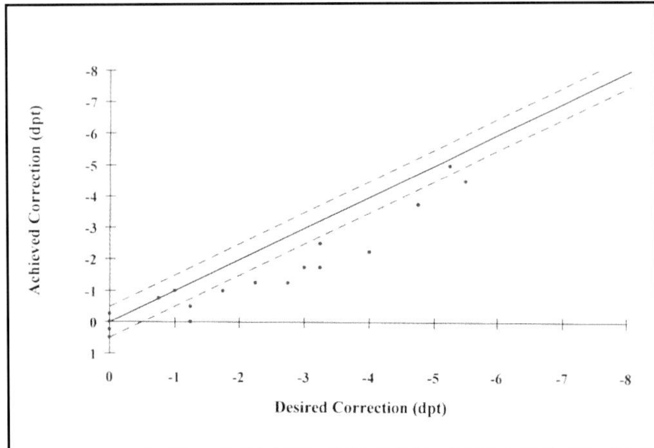

Figure 16-24.
Comparison of desired and achieved myopic cylindrical correction in combination with hyperopic treatments of 6-month postoperative examination.

cal averages of these two groups are +2.06 D and +6.00 D, respectively. The 6-month follow-up data show a postoperative average of 0.32 D and 0.82 D.

In analogy to the scattergrams of the spherical correction, an analysis for the astigmatic correction follows. Figures 16-22 through 16-24 show the follow-up results for 1, 3, and 6 months.

The analysis of the spherical component of mild hyperopic treatments yields a standard deviation of 0.75 D for the 1-month data. The 90% confidence interval is 0.66 D to 0.88 D. The corresponding values for the 3- and 6-month follow-up data are 0.86 D with 0.73 D to 1.04 D and 0.80 D with 0.55 D to 1.53 D, respectively. The graphical representation of these results is shown in Figure 16-25.

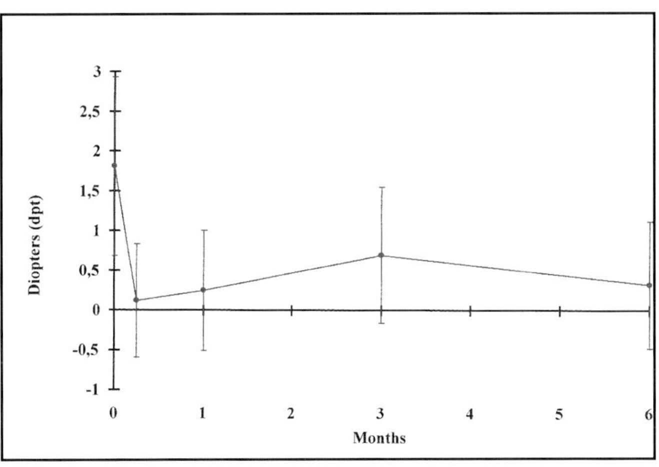

Figure 16-25.
Time development of the mean spherical refraction and standard deviation for corrections less than +4 D.

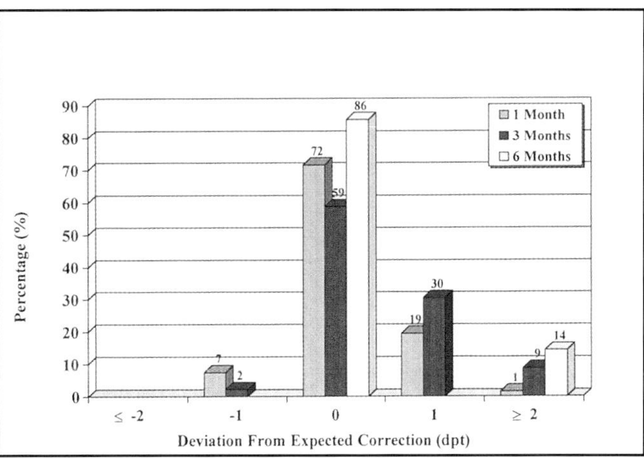

Figure 16-26.
Predictability of the spherical correction for refractions less than +4 D.

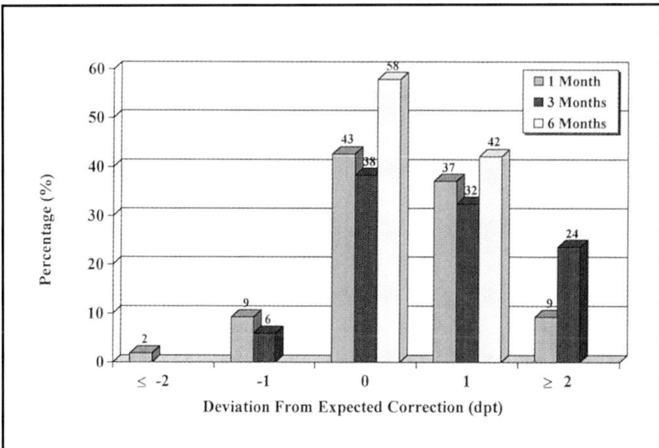

Figure 16-27.
Predictability of the spherical correction for refractions greater than +4 D.

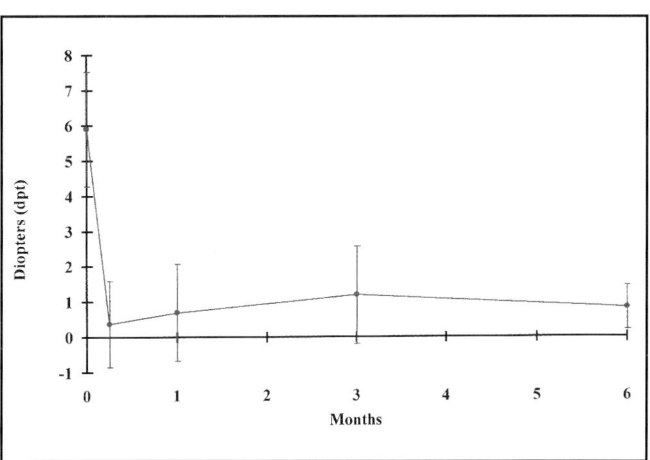

Figure 16-28.
Time development of the mean spherical refraction and standard deviation for corrections greater than +4 D.

As presented in Figure 16-26, 86% of all patients achieved the desired refraction 6 months after the treatment. Only 14% show an undercorrection of 2 D (see Figure 16-26).

In the case of spherical corrections greater than +4 D, 42% of the patients show an undercorrerction of 1 D (Figure 16-27). By taking the preoperative mean value of +6.00 D into account (Figure 16-28), this undercorrection is a 17% fraction of the mean refraction.

In Figures 16-29 through 16-31, the analog presentation for the astigmatic data has been given. In total, 69% of all patients are plano after 6 months. In 31% of all cases, an undercorrection of 1 D was observed.

The treatment of hyperopic eyes with the PlanoScan-LASIK algorithm seems to produce predictable and sta-

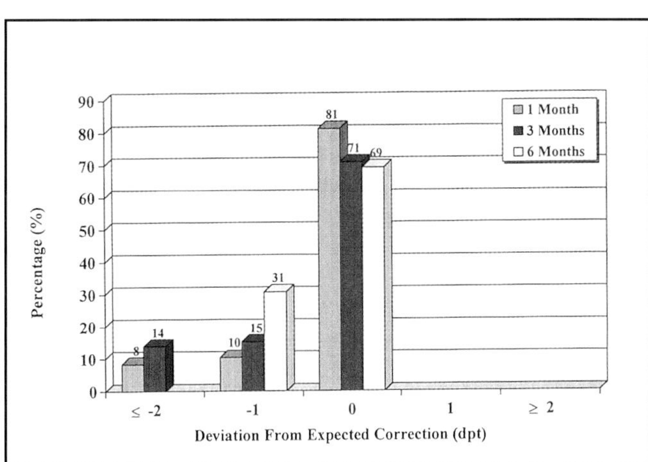

Figure 16-29.
Predictability of the astigmatic treatments in combination with the hyperopic correction.

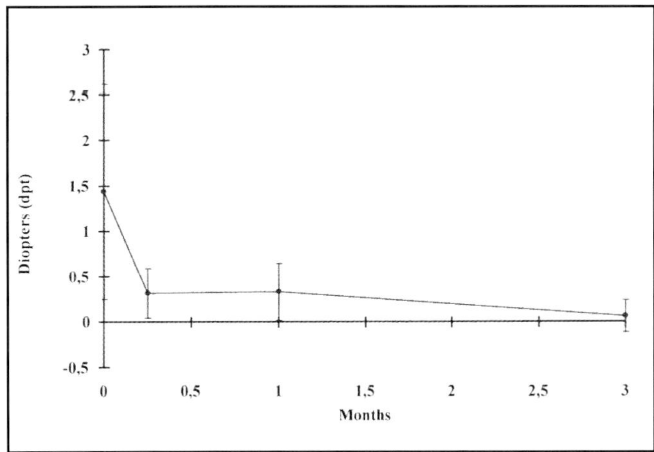

Figure 16-30.
Time development of the mean cylindrical refraction and standard deviation for corrections with hyperopic cylinder.

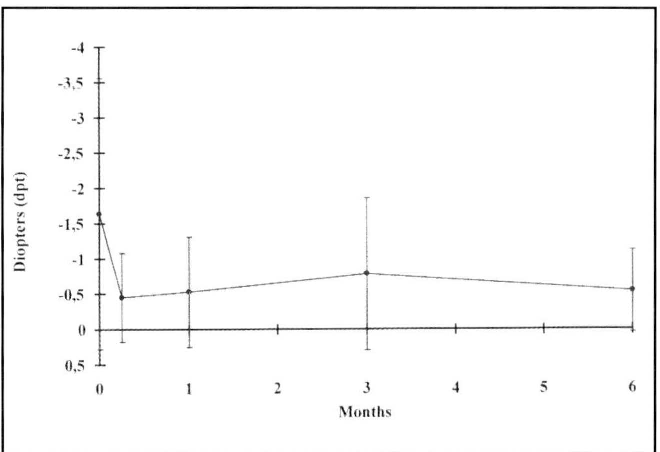

Figure 16-31.
Time development of the mean cylindrical refraction and standard deviation for corrections with myopic cylinder.

ble results. Even if there is evidence of a slight undercorrection both in sphere and cylinder, the stable results show the possibility of achieving the desired refraction.

The undercorrection of the astigmatic component (independent from the sign of the cylinder) is done on purpose to avoid an axis rotation by a slight overcorrection. Thus, the postoperative mean includes a shift, which can easily be seen in the scattergrams. Also, the standard deviation indicates a high level of stability during the whole follow-up time and there is no reason to suggest changes in this tendency for the future.

References

1. Couderc JL, Lozano-Moury F, De Charnace B. Comparative results of myopic keratomileusis with and without freezing. *Ophthalmology*. 1988;2(4):293-296.

2. Cherry PM. Holmium:YAG laser to treat astigmatism associated with myopia or hyperopia. *J Refract Surg*. 1995;11(suppl).

LASIK vs Multizone PRK: Summit High Myopia Study

STEPHEN F. BRINT, MD, FACS

TABLE 1

LASIK: Summit High Myopia Study

Postoperative eyes	n = 56 (33 patients)
Mean refractive error	-9.56 D
Range of myopia	-6.25 D to -22.00 D
Average age	37 years
Age range	22 to 53 years

TABLE 2

PRK (Multizone): Summit High Myopia Study

Postoperative eyes	n = 44 (27 patients)
Mean refractive error	-8.7 D
Range of myopia	-6.00 D to -13.63 D
Average age	36 years
Age range	22 to 49 years

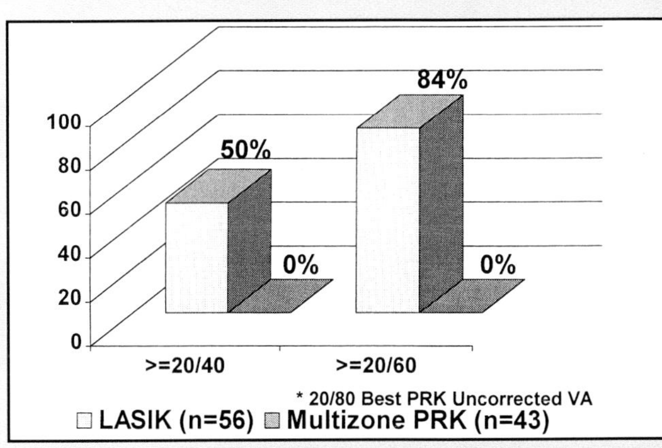

Figure 1.
One-day uncorrected visual acuity.

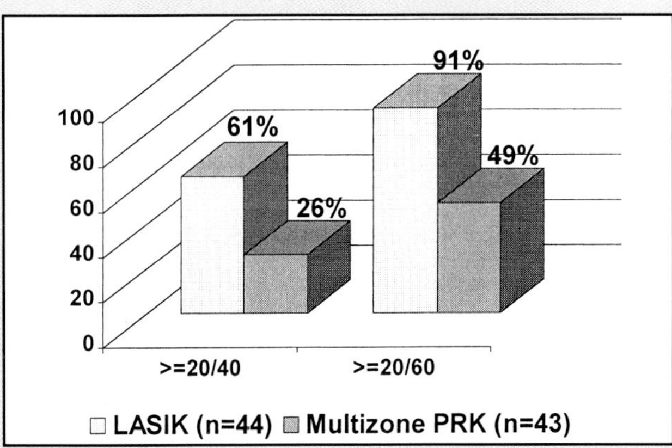

Figure 2.
Three- to 5-days uncorrected visual acuity.

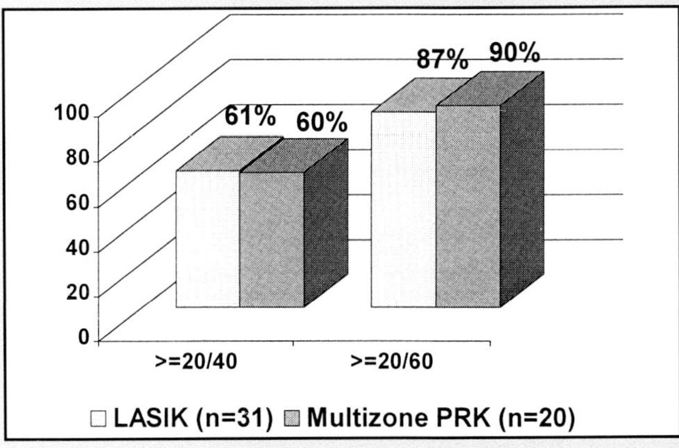

Figure 3.
Eight- to 12-days uncorrected visual acuity.

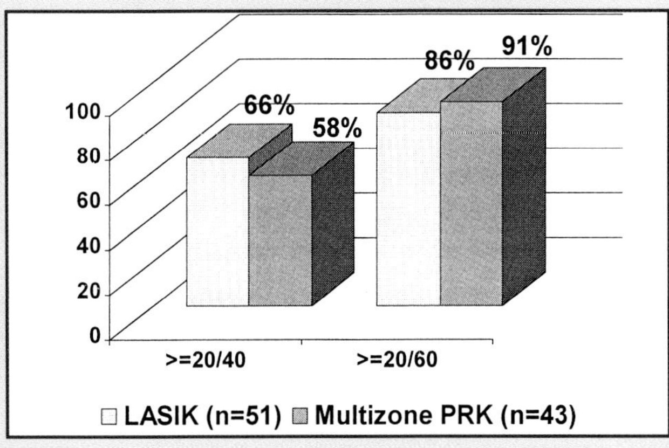

Figure 4.
One-month uncorrected visual acuity.

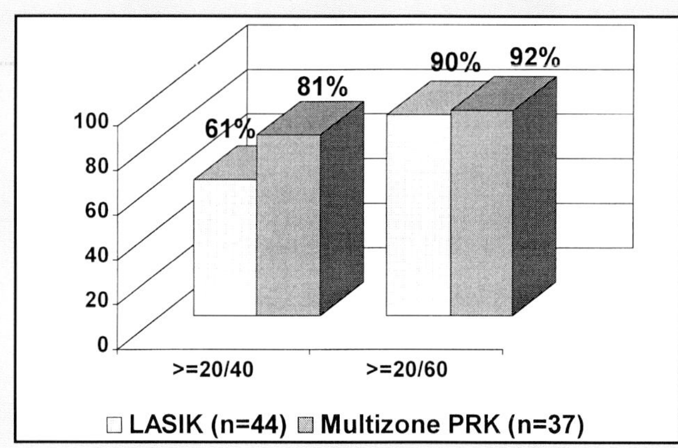

Figure 5.
Three-month uncorrected visual acuity.

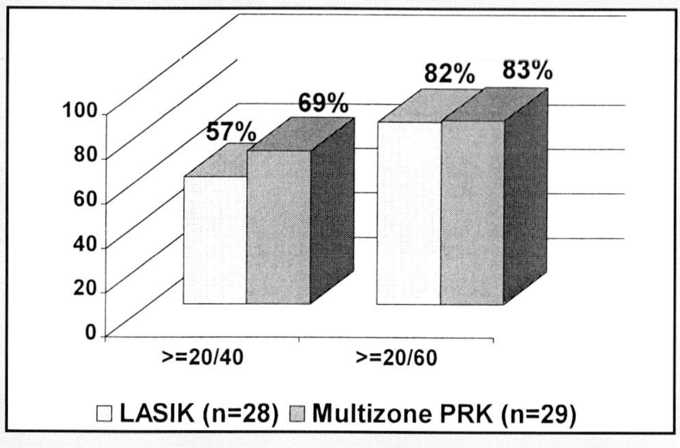

Figure 6.
Six-month uncorrected visual acuity.

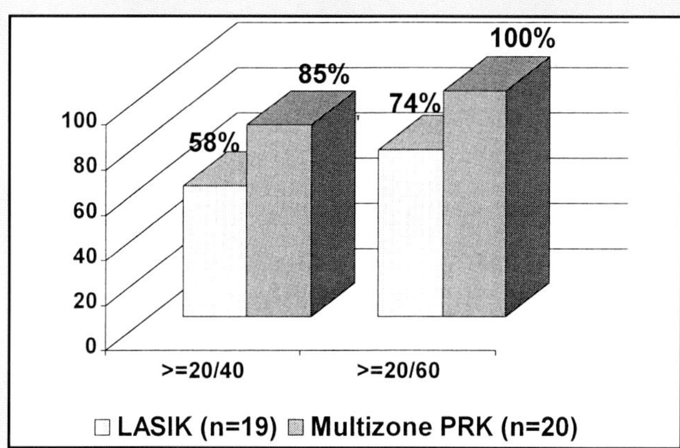

Figure 7.
Nine-month uncorrected visual acuity.

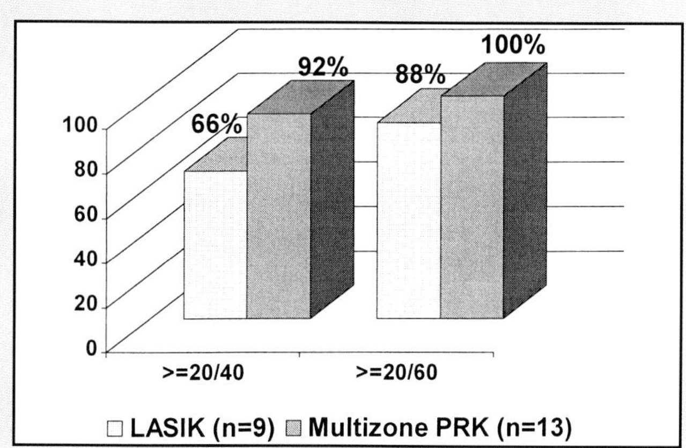

Figure 8.
One-year uncorrected visual acuity.

TABLE 3

LASIK: 3-Month Postoperative (N=45)

Complication Type	No. of Eyes
Dislocated or free flap	0
Epithelial ingrowth	0
Infection	0
Central islands	3
⇦Best corrected visual acuity with central islands	3

TABLE 4

PRK: 3-Month Postoperative (N=37)

Complication Type	No. of Eyes
Decentered ablation	0
Epithelialization problems	0
Infection	0
Central islands	21
⇦Best corrected visual acuity with central islands	10

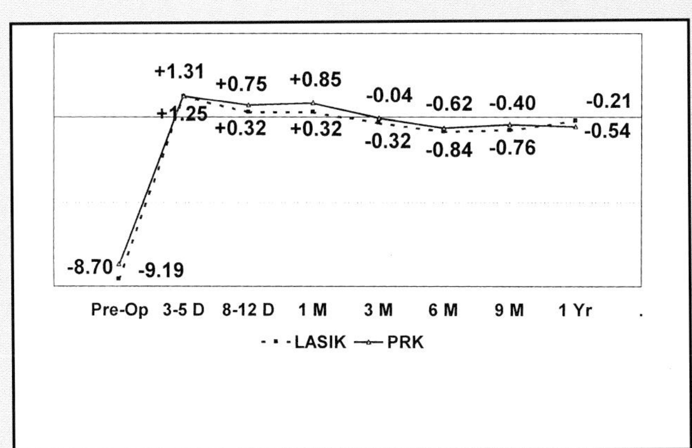

Figure 9.
Mean spherical equivalent vs time.

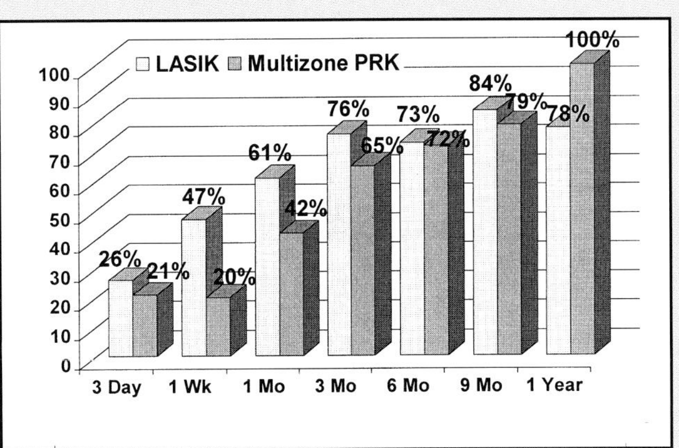

Figure 10.
Postoperative return to preoperative best corrected visual acuity.

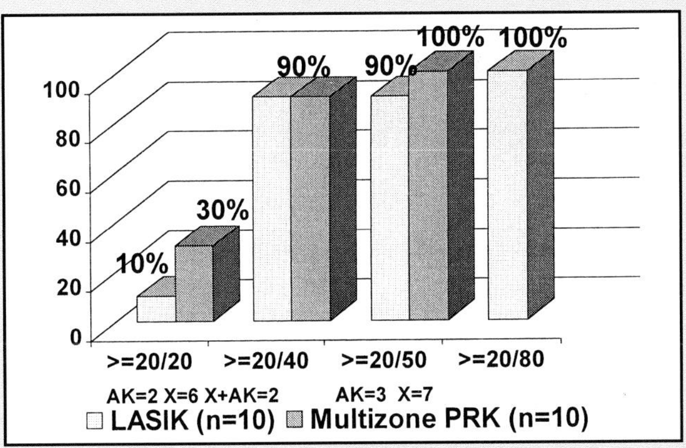

Figure 11.
Uncorrected visual acuity 1-month post-enhancement (100% returned to best corrected visual acuity ± 1 line).

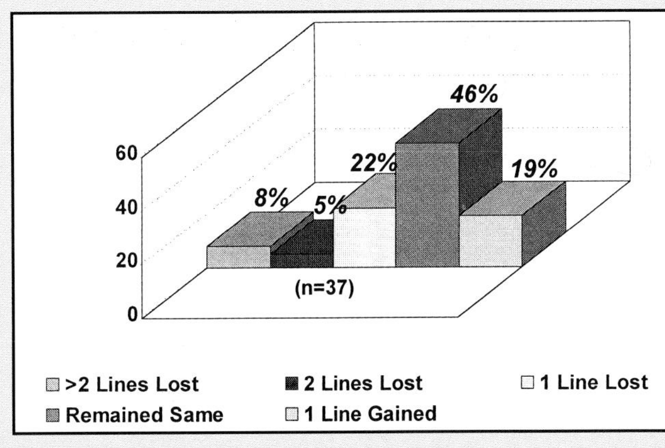

Figure 12.
Multizone PRK change in best corrected visual acuity at 3 months.

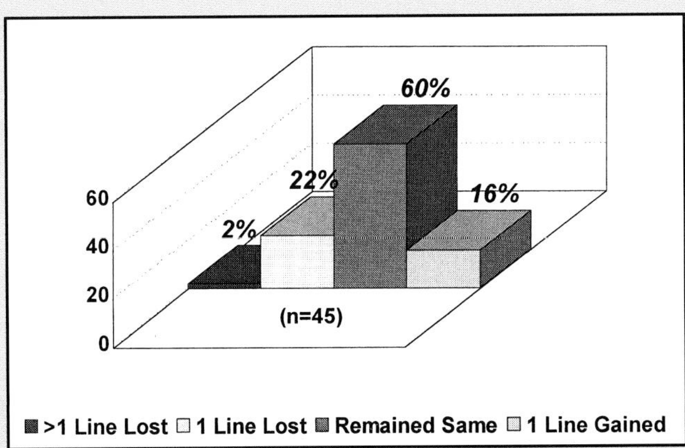

Figure 13.
LASIK change in best corrected visual acuity at 3 months.

TABLE 5

LASIK Patient Evaluation

Best Spectacle Corrected Visual Acuity **Best Corrected Visual Acuity/Central Islands**

Patient XX: LASIK 9-20-95, ReTx 6-25-96

Exam	*Best Corrected Visual Acuity*	*Best Spectacle Corrected Visual Acuity*	*Refraction*
Preop	CF3′	-12.00 +1.00 x 100°	20/20
3 to 5 days	20/50	-0.75 +1.00 x 105°	20/40
1 month	20/100	-2.25 +1.75 x 95°	20/25
3 months	20/80	-2.25 +1.75 x 90°	20/25
6 months	20/70	-2.50 +1.75 x 90°	20/25
9 months	20/100	-2.25 +2.00 x 90°	20/20
1 year	20/30	-0.75 +1.50 x 95°	20/20

TABLE 6

Mean Spherical Equivalent vs Time

LASIK			Multizone PRK	
Mean Sph Eq	*No.*	*Exam*	*No.*	*Mean Sph Eq*
-9.56	(n=56)	Preop	(n=44)	-8.7
1.25	(n=32)	1 to 5 days	(n=14)	1.31
0.32	(n=29)	1 week	(n=15)	0.75
0.32	(n=51)	1 month	(n=43)	0.85
-0.32	(n=43)	3 months	(n=37)	-0.04
-0.84	(n=28)	6 months	(n=29)	-0.62
-0.76	(n=19)	9 months	(n=19)	-0.40
-0.21	(n=9)	1 year	(n=9)	-0.54

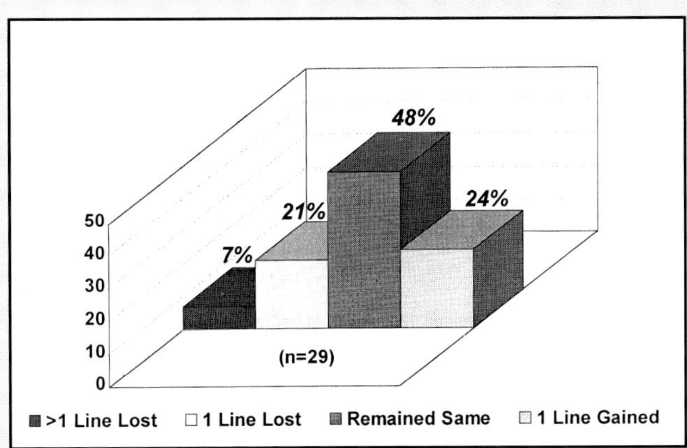

Figure 14.
Multizone PRK change in best corrected visual acuity at 6 months.

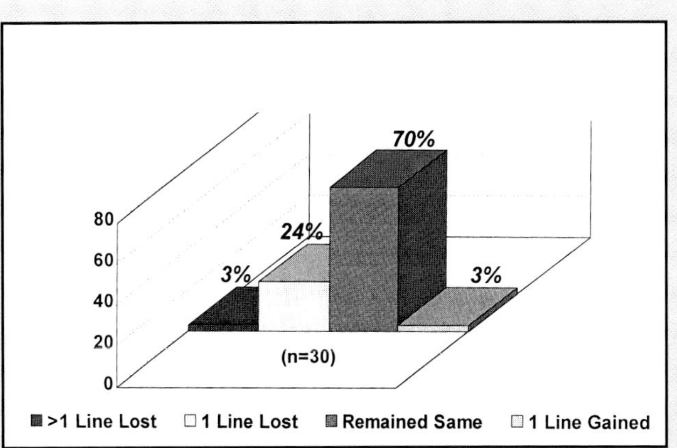

Figure 15.
LASIK change in best corrected visual acuity at 6 months.

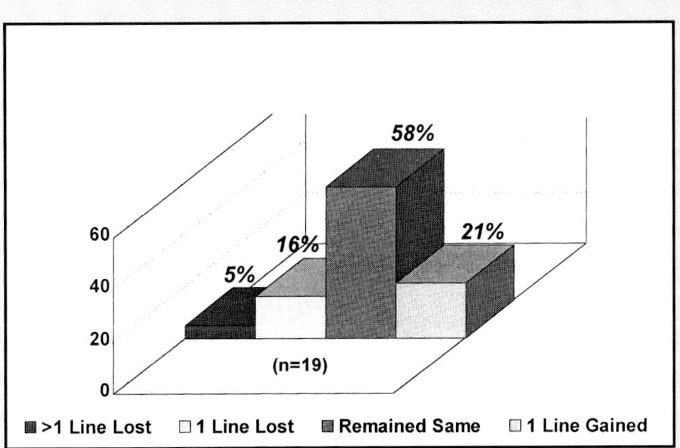

Figure 16.
Multizone PRK change in best corrected visual acuity at 9 months.

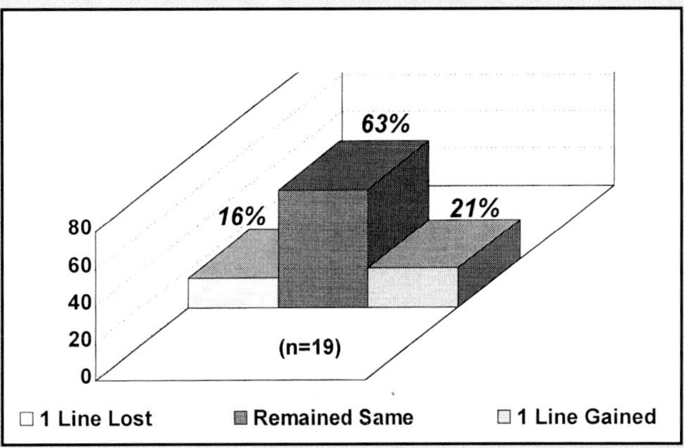

Figure 17.
LASIK change in best corrected visual acuity at 9 months.

TABLE 7

LASIK

Postoperative Period	Eyes With Central Islands
1 month (n = 49)	7 (14.3%)
3 months (n = 45)	3 (6.7%)
6 months (n = 30)	2 (6.7%)
9 months (n = 19)	0

TABLE 8

MULTIZONE PRK

Postoperative Period	Eyes With Central Islands
3 months (n = 37)	21 (56.8%)
6 months (n = 29)	10 (34.5%)
9 months (n = 19)	5 (26.3%)
1 year (n = 9)	3 (33.3%)

At 3 months, 52% of eyes with central islands had decreased best corrected visual acuity from preoperative status.

TABLE 9

LASIK 23% ENHANCEMENTS (N=56)

Postoperative Interval from Initial Tx	13 Eyes Enhanced	Type Enhancement
Range:	2 (15%)	LASIK and AK
9 to 11 months		Excimer (lifted flap)
12 to 14 months		AK
Range:	6 (46%)	LASIK ReTx
6 to 9 months		3 new flap, 3 lifted
Range:	5 (39%)	AK ReTx
1 day to 8 months		

TABLE 10

PRK 23% Enhancements (N=44)

Postoperative Interval from Initial Tx	10 Eyes Enhanced	Type Enhancement
7 to 9 months	7 (70%)	Excimer ReTx
6 to 15 months	3 (30%)	AK

Multicenter Data

TABLE 11

LASIK

Postoperative eyes	n = 106
Mean refractive error	-10.10 D
Range of myopia	-6.00 D to -22.63 D
Average age	38.04 years
Age range	21 to 64 years

TABLE 12

PRK (Multizone)

Postoperative eyes	n = 99
Mean refractive error	-9.28 D
Range of myopia	-6.00 D to -14.38 D
Average age	38.80 years
Age range	21 to 58 years

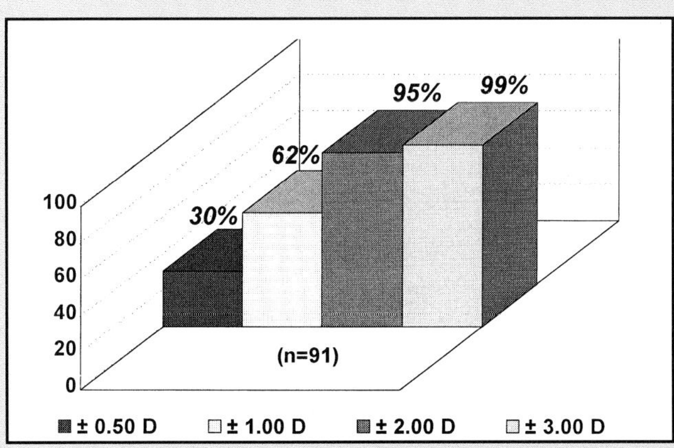

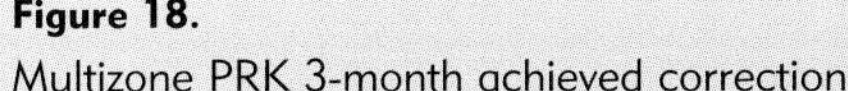

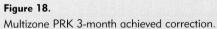

Figure 18.
Multizone PRK 3-month achieved correction.

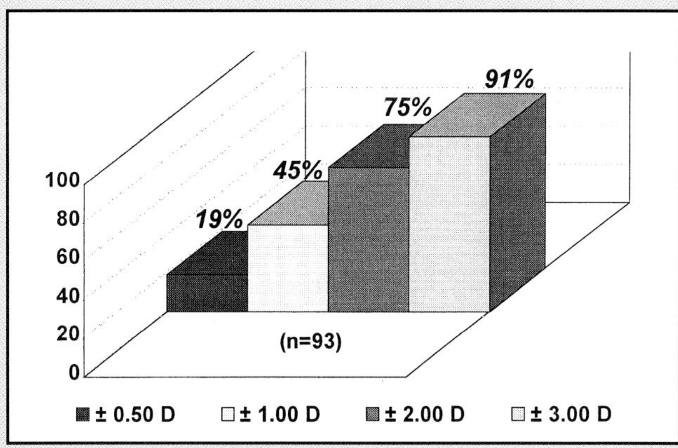

Figure 19.
LASIK 3-month achieved correction.

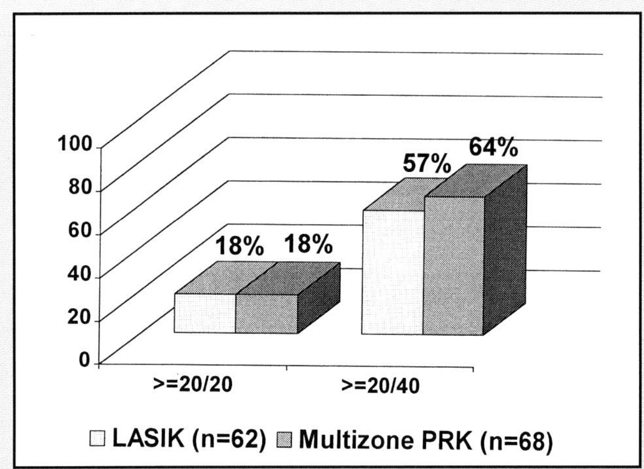

Figure 20.
Six-month uncorrected visual acuity.

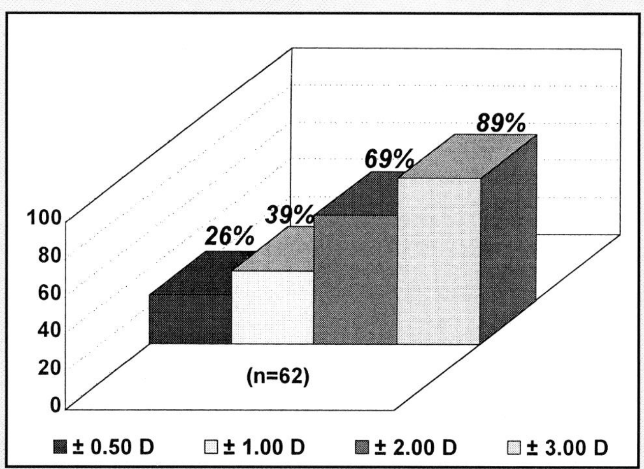

Figure 21.
LASIK 6-month achieved correction.

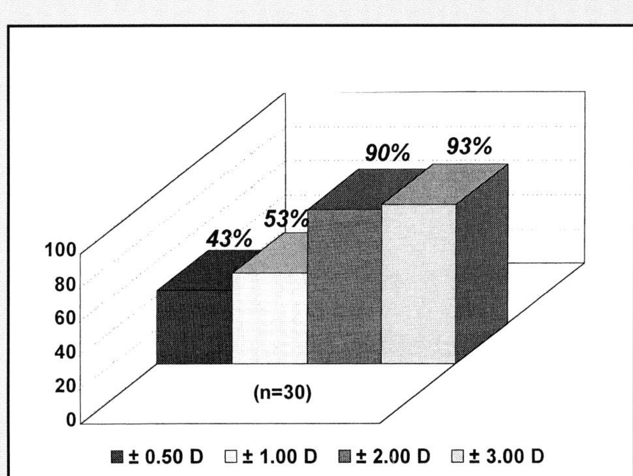

Figure 22.
Multizone PRK 1-year achieved correction.

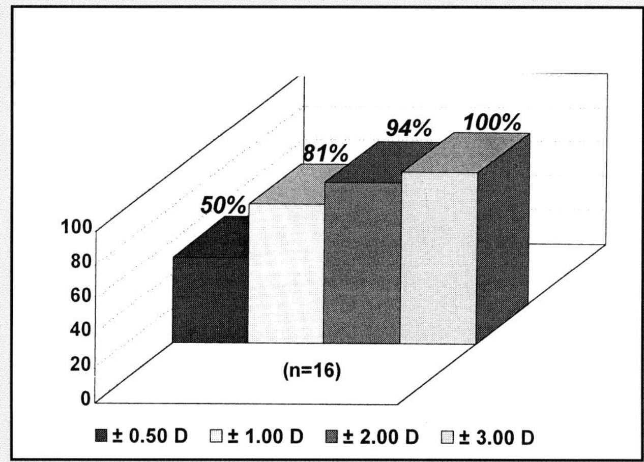

Figure 23.
LASIK 1-year achieved correction.

Chapter 17

LASIK: A COMPARISON WITH OTHER TECHNIQUES

Richard L. Lindstrom, MD

INTRODUCTION

Refractive surgery has undergone such a rapid gain in popularity that it some day could be as big as or bigger than cataract surgery is today in ophthalmology. A fax poll conducted in *Ocular Surgery News* stated that 62% of a small random sample of ophthalmologists said they intended to perform photorefractive keratectomy (PRK).[1] In 1994, an audience poll at the Pre-Academy meeting of the International Society of Refractive Surgery revealed that 97% intended to perform PRK.

Is it acceptable to perform refractive surgery as an ethical physician? I have debated this point with ophthalmologists who do not believe that refractive surgery is ethical and appropriate, but the word "handicap" helps place the issue in perspective. Ethical physicians should help patients overcome handicaps. During the Prospective Evaluation of Radial Keratotomy study (PERK) it was said that "The desire to have normal bodily function without dependence on external prosthetic devices is normal."

With that in mind, I have performed refractive surgery. But in the past 3 years, my own practice has undergone a tremendous transition in the preferred surgical technique to correct myopia. In 1995, radial keratotomy (RK) dominated my practice. The following year, PRK dominated. Now, we primarily perform laser in situ keratomileusis (LASIK).

PATIENT DEMOGRAPHICS

Much of the discussion about how many patients could benefit from myopic surgery has been inaccurate. First, consider that about half the population is emmetropic between -0.87 D and +0.87 D. There are many presbyopic patients, particularly now that the baby boomers are aging into their 40s; a good surgical option does not exist for this group. Interestingly enough, the smallest group of patients who need vision correction is the myopic group, particularly those with clinically significant myopia. Much of the analysis of the incidence and prevalence of myopia has not taken into account that the majority of myopes are between plano and -1 D. The lowest myope I have ever operated on was -1.50 D. So, nearly half of myopic patients fall outside the surgical range because they have so little myopia. About 18% of the population need between -1 D and -5 D, and it is with these low myopia patients that ophthalmologists make their bread and butter. Only about 3% of patients have between -5 D and -10 D. High and extreme myopia of greater than -10 D is relatively rare. Thus, the market is smaller than initially thought.[2]

The easiest way to analyze market size is by the number of patient eyes per thousand population. The average comprehensive ophthalmologist cares for 20,000 people. If you take an average of two eyes per thousand undergoing a refractive procedure, the average ophthalmologist taking care of his or her own patients could do about 40 eyes annually. By the year 2000, this will grow to compare with the rate of cataract surgery, which is six eyes per thousand. As the public educates itself, market penetration will increase. As patients continue to educate themselves about refractive procedures, they will become even more significant to our practices. Even at relatively low volumes, this can be important to the ophthalmologist. So, any comprehensive ophthalmologist with any interest at all should participate in refractive surgery. But, ophthalmologists should not buy their own excimer laser unless they can operate on between 750 and 1000 eyes annually.

MINI-RK AND PRK

Before discussing LASIK, it is important to understand the refractive techniques that led up to it and how each one can be used to correct refractive problems. I started performing RK with the PERK study in 1980. The 10-year data show that 53% of our patients are 20/20 and 85% are 20/40.[3] This means that 85% are legal to drive without glasses, and that seven out of 10 are independent of spectacles even 10 years after surgery.

However, there is less potential to treat high degrees of myopia because progressive hyperopic shift occurred. If surgeons performed about 1 million overly aggressive RKs in the 15 years from 1980 to 1995, the profession could have about 200,000 consecutive hyperopes to treat. And, if the average RK patient was 35 to 40 years old, now they are 45, presbyopic, hyperopic, and unhappy.

To correct this problem, I developed mini-RK to maximize corneal flattening with the minimum number and length of incisions to try and stay inside the range where we do not destabilize the cornea. We know that the way RK works is that you make some weakening incisions in the mid-periphery in a cornea that is steep peripherally to get a compensatory central flattening. I developed a concept that I call the zone of maximum benefit, a 2-mm zone between my smallest preferred optical zone of 3 mm and 7 mm.

When I perform mini-RK now, I can tell patients that I do not weaken their eye, and it is not more susceptible to trauma than a normal eye, based on two independent laboratory studies. In addition, we are starting to develop evidence that it may not be as susceptible to hyperopic shift. Mini-RK does not excessively weaken the eye, and it can be used in the low to moderate myopic group of patients. So, some RK is acceptable, even in the LASIK era.

The advent of the excimer laser for myopia led to PRK. I became involved with PRK quite early. However, while I used RK for 14 years in my practice, I relied on PRK for only 1 year for a variety of reasons. We can tell patients that about one in a thousand in the -1 D to -6 D range who undergo two treatments will have significant loss of vision from haze. Patients did not like the visual recovery period of between 3 and 6 months. About one in a thousand experienced infections.

In addition, we have not been successful treating higher levels of myopia with PRK. In our study of treating patients with more than -8 D, 12% of patients lost best corrected visual acuity. For PRK greater than 8 D of correction, only 30% of patients achieved 20/25 or better. Even our 1-year results showed a significant number of patients who had lost best corrected visual acuity. Some of these have since regained their visual acuity, and a few

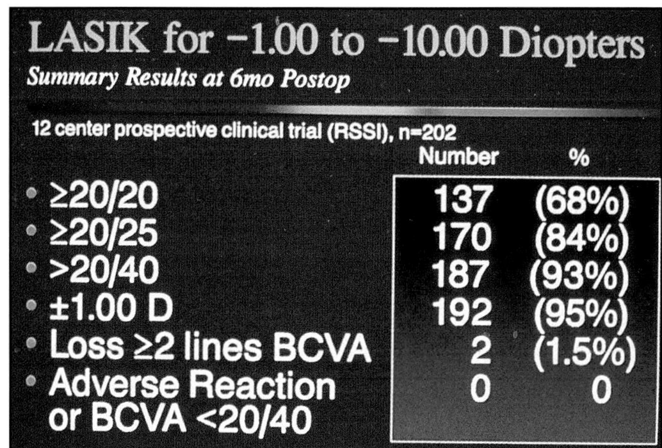

LASIK for -1.00 to -10.00 Diopters
Summary Results at 6mo Postop

12 center prospective clinical trial (RSSI), n=202

	Number	%
≥20/20	137	(68%)
≥20/25	170	(84%)
>20/40	187	(93%)
±1.00 D	192	(95%)
Loss ≥2 lines BCVA	2	(1.5%)
Adverse Reaction or BCVA <20/40	0	0

Figure 17-1.
LASIK for -1.00 D to -10.00 D.

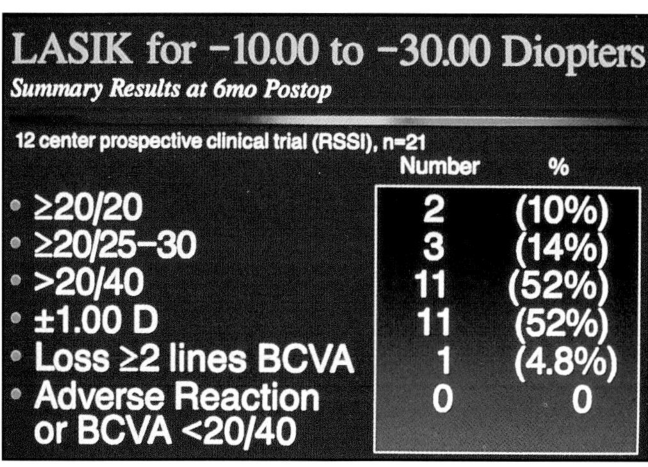

LASIK for -10.00 to -30.00 Diopters
Summary Results at 6mo Postop

12 center prospective clinical trial (RSSI), n=21

	Number	%
≥20/20	2	(10%)
≥20/25-30	3	(14%)
>20/40	11	(52%)
±1.00 D	11	(52%)
Loss ≥2 lines BCVA	1	(4.8%)
Adverse Reaction or BCVA <20/40	0	0

Figure 17-2.
LASIK for -10.00 D to -30.00 D.

who had significant hyperopia and haze for 3 or more years have corneas that have since cleared. Still, we were unhappy that so many patients were losing visual acuity and requiring so much reassurance time. Also, telling patients preoperatively that they had a one in 10 chance of losing vision was uncomfortable. When correcting up to 8 D of myopia, I perform PRK, but the data have led us to believe that correcting refractive errors between 8 D and 18 D requires lamellar surgery.

COMPARATIVE RESULTS OF MINI-RK, PRK, AND LASIK

About the same time we came to this conclusion, automated lamellar keratoplasty (ALK) resurged in popularity. Data from our first 289 cases showed that ALK was not competitive with RK and PRK for patients requiring less than 10 D of correction. Two years later, LASIK was developed by marrying lamellar refractive surgery to the excimer laser, which offered the advantage of removing tissue in the corneal bed instead of the surface.

LASIK is patient-friendly surgery that provides patients with rapid visual recovery with little or no pain. Unfortunately, it is surgeon-unfriendly because it requires expensive disposables and significant surgical skill. Nonetheless, patients are going to drive refractive surgeons from PRK to LASIK, and the data support that movement.

In a 12-site study of LASIK centers for between -1 D and -10 D of myopia, 68% of patients achieved 20/20 vision, 84% achieved 20/25, and 94% achieved 20/40 with less than 5% loss of best corrected visual acuity (Figures 17-1 and 17-2). This is reasonable data even in the extreme myopes, who are not all capable of 20/20 preoperatively.

In breaking down the data, we find that the competitive data sets of RK, PRK, and LASIK are comparable for low myopes between -1 D and -3.75 D. Any operation is appropriate for low myopes, so patient and surgeon preferences indicate which technique to use. However, I no longer offer my younger, moderately myopic (between -4 D and -6 D) patients the choice of RK unless it is an unusual and special situation. High myopia of between -6 D and -10 D is the frontier (Figures 17-3 through 17-6). Although the data from our investigation of LASIK are incomplete, we do have some interim results worth noting. The adverse reaction rate for LASIK begins to taper in moderate myopes between -4 D and -6 D, but RK and PRK are still equivalent. Of the LASIK patients, 0.5% lost best corrected visual acuity, mainly due to irregular astigmatism. Again, patient and surgeon preferences should dictate which procedure to use.

LASIK outperforms PRK for the high myopic patients between -6 D to -10 D. More patients achieve 20/20 and 20/40 vision with fewer patients losing best corrected visual acuity. Finally, for extreme refractive errors of -10 D to -30 D, LASIK is the only operation. Several LASIK studies have been performed. [4-12] A study on partially sighted eyes[7] found that four of eight eyes achieved within 1 D of intended correction at 6 months. A FDA study showed that 91% of patients achieved a best corrected

Low Myopia (−1.00 to −3.75D)

	PRK 1yr Lindstrom, n=28	Mini RK 1yr Lindstrom, n=47	LASIK 6mo Multictr, n=123
20/20	73%	76%	78%
20/25	91%	88%	87%
20/40	100%	100%	93%
±1.00D	97%	100%	98%
Loss ≥2 lines BCVA	0	0	0
Adv.Reaction (or BCVA <20/40)	0	0	0

Figure 17-3.
Low myopia (-1.00 D to -3.75 D).

Moderate Myopia (−4.00 to −6.00D)

	PRK 1yr Lindstrom, n=61	LASIK 1yr Lindstrom, n=177	Mini RK 6mo Multictr, n=53	ALK 6mo Multictr, n=97
20/20	73%	71%	64%	41%
20/25	85%	85%	76%	62%
20/40	99%	92%	100%	77%
±1.00D	92%	96%	87%	72%
Loss ≥2 lines BCVA	0.5%	0.6%	0%	5.2%
Adv.Reaction (or BCVA <20/40)	0	0	0	0

Figure 17-4.
Moderate myopia (-4.00 D to -6.00 D).

High Myopia (−6.25 to −10.00D)

	LASIK 6mo Multictr, n=25	PRK 1yr Lin, n=95	ALK 6mo Multictr, n=289
20/20	48%	39%	20%
20/25	76%	54%	37%
20/40	96%	86%	70%
±1.00D	88%	76%	56%
Loss ≥2 lines BCVA	4.0%	6.0%	5.9%
Adv.Reaction (or BCVA <20/40)	0	0	1.0%

Figure 17-5.
High myopia (-6.25 D to -10.00 D).

Extreme Myopia (−10.25 to −30.00D)

	LASIK 6mo Multicenter, n=21	ALK 6mo Lindstrom/Hardten n=168	PRK 1yr Linstrom–Taylor–Lins n=148
20/20	10%	11%	–%
20/25	24%	30%	–%
20/40	52%	62%	52%
±1.00D	52%	58%	54%
Loss ≥2 lines BCVA	4.8%	8.9%	13.5%
Adv.Reaction (or BCVA <20/40)	0%	1.2%	10%

Figure 17-6.
Extreme myopia (-10.25 D to -30.00 D).

visual acuity of 20/40 or better 6 months postoperatively.[9] Also, 71% of patients fell within 2 D of their intended correction 6 months postoperatively. A prospective single-center trial in Bogota, Colombia, found that 89% of patients achieved 1 D less of myopia or hyperopia 6 months postoperatively.[10] No eyes lost more than two lines of best corrected visual acuity at 6 months.

The Phillips Eye Institute conducted two prospective studies between March and November 1996. The first study had 101 eyes with between 0.75 D and 6 D of myopia with less than 1 D of astigmatism. The second had 98 eyes with high myopia of 6 D to 20 D with astigmatism of up to 4.5 D. In the low myopia group, 48% achieved 20/25 acuity and 90% achieved 20/40. One month postoperatively, 89% were within 1 D of emmetropia. For the high myopia group, 17% achieved 20/25 or better and 61% were 20/40 or better 1 day postoperatively, with 58 within 1 D of emmetropia. One month postoperatively, 35% achieved 20/25 acuity and 71% achieved 20/40 and 63% were within 1 D of emmetropia. Patients with less than 4 D myopia typically achieve 20/25 or better visual acuity 1 day postoperatively. Patients with up to 8 D of myopia typically achieve 20/40 or better 1 day postoperatively, while recovery takes longer with the higher myopes. Most patients will be slightly hyperopic on the first day. At 1 month they will fade 0.5 D and by 1 to 3 months they will fade another 0.5 D and stabilize.

ADVANTAGES OF LASIK

LASIK is easier to learn than phacoemulsification. It has a shorter learning curve and a lower complication rate. At the Phillips Eye Institute, surgeons who performed 1500 microkeratome passes experienced only a 1% complication rate. This is a lower complication rate than with phaco. In comparison with LASIK, every PRK every case is complicated. Each one has an epithelial defect, and sometimes significant haze. With LASIK, these would be major complications.

Patients are more comfortable postoperatively because LASIK induces less pain than PRK. LASIK is the only operation that can safely be performed bilaterally, because it is the only operation that offers visual recovery within a few hours. Bilateral RK was too unpredictable, but bilateral LASIK is predictable to within ±0.75 D.

Also, enhancements are easy and can be done 1 month postoperatively with LASIK, whereas PRK requires 1 year or more of healing because the cornea is still remodeling. LASIK enhancements run less than 5%, so I tell patients that 95 out of 100 patients achieve good results and the rest can undergo enhancement as early as 1 month.

ISSUES FOR DISCUSSION

There are a few disadvantages to LASIK. As mentioned previously, LASIK requires more skill. Extreme myopes of greater than -15 D are poorer candidates because if the cornea flattens too much patients lose vision. Patients with thin corneas and keratoconus are poor candidates because of the difficulties of attaching the suction ring. However, these are concerns with any refractive surgery.

LASIK requires more expensive equipment, but it is more cost-effective in terms of surgeon time. PRK requires an average of six postoperative visits of 10 to 15 minutes, while LASIK requires an average of two 5-minute visits. Cataracts require a 30- to 60-minute preoperative exam and 10 to 20 minutes of surgery. On average that calculates out to 1.5 hours of work for $1000 reimbursement. Reductions in the practice expense reimbursement component of Medicare could lower this to $500 by 1998. PRK has the same amount of pre- and postoperative work, and requires spending more reimbursement time with patients. It works out, on average, to 2.5 hours of work for $1000. Bilateral LASIK needs the same amount of preoperative and surgical time, but it is a more stable and complication-free procedure that reduces the amount of follow-up required. So, 1.5 hours of work can reap $2000. This is the most lucrative surgery per unit time in ophthalmology.

Before taking up LASIK in their practices, surgeons should consider some technical and regulatory aspects of the procedure. First, the FDA has not approved the procedure, except as mentioned previously. Second, the laser and microkeratome require training. Third, surgeons should participate in a clinical trial with one of the investigational groups underway.

Also, the FDA and Federal Trade Commission have issued marketing guidelines that restrict advertising and the claim that LASIK is better than other procedures.[13] Next, although performing LASIK under the auspices of an investigational review board is not required for collecting informed consent and data, that is the ideal route to follow. Finally, your insurance carrier needs to be told that you are performing LASIK, and if the company will not cover you then you need to find one that will.

CONCLUSION

Mini-RK is an acceptable treatment for low and occasionally moderate patients, and PRK and LASIK help the low, moderate, and high myopes. LASIK represents the future for high and extreme myopia and may well push on down into the moderate and low myopia as well. The FDA has approved the investigational device exemption (IDE) of CRS-USA Inc allowing any surgeon willing to invest in the study the ability to perform LASIK within the confines of an approved IDE.[14] And, on July 11, 1997, the FDA ophthalmic devices panel recommended for approval with conditions a LASIK software package and nomogram developed by Drs. George O. Waring III, Keith Thompson, and R. Doyle Stulting, all of the Emory Eye Center in Atlanta, Ga.[15]

Ophthalmologists have asked me if I promote LASIK too aggressively. I do, because LASIK is worth learning about. I trained as an intracapsular cataract surgeon who learned extracapsular techniques within a year of completing my residency. By 1978, I had embraced phaco. LASIK represents the same type of advance. And once again, ethical physicians should help patients overcome handicaps, because the desire to function without depending on prosthetic devices is normal. LASIK is good for the patient, good for the surgeon, and a driving force in today's refractive market.

References

1. FaxPoll. *Ocular Surgery News*. 1995;13:13.
2. McCarty CA, Livingston PM, Taylor HR. Prevalence of myopia in adults: implications for refractive surgeons. *J Refract Surg*. 1997;13:229-234.
3. Waring GO, Lynn MJ, McDonnell PJ, the PERK Study Group. Results of the Prospective Evaluation of Radial Keratotomy (PERK) study 10 years after surgery. *Arch Ophthalmol*. 1994;112:1298-1308.
4. Salah T, Waring GO III, El Maghraby A, Moadel K, Grimm S. Excimer laser in situ keratomileusis under a corneal flap for myopia of 2 to 20 diopters. *Am J Ophthalmol*. 1996;121:143-155.
5. Buratto L. Excimer laser intrastromal keratomileusis: case reports. *J Cataract Refract Surg*. 1992;18:37-41.
6. Buratto L, Ferrari M, Genisi C. Myopic keratomileusis with the excimer laser: one year follow-up. *Refract Corneal Surg*. 1993;9:12-19.
7. Siganos DS, Pallikaris IG. Laser in situ keratomileusis in partially sighted eyes. ASCRS abstracts. 1993.
8. Ferrari M, Buratto L. Intrastromal keratomileusis with the excimer laser (Buratto's technique). ASCRS abstracts. 1993.
9. Slade SG, Brint SF. Initial clinical results of FDA phase 1 multicenter study of keratomileusis using the Summit UV 100 LA excimer laser. ASCRS presentation, 1994.
10. Ruiz L, Slade SG, Updegraff SA. Excimer myopic keratomileusis: Bogota experience. In: Salz JJ, ed. *Corneal Laser Surgery*. St. Louis, Mo: Mosby-Year Book Inc; 1995:195.
11. Liu JC, McDonald MB, Varnell R, Angotti HA. Myopic excimer laser photorefractive keratectomy: an analysis of clinical correlations. *Refract Corneal Surg*. 1990;6:321-328.
12. Lindstrom RL, Chu YR, Hartden DR. An evaluation of the efficacy, safety and predictability of laser in situ keratomileusis (LASIK) in the treatment of low, moderate and high myopia. American Ophthalmological Society abstract. 1997.
13. Throw away your...ad campaign. *Ocular Surgery News*. 1996;18:12-13.
14. NewsFlash: physician-led company gets IDE for LASIK. *Ocular Surgery News*. 1996;21.
15. Intelligence report: FDA panel conditionally approves Emory's LASIK package. *Ocular Surgery News*. 1997;July 21.

Chapter 18

LASIK FOR THE CORRECTION OF HYPEROPIA

Patrick I. Condon, MCh, FRCOphth, Till Anschuetz, MD, Klaus Ditzen, MD, Jose L. Güell, MD, Michael C. Knorz, MD

LASIK, or laser in situ keratomileusis, for hyperopia involves the cutting of a superficial lamellar flap of cornea involving the epithelium, Bowman's membrane, and a 160-µm thick flap of anterior stroma with a microkeratome exactly the same way as for myopia. This is followed by excimer laser ablation of the peripheral part of the underlying stroma. It is different from the ablation profile produced in myopia in that minimal ablation occurs in the center of the cornea.

ANESTHESIA

While topical application of 0.4% Oxybuprocaine, 0.5% tetracaine (amethocaine), or an equal mixture of 4% Xylocaine and 0.5% Marcaine may be used on their own, the relatively small hyperopic eye together with small palpebral aperture may make it extremely difficult for the vacuum ring and the microkeratome to fit to the globe and may even precipitate a sudden loss of vacuum during the passing of the microkeratome across the cornea. This could result in the potentially disastrous complication of an excessively thin flap, which may result in scarring and irregular astigmatism, and the need for a corneal graft at a later stage. In smaller eyes, therefore, it is essential to propose the eye forward by giving a retrobulbar injection of 5 cc of 2% Xylocaine using a longer needle and depositing the bulk of fluid as far back in the orbit as possible. This helps to avoid the tracking forward of fluid anteriorly with perilimbal conjunctival chemosis, which can

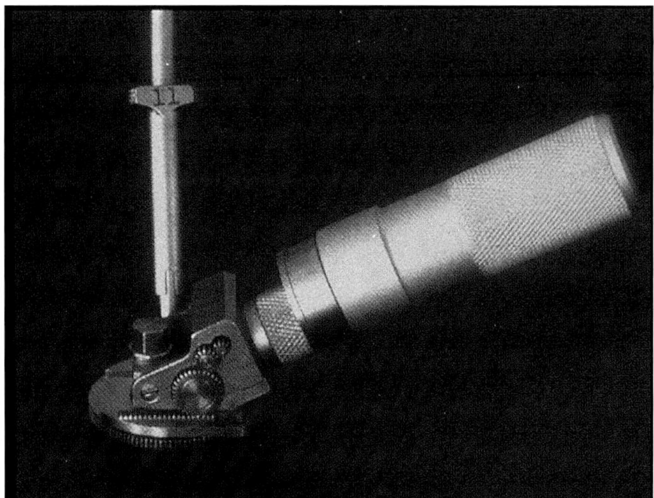

Figure 18-1.
The Automated Corneal Shaper is used to perform LASIK.

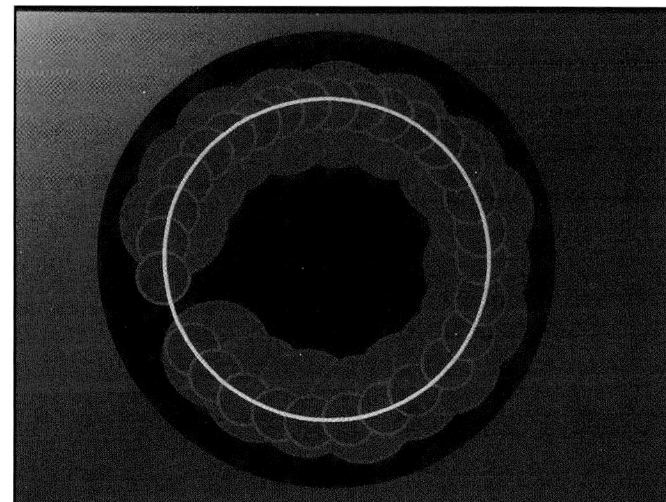

Figure 18-2.
Annular ablation profile used to correct hyperopia. The ablation is concentrated in a donut shaped ring extending from 4.5 to 9 mm from the center of the cornea (Chiron).

result in blockage of the suction part of the vacuum ring and may prevent an adequate rise in IOP necessary for an accurate flap cut. In order to prevent this from occurring, verification of the IOP with the tonometer after the vacuum ring has been fixed to the eye, but before the microkeratome cut is performed, cannot be overemphasized. Preoperative topical 4% pilocarpine is useful to counteract the mydriasis which may occur with a retrobulbar injection and may confuse the antitracking devices of the laser, some of which depend on the presence of a normal pupil with which they retain centration. One author (PC) has found the use of a Nevyas speculum (Katena) to augment the proptopic effect of the retrobulbar injection helpful, while another (KD) prefers not to use any speculum but hold the eyelids apart manually while applying the vacuum.

MICROKERATOME

Any of the available microkeratomes can be used for making the flap cut. Apart from a few cases in which the lamellar rotor microkeratome by Storz Ophthalmics (St. Louis, Mo) was used, and the Barraquer-Krumeich instrument by TA, all cases carried out utilized the Chiron Automated Corneal Shaper with a 160-µm plate and hinge stop (Figure 18-1). The microkeratome is fitted to the cornea with the LASIK-designed fixed vacuum ring which results in a 9.0- to 9.5-mm diameter flap suitable for hyperopia. On no account should the adjustable vacuum ring used for ALK be used as it only gives a maximum size flap of 7.5- to 8.0-mm diameter, which is unsuitable for LASIK hyperopia.

The corneal flap is then displaced nasally with a blunt spatula.

EXCIMER LASER ABLATION

The ablation profile for hyperopia is completely different from that of myopia in that the tissue is ablated from the periphery of the stroma underlying the flap in a donut-type configuration. By ablating this annular zone of the paracentral cornea, the central cornea is steepened and the refractive power of the central corneal increased.

The lasers used were the Aesculap-Meditec MEL 60 and the Chiron Keracor 116. The Meditec (PC, KD, TA) utilized a linear scanning technique, the eye being fixated by a horseshoe-shaped suction ring to accommodate the nasally reflected hinged flap. Chiron Keracor 116 (JG, MK) employed a circular scanning beam which traversed the cornea in a circular manner (Figure 18-2). In the case of the Aesculap-Meditec, the resulting donut-shaped ablation extended from 5 to 7.5 mm from the center of the cornea. The Chiron produced a similarly shaped ablation zone extending form 4.5 to 9 mm into the periphery of the cornea. A scanning electron microscopy (SEM) scan of a porcine cornea treated with the hyperopia software of the Keracor 116 is shown in Figure 18-3.

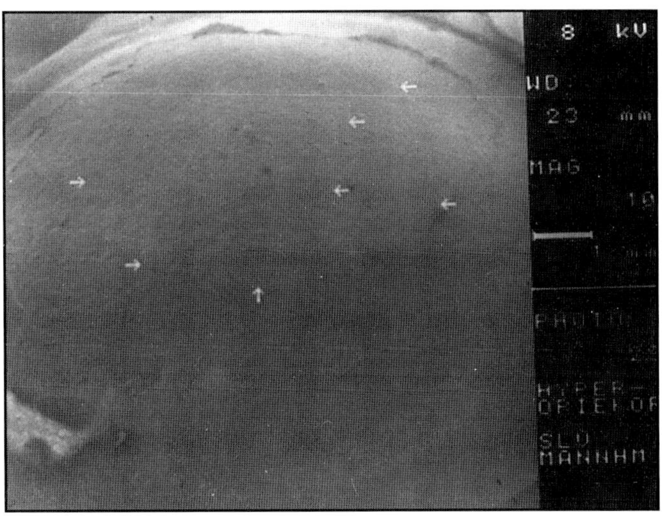

Figure 18-3.
SEM of porcine cornea after hyperopia ablation. The edges of the central optical zone (4.5 mm) and of the ablation zone (9 mm) are outlined by arrows (Knorz).

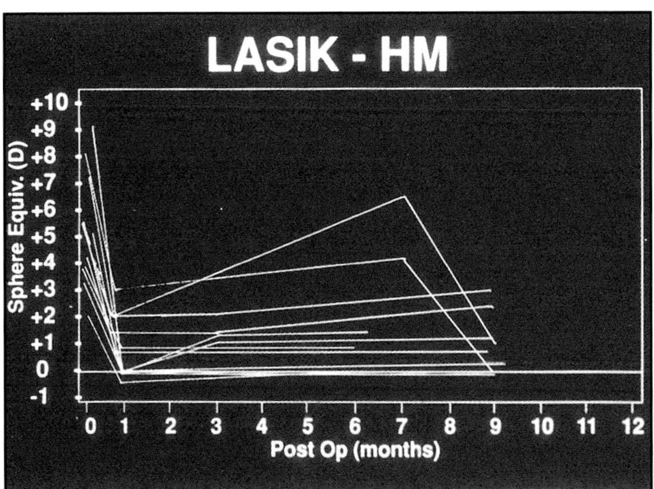

Figure 18-4.
Results in 10 cases treated with the Aesculap-Meditec laser showing immediate effective response followed by a regressive period with retreatment of two eyes successfully at 7 months (Condon).

Because of the need for accurate centration of hyperopic excimer laser ablation, the benefits of the vacuum ring for fixation of the eye with the Aesculap-Meditec system were considered an advantage. However, the use of the active autotracker system of the Chiron was considered to be most effective and was utilized in all cases treated with the Keracor.

Protection of the hinge from aberrant laser exposure was prevented during treatment by shielding the base of the flap with a spatula. Dissipation of foreign body fragments into the operation site were found to be a possible complication of the use of a Merocel sponge to protect the flap during laser treatment. It has been recently found that the use of ordinary transparent glass can be used to shield the flap and at the same time monitor the flap behavior during treatment. This will protect the flap from damage by the laser.

In order to avoid undercorrections, the stroma was maintained in a completely dry state during laser treatment and any excess of water into the treatment area was immediately wiped away while the laser was in progress.

Repositioning of the Corneal Flap

The maneuver is exactly the same as in myopic LASIK. However, because of the increased curvature of the hyperopic treated cornea, there is an increased danger of cap displacement and greater attention should be paid to replacement of the flap. In order to avoid the ingress of foreign material to the interface preoperatively, with subsequent trapping of conjunctival and eyelid debris postoperatively, the hinged corneal flap is washed extensively by flushing with BSS while simultaneously using suction to rapidly remove the excess fluid from the area. Whereas one author (PC) prefers to replace the heavily hydrated flap onto a dry stromal bed in order to encourage adherence of the flap, others irrigate the stromal bed with BSS in an effort to remove any contaminated foreign material that may have inadvertently been introduced onto the surface. The flap is then either brushed back into place with a wet Merocel sponge or rolled from beneath with a fine Rycrofts attached to a syringe. The eye is then allowed to dry for 2 minutes in order to allow the flap to adhere. Two drops of 50% diluted aqueous solution of Betadine as a disinfectant and gentamicin as an antibiotic are then instilled topically into the conjunctival sac and the speculum gently removed from the eye without disturbing the flap. Postoperatively topical antibiotics are used for 5 days but corticosteroids are also occasionally used when there is aggravation of preexisting blepharitis induced by the local trauma of the operative procedure.

RESULTS

Aesculap-Meditec MEL 60

Ten eyes ranging from 2 D to 9 D (average: 5.25 D)

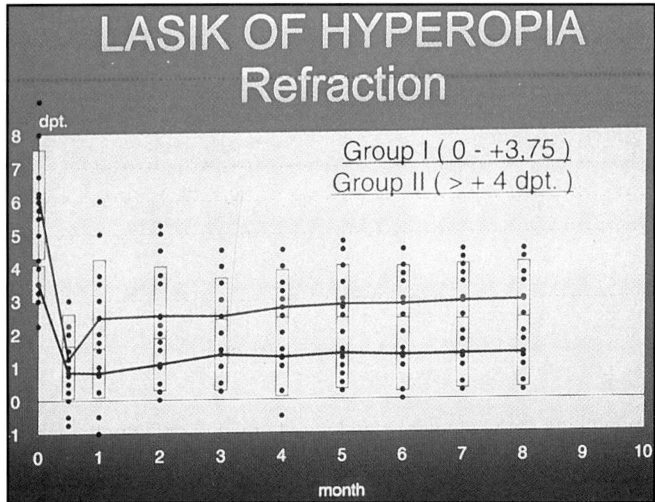

Figure 18-5.
Mean results in two groups 0 to 3.75 D and 4.0 D and above showing decreased effectiveness of treatment in the higher refractive error group (Ditzen).

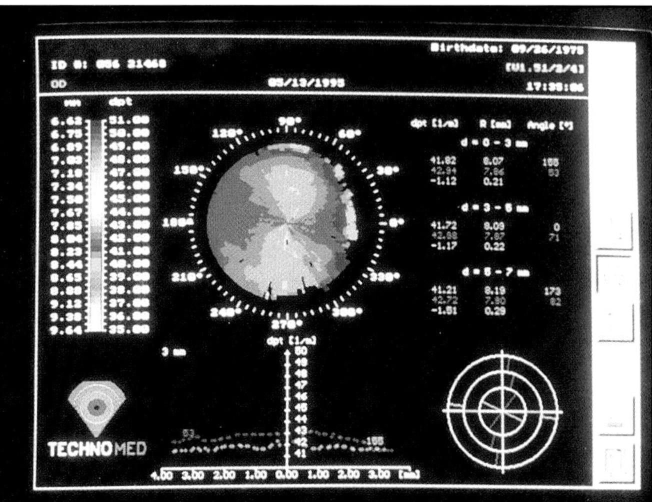

Figure 18-6.
Preoperative topography with Technomed C Scan of eye with 9 D error (Condon).

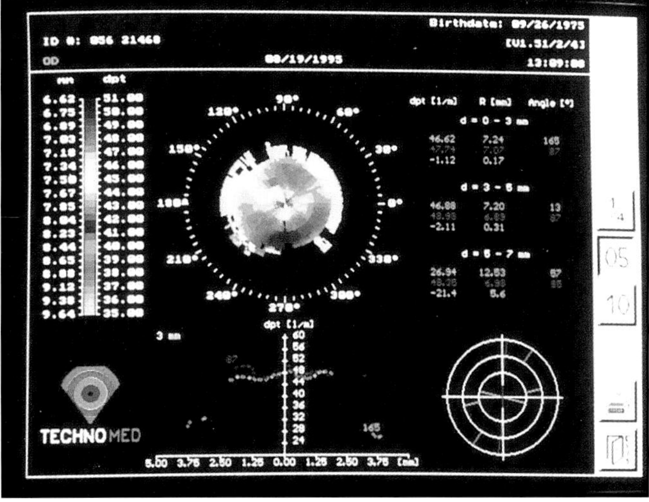

Figure 18-7.
Postoperative topography with Technomed C Scan of eye resulting plano correction. This resulting correction and topographical appearance have shown no change over a 9-month period (Condon).

(PC), 41 eyes ranging from 2.5 D to 7 D (average: 4.8 D) (KD), and 11 eyes ranging from 4 D to 10 D were treated. Treatment was followed by an immediate improvement which lasted 2 to 4 weeks (Figure 18-4) and was followed by a regressive trend more obvious with preoperative correction greater than 4 D (Figure 18-5) (KD). Average correction achieved at 6 months was 1.5 D (PC) and 2.5 D (KD). Regression occurred more commonly in the higher degrees of hyperopia and was a mean of 0.7 D in the 4 D to 6 D group as compared to a mean of 2.0 D in the 7 D to 10 D group (TA). Two eyes with 7 D and 9 D preoperatively that were initially undercorrected and who regressed to 5 D and 3 D, respectively, were retreated and achieved a final correction of plano and 1 D, respectively (PC).

Chiron Keracor 116

Eighteen eyes ranging from 2.25 D to 9 D (average: 6.21 ± 2.25 sphere; -1.79 ± 1.86 cyl) (JG) were treated. Average correction achieved at 3 months was 1.9 ± 1.8 sphere, -0.33 ± 0.58 cyl (JG). In the five eyes out of 11 that were followed up for a 6-month period, the average was 0.2 D. In the 11 eyes ranging from 2.5 D to 8 D (average: 6.6 D) treated by MK, five of which were followed up 12 to 14 months postoperatively, the mean postoperative refraction was 0.5 D.

Visual Acuity

Uncorrected visual acuity 6 months after surgery was comparable to the preoperative values with correction in most cases. Three eyes lost one line of visual acuity (MK) and two eyes lost two lines of visual acuity (TA). In the larger series of 41 cases (KD), 50% of eyes had an unchanged visual acuity result, 39% improved, and 11% were worse, 7% losing one line and 5% two lines of visual acuity. This was due to a combination of flap problems ranging from epithelial ingrowth and interface debridement with or without associated flap displacement to postoperative problems.

Corneal Topography

The remarkable change in contour of the cornea can be easily visualized in Figures 18-6 and 18-7 which have comparable color scales and illustrate the central steepening of the cornea achieved LASIK in a patient with 9 D preoperatively and who achieved a plano correction postoperatively. The steepening causes an increase in dioptric power which is expressed by the red colors on the color map, which is also confirmed by the contour map in the vertical scale. It is also interesting to note that no astigmatism has been induced by the treatment and the subsequent topographic tests showed no change in this eye. The second eye of this patient has since been treated with a similar result, the first eye showing no regression or change over a 9-month postoperative period.

Subjective Symptoms

Subjective symptoms of glare and halos around lights at night, which were more common in the immediate postoperative period, were considered to be due to settlement of the corneal interface, settled within a period of 3 months. The relative lack of symptoms 6 to 9 months postoperatively when compared to PRK patients is probably related to the size of the central optical zone, which measures 4.5 mm in diameter and is larger than the entrance pupil, and the fact that the central steepening effect is well-centered with reference to the entrance pupil.

Complications

In general there were few complications, undercorrections and regression being the main ones, which would be expected with a new procedure and using PRK algorithms. Retreatments by lifting the flap and retreating the stroma were carried out 3 months postoperatively in two eyes for undercorrections and in one case a marked regression to the original preoperative refraction of 7 D. In one patient with 9 D preoperative error, dislocation of the flap occurred in the first 24 hours which necessitated resuturing with two 10-0 nylon sutures which stabilized it completely, allowing it to heal. Despite the presence of two cap stress lines across the cornea in line with these suture positions, the resultant visual acuity of 20/20 unaided and no significant refractive error was most satisfactory.

SUMMARY

LASIK for hyperopia is a relatively new technique. A total of 91 eyes were treated with the Aesculap-Meditec MEL 60 and Chiron Keracor 116 lasers. Apart from one flap dislocation, which achieved excellent vision with resuturing the flap, there were no significant complications. Loss of visual acuity of two lines varied from 5% (KD) to 18% (TA) and was mainly due to preoperative difficulties encountered with the flap at surgery and interface opacities of debris and epithelial ingrowth postoperatively. Whereas the reversal of hyperopia was immediate, a number of eyes were undercorrected and regression occurred in some of the higher hyperopic eyes. This was reasonable to expect in view of the algorithms used which were designed for surface PRK. Adjustments are currently being made to counteract this problem and more accurate algorithms are being designed. In comparison with the relatively poor results on PRK for hyperopia reported, results to date with LASIK showed it to be a more reliable technique, which may be related to the placing of the ablation at a deeper level in the cornea. Further evaluation will have to continue before LASIK can be classified as a definitive treatment for hyperopia.

Chapter 19

LASIK: THE LATIN EXPERIENCE

Antonio Mendez Noble, MD,
Antonio Mendez G., MD

INTRODUCTION

I started with lamellar refractive surgery in 1990 under the supervision of Drs. Tito Ramirez, Raul Suarez, and Enrique Graue in Mexico City with keratomileusis in situ, or KMIS. At this time, KMIS was evolving very fast going from a five-point anti-torch suture to a suture that did not penetrate the cap and finally to a sutureless flap. The equipment evolved, too. Electric motors changed, turbines fine-tuned, and from a manual pass to the automated lamellar keratoplasty. Through all this time the refractive cut, the second pass, was always unpredictable. Blade quality is still one of the most important factors of this unpredictability. The edge of the blade has to be exactly at the right angle of attack, and this has to be maintained on every production line. Remember, we were removing microns out of the cornea mechanically.

Gaining access to an excimer laser in August 1993, and recognizing its advantages in regard to the precision of a refractive correction (and the refractive stability and rapid rehabilitation in patients with KMIS on the other hand), the combination of both procedures came naturally and was inevitable. In September 1993, we performed our first laser in situ keratomileusis (LASIK) procedure. We started initially with high myopic patients, moved to high hyperopia, and soon started treating moderate and low myopia and hyperopia. The rapid visual rehabilitation of the patients, low dependence of steroids, absence of haze, preservation of Bowman's layer, and shorter follow-up were great advantages. Currently, we perform LASIK on almost all our patients. The low percentage who are not being treated with LASIK have undergone conductive keratoplasty (low hyperopia) with the MCS unit (Refratec Inc).

SITES AND EQUIPMENT

We are currently working in two sites in Baja California, Tijuana and Mexicali, Mexico, using an Aesculap-Meditec MEL 60 excimer laser in each office and two Chiron ALK Systems per site, and also using the Moria (Microtech) at the Tijuana office. It is very important to have more than one microkeratome accessible because of the possibility of breakdown or necessary maintenance.

The Aesculap-Meditec MEL 60 excimer laser is a scanning laser that uses computer-driven motorized masks that fit over the eye, fixated with a suction ring. The mask is computer-driven and controls the pattern of ablation of the corneal tissue as it rotates (Myopia II and Hyperopia masks) or opens and closes (Myopia I and III masks). Four different masks may be used in LASIK depending on the treatment required:

- Myopia I—Corrects myopic spherical component.
- Myopia II—Corrects a combination of myopia and astigmatism.
- Myopia III—For the correction of minus cylinder.
- Hyperopia—Corrects a combination of hyperopia and hyperopic astigmatism.

The excimer laser's suction ring is also designed specially for LASIK. Suction is present only in three quarters of the ring. The primary function of the remaining quarter of the suction ring is to hold the flap in place away from the ablation area. No suction is required in this area; the edges of the suction ring are smooth so that the flap is not damaged.

TECHNIQUE

Patient Preparation

We premedicate our patients with 5 mg of Valium 30 minutes before the procedure. The patient is given a facial wash with iodine solution. Wearing a cap and gown, the patient is taken and placed under the excimer laser. The eye that is not going to be treated is closed with Transpore (3M) tape. A disposable plastic drape (40 X 40 cm) with fenestration is placed over the patient's face. Transpore tape is used to separate and open the patient's eyelids; the objective being to keep the eyelashes away from the surgical area and to have a large comfortable surgical area.

I use a Barraquer wire speculum, and place it over the taped eyelids. I have found that this combination of taped lids with a simple wire speculum works very well. The patient feels comfortable, and I have a large enough area to do my procedure—no need for bulky specula.

Procedure

I believe that marking is very important. The mark should:

- Help you to determine which side is the epithelium side in case of a free cap.
- Assist you in determining the patient's visual axis.
- Indicate where to place the microkeratome suction ring in order to have a large enough area to produce the ablation.
- Give you enough guide for perfect apposition of the flap.

For all these reasons I have designed a marker that consists of four lines: three help determine the visual axis, the vertical marks align with the suction ring handle for proper centration of the flap with the ablation, and the fourth line helps in case a free cap is obtained to determine which is the epithelium side.

The microkeratome has already been assembled and checked. The microkeratome suction ring is placed over the patient's eye while the middle and index finger of the other hand hold the wire speculum down to protrude the globe. Once good suction is obtained, the IOP is checked with the Barraquer tonometer, a couple of drops of BSS are placed over the cornea, and the microkeratome pass is made.

The flap has to be centered on the visual axis and not on the anatomical center of the cornea. If the flap is not centered on the visual axis, the hinge may be in the way of the excimer laser when the ablation takes place. This may induce irregular astigmatism, especially when working with a large optical center or in hyperopic patients. The flap may look decentered anatomically, but the first cut is not a refractive cut. The patient will have much better vision if the hinge of the flap is not ablated.

I use a McFerson's forceps to find the groove and lift

the flap. I have designed a forceps for LASIK (Mendez Jr. LASIK Forceps, Katena Instruments) and use it closed to find the groove and lift the flap. The same forceps is used to mark the visual axis with a very light depression. Once the flap is lifted, it is very hard for the patient to determine the position of the fixation light with the same precision as before lifting the flap. The mark from Mendez Jr. Marker (Katena Instruments) helps confirm that the patient is still at the right position for the ablation. An imaginary line is drawn between the vertical and one of the horizontal lines. The intersection shows the visual axis. Care has to be taken after lifting the flap that no liquid goes into the corneal stroma. The liquid will be absorbed almost immediately by the stroma and produce corneal swelling. The ablation over this area may induce irregular astigmatism.

The excimer laser's suction ring is placed over the patient's eye, taking special care in centration. The programmed refraction of the patient is checked in the computer of the excimer laser before starting the ablation.

During the ablation we must make sure that the patient does not move and keeps centered. Homogeneity in the surface being ablated is very important since the laser copies the surface. If any detritus-like filaments appear during the ablation, you must stop and remove them or the laser will not ablate under the particles, producing an irregularity. Another important factor is humidity. As the tissue evaporates, water is formed in the ablated area thus producing irregularity in the rate of ablation. The Aesculap-Meditec MEL 60 excimer laser has a built-in aspirator in the suction ring. This maintains a humidity-controlled area, but if the aspiration is too high, dryness of the cornea may be the cause of overcorrection.

Once the ablation is finished, thorough cleaning of the interface is important. The assistant irrigates with BSS. During this procedure aspiration is done through an 18-gauge cannula connected to an aspirator being held in one hand and a microsponge in the other. With this procedure the area is eliminated of floating particles and other detritus, loosened with the microsponge, and aspirated through the cannula. Aided by the same microsponge, the flap is replaced over a bed of solution. The flap is not touched any more. Using the tip of the cannula that is connected to the aspirator, the solution in the interface is eliminated when the tip is placed in the groove. The flap will stick into place immediately. I check that the four lines are aligned and wait 2 minutes before removing the speculum and the tapes. It is a good idea to lubricate the epithelium at this moment. The adherence of the flap does not seem to be affected by this extra humidity.

No more than 3 cc of BSS should be irrigated to the stroma or flap. It is not necessary to induce much pressure during the irrigation. The washing movements that are done with the microsponge should also be gentle. If these simple rules are not followed, it is my experience that generalized infiltrates may appear the next day in the interface and worsen by third day in susceptible patients. Prednisolone 1% every 2 to 3 hours tends to remedy these cases usually by the first week.

Sterility is one important factor as in any surgery performed on the eye. We do LASIK under sterile conditions. We sterilize the microkeratome head for every patient. The excimer laser is placed in a surgical suite.

Postoperative Management

I use one drop of diclofenac sodium and tobramycin after the procedure. The patient is asked to continue with the tobramycin every couple of hours for the rest of the day. I see my patients the day after surgery and check that the flap is in place, that the interface is clean, that the new epithelium has covered the groove of the flap, and that no epithelial defects are present. If all this is correct, I add a prescription of prednisolone 0.5% three times a day for 5 days.

The next scheduled visit is at 1 week. I check visual acuity, refraction, and computer-assisted corneal topography, and repeat these exams at 1, 3, and 6 months. After 6 months, we ask our patients to visit every year for a complete eye exam.

An enhancement is done on patients who have under- or overcorrection higher than 2 D that is maintained for over 2 weeks on the third week. The flap is lifted using the Mendez Jr. LASIK Forceps.

For under- and overcorrections of under 1.5 D, I wait 3 months for an enhancement and usually make a new flap with the microkeratome.

For overcorrections, it is very important to treat only one third of the residual refraction. The hyperopia mask not only increases the central curvature but also increases the diameter of the previous myopic treatment, therefore, increasing the capability of correcting residual hyperopia.

LASIK IN ASTIGMATISM

Using the excimer laser, astigmatism is corrected more easily and with much better results than with any type of incisional surgery. When combined with keratomileusis, the stability and absence of haze is a definite advantage.

The basic LASIK technique described before works well with the correction of astigmatism. It is very important to remember when performing surgery that the sclera of patients may be as irregular as the cornea, especially in high astigmatism. This may produce a sudden loss of suction during the microkeratome pass.

In cases of high astigmatism, it is very important to mark the axis in the slit lamp before proceeding to surgery since some patients may present rotation of the globe while lying under bright light under the excimer laser. You must compensate the change of axis in case this happens.

With the Aesculap-Meditec MEL 60 excimer laser, when using the Myopia II mask (patients with myopic and astigmatic correction) or the Hyperopia mask (patients with hyperopic and astigmatic correction), in patients with high astigmatic component, a mark must be made on the axis of 180° at the slit lamp with the patient sitting down. The mask must be oriented in the same direction as the mark and the correction of the astigmatism will be corrected as programmed in the computer.

When the Myopia III mask is used (pure astigmatic correction), it is very important to mark the patient previously to the treatment at the slit lamp, this mark should be made on the axis of the astigmatism using negative cylinder (the flatter meridian). The mask should be oriented according to the marks. This procedure eliminates the possibility of treating the wrong axis due to involuntary rotation of the globe. With the large diameters used to correct pure astigmatism it is possible that in some treatments the hinge of the flap may be in the way of the ablation. In this case, the scanning of the excimer laser must be stopped before reaching the hinge. Another alternative is to make the flap so that the hinge is 90° away from the largest diameter of the ablation. For example, if the patient is plano -3.00 x 180, then the flap may be made from 6:00 to 12:00, leaving a superior hinge and reducing the possibility of inducing irregular astigmatism. The flap may also be made oblique with no changes in refraction at least after 1 year. The laser may ablate some epithelium in the edge of the stromal bed without any repercussions.

LASIK IN HYPEROPIA

One of the greatest advantages of LASIK is its refractive stability. This is also true in hyperopia. Increasing the curvature of the cornea using a mask that ablates from 2.5 mm up to 7.5 mm around the visual axis has given results up to 7 D correction.

The procedure for the correction of hyperopia is similar. Some characteristics of hyperopic patients are important to remember. Patients with hyperopia tend to have flatter corneas; this translates to smaller diameter flaps. Also patients with hyperopia usually have the visual axis nasally very close to the pupil's edge. All this, plus the fact that these patients also have small eyes and small lid apertures, makes the hyperopic patient difficult to perform surgery on. It is very important in these patients to place the suction ring centered in the visual axis of the patient. In these cases, the flap may look very decentered anatomically but this will facilitate the ablation of the stromal bed without touching the hinge of the flap.

Good centration in these patients is also very important since the ablation should be around the visual axis. The greatest effort must be made to ensure the ablation is always centered.

Once the flap is replaced it may seem smaller, especially when treating a high hyperopia. This is because of the central increased curvature. Special attention has to be paid not to stretch the flap to compensate.

Hyperopic patients once corrected will give you the best surprises; some older presbyopic patients may achieve a multifocal effect and see 20/20 and a J2.

COMPLICATIONS

One of the most common complications is detritus in the interface. We discovered that this is managed quite well by using the aspirator and irrigation with BSS. Decentration is also a common complication; this is more frequent than in PRK. The reason for this is that once the flap is removed, the surface through which the patient has to see is very rough compared to the untouched epithelium, and a light scattering effect is obtained. Some patients more frequently with high myopia will refer to seeing the fixation light but not knowing where the center is. Good orientation and patient education has to be given in this matter prior to the procedure. The Mendez

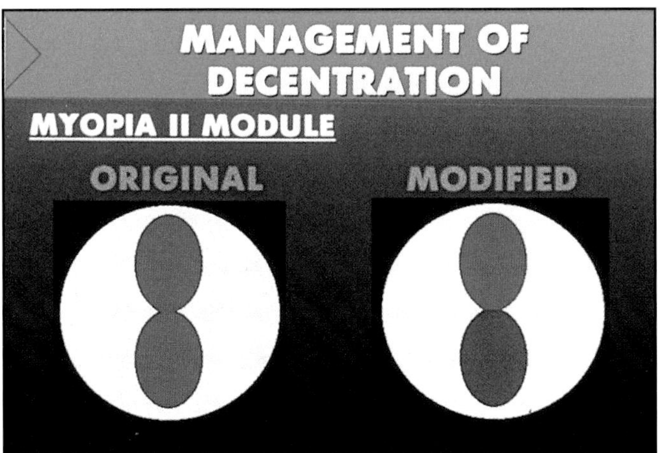

Figure 19-1.
Modified mask for correction of decentration.

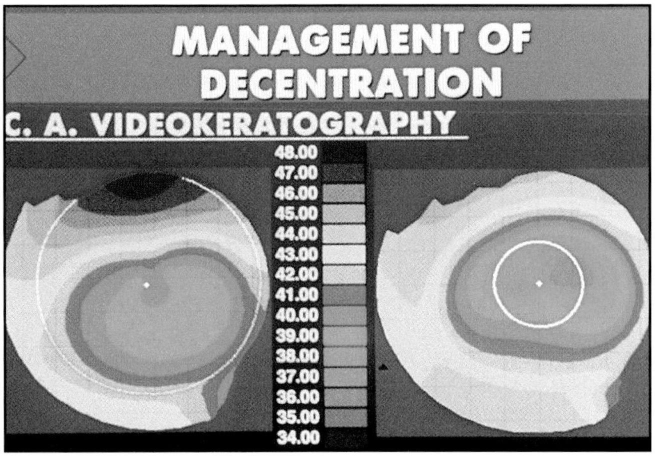

Figure 19-2.
Pre- and postoperative topographies.

Jr. Marker was developed for this reason.

Most of the other complications are related to the microkeratome, incomplete pass, damaged flap, thin cap, thick flap, irregular flap, or, worst of all, penetration to the anterior chamber. Most of the time, all of these complications are related to poor maintenance, loss of suction, or improper assembly of the microkeratome. As microkeratomes evolve, there will be much less possibility of having these complications.

I do not consider a free cap a complication, since this is how early KMIS procedures were done. The excimer laser may be applied and a corneal and refractive surgeon should be able to handle this without any problem.

In regard to incomplete pass, damaged flap, and irregular flap, the procedure should be aborted and rescheduled for another day. The repositioning of the cornea is easy and 98% of the time there will be no significant scarring tissue.

When a thin cap occurs, the possibility of developing haze is high, especially if the cut went through Bowman's layer. In case a thick cap occurs, it is very important to calculate how much of this untouched cornea will be left after the ablation in order to prevent uncontrolled ectasia.

The presence of a diffuse infiltrate (with the distribution of sand dunes) in the interface that may be present between 50% to 100% of the cornea with a quite eye that appears 24 hours postoperatively with relative good vision may be seen in susceptible patients from excess trauma (either by irrigation or by cleaning with the sponge), or may be caused by extreme sensitivity to a chemical present during the procedure, maybe even secretions of the Meibomian glands. Generally, these patients respond very well with intense administration of prednisolone 1%. Washing the interface immediately after the case has been noticed also helps improve the long-term rehabilitation in the worst patients. These patients may have after 3 months moderate to high hyperopia that may be treated after 3 months.

MANAGEMENT OF DECENTRATION

The Myopia II mask of the Aesculap-Meditec MEL 60 excimer laser may be modified to correct decentration. One side of the figure eight of the mask is covered (Figure 19-1). Guided by a corneal topography map we can detect the area of decentration and the area that needs to be treated. The technique consists of lifting the flap, locating the real visual axis, and completing ablation. The same preoperative refraction of the first laser treatment is programmed into the computer except for the axis. The axis of the area where the ablation needs to start is programmed instead. Only one pass is necessary to obtain the ideal correction (Figure 19-2).

Chapter 20

THE COMPREHENSIVE REFRACTIVE SURGERY LASIK STUDY

Guy M. Kezirian, MD, FACS, J. Charles Casebeer, MD,
Jeffery B. Robin, MD, Daniel Durrie, MD,
George O. Waring III, MD, FACS, FRCOphth,
Greg Hanson, PA

The Comprehensive Refractive Surgery (CRS) LASIK Study is a large, multicenter trial organized by clinicians to better understand LASIK, or laser in situ keratomileusis. It differs from most trials in several respects.

Perhaps the most unusual feature is the spontaneous manner in which the study came to be organized—it was established by and for physicians, without the usual input from industry, government, or universities. All funding to support the study is derived from the participating surgeons. Financial independence permits the comparison of technologies, something which is not always possible with industry funding.

The study design allows surgeons to access data as they are generated, expediting the application of results into clinical practice. This is quite different from most trials, where results are hidden from investigators to avoid potential bias. Because the CRS LASIK Study is a clinical outcomes trial designed to gain a better understanding of the procedure, it is beneficial to permit surgeons to access results and improve their techniques as the study progresses. This feature is enhanced by the use of electronic "online" data reporting.

Open access to results provides an immediate benefit to participating surgeons. By using special software developed specifically for this project, surgeons report their results from their offices directly into a central database located in Kansas City, Mo. In turn, they can obtain reports of the results in a computer-generated format that is tailored to their needs. For example, surgeons wishing to examine their refractive results for patients between -5.00 D and -7.00 D for the previous 3 months can do so online, on command. The reports compare individual results to the grouped results of all the investigators, allowing surgeons to grade their own performance.

The potential benefits of this design are particularly appropriate to LASIK. It is well recognized that two LASIK surgeons doing the same procedure with the same equipment can achieve very different results, due to a variety of individual variations in their technique. Corneal hydration, management of surface fluid, centration techniques, and tissue handling can all affect a surgeon's outcomes. The study permits surgeons to adjust their techniques to improve their results, providing an immediate benefit to their practice of medicine.

Another unusual feature of the CRS LASIK Study is the participation of a professional society. The International Society of Refractive Surgery (ISRS) provides a professional forum for meetings about the study, and has taken an innovative role by supporting a clinical trial among its members. This is a departure from the usual function of professional groups, and may set a precedent for greater involvement of societies in the evaluation of clinical procedures.

The CRS LASIK Study provides a new model for performing clinical trials. It is worthwhile to review how this study came to be, as a new paradigm for surgeon-controlled clinical trials.

BACKGROUND

Since its introduction, refractive surgeons have greeted LASIK with enthusiasm. The appeal of LASIK is intuitive. LASIK offers better accuracy than keratomileusis performed with a microkeratome, while preservation of the epithelium and Bowman's layer permits more rapid healing and better stability than can be achieved with surface PRK. However, the risks of LASIK were poorly understood. Lamellar surgery introduced a new set of potential complications, and existing keratomes were complex and as yet unperfected.

Consistent with its mandate to guard public safety, the US FDA has tempered the enthusiasm of LASIK surgeons with regulatory controls. In late 1995, the FDA released the Summit Apex laser for correction of myopia between 1.50 D and 7 D. This was followed in early 1996 with the release of the VisX Star laser for correction of myopia between 1 D and 6 D. Neither laser was released for astigmatic correction, and neither laser was labeled for use in LASIK—two restrictions that severely limited their use.

Meanwhile, refractive surgery in other parts of the world continued to advance rapidly. Multizone/multipass ablations were developed, providing smoother and more consistent surfaces than was possible with single zone methods. New scanning spot lasers permitted greater control of the ablation profile, along with the promise of smoother ablations. In the United States, these technologies were available to only a few investigators and limited numbers of eyes due to regulatory controls.

Many refractive surgeons were comfortable using the approved lasers to perform surface PRK for low myopia. However, most were not enthusiastic about surface photorefractive treatment for higher ranges of myopia. Further, there was no accepted medical justification for the de facto regulatory requirement to perform incisional keratotomy for astigmatism in the setting of excimer surgery. LASIK offered clear advantages to these options, as did excimer corrections for astigmatism. However, regulatory barriers kept the lasers and software to perform these procedures out of reach.

In this setting, the American refractive surgeon was forced to choose between the Scylla of outdated technology and the Charybdis of off-label procedures. Either option raised difficult concerns from ethical and liability perspectives.

Surgeon response was varied. Some chose to do nothing, advising patients to wait until better technology became available. Others entered comanagement relationships with surgeons in Canada and Mexico who had access to state-of-the-art lasers. Still others experimented with approved technology, adding multiple single zone ablations to reach higher corrections, and combining incisional correction for astigmatism with photoablation for myopia. A few surgeons built "custom" lasers that were able to perform a greater range of treatments outside of FDA scrutiny.

The end result was to expose the public to new risks in the name of regulatory control, exactly contrary to the FDA's mission.

The Role of International Society of Refractive Surgery in the LASIK Study

JEFFERY B. ROBIN, MD

The International Society of Refractive Surgery (ISRS) has played a pivotal role in the inception, formulation, and development of the LASIK Study. Throughout its history, ISRS has had a strong connection with lamellar refractive surgery. The Society was founded in 1978 by three American ophthalmologists—Drs. Richard Troutman, Miles Friedlander, and Casimir Swinger—all of whom had spent considerable time in Bogota, Colombia, learning lamellar refractive techniques from Prof. Jose I. Barraquer. In fact, soon after its founding, ISRS made Prof. Barraquer an honorary co-founder and its Honorary President. Nearly every president of ISRS has spent time in Bogota at the Barraquer Institute of America.

From its inception, ISRS has been the natural home for dedicated refractive surgeons. At that time, only a few refractive techniques were in use, such as RK and the Barraquer lamellar procedures. The small number of ophthalmologists who comprised ISRS were the world's leaders in these procedures.

By providing a venue for refractive surgeons to meet, the ISRS has been a catalyst for the development of refractive surgery. Its 2000 members represent more than 60 countries from around the globe, and its political and administrative leadership reflects this diversity. This impact has been particularly felt in LASIK, which owes its development to the contributions of surgeons from several continents. One of our prominent members, Dr. Ioannis Pallikaris, presented his initial experience with the procedure in 1989 at an ISRS refractive surgery symposium in New Orleans, La. Drs. Luis Ruiz of Bogota and Lucio Buratto of Milan, Italy, have also made significant contributions, and have presented their results at meetings of the ISRS.

Over the last several years, presentations devoted to LASIK have taken an increasingly predominant role in ISRS's major professional symposia. Additionally, ISRS actively co-sponsors regional refractive surgery meetings around the world, many of which have recently been almost entirely devoted to LASIK.

Given this background, it is not surprising that the CRS LASIK Study developed as a brainchild of prominent ISRS figures. The idea was conceived at a LASIK educational event in early 1996 and involved J. Charles Casebeer, MD, Greg Hanson, and this author. Recognizing that LASIK would rapidly become the predominant refractive surgical procedure worldwide, there was a clear need for a prospective evaluation of the efficacy, stability, and safety. This need was compounded in the United States, where LASIK had not received regulatory approval. It was decided that ISRS—because of its ties to state-of-the-art refractive surgical techniques and technologies, its membership of dedicated refractive surgeons, as well as its international character—would be the natural vehicle by which this study could progress.

That a professional society would assist in the organization of a study for its members is unique. It seems particularly appropriate for this project, given the international origin of LASIK and the demonstrated technical innovations of the ISRS membership. However, in today's setting of expanding knowledge and rapid introduction of new techniques, it may be a model for other societies to follow. The members of professional societies have a deep commitment to their profession, and the societies themselves provide a vehicle for communication. To act as an intermediary in collaborative research efforts would seem to be a natural extension of their raison d'être.

As the LASIK Study has developed, ISRS continues to play an important role. All of the study's medical monitors are ISRS board members or officers. Furthermore, because of its many vehicles to educate and communicate with refractive surgeons worldwide, it was decided that all participants (investigators) in the study would need to be members of ISRS, and that the ISRS would provide a venue for meetings of the study participants. As the CRS LASIK Study progresses to involve refractive surgeons from around the world, it is expected that the ISRS will continue as a central figure in this groundbreaking exercise in practical assessment of a refractive surgical technique.

ADMINISTRATIVE ORGANIZATION

In April 1996, three groups of ophthalmologists entered discussions in an effort to find a solution to the regulatory dilemma, with an eye toward improving their understanding of the risks and limitations of the LASIK procedure. The group included representatives from CRS USA Inc, the ISRS, and Data.site Inc. Together, they defined three goals:

1. A desire to better understand the clinical outcomes of using available technology to perform LASIK.
2. A common interest to promote safe practices in refractive surgery, protecting patients and surgeons alike.
3. A need to evaluate technologies independent of industry and manufacturer control.

The group decided to develop a study of LASIK using the technologies that were currently available. To maintain independence from industry, the project would be financially supported by the participating surgeons. As a collegiate effort, any qualified ophthalmologist interested in participating would be invited to join. They created a protocol for performing LASIK using the FDA-approved lasers that were available to US surgeons, with provisions for including other technologies available in other countries.

CRS USA Inc plays the role of administrating sponsor of the study. CRS USA Inc is a teaching and research company located in Scottsdale, Ariz. The chairman of CRS USA Inc is J. Charles Casebeer, MD, a long-time teacher of refractive surgery and professor at the University of Utah. Other faculty members of CRS USA, Inc., include Stephen Slade, MD, of Houston, Tex, Luis Ruiz, MD, of Bogota, Colombia, Marguerite McDonald, MD, of New Orleans, La, Richard Lindstrom, MD, of Minneapolis, Minn, and George O. Waring III, MD, FACS, FRCOphth, of Atlanta, Ga.

A second group, the ISRS, is the participating peer group affiliated with the study. The president-elect of the ISRS, Jeffery B. Robin, MD, of Cleveland, Ohio, became involved early in the project and suggested that involving the ISRS would bring added credibility to the grass roots effort. As a large, international professional society, the ISRS provides an institutional presence and a forum for communication. Meetings for investigators are often held in conjunction with meetings of the ISRS, and the ISRS has offered its *Journal of Refractive Surgery* as an avenue for publication of study reports.

Finally, Data.site Inc (formerly RSS) of Kansas City, Mo, was contracted to provide online databasing services for the project. Data.site is run by Ram Rao, formerly of Tomey Technologies, and is chaired by Dan Durrie, MD. The involvement of Data.site provides the study with state-of-the-art online communications, permitting online data entry and custom generated reports. In addition, the service includes online discussion forums for investigators to share information among themselves using an electronic bulletin board.

To coordinate communication between these groups and to facilitate interaction with investigators, CRS USA Inc retained the services of SurgiVision Consultants Inc, a refractive surgery consulting firm located in Scottsdale, Ariz. SurgiVision Consultants Inc is run by this author.

Rounding out the administrative group is George O. Waring III, MD, FACS, FRCOphth, who provides consulting services to the study.

THE MEDICAL MONITORS

The study has five medical monitors: Drs. Casebeer, Durrie, Robin, Slade, and Lindstrom. The monitors are responsible for oversight of the study. They participate in the development of study protocols, and determine the treatments to be included in the study. They moderate the online forums, guiding discussion among investigators, and participate as faculty at the LASIK symposia that are held for investigators.

FROM STUDY TO INVESTIGATIONAL DEVICE EXEMPTION

Consistent with the original purpose of the study—to accelerate the understanding of LASIK performed using available technologies—the medical monitors and CRS USA Inc, wrote a study protocol in May 1996. As defined by the study consultant, George O. Waring III, MD, FACS, FRCOphth, the protocol design differs from conventional protocols in several respects. It standardized the clinical observations that are made and the intervals at which they are made, but not the details of the proce-

DATA.SITE INC CLINICAL OUTCOMES ANALYSIS AND ONLINE COMMUNICATION

DANIEL DURRIE, MD

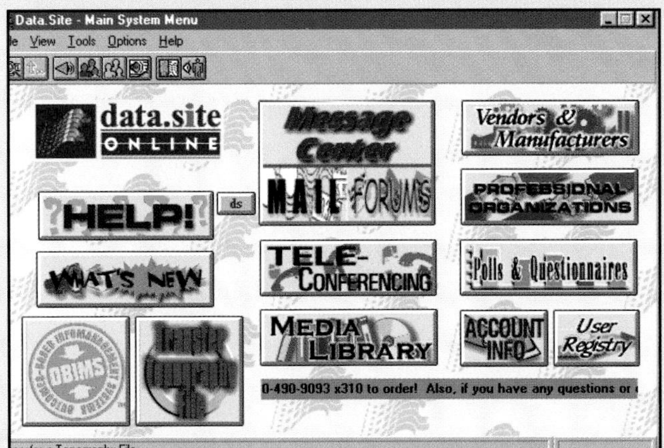

Figure 1.
Newer technological options.

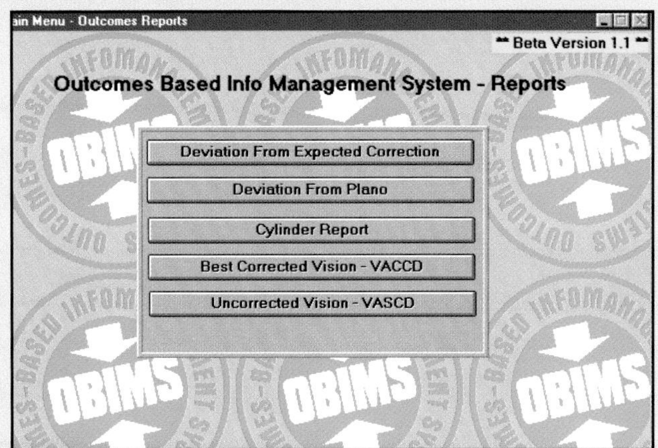

Figure 2.
Data entry forms and reports.

Today, a major focus in health care is to reduce costs without compromising the quality of care. Physicians, as care providers and often as "risk bearers," must increase their productivity while maintaining patient satisfaction. Eye care specialists throughout the world are focused on optimizing quality outcomes, productivity, and marketing efficiency.

Participation in the CRS LASIK Study combines these objectives. Use of online data reporting and analysis provides a unique element to their participation.

At the core of any good data analysis system is a single question: How can the system combine maximum utility while maintaining confidentiality? The role of Data.site in this project is to provide surgeons with a global database for comparison of individual results. Participation therefore provides an opportunity for surgeons to improve their outcomes, while contributing data into the general pool. Online access expedites the sharing and utilization of information.

Data.site is an international leader in ophthalmic data collection and analysis. The company mission is to provide accurate, relevant, and standardized medical outcomes analysis for medical professionals. This in turn facilitates their understanding of the strengths and weaknesses of surgical procedures. Data.site's participation in this project permits surgeons to incorporate newer technologies as their advantages become apparent (Figure 1).

IMPORTANCE OF THE STUDY

In a medical environment where new technologies are emerging daily, it is rare for a study to be proposed and designed by surgeons. The potential impact on the future of technological developments is immeasurable. While the study may or may not support the goals that the surgeons have set forth, the process will have profound effects. Their voluntary participation and support reflect their commitment to promoting the development of refractive surgery.

CENTRALIZED DATA COLLECTION

Data standardization is essential to careful tracking of patient surgical outcomes. The Data.site system permits the collection of data in a centralized, secure environment. Each client's data is protected by a unique password. Multiple levels of access can be programmed to allow data entry by surgeons and referring and postoperative care doctors. The data entry forms replicate the surgeon's practice to facilitate accurate reporting, while standardizing the entry fields (Figure 2). These fields create the data needed to compile basic statistical data for clinical reports centered on the surgical and postoperative care for every patient in the system. Validation occurs at the entry of data into the system (Figure 3).

A secured online bulletin board system (BBS) provides a mechanism for surgeons to communicate among them-

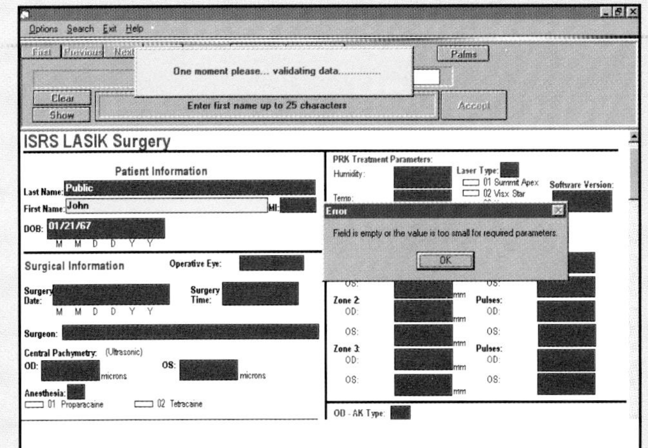

Figure 3.
Validation upon data entry.

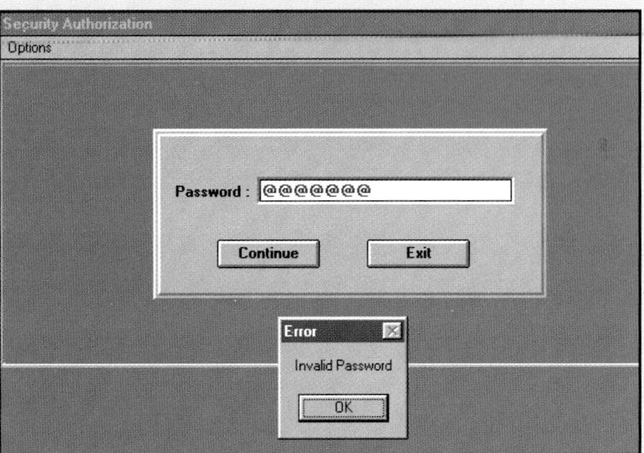

Figure 4.
Access to an individual surgeon's data is limited to the surgeon.

selves. Like the database, the BBS is password protected. Data is stored in a complex array of databanks which immediately transfer new data to safe and inaccessible data reserves. Data are carefully encrypted. Databases queries can be performed by those with password access only. In the CRS LASIK Study, individual results may be compared to the global database (a blind database with no names identified for surgeons or patients) for the study, but access to an individual surgeon's data is limited to the surgeon (Figure 4).

An important outcome parameter of this study is the patient satisfaction survey. This survey translates the subjective impressions of the patients into a quantifiable score. Patients are asked to respond to a standardized set of questions about the quality of eyesight prior to the surgery and at regular intervals after the surgery. They also answer questions about the surgery in relationship to key quality of life issues. Questions are answered on a gradient scale that is scored by a technician and the results are entered into the data report forms. Scores are compared automatically by the electronic system.

All reports are formatted regularly and the report generator system is applied to the data to create critical reports at predetermined intervals. The reports are available to surgeons online.

REPORTS

Each of the basic reports provides critical data that can be reviewed and interpreted to meet a variety of goals. The system allows surgeons to review the details of individual records that contributed to the report. It also allows surgeons to generate reports to meet their own needs. Some examples of the diverse information that can be obtained include:

- Refractive outcomes to assist in the development of a surgical nomogram.
- A report of missing information to generate the names and phone numbers of patients who need to schedule follow-up visits.
- The results of patient satisfaction surveys by specific topics provide feedback, comanaging physicians or doctors from other specialties.
- Marketing information.
- Reports to document outcomes success to managed care groups.
- Visual outcomes to assist in patient counseling.

THE PROCESS

Prior to beginning the surgeries for the IDE, each center receives a master set of clinical forms and a set of patient satisfaction questionnaires. These forms become part of the medical record and record information gathered at each patient visit, including surgery. Schematics of eye conditions, corneal topography, or other fields required in each individual practice may be kept along with the forms.

Although these forms are standardized, information about the center is gathered to customize the database for each surgeon. Software diskettes are created and distributed by mail, and permit entry from each of the center's doctors who will be caring for patients treated under the protocol.

To expedite data entry, the forms provide pop-up menus with information relevant to each field. The user can click on

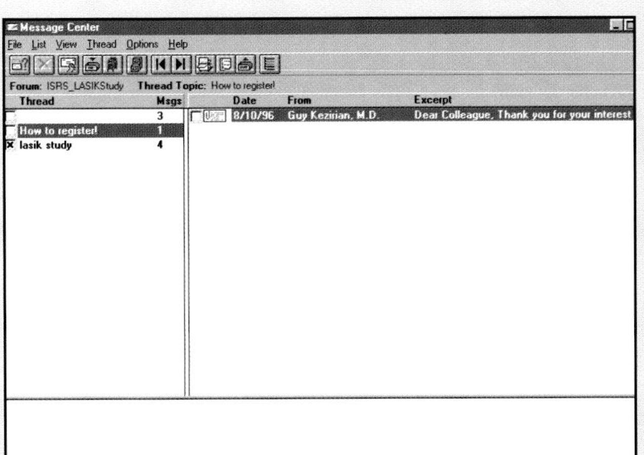

Figure 5.
BBS forums allow immediate communication.

an item and the information will be copied automatically onto the form. This process eliminates the time taken to enter data. Doctors' names, visual field values, and other common data sets are available in these pop-up menus so that input does not need to be re-entered every time it appears. This process also increases the accuracy of the data entered.

During the process of creating the database, each center receives online disks that allow multiple users from each center to log on to the Data.site online system. An online communications module provides email communications. Different centers may communicate with each other, medical monitors may communicate with surgeons, doctors working with the same patients can use the system for clinical communication, and investigators can participate in online forums to discuss surgical issues.

The BBS forums provide a key feature to the study. The forums are password protected to limit access to investigators. Participants may choose only to monitor the forum or may post responses to the questions and philosophies that are expressed. The forums may be thought of as a long-term conversation where a question is posed electronically and responses may be posted over a period of time.

This provides for the kind of exchange that formerly existed only through attending panel discussions at meetings or by participating in expensive teleconferencing. It also creates a mechanism for immediate communication that is generally not available in traditional studies (Figure 5).

The online system is the pipeline for providing clinical reports to the investigators involved in the study. It also serves as a communication tool through which surgeons study monitors, and follow-up doctors can communicate—a necessary feature of this large project. Email is delivered without the time limitations of phone calls and faxes. Participants can access their messages at any time during the day or night despite time zone differences.

In this atmosphere of communication and access to data, the potential for improving techniques and patient care is great.

Data.site recommends that each center purchase a computer system that will be dedicated for the Data.site system. Minimum hardware requirements are a 486 or Pentium processor computer with a 28.8 modem, with at least 16 MB RAM and a 1.6 GB hard drive.

dure. As such, the "study" is better termed a "clinical outcomes trial," and the term "protocol" can be replaced by "guideline."

The original intent was to study LASIK for the correction of myopia in the low myopia ranges that could be treated by the approved software for the Summit Apex (-1.50 D to -7.00 D) and VisX Star (-1.00 D to -6.00 D) lasers. The guidelines called for the manufacturer's software for surface PRK to be used beneath a flap. As an initial trial, the Chiron Automated Corneal Shaper was selected as the keratome to standardize that aspect of the trial. Astigmatic corrections using incisional keratotomies would be permitted at the discretion of the investigator.

Once the administration was in place and the protocol written, it was time to enroll investigators. An organizational meeting was held in Seattle, Wash, on May 31, 1996 to present the project to invited surgeons who had expressed interest in participating.

The outcome of that meeting was the establishment of a core group of approximately 30 investigators who would submit their results into a reference pool, against which individuals could compare their results. Through the power of electronic databasing, this could be automated during data processing, providing information that could be accessed by each of the investigators, while preserving the confidentiality of the data.

Additionally, it was decided that each investigator would submit 50 eyes into the reference pool that underwent spherical corrections only, within the ranges of the

Clinical Trials: Formal vs Informal

GEORGE O. WARING III, MD, FACS, FRCOPHTH

INTRODUCTION

In clinical medicine, there are many sources of information: the experience of an individual case, an individual physician's cumulative experience, an informal case series, a retrospective review, an informal evaluation, a formal prospective trial, and a prospective randomized clinical trial. Along this spectrum, the quality of the information generally improves and the confidence that physicians have in the results increases. Of course, the complexity, expense, time, and effort also increase.

When new surgical techniques emerge, many surgeons often utilize them early, contributing to the evolution and development of the techniques. If the technique seems useful, a formal trial may be set up. A good example is the emergence of RK in the United States in the early 1980s, where hundreds of ophthalmologists studied and refined techniques in a rather helter skelter way, but with a generally useful amount of cumulative knowledge. At the same time, a formal prospective trial of RK, the United States National Eye Institute's PERK study, was conducted. Both the informal and the formal approaches contributed useful information to the overall advancement of refractive keratotomy. The PERK study published more than 30 papers about its results—a major advantage—but studied only one technique—a disadvantage.

The situation is now similar for LASIK. Keratomileusis itself has evolved over 30 years and ophthalmologists from around the world have applied the excimer laser to keratomileusis. In the United States, formal industry-sponsored and privately sponsored clinical investigations are being done under the auspices of the FDA. At the same time, a large number of ophthalmologists are utilizing different lasers and different techniques of LASIK in an informal manner.

To capture as much useful information as possible from this informal approach, the CRS group, an educational consortium of ophthalmologists with the help and support of the ISRS, Data.site Inc, and SurgiVision Consultants Inc has mounted an informal evaluation of LASIK.

In order to clearly communicate among ourselves, it is important to define the terms that we use. I have previously referred to this as "keratospeak" in the context of refractive surgery. Here, I wish to contrast formal and informal clinical evaluations, to better delineate what is being undertaken in this project.

FORMAL VS INFORMAL

This project is best described as informal. A formal approach is usually designated an investigation or a clinical trial. An informal approach is better called an evaluation or simply an informal study. In a formal evaluation, a fixed surgical protocol is usually followed to control as many variables as possible. In an informal evaluation, techniques currently used in clinical practice are studied—usually with many variations.

STUDY DESIGN: PROTOCOL VS GUIDELINES

A formal investigation has a rigid protocol that specifies patient entry criteria, preoperative measurements, surgical technique, outcome variables, statistical methods, and monitoring procedures. Informal evaluations have guidelines that indicate the type of patient, surgery, and clinical assessments to be studied. The formal investigation is characterized by a rigid set of parameters, the informal evaluation by the practical reality of current usage. The methods outlined in this project are best described as guidelines.

PARTICIPANTS

A formal study involves investigators, a data and safety monitoring committee, clinical monitors, and biostatisticians. The informal evaluation involves participants in the form of clinical practitioners and advisors to help guide the trial and individuals to collect the resultant information. Those responsible for carrying out a formal trial are usually designated investigators, their number is limited, they participate in uniform training for the investigation, and they sign agreements to adhere to the study directives and protocol. An informal trial involves participants, who generally follow their own style of practice and often their own surgical techniques, but put forth the extra effort to document and report their findings. The surgeons in this study are best described as participants.

MONITORING

Formal trials have multiple monitoring mechanisms that include an independent institutional review board, a human investigations committee, a data and safety monitoring board that reviews periodically the results of the investigation, and individual physicians or staff who visit clinical centers to ensure adherence to the protocol. Informal trials have minimal monitoring, because there is not a requirement for strict adherence to a detailed protocol; advisors with experience in the field may help oversee and direct the project. The medical administrators (monitors) in this study are best described as advisors.

EQUIPMENT

In a formal investigation, important equipment is standardized. For example, a surgical laser is standardized among centers with the same software and clinical nomograms; measurement of visual acuity might use a standardized chart such as the National Eye Institute's vision charts. In an informal trial, each surgeon uses the equipment available to the practice, so a variety of surgical lasers using disparate software, nomograms, and treatment algorithms, as well as different methods of clinical measurements, are all reported together.

INFORMATION COLLECTED AND REPORTED

A formal investigation uses standardized data sheets to record uniform information before, during, and after surgery, with multiple layers of data validation built into the reporting process. Analysis of data is often done by trained staff and biostatisticians. While an informal study may collect information on standardized forms, it usually lacks the means to perform in-depth data validation.

BLINDED VS OPEN

The interim results of a formal investigation are usually blinded to the investigators. This project permits investigators not only to access reports of their results, but to compare them with the results of other surgeons in the interest of improving their outcomes. This introduces a potential for bias that would be intolerable to a formal trial. However, in the context of this project, it is an appropriate measure.

IDE VS PRIDE

Clinical trials of new devices carried out under the auspices of the US FDA are commonly done under the process of an IDE, an extremely strict set of rules guiding the evaluation of new instruments. This entails a formal protocol, compliance with FDA regulations, meticulous execution of the trial and reporting of data, enduring FDA site inspections, and in many cases, presenting data to the FDA Ophthalmic Devices Panel and FDA staff. The CRS LASIK Study is carried out in conjunction with the FDA (at the FDA's request), probably one of the first times the FDA has been involved in an informal study. The CRS staff have dubbed their relationship with the FDA as a "practical reality investigational device exemption (PRIDE)," a term coined by Dr. J. Charles Casebeer, a term not included in the standard FDA vocabulary. This was done to distinguish the formality of the standard IDE from the informality of the PRIDE characterizing the study described here. Both CRS and the FDA deserve kudos and encouragement in their attempts to harness the valuable information achieved through informal clinical studies and, at the same time, to adhere to reasonable protections for the American public.

approved software. It was decided that adjunct investigators would be enrolled, and would be permitted to participate in the same capacity as core investigators, except that their data would not be submitted into the reference pool.

Following this meeting, the goals of the study were expanded beyond the original purpose of simply accelerating the understanding of LASIK to include the following:

- Provide a communications forum to disseminate advances among surgeons.
- Standardize the procedure by creating guidelines that are acceptable to participating surgeons, through consensus.
- Minimize surgical complications and surgeon liability through standardization.
- Provide a mechanism for self-evaluation through the development of a reference pool of results generated by the core investigators.

Interest in participating grew rapidly. Within a few weeks more than 60 surgeons enrolled as investigators. The electronic database was established, and surgeons began submitting their results. It quickly became apparent that surgeons were willing to invest their time and resources into a project that brought better technology to their patients.

What began as an effort to make the best use of the limited approvals became a vehicle for accessing state-of-the-art technology. At best, it represents a public-private partnership between regulators and practitioners that will protect the public from unregulated procedures, while providing them access to up-to-date care. At worst, it represents an intrusion of bureaucrats into the practice of medicine and places limits on access to technology. Which view prevails will depend largely on the success of the project, and the continued cooperation of the parties involved.

FINANCIAL SUPPORT

To the point of IDE approval, the project has been totally supported by the participating surgeons. Financial independence from outside agencies and from industry has permitted free comparison of technologies, without censoring. However, new technology is expensive, and the advantages of new methods are often uncertain. As the project grows, it may be necessary to supplement surgeon funding with industry support, as long as support can be provided without censoring of results.

CLINICAL FEATURES

The basic feature of LASIK—refractive photoablation beneath a hinged flap—is fairly well established. However, there are many differences in the way LASIK is performed, and techniques are changing rapidly. Different keratomes are being developed. Surgeons vary in their preference for flap thickness and diameter. Photoablation patterns vary. Techniques for enhancements are being introduced.

In the design of the study, it was necessary to accommodate these variations while still allowing for meaningful comparisons of results. This was done by standardizing certain features of the study, while leaving details of the technique up to the surgeon. Use of electronic databasing permits cataloging the results into similar cohorts, and the large numbers of eyes being submitted preserves the statistical validity of the results.

The clinical procedures that were standardized are:

- Inclusion and exclusion criteria for patient entry into the study.
- The clinical observations that are made, such as vision, refraction, slit lamp examination, etc.
- The timing of clinical examinations (preoperative, 1 day postoperative, 1 and 3 months postoperative).
- The general elements of the surgical procedure.
- Requirements for study completion.
- The computerized reporting forms and methods.

A general principal in designing the protocol was to minimize interference with the surgeon's normal office routine. Another principal was to collect data that were used in the routine practice of refractive surgery. Through informal surveys of participating surgeons, it was learned that most practices do not routinely measure glare and contrast sensitivity, and there is significant disagreement about the interpretation of these findings. As a result, these examinations were not included in the protocol. Since many surgeons reported using the visual and refractive measurements made at the 3-month postoperative visit as the basis for further surgical decisions, required follow-up ends at 3 months. Cycloplegia was most commonly used for refractive measurements and was included in the protocol.

ADMINISTRATIVE CHALLENGES

Any large clinical trial poses administrative challenges, and the CRS LASIK Study is no exception. To date, the most common problems have been in the assimilation of the online reporting technology and in achieving investigator compliance.

Remarkably, despite the technological nature of refractive surgery, many of the clinical investigators were not computer literate when they entered the study. While many surgeons had computers in their practices, the majority were unfamiliar with how to use them and had delegated computer tasks to staff members. Some practices actually had no computers at all. Familiarity with online computing was even less common—only 25% of participants reported having email addresses when they enrolled.

Since the study requires online access for participation, computer illiteracy was a major hurdle for many surgeons. Most were able to overcome this obstacle in a few weeks, but some did not, and opted for paper reporting instead. This has limited the benefit of their participation, as it precluded online access to data reports and communication forums.

Obtaining follow-up reports has been the most challenging aspect of achieving investigator compliance. To address this problem, a policy was developed to require at least 75% follow-up at 3 months, within 120 days of surgery. Surgeons who fell below this rate were issued a warning letter advising them of the need to comply. If compliance was not obtained within 30 days, they were dropped from the study and their results were removed from the database.

INVESTIGATOR SYMPOSIA

Once the project was established, it became clear that the participating surgeons were anxious to discuss their experiences among themselves. To meet that demand, Investigator Symposia were organized in conjunction with major refractive surgery meetings. By consensus, the Symposia are didactic in nature, with invited speakers presenting their methods of managing certain aspects of the procedure. In keeping with the collegiate intent of the study, all interested surgeons are invited to attend these meetings, whether or not they participate as investigators.

The response to these Symposia has been enthusiastic, and they will be continued as long as interest warrants. (Figure 1 of Dr. Durrie's boxed aside features a sample agenda for an Investigator Symposium that was held at the 1996 Pre-Academy meeting of the ISRS in Chicago, Ill.)

EARLY RESULTS

Data to date are very limited, as the study is just getting underway. However, some of the early impressions are interesting.

Contrary to expectations, it appears that it may not be possible to develop a universal "nomogram" for LASIK ablations—each laser, and indeed each surgeon, may have to develop his or her own. This is due to variations that exist between lasers, and the sensitivity of lasers to environmental conditions such as room humidity. Surgeon technique is also important, particularly as it relates to the management of tissue hydration. Slower surgery may lead to drier stroma, and therefore to greater amounts of correction. A surgeon who interrupts the ablation to remove surface moisture may also experience greater amounts of correction. These and other factors suggest that a single "nomogram" for laser ablation may not be feasible, and speak for the importance of surgeon databasing as occurs in this study.

These features also exist in surface ablation, but are more apparent in LASIK because of the lack of any ability to modulate the refractive outcome during the postoperative period. With surface PRK, topical medications can be used to slow or accelerate healing. With LASIK, results are sealed once the corneal flap is back in position. The finality of the results in LASIK highlights the importance of technical consistency.

Corneal thickness is of paramount importance in LASIK. It is well recognized that deep lamellar dissections of the cornea result in central ectasia and corneal instability—this observation is the basis for hyperopic ALK. Since LASIK ablations begin at a stromal depth of 130 to 160 µm, ablations for higher amounts of myopia run the risk of going too deep and causing central corneal steepening. The margin of safety is poorly defined but appears to be in the range of 50% of overall thickness, or at least 250 µm from the endothelium.

Related to concerns about depth are concerns about glare. One solution to limiting ablation depth is to decrease the diameter of the ablation zone. However, this may result in increased symptoms of glare, especially in single zone ablations that do not have the blended transition zones of multizone or scanning spot treatments. Therefore, it is important to consider the patient's pupil diameter in mesoptic conditions during surgical planning. If it is larger than the diameter of the planned ablation, night glare may be expected postoperatively.

While these general observations seem valid, their relevance to clinical practice will be determined by the data. The collaborative nature of this project will greatly accelerate that process.

FUTURE EXPANSION

Whether the CRS LASIK Study expands beyond its current form depends on several factors. Clearly, much of the impetus for surgeon enrollment has been the hope of obtaining access to technologies that are otherwise unobtainable in the United States by virtue of being an investigator in this study. Interest may wane if the US FDA removes the regulatory obstacles that block surgeon access to new lasers. Should this occur, the study may languish from lack of interest.

However, there is some hope that surgeons will see the benefits of online databasing and sharing results, and that these benefits may spark interest in further studies. The communication of results among surgeons may prevent the repetition of costly mistakes, saving eyes and reducing surgeon liability. The rapid generation of a large database will speed the understanding of new procedures, which should directly improve clinical practice. The surgeons who have participated in this study have become accustomed to receiving these benefits, and may desire to maintain them as they introduce new procedures into their practices.

Many participants report that the bulk of their work was encountered in the early phase of their involvement, setting up the computers and training their staff to complete the reporting forms. Now that the infrastructure is in place, surgeons may be willing to continue the effort.

Refractive surgery is rapidly developing, and we can expect many new procedures to appear in the coming years. LASIK for hyperopia is already being performed in many centers, and many unanswered questions remain about the use and limits of this procedure. New lasers permit increased surgeon control of ablation patterns. IOL implants may offer advantages over cornea-based techniques. Even without the regulatory challenges of the FDA, there may be enough interest among surgeons to study clinical outcomes with these technologies.

There appears to be sufficient interest among surgeons outside the United States to warrant geographic expansion around the world. There is a current effort to form regional associations to accommodate this interest. Dividing the globe into regions makes sense because of differing access to technology. It will also facilitate communication and decrease travel distances to meetings. With careful planning to ensure that databases are compatible, regional differences in outcomes could be compared and analyzed.

The CRS LASIK Study permits broad-based collaboration of clinical results between surgeons. It has been made possible by the efficiency of electronic communications and the desire of ophthalmologists to advance their profession. The ultimate success of the study will depend on the commitment of the participants to see the project through. Early indications are promising.

Chapter 21

LASIK: THE PRELIMINARY AMERICAN EXPERIENCE

Keith P. Thompson, MD,
Jonathan D. Carr, MD, MA, FRCOphth,
George O. Waring III, MD, FACS, FRCOphth,
R. Doyle Stulting, MD, PhD

INTRODUCTION

Although laser in situ keratomileusis (LASIK) is rapidly gaining favor with many refractive surgeons worldwide, there is a lack of published data from prospective clinical trials with the new procedure.[1-4] This chapter summarizes the preliminary experience of LASIK in treating -2.00 D to -22.00 D of myopia at the Emory Vision Correction Center in Atlanta, Ga, from September 1 to December 31, 1995.

PATIENTS AND METHODS

Investigation of LASIK at Emory Vision Correction Center

In May 1995, an institutionally sponsored investigational device exemption (IDE) was conditionally approved by the US FDA to initiate a study of LASIK at Emory utilizing the Summit OmniMed excimer laser (Summit Technology, Waltham, Mass) and the Chiron Automated Corneal Shaper (Chiron Vision Corp, Claremont, Calif). The study was based upon experience with LASIK obtained by Waring and colleagues at the El-Maghraby Eye Hospital in Jeddah, Saudi Arabia.[4] The objectives of the LASIK study were to evaluate the safety and efficacy of LASIK in treating myopia (low, moderate, and high myopia), a single-zone vs multizone laser algo-

TABLE 21-1

Inclusion Criteria for Entry into the Emory LASIK Study

- 18 years of age or older.
- Myopia of -2.00 D to -30.00 D with 4.00 D or less of refractive astigmatism.
- Stability of refraction.

The following criteria were used to document stability of refraction in all eyes:

1. Measurement of present spectacles and comparison of that correction with the present refraction.
2. Inspection of records of previous refractions.
3. In eyes with pathological degenerative myopia, stability of refraction within the preceding 1 to 2 years. This eliminated patients with rapidly progressing myopia but included those patients who might subsequently have only mild progression of their myopia in the years after surgery.

- No previous ocular surgery for at least 12 months before enrollment.
- Normal videokeratography with absence of sign of keratoconus and contact lens-induced warpage. (Patients demonstrating contact lens warpage were required to show restoration of normal topography before enrollment into the study.)
- Normal anterior ocular segment by slit lamp microscopy.
- Absence of glaucoma or ocular hypertension.
- Absence of systemic collagen vascular disease, pregnancy, or the use of systemic corticosteroids.
- Realistic understanding of refractive surgery, its risks and benefits, and its level of predictability.
- Patients capable of returning for follow-up examinations.

rithm for treatments less than 7.00 D (all treatments over 7.00 D were multizone), and a comparison of the safety and efficacy of bilateral simultaneous vs sequential surgery (2 weeks apart) for patients desiring to have both eyes treated at the same surgery.

Patients were selected from the clinical practice of the 14 participating surgeons. During the course of the consultation, appropriate patients were introduced to the LASIK procedure and it was offered as an alternative in the management of their myopia.

Three hundred twenty consecutive eyes are the subject of this study. Three hundred nineteen eyes received LASIK; laser ablation was aborted in one eye after a hole was noticed in the corneal flap. Fifty-seven eyes had simultaneous arcuate transverse keratotomy (Arc-T) for reduction of astigmatism. All primary surgeries were performed between September 1 and December 31, 1995. All patients were followed for 3 months before being considered for either repeat LASIK or Arc-T. Patients ranged in age from 18 to 65 years with a mean of 40.9 years ± 9.2 standard deviation (SD). Mean preoperative spherical equivalent refraction was -7.2 D ± 3.1 SD.

All patients underwent an informed consent approved by the Emory University Human Investigations Committee prior to commencing the study. Inclusion criteria for the study are shown in Table 21-1. Patients wearing soft contact lenses were required to remove their lenses at least 3 days, and those wearing hard contact lenses for at least 2 weeks, before their baseline preoperative measurements. Patients who demonstrated contact lens warpage on videokeratography could not enter the study, unless prolonged cessation of contact lens wear restored corneal topography to normal.

Patients requesting bilateral simultaneous surgery (approximately two thirds of patients) were randomized to receive surgery either at the same sitting (simultaneously) or sequentially (at least 2 weeks apart). A random number table was used for patient assignments. Patients

TABLE 21-2

PREOPERATIVE EXAMINATION PROTOCOL

- Manifest and cycloplegic refractions.
- Distance visual acuity without correction and with manifest and cycloplegic refractions using a Snellen chart and the NEI Lighthouse chart. Near visual acuity measured with and without correction at 14 inches using the Lighthouse NEI near vision card.
- Slit lamp microscopy of the anterior segment.
- Diameter of pupils measured at approximately 300 Lux.
- Measurement of IOP.
- Ultrasound pachymetry using a Mastel KSX-1000, set at 1640 m/sec.
- Videokeratograpy with EyeSys System Model 3B using the current software edition.
- Contrast sensitivity testing with Pelli Robson charts with the pupils undilated and dilated.
- Ocular dominance.
- Specular microscopy.

requesting sequential surgery received LASIK at least 2 weeks apart. Two ablation algorithms were used: a 6.0-mm single-zone ablation and a three-zone (5.5, 6.0, and 6.5 mm) multizone ablation. In order to determine if there was a difference in outcome between the 6-mm single-zone laser algorithm and the multizone laser algorithm, patients undergoing simultaneous surgery were randomized to receive single-zone treatment in one eye and multizone treatment in the fellow eye. The patient's more myopic eye was used as the basis for assignment using a random number table.

Patients satisfying the inclusion criteria for entry into the study received a full ophthalmic examination as defined in Table 21-2. A consensus refraction was obtained, which was the surgeon's average of two manifest refractions performed on different days, and one cycloplegic refraction. A consensus refraction was used to determine the laser setting using a nomogram that was based on results from a pilot series of 25 eyes followed for 2 weeks. The nomogram was calculated such that only 5% of eyes would achieve a postoperative spherical equivalent refraction of greater than +0.50 D.

The Summit OmniMed excimer laser was used throughout the study, and was calibrated and operated in the fashion described in the Summit *User Manual*. Briefly, at the beginning of each operating day, the laser was calibrated by using the laser's internal calibration check and then performed an ablation through a 100-µm thick piece of wratten gel filter (Eastman Kodak Co, Rochester, NY). If the filter perforated within 530 and 630 pulses, and the breakthrough pattern met specifications, the laser was deemed calibrated.

Lamellar keratotomy was performed with the Chiron Automated Corneal Shaper using a flat, non-adjustable suction ring. The microkeratome was cared for and assembled by trained and dedicated technical personnel and inspected personally by the surgeon, who followed a checklist prior to each procedure.

Surgical Technique

PRIMARY TECHNIQUE

Typically, a sedative medication was not used preoperatively. For cases in which LASIK only was performed, the patient was prepped and draped for the surgical procedure with a plastic lid drape taped over the eye. Topical anesthesia was obtained using several drops of 1.0% proparacaine and additional conjunctival anesthesia was obtained by soaking Weck-cel sponges in proparacaine and applying them to conjunctiva for several seconds.

After the patient was positioned and the eye well anesthetized, the cornea was aligned under the excimer laser by centering the two helium-neon laser alignment beams on the corneal apex such that they intersected the apex and impinged on the iris to either side of the pupil at 3:00 and 9:00. At this time, the cornea was dried slightly, and eight fiduciary marks were made with an RK marker stained with methylene blue dye. The suction ring was then positioned on the cornea with careful attention to decenter the suction ring slightly nasally. Suction was then activated with the footswitch while simultaneously pressing the suction ring posteriorly in order to avoid rotation of the globe as suction was applied. Suction was maintained at 28 inches of mercury by the Chiron ALK system suction pump.

To verify that adequate IOP was achieved, a handheld applanation lens was held in position over the cornea, allowing the surgeon to personally observe that the diameter of applanated cornea was equal to or less than the inscribed circle, indicating an IOP of approximately 65 mmHg. After adequate IOP was verified, several drops of BSS were placed on the cornea and the microkeratome head was engaged into the suction ring tracks and slid forward until the gear on the microkeratome head engaged the track of the suction ring. The surgical assistant then paid careful attention to the patient's lids and ensured that the track of the microkeratome would be clear and not catch the patient's eyelids or bulbar conjunctiva. Once clearance was verified, the surgeon translated the microkeratome by means of a footswitch. The translation stopped when the stopper on the microkeratome head hit the suction ring housing. The microkeratome was then reversed and removed from the tracks. The suction ring was then removed. The patient was then realigned under the laser and the flap was reflected using either smooth forceps or an iris sweep. Any accumulating fluid was removed from the bed before laser ablation. At this time, the patient was asked to fixate on the green fixation light which was coaxial with the excimer laser. The globe was not stabilized by the surgeon during the ablation. Once adequate fixation was achieved under direct observation of the surgeon, the ablation was commenced and fixation was monitored by the surgeon. If any loss of fixation occurred, the treatment was interrupted until the patient was able to re-establish steady fixation. Following ablation, the flap was rolled into position using the end of an irrigation cannula or an iris sweep. The flap was then allowed to dry in position for approximately 5 minutes. The lid speculum was then removed and the patient's lids were allowed to gently cover the edge of the flap. One drop of a combination preparation of tobramycin and dexamethasone (0.1%), and one drop of ketorolac were placed in the eye at this time. The patient was encouraged to blink gently for several minutes and then was placed in an exam room chair where the flap position was checked at the slit lamp. If the fiduciary lines aligned properly and there were no visible striae or wrinkles in the flap, the patient was discharged.

Postoperative Medications

No postoperative medications were used on the day of surgery. The patient was instructed to sleep with a metal shield taped into position at bedtime. On the first postoperative day, the patient was instructed to begin placing one drop of a combination preparation of tobramycin and dexamethasone (0.1%) in the operated eye four times daily for 1 week. Nonpreserved artificial tears were recommended for symptoms of mild irritation.

Postoperative Examinations

Postoperative examinations were made at 24 hours, 2 weeks, and 3, 6, and 12 months. On the first postoperative day, flap position, unaided vision, and manifest refraction were recorded. At all other testing intervals, uncorrected visual acuity and best spectacle corrected manifest and cycloplegic refractions were recorded (Table 21-3), as well as glare testing and contrast sensitivity testing in selected subsets of patients. Corneal topography was routinely performed at each examination except the first day.

Enhancement Technique

Prior to enhancement, the patient was examined at the slit lamp in order to identify the edge of the flap. Once in the operating room, a Sinskey hook was used to define the edge of the flap that was created at the time of primary LASIK. The flap was then reflected, exposing the stromal bed. As with the primary LASIK procedure, the patient was asked to fixate on the green light which was coaxial with the excimer laser. Excimer laser ablation then followed after which the flap was repositioned in the same way as with the primary technique.

TABLE 21-3

Postoperative Examination Protocol

- Manifest and cycloplegic refractions. Each eye is refracted on each examination whether or not surgery has been done.
- Distance visual acuity without correction and with manifest and cycloplegic refractions using a Snellen chart and the NEI Lighthouse chart. Near visual acuity was measured with and without correction at 14 inches using the Lighthouse NEI near vision card.
- Slit lamp microscopy of the anterior segment. The cornea is examined with regard to corneal clarity, density of scar at flap edge, opacities in the lamellar bed. Each variable is graded on a 0 to 4 scale: 0=clear, 0.5=barely visible, 1=trace, 2=mild, 3=moderate, 4= severe.
- Measurement of IOP.
- Videokeratograpy with EyeSys System Model 3B using the current software edition.
- Contrast sensitivity testing with Pelli Robson charts with the pupils undilated and dilated.
- Glare testing with the Mentor Brightness Acuity Tester (visual acuity was recorded as the total number of letters read) with the pupils undilated and dilated.
- Change in spectacle corrected visual acuity. If the visual acuity with spectacle correction is two lines or less than that obtained preoperatively, a hard contact lens overrefraction will be performed to detect the effect of irregular astigmatism and to estimate the best possible corrected visual acuity.
- Specular microscopy.

RESULTS

Figure 21-1 shows a primary LASIK scattergram, with achieved change in spherical equivalent as a function of attempted correction. Patients were followed for a minimum of 3 months following primary LASIK before repeat surgery was considered. Fifteen percent (49 of 319) of eyes received repeat surgery. Eighteen eyes received repeat LASIK alone, nine eyes received repeat LASIK with Arc-T, and 22 eyes received Arc-T alone. The mean follow-up period for all patients including repeat surgeries was 5.2 months ± 1.3 SD.

Those eyes receiving repeat LASIK with and without Arc-T are shown in Figures 21-2 and 21-3, respectively. When enhancement data and 6-month postoperative data from eyes not receiving enhancement were included, the overall mean follow-up of eyes was 5.3 months ± 1.3 SD. At a mean follow-up of 5.3 months, 62.1% (198 of 319) of eyes were within ± 0.50 D of intended correction, 78.4% (250 of 319) were within ± 1.00 D, and 95% (303 of 319) were within ± 2.00 D.

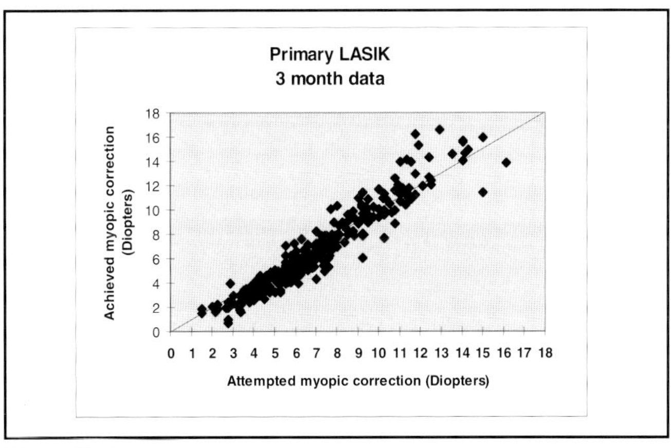

Figure 21-1.
Primary LASIK scattergram showing 3-month postoperative data. Attempted myopic correction (diopters) is shown on the x-axis, and the achieved change in spherical equivalent refraction on the y-axis. There is good predictability for the lower range of myopic corrections, but there is a tendency toward overcorrection for the higher myopes.

Figure 21-4 shows uncorrected visual acuity data after LASIK including enhancements with 26 monovision eyes excluded. The percentage of eyes that achieved uncorrected visual acuity of 20/40 or better was 85.3% (250 of

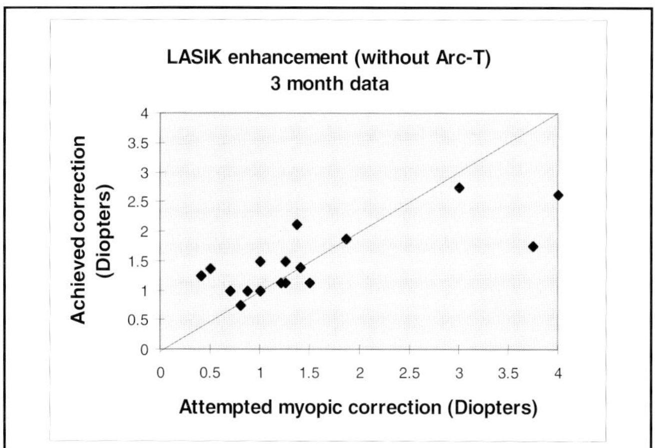

Figure 21-2.
Scattergram showing the 22 eyes that received repeat LASIK. The mean outcome was an overcorrection of 0.19 D ± 1.20 SD.

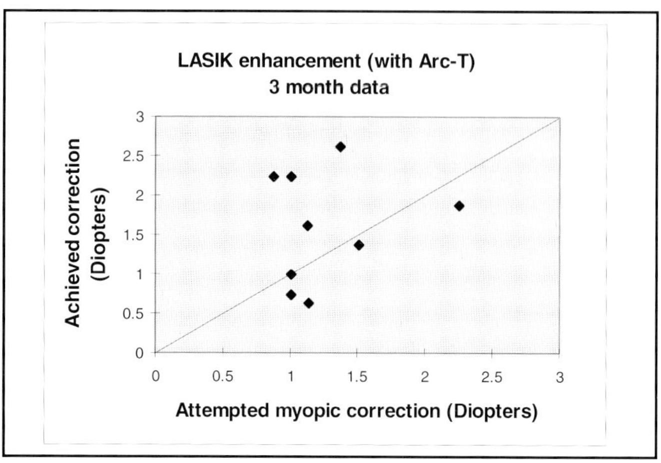

Figure 21-3.
Scattergram showing the nine eyes that received repeat LASIK with simultaneous Arc-T. The mean outcome at 3-month postoperative enhancement was an overcorrection of 0.35 D ± 0.76 SD.

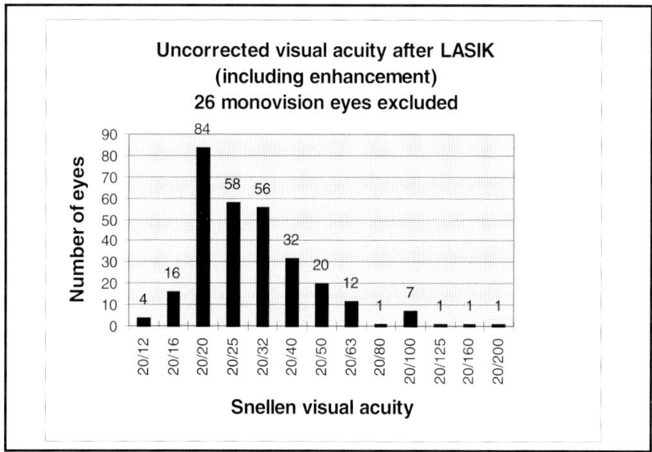

Figure 21-4.
Bar graph showing uncorrected visual acuity after LASIK including data from enhanced eyes. Eighty-five percent of eyes achieved uncorrected visual acuity of 20/40 or better.

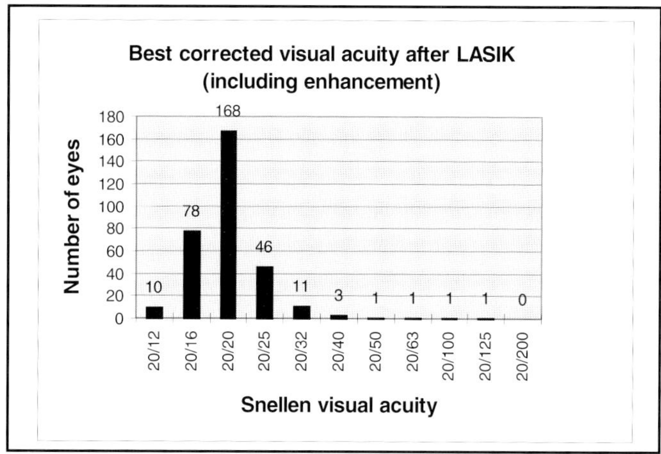

Figure 21-5.
Bar graph showing best corrected visual acuity after LASIK including data from enhanced eyes. Only four eyes had acuity worse than 20/40.

293), and 35.5% of eyes (104 of 293) saw 20/20 or better. This is a considerable improvement over primary LASIK data for uncorrected acuity, where 80.5% (236 of 293) of eyes achieved uncorrected acuity of 20/40 or better, and 21.8% (64 of 319) saw 20/20 or better.

Best corrected visual acuity for all patients including enhancements is shown in Figure 21-5. Only four of 320 eyes had best corrected acuity worse than 20/40 at a mean follow-up of 5.3 months. Figure 21-6 shows the change in best corrected visual acuity after LASIK including enhancements. Nineteen of 320 eyes gained two or more lines of best corrected vision, the vast majority of eyes changing by less than two lines. There were eight eyes that lost two or more lines of best corrected visual acuity, and they are described in Table 21-4. The loss of three lines of best spectacle corrected visual acuity to 20/60 in one eye occurred after the laser ablation was aborted due to a buttonhole in the corneal flap; this eye also developed a macular epiretinal membrane presumably related to a retinal detachment that occurred before entry into the study. The remaining seven eyes all had best corrected vision of 20/40 or better despite a loss of two or more lines of best corrected visual acuity.

There were 13 complications from the study of 320 eyes; four were intraoperative and nine were postoperative (Table 21-5). Six of the 13 complications developed in patients of the three investigators with prior experience with lamellar surgery (GOW, RDS, KPT), the remaining seven complications developed among the 11 surgeons with little prior experience with lamellar surgery. As a percentage of total cases performed in the study, the complication rate for the experienced surgeons was 2.8% (six of 214), and that for the less experienced LASIK surgeons was 6.7% (seven of 105).

Of the four intraoperative flap complications, one case was aborted after a buttonhole flap. The procedure was aborted without laser treatment and the flap repositioned. There were two free flaps and one eye in which the flap was too thick. The free flaps were repositioned uneventfully without suture. In these latter three eyes, laser ablation proceeded uneventfully with good visual outcome.

Postoperative complications consisted of five partially slipped flaps which were repositioned with no loss of best spectacle corrected visual acuity of greater than one line. Similarly, two eyes with flap folds were successfully managed with repositioning of the flap without suture. The two cases of epithelial ingrowth received flap revision which consisted of epithelial removal from the stromal bed.

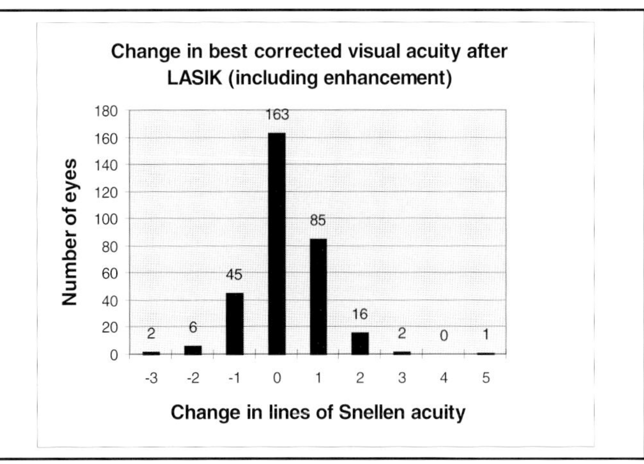

Figure 21-6.
Bar graph showing the change in level of best corrected visual acuity as a result of LASIK (including enhancement data). Eight eyes lost two or more lines of best corrected acuity, only one of which had best corrected visual acuity worse than 20/40 due to a macular epiretinal membrane.

DISCUSSION

LASIK is a very promising technique capable of correcting low, moderate, and high degrees of myopia.[1-6] It can be combined effectively with astigmatic keratotomy (AK) in the same surgical setting. There are four major advantages of LASIK over PRK:

1. Negligible postoperative discomfort.
2. Rapid recovery of visual acuity postoperatively.
3. Minimal postoperative care and monitoring are required.
4. LASIK is an adjustable procedure.

Following enhancement, 85.3% of eyes achieved uncorrected acuity of 20/40 or better in this series of highly myopic patients. This compares favorably with the currently available literature for correction of moderate and high myopia.[6-11] The percentage of eyes with uncorrected visual acuity of 20/40 was 80.5% after primary LASIK, and 85.3% after enhancements and 6-month postoperative data from eyes not receiving enhancements were included. Twenty-two percent of eyes had uncorrected acuity of 20/20 or better after primary LASIK, and this increased substantially to 35.5% after inclusion of enhancement data.

The striking feature of this highly myopic patient group is that so many eyes actually gained lines of best corrected visual acuity. At a mean follow-up of 5.3 months, 32.5% (104 of 320) of eyes gained one or more lines of best spectacle corrected visual acuity. Of the eight eyes that lost two or more lines of best spectacle corrected visual acuity, the only case with acuity of worse than 20/40 was attributable to a macular epiretinal membrane that preceded LASIK. All other patients retained 20/40 best corrected visual acuity despite the two or more line loss of vision.

In conclusion, LASIK is a promising technique that can treat low, moderate, and high levels of myopia. In comparison to PRK, LASIK is associated with less postoperative discomfort and a more rapid recovery of visual acuity. LASIK is an adjustable procedure whereby enhancement can be safely performed as early as 3 months after the primary LASIK procedure. This adjustability allows LASIK to accurately correct high levels of myopia while at the same time minimizing the likelihood of overcorrection. The ability of LASIK to correct higher levels of myopia must be weighed against the possibility of adverse events related to the use of the microkeratome. Fortunately, the complication rate appears to decrease as the surgeon gains experience with the procedure (data not shown). Continued improvement in both excimer and microkeratome technology should help to further improve the outcome of the LASIK procedure.

TABLE 21-4

Clinical Information Relating to the Eight Eyes Losing Two or More Lines of Best Corrected Visual Acuity

Preoperative BCVA	Final BCVA	Change in BCVA	Comment
32	63	-3	Buttonhole in flap, laser ablation aborted pre-existing epiretinal membrane
20	40	-3	Irregular astigmatism
25	40	-2	Irregular astigmatism
25	40	-2	Etiology of loss of BCVA unknown
20	32	-2	Etiology of loss of BCVA unknown
12	20	-2	Etiology of loss of BCVA unknown
20	32	-2	Irregular astigmatism
20	32	-2	Etiology of loss of BCVA unknown

TABLE 21-5

Complications

Eye	Time of Complication	Type of Complication	Management
1	Intraoperative	Buttonhole in flap	No ablation; three lines of BCVA lost
2		Free flap	Ablated; flap repositioned
3		Free flap	Ablated; flap repositioned
4		Thick flap	Ablated; flap repositioned
5	Postoperative	Partial flap slip	Ablated; flap repositioned
6		Partial flap slip	Ablated; flap repositioned with suture
7		Partial flap slip	Ablated; flap repositioned with suture
8		Dislocated flap	Ablated; flap repositioned
9		Dislocated flap	Ablated; flap repositioned
10		Epithelial ingrowth	Epithelial removal
11		Epithelial ingrowth	Epithelial removal
12		Folds in flap	Flap repositioned
13		Folds in flap	Flap repositioned

References

1. Fiander DC, Tayfour F. Excimer laser in situ keratomileusis in 124 myopic eyes. *J Refract Surg*. 1995;11:S234-S238.

2. Güell JL, Muller A. Laser in situ keratomileusis (LASIK) for myopia from -7 to -18 diopters. *J Refract Surg*. 1996;12:222-228.

3. Knorz MC, Liermann A, Seiberth V, Steiner H, Wiesinger B. Laser in situ keratomileusis to correct myopia of -6.00 to -29.00 diopters. *J Refract Surg*. 1996;12:575-584.

4. Salah T, Waring GO III, El Maghraby A, Moadel K, Grimm SB. Excimer laser in situ keratomileusis under a corneal flap for myopia of 2 to 20 diopters. *Am J Ophthalmol*. 1996;121:143-155.

5. Pallikaris IG, Papatzanaki ME, Siganos DS, Tsilimbaris MK. A corneal flap technique for laser in situ keratomileusis. Human studies. *Arch Ophthalmol*. 1991;109(12):1699-1702.

6. Pallikaris IG, Siganos DS. Excimer laser in situ keratomileusis and photorefractive keratectomy for correction of high myopia. *J Refract Corneal Surg*. 1994;10(5):498-510.

7. Heitzmann J, Binder PS, Kassar BS, Nordan LT. The correction of high myopia using the excimer laser. *Arch Ophthalmol*. 1993;111(12):1627-1634.

8. Sher NA, Hardten DR, Fundingsland B, et al. 193-nm excimer photorefractive keratectomy in high myopia. *Ophthalmology*. 1994;101(9):1575-1582.

9. Menezo JL, Martinez CR, Navea A, Roig V, Cisneros A. Excimer laser photorefractive keratectomy for high myopia. *J Cataract Refract Surg*. 1995;21(4):393-397.

10. McCarty CA, Aldred GF, Taylor HR, the Melbourne Excimer Laser Group. Comparison of results of excimer laser correction of all degrees of myopia at 12 months postoperatively. *Am J Ophthalmol*. 1996;121:372-383.

11. Price FW Jr, Whitson WE, Gonzales JS, Gonzales CR, Smith J. Automated lamellar keratomileusis in situ for myopia. *J Refract Surg*. 1996;12:29-35.

Chapter 22

LASIK RESULTS

Laurent Gauthier-Fournet, MD

The intrastromal photoablation is the present and logical solution to several problems of refractive surgery. Nowadays, only some technical difficulties, which probably can be solved, have stopped a more important diffusion of these problems.

THE MYOPICS

Different questions must be answered:

- What is the ideal thickness of the flap?
- What is the ideal diameter of it?
- Which ablation shape is better?
- What are the results?
- What are the complications?

Thickness of the Flap

Flaps often used are 130 to 160 µm. A certain consensus seems to emerge to use a flap of 160 µm for myopias less than -10 D and one of 130 µm for myopias higher than -10 D.

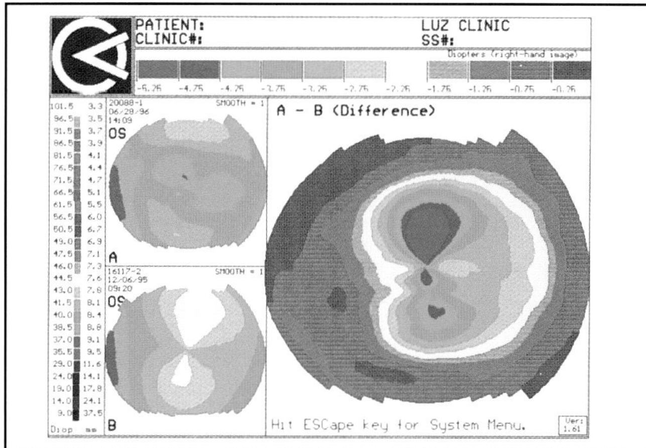

Figure 22-1.
A differential topography showing high astigmatism associated with a low myopia.

Diameter of the Flap

This is dependent on the size of the photoablation performed, on the control of the long hinge. A bigger flap does not damage, whereas a shorter flap can be embarrassing. An 8- to 9-mm diameter is ideal.

What is the Better Profile Ablation?

For low myopias (inf-10), maximal depth of ablation is not reached so do we have to favor high diameters of ablation, often 6 mm (Figure 22-1). Also, 7-mm diameters can be used to correct myopias lower than 5 D. The interest of a peripheral zone of transition must be examined because the observed regression is slight.

For high myopias (sup-10), the maximal ablation that is acceptable presents a problem. This ablation is around 150 µm. However, it is dependent on initial pachymetry. Under the flap, it is probably necessary to have a cornea around 200 µm at least to avoid a secondary corneal ectasia.

This maximal depth of ablation requires one to increase the proportion of correction performed on a 5-mm diameter. Concerning high myopias, a reduction of ablation diameter leads to reduce the useful optical zone.

Results

Tables 22-1 through 22-4 show the results of 765 cases performed and followed-up for 3 months. We used the Aesculap-Meditec MEL 60 excimer laser and an ALK microkeratome from Chiron.

Comments

Laser in situ keratomileusis (LASIK), as with all techniques of refractive surgery, gives better precision for low myopias than for higher myopias. For higher myopias, lower precision is dependent on a repercussion more important of an error percentage (eg, 10% error on -7 = 0.7 D, 10% error on -15 = 1.5 D) on the most important effect of possible decentrations as well.

Unlike photorefractive keratectomy (PRK), there is not a superior and theoretical limit to LASIK, seeing that in our series we performed a case with -26 D in preoperative with a final result at +0.50 D. However, for these myopias higher than 15 D, other techniques of refractive surgery (ie, IOLs) permit a notable gain of visual acuity, whereas with LASIK these corrected visual acuities are retained at the very most.

Moreover, for these high myopias, the optical zone that is created is too short and produces a monocular diplopia as well as parasite effects at night. Now these disadvantages are leading us to limit LASIK indication to myopias lower than 15 D.

When there is an over- or undercorrection, the flap will be held up without any problem 3 months after the initial surgery, that is to say after the stabilization of the refraction. A second photoablation is possible whenever it is myopic or hyperopic. These photoablations give excellent results since 75% of patients treated again present a refraction between +1 D and -1 D in the postoperative.

ASTIGMATISM TREATMENT

We have to consider two cases:

1. For astigmatism higher than myopia, it is pure myopic astigmatism. A "photoablation like slit" will be performed on the flattest axis and possibly completed by an associated myopic treatment (Table 22-5).
2. Myopia and astigmatism included in the sphere that is higher than the cylinder. Then, an elliptical photoablation will be performed (Table 22-6).

So, treatment of associated astigmatism is possible. It is more difficult to perform an astigmatism as a rule because the long axis of ablation is horizontal and at the same time the hinge is going to disturb the photoabla-

TABLE 22-1

MYOPIA ONLY: SPHERICAL EQUIVALENT LOWER THAN -5 D (18 CASES)

Mean	Preoperative	Postoperative
Spherical equivalent	-4.465	0.083
Spherical equivalent SD	0.510	0.701
Best corrected visual acuity	9.88	9.77
Uncorrected visual acuity	0	9
Spherical Equivalent	**No.**	**%**
Between +1 and -1	16	88.90
Between +1 and +2	1	5.55
Between -1 and -2	1	5.55
	No.	**%**
±1 line of preoperative visual acuity	18	100

tion. The primary cut may be slightly decentered temporally.

As for myopia, a wide ablation will produce better optical qualities. In the future, a more accurate topographic analysis will probably permit the treatment of asymmetric astigmatisms.

By themselves, decentered photoablations can produce astigmatism, so they disturb the result of astigmatism treatment.

COMPLICATIONS

Losing or Moving of the Lenticles

In our series, we did not note any lenticle lost. It is important to observe that most cases had a suture. In two cases, the patient rubbed his or her eye 2 days after surgery. The flap was wrinkled and we had to set it again without any later consequences resulting.

Epithelial Invasions

In our first 60 cases, we observed seven cases of epithelial invasions (12%) which required the removal of the lenticle, washing it, and putting it back again with suture.

The following 700 cases were sutured systematically. Only one epithelial invasion appeared and we had to wash and suture the lenticle.

The next 150 cases did not have suture but we took care to wash the interface meticulously and to have a good alignment of the edges. We did not note any case of epithelial invasion. It confirms that these complications declined with the surgeon's experience.

If they are central or paracentral, these epithelial invasions are potentially serious complications because they can lead to perforations of the lenticle under effect of the collagenases produced by epithelial cells.

The washing is not a simple thing because the lenticle is thin and cannot be easily scratched.

Decentrations

Decentrations can have serious consequences when the myopia we have to correct is high. They induce astigmatism, monocular diplopia, and parasite effects at night.

Their reason is varied, whether it is the bad fixation of the patient through the corneal stroma, the agitation or

TABLE 22-2

Myopia Only: Spherical Equivalent Between -5 D and -10 D (257 Cases)

Mean	Preoperative	Postoperative
Spherical equivalent	-7.51	0.315
Spherical equivalent SD	1.96	1.10
Best corrected visual acuity	8.96	8.82
Uncorrected visual acuity	0	7.49
Spherical Equivalent	**No.**	**%**
Between +1 and -1	185	71.42
Between +1 and +2	46	17.76
Between -1 and -2	18	6.94
Greater than +2	8	3.08
Less than -2	2	0.77
	No.	**%**
±1 line of preoperative visual acuity	227	88.32
2 lines gained	6	2.33
More than 2 lines gained	2	0.77
2 lines lost	16	6.22
More than 2 lines lost	6	2.33

the failure to understand, the sliding of fixation rings (lasers which use them), or the eyetrackers used that do not work.

The treatment of decentrations is difficult and can consist of making an asymmetric incision or making an asymmetric photoablation.

HYPERMETROPIC LASIK

An ablation in a ring around the optical axis permits an increase of the central curve. This surgery presents some specifics:

- The total diameter of photoablation must be the widest possible. An 8.5- to 9-mm zone is essential. Present microkeratomes have difficulty cutting so wide a diameter. Moreover, a diameter can change from one eye to another using the same machine.
- Because of this wide ablation diameter, the hinge must usually be protected during surgery.
- Curve rays of hypermetropic eyes are not adjusted well to current microkeratomes. Thus, fixation is sometimes difficult.
- Highest photoablation requires either a mechanical fixation or an efficient eyetracking.

RESULTS

Table 22-7 shows our results for our first 53 cases of hypermetropia between +1 D and +7.25 D.

TABLE 22-3

MYOPIA ONLY: SPHERICAL EQUIVALENT BETWEEN -10 D AND -15 D (141 CASES)

Mean	Preoperative	Postoperative
Spherical equivalent	-12.46	0.315
Spherical equivalent SD	1.48	
Best corrected visual acuity	7.46	7.54
Uncorrected visual acuity	0	5.70
Spherical Equivalent	**No.**	**%**
Between +1 and -1	73	51.77
Between +1 and +2	14	9.92
Between -1 and -2	30	21.27
Greater than +2	16	11.34
Less than -2	8	5.67
	No.	**%**
±1 line of preoperative visual acuity	112	79.43
2 lines gained	6	4.25
More than 2 lines gained	10	7.09
2 lines lost	11	7.80
More than 2 lines lost	2	1.41

Characteristics of Hypermetropic PRK

- Regression around 20% of the initial effect obtained with stabilization at 3 months.
- Refractive precision lower than myopic LASIK.
- Loss of the best corrected visual acuity.

For high myopia, straight optical zones produce parasite effects at night, astigmatism when there is decentration, and a decline of visual acuity.

Now that we are treating 9 mm of cornea, results are much better than they were with the old 7-mm zones. Nevertheless, it will be necessary to try to increase this optical zone more either by extending the treatment zone or by changing ablation profiles.

Hypermetropic LASIK is the only technique that can correct hypermetropias with reliability (Figures 22-2 and 22-3). Results about spherical hypermetropias until 5 D are excellent. Beyond, the small optical zone created produces visual discomfort.

TABLE 22-4

MYOPIA ONLY: SPHERICAL EQUIVALENT HIGHER THAN -15 D (32 CASES)

Mean	Preoperative	Postoperative
Spherical equivalent	-18.58	1
Spherical equivalent SD	±3.20	±2.43
Best corrected visual acuity	5.98	5.70
Uncorrected visual acuity	0	4.03
Spherical Equivalent	**No.**	**%**
Between +1 and -1	4	12.5
Between +1 and +2	15	46.87
Between -1 and -2	4	12.5
Greater than +2	1	3.12
Less than -2	8	25
	No.	**%**
Between ±1 line of preoperative visual acuity	24	75
2 lines gained	3	9.37
2 lines lost	3	9.37
More than 2 lines lost	2	6.25

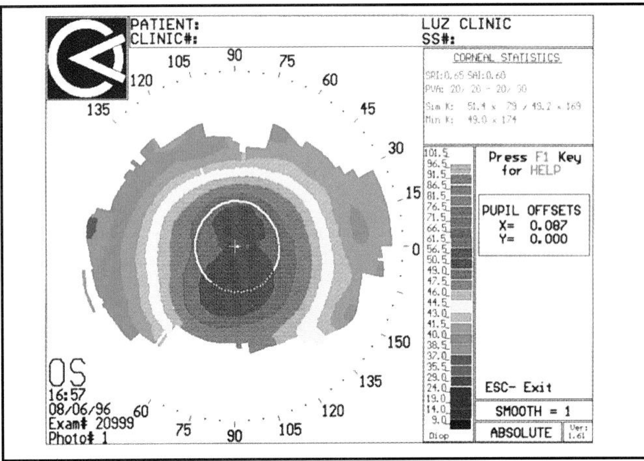

Figure 22-2.
Topography of a corrected hyperopia (+7 D) by LASIK.

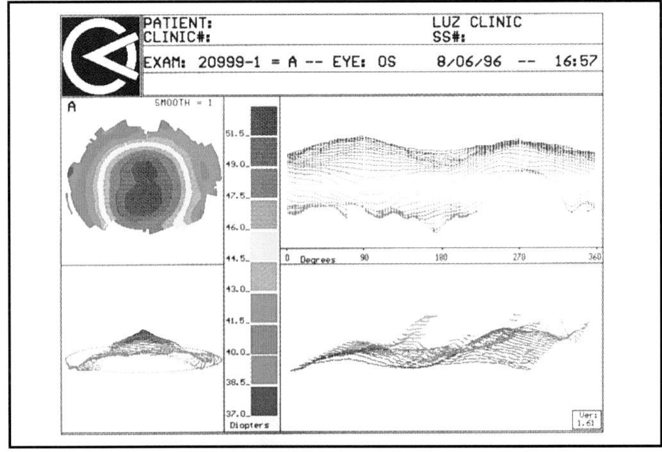

Figure 22-3.
Topography of hyperopia from Figure 22-2 in composite vision. The shape vision shows the straight side of this optical zone.

TABLE 22-5

Astigmatism Higher Than Myopia/Pure Myopic Astigmatism (13 Cases)

Mean	Preoperative	Postoperative
Spherical equivalent	-3.23	0.04
Spherical equivalent SD	±1.35	±0.67
Astigmatism	2.98	0.98
Best corrected visual acuity	8.61	8.69
Uncorrected visual acuity	0	6.84
Spherical Equivalent	**No.**	**%**
Between +1 and -1	12	
Between -1 and -2	1	
	No.	**%**
±1 line of preoperative visual acuity	11	84.61
More than 2 lines gained	1	7.69
2 lines lost	1	7.69

TABLE 22-6

Myopia and Astigmatism Included in the Sphere (Which is Higher Than the Cylinder) (251 Cases)

Mean	Preoperative	Postoperative
Spherical equivalent	-8.57	0.12
Spherical equivalent SD	±2.57	±1.32
Astigmatism	2.055	0.75
Best corrected visual acuity	7.92	8.16
Uncorrected visual acuity	0	6.60
Spherical Equivalent	**No.**	**%**
Between +1 and -1	178	70.91
Between +1 and +2	30	11.95
Between -1 and -2	19	7.56
Greater than +2	14	5.57
Less than -2	10	3.98
	No.	**%**
±1 line of preoperative visual acuity	171	68.12
2 lines gained	18	7.17
More than 2 lines gained	31	12.35
2 lines lost	18	7.17
More than 2 lines lost	13	5.17

TABLE 22-7

HYPERMETROPIA (53 CASES)

Mean	Preoperative	Postoperative
Spherical equivalent	4.03	0.246
Spherical equivalent SD	±1.50	±1.23
Best corrected visual acuity	9.49	8.77
Uncorrected visual acuity	4.64	7.62
Spherical Equivalent	**No.**	**%**
Between +1 and -1	32	60.37
Between +1 and +2	12	22.64
Between -1 and -2	2	3.77
Greater than +2	6	11.32
Less than -2	1	1.88
	No.	**%**
±1 line of preoperative visual acuity	47	88.67
2 lines gained	1	1.88
2 lines lost	5	9.43

LASIK vs PRK in Moderate Myopia

ANTÓNIO MARINHO, MD

INTRODUCTION

Photorefractive keratectomy (PRK) is generally accepted as a good way to correct low myopia (less than -6.00 D) in myopia above -10.00 D. Laser in situ keratomileusis (LASIK) is usually preferred, but in moderate myopia (-6.00 D to -12.00 D) controversy between the merits of both techniques still persists.

We selected two similar groups of patients with moderate myopia and evaluated the results at 1, 3, and 6 months and 1 year in order to establish which technique is better to deal with these patients.

MATERIALS AND METHODS

We divided the patients into two groups. Group 1 (PRK) had 325 eyes (227 female and 98 male) with a mean myopia of 8.63 D ± 1.79 (-6.00 D to -12.00 D) (Figure 1). In this group, PRK was performed using the Summit OmniMed laser with a single ablation zone (4.7 mm) in 53 eyes and two ablation zones (4.5 and 5.0 mm) in 272 eyes. In these eyes, 70% of the total correction was done at a 4.5-mm optical zone and 30% with a 5.0-mm optical zone. The correction used was 100% of vertex corrected myopia in all cases.

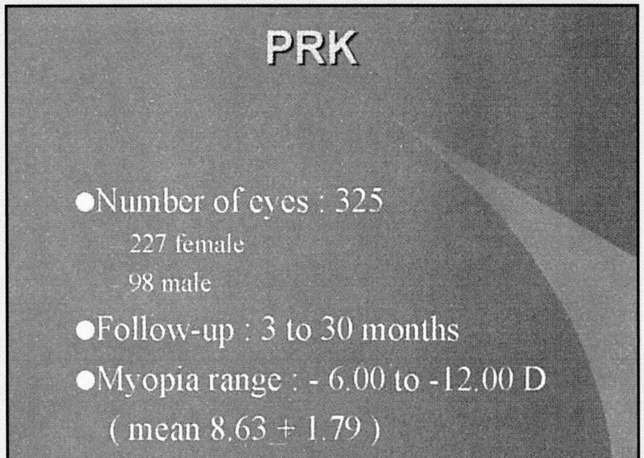

Figure 1.
PRK group.

Group 2 (LASIK) had 58 eyes (36 female and 22 male) with a mean myopia of 9.84 D ± 1.49 (-6.00 D to -12.00 D) (Figure 2). In this group, LASIK was performed using a Chiron microkeratome to create a flap of 160 µm with a diameter of 7.2 mm. The laser ablation was done using the same Summit laser at a single zone of 5.00 mm in 37 eyes and 4.5 mm in 16 eyes. A personal nomogram was used. This nomogram uses 100% of vertex corrected myopia below -6.00 D, 95% from -6.00 D to -8.00 D, 90% from -8.00 D to -10.00 D, and 85% from -10.00 D to -12.00 D.

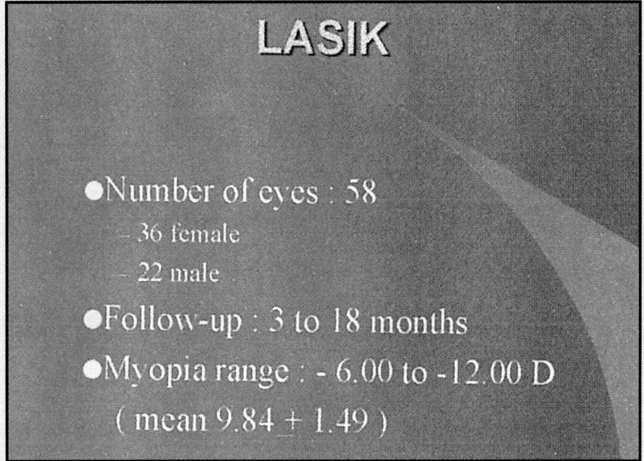

Figure 2.
LASIK group.

As postoperative medications, topical tobramycin was used for 4 days in both groups and topical corticosteroids were used up to 6 months in PRK and up to 7 months in LASIK. The duration of steroids depended on the refraction achieved at 1, 3, and 6 months, retaining the steroids if a tendency toward regression was observed.

RESULTS

We were primarily concerned with the refractive efficacy of PRK and LASIK, but also with the safety of the procedures and patient satisfaction, as well as the quality of vision.

At 1-month follow-up, 75% of LASIK eyes (Figure 3) were in the optimal range (-1 to +1) compared to only 43% of PRK (Figure 4). Half of PRK eyes (52%) were still hyperopic compared to only 19% of the LASIK group. The undercorrections were few in LASIK (7%) and in PRK (5%) at 1 month.

At 3 and 6 months, LASIK had 83% of eyes between -1 and +1 compared to 73% in PRK, but in this PRK group undercorrections began to increase showing 18% at 6 months.

At 1 year, the best cases were similar (78% with LASIK [Figure 5] and 73% with PRK [Figure 6]), but there were already 25% of eyes in PRK more myopic than -1.00.

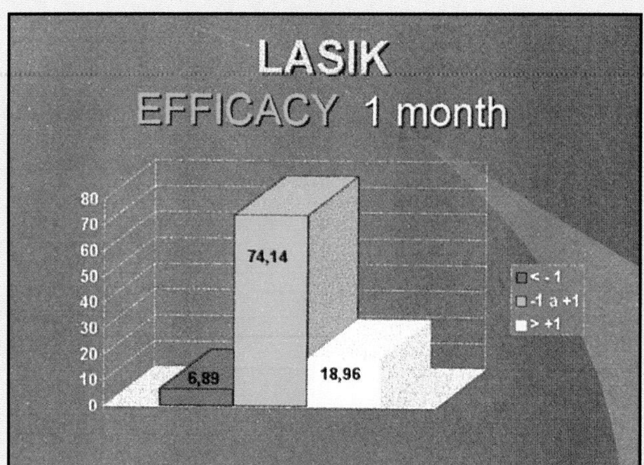

Figure 3.
LASIK efficacy at 1 month.

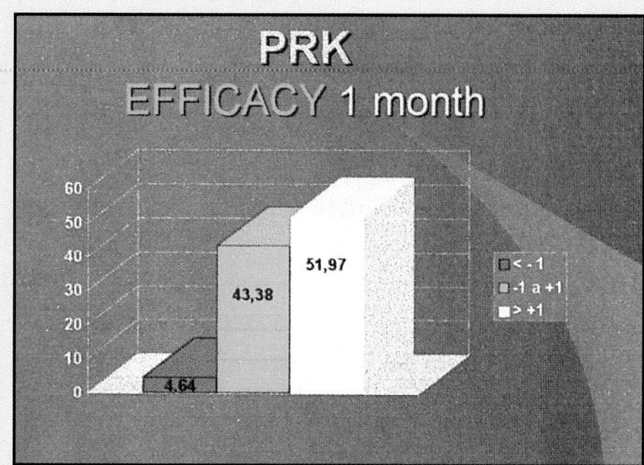

Figure 4.
PRK efficacy at 1 month.

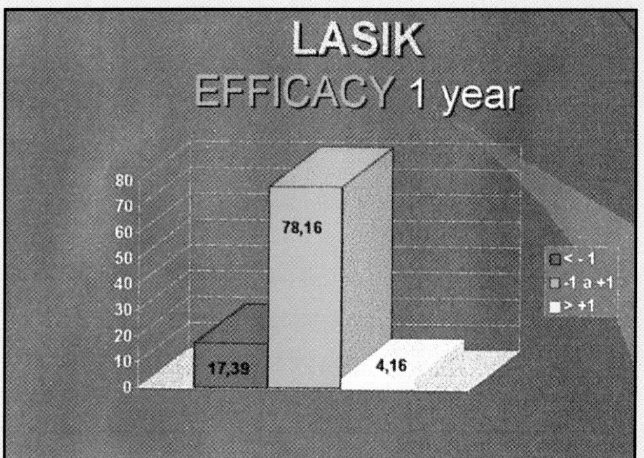

Figure 5.
LASIK efficacy at 1 year.

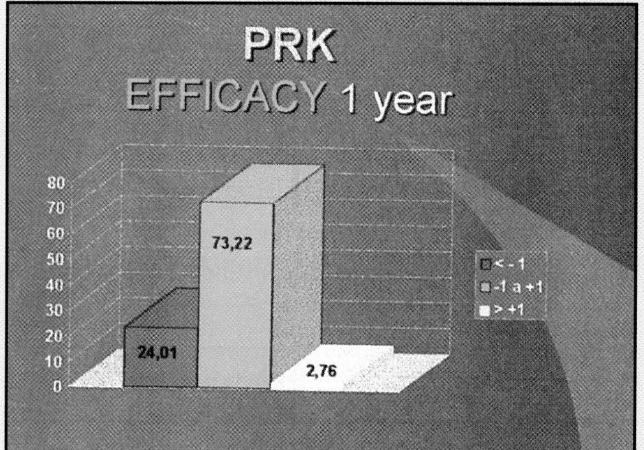

Figure 6.
PRK efficacy at 1 year.

These results show very clearly that regression is much more intense with PRK. In fact, the regression with LASIK from 1 month to 1 year is only -0.50 (Figure 7) while with PRK it is about -3.00 (Figure 8).

To evaluate safety of these procedures, we used best corrected visual acuity and expressed its variations in gains and losses of Snellen lines. In the LASIK group, 62% retained best corrected visual acuity, 28% improved best corrected visual acuity, and only 8% lost one or two lines. In the PRK group, 62% retained best corrected visual acuity, while 14% lost one or two lines. We also see here better performance of LASIK because of the total absence of corneal haze that caused most cases of loss of best corrected visual acuity in PRK.

Patient satisfaction was judged by a simple questionnaire on how the surgery had met each individual's expectations and his or her willingness to do the second eye or do the surgery again. The results were similar in both groups with 94% of the patients happy with their procedures.

Besides the refractive result, it is very important in refractive surgery to evaluate the quality of vision. In order to achieve this goal, we selected 36 eyes of Group 1 and 30 eyes of Group 2, as well as 25 control eyes, and studied contrast sensitivity using a Nicolet Optronics graphic processor studying the 0.5, 1, 3, 6, 11.4, and 22.8 cycles/degree frequencies repeated three times. The results showed no difference between the two groups, although at 6 cycles/degrees, PRK had better results. Although these results are preliminary, it seems that some not perfect interfaces in LASIK may be responsible for these findings.

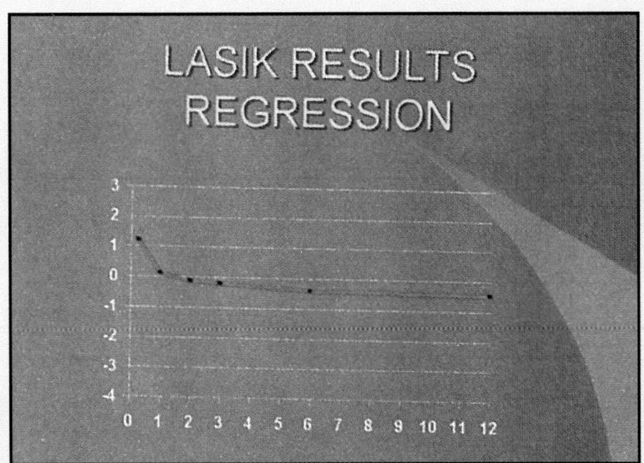

Figure 7.
LASIK regression results.

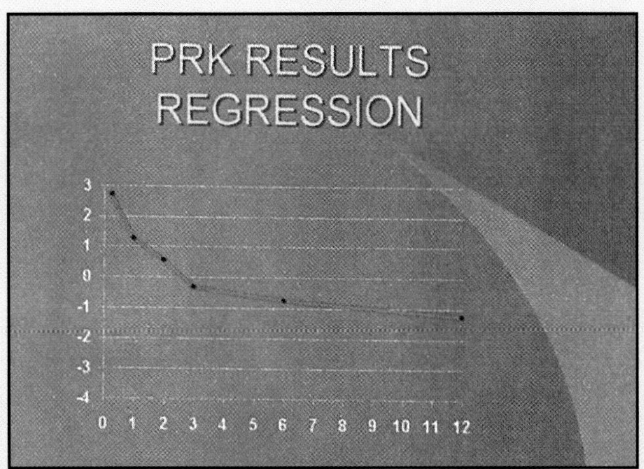

Figure 8.
PRK regression results.

DISCUSSION AND CONCLUSION

As we see from the above results, both PRK and LASIK are effective at 1-year follow-up to correct myopia between -6.00 D and -12.00 D. Nevertheless, LASIK has a much more rapid visual recovery (74% of cases between -1 and +1 at 1 month) than PRK. The results of LASIK at 1 month are only comparable with PRK at 6 months (74% of eyes between -1 and +1).

Regression is almost nil with LASIK after 3 months while in PRK it is still continuing at 1 year, and we know that in some cases it can continue up to 2 years or even more.

Both PRK and LASIK are reasonably safe, although in PRK we had in our series 4% of significant haze with loss of best corrected visual acuity (still present at 1 year).

The quality of vision (measured by contrast sensitivity) is similar in both techniques.

In summary, we think that LASIK should be used as the first choice for moderate myopia because of its following characteristics:

- Very effective and predictable.
- Rapid visual recovery.
- Good quality of vision.
- No noticeable regression.

Chapter 23

CORRECTION LIMITS WITH LASIK

Jose L. Güell, MD

After reviewing the scarce literature published on laser in situ keratomileusis (LASIK), as referred to myopia correction between 0.5 D to 24 D, while at the same time revising the results obtained with other surgical techniques capable of correcting low, medium, and high myopia, we may conclude that LASIK is an excellent procedure with regard to predictability, safety, and stability. In fact, if we only consider the classical parameters used to describe the results after refractive surgery (eg, uncorrected visual acuity, best spectacle corrected visual acuity, deviation from emmetropia [± 0.50 D from intended correction], and loss of two or more lines of visual acuity), LASIK is an excellent procedure for 0.50 D to 20 D of myopia and astigmatism correction, according to my 4 years' experience with this technique. Yet, as all refractive surgery specialists do, we know that these parameters do not suffice to describe our patients' visual capacity. Many of them present visual capacity decrease under low illumination conditions, while one of them is entirely unable to drive or to carry out any activity requiring good visual acuity under these conditions.

We will now consider some factors I believe to be extremely important at the time to decide which are the LASIK, as far as surgical procedure, correction limits.

Any corneal ablational procedure, whether photorefractive keratectomy (PRK) or LASIK, when it attempts to sculpt a lens over the cornea, must follow some rules related to ablation diameter and depth. As Munnerlyn et al described it, the relationship between the optical diameter desired and the "ablation central depth" in

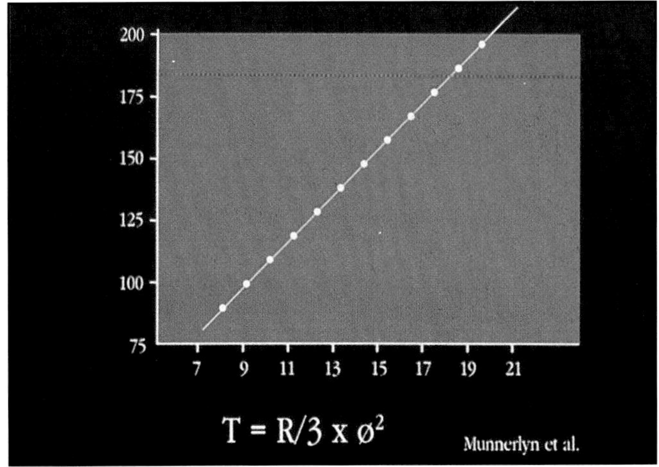

Figure 23-1.
Relation between number of diopters to be corrected and central corneal ablation depth for a 6-mm optical zone.

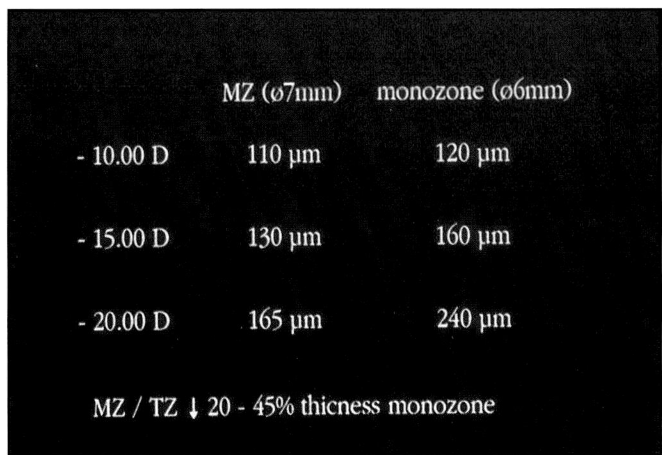

	MZ (ø7mm)	monozone (ø6mm)
- 10.00 D	110 µm	120 µm
- 15.00 D	130 µm	160 µm
- 20.00 D	165 µm	240 µm

MZ / TZ ↓ 20 - 45% thicness monozone

Figure 23-2.
With these ablation profiles we are, in fact, reducing the real basic optical zone.

myopia correction is evident (Figure 23-1). In order to attempt to diminish the ablation central depth, some units started programs variously named as "transition area," "transition zone," and "multizones"(Figure 23-2). In fact, these ablation profiles manage to reduce the real optical area, despite that a large ablation diameter (transitional area) was apparently maintained. This can be clearly noticed when postoperatively studying the topographical map. Despite the fact that we work with, for example, a multizone whose final ablation area reaches 7 mm in diameter, it is noticed also that the real optical area (such as we have topographically and clinically verified) in a 15 D correction is about 4.0 mm (approximately 90% of the correction is in this small area).

In our early LASIK experience, the use of thinner lenticles to reduce the last ablation impact depth was another of the foreseen methods we had thought of. In fact, in late 1993 and early 1994, we only used the 130-µm plate. We thought that aside from moving a little further away from the endothelium, it could probably transmit better to the surface the induced curvature change of the cornea, particularly on the cylindrical correction. As a matter of fact, what we observed was that both the sphere as well as the cylinder were equally corrected using the 130- or 160-µm plate (personal communication). What took place was that the complications rate related to the flap, though insignificant, was in any case higher in those eyes that had been operated with the 130-µm flap, as compared to the 160-µm flap. Regarding this, I would like to remind one of the lenticle low thickness predictability with the microkeratome with which we have the most experience (ALK, Chiron Vision Corp).

In our experience, on the desired thickness we found a +5 / -35 µm slippage. In any case, every time we used the 130-µm plate, it was evident that the lenticle was smaller than when we used the 160-µm plate and thus we were able to compare our results with both plates.

On the other hand, we must also take into account that, through the published research regarding endothelium damage, excimer laser ablation is safe providing we uphold a distance of between 220 and 250 µm from the last laser shut. Possibly we could reach more deeply without any damage, but we cannot ascertain this fact for the time being (Figure 23-3).

Finally, we must never forget the possibility of a progressive corneal ectasia after a corneal ablation procedure. According to the studies carried out a long time ago by Dr. Jose I. Barraquer, and providing we retain a minimal thickness of 300 corneal residual microns, we would remain within the certainty range that no ectasia would occur. Especially after carrying out a lamellar cut and a 360° sectioning of the Bowman's membrane, it would probably be more adequate to maintain 350 µm. In any case, we also find here another limitation we cannot surpass without assuming the risk of a possible progressive problem (see Figure 23-3).

Regarding the "ablation diameter," perhaps the factor that should be best understood is what we have already discussed. That is the "multizone" and "transition zones" methods carried out by some units enable us not to have

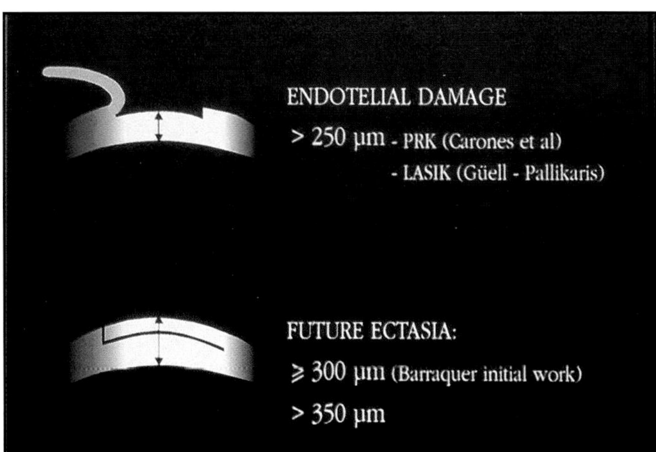

Figure 23-3.
Approximate values for maximum central ablation.

MULTIZONE ABLATION:	65%	80% (entrance pupil)
- 10.00 D	4.5	5.5
- 15.00 D	4.0	5.0
- 20.00 D	3.5	4.6

Figure 23-4.
Theoretical relation between real pupil diameter and refractive correction. We must take into account that the "entrance pupil" is always larger than the real pupil, especially in those highly myopic eyes with deep anterior chamber. In that case, the disparity between both values is still larger.

such a distinct change between the non-treated cornea and the treated cornea. This change was very noticeable when we tried to get high corrections with the so called first-generation units. With all these new ablation profiles, visual complaints such as halos or monocular diplopia are much less frequent. However, it must be remembered that whenever we use an ablation pattern of this type, the ablation real diameter is much smaller than the ablation maximal zone (see Figure 23-2). This means that, and provided we do not reach any further than a 120-μm depth but use an ablation maximal diameter of 6.5 mm in the transition area, 80% of our treatment is found in an approximately 4.5-mm diameter area.

As we have already commented, this can be clearly observed on the postoperative topographical analysis, so whatever the ablation pattern our unit might be using, the real ablation area is an area much smaller than the one we had imagined. Once again, it is important to remember the concept described by Peyman et al about the "entrance pupil," that is, the projection of the pupil over the cornea (Figure 23-4). Ideally, this is the area that should be totally occupied by the real ablation area, in order to prevent any type of visual quality problem. Practically speaking, this could be difficult in the presence of a dilated pupil (ie, under low illumination conditions). It should also be remembered that the projection of the pupil over the cornea or entrance pupil is always larger than the real pupil. This is still more significant in those eyes presenting a deep anterior chamber, where there is a large distance between the iris plane and the anterior corneal surface, as characteristic in most myopic eyes, especially in highly myopic patients.

Clinically, this is not true either as we know that, except on corrections higher than 10 D, it is very rare to find patients presenting night vision problems. Despite this fact, these problems might be discovered through a more detailed study of the visual conditions, through the contrast sensitivity tests and with more reliable methods than those existing now.

Finally, and from the corneal curvature concept and despite the available technology clear limitations to evaluate this corneal curvature, in particular on the postoperative period (both obtained from keratometers as well as from videokeratographs, whether based on a Placido ring projection as well as with the new slit systems or on other corneal height measuring systems), we should clearly consider certain points.

On one hand, the induced change on corneal curvature obtained with the ablation should at least theoretically be in proportion to the number of diopters to be corrected, and which we verify refractively. We know perfectly well that this is untrue and that we can frequently have similar final K's on two patients with similar preoperative keratometric readings, even if we have made a 7.00 D correction to one and a 12.00 D correction to the other. In second place, and maybe even more important-

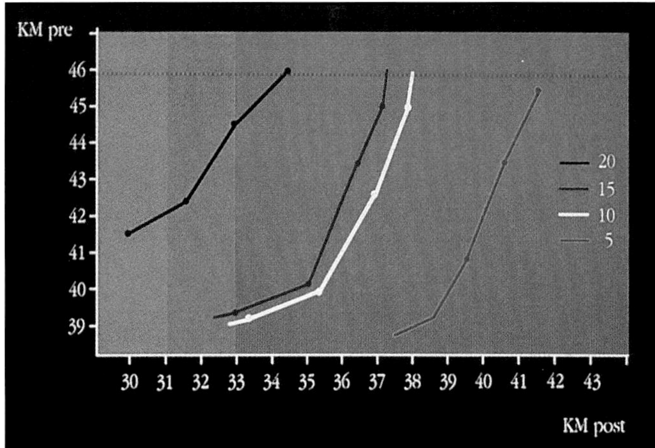

Figure 23-5.
Relationship between pre- and postoperative K's for different degrees of correction (5,10,15, and 20 D). Residual K's under 33 D are in high risk of distorted vision, especially under dim illumination conditions because of a larger pupil.

ly, is the fact that there must be a corneal curvature change limitation present that we can induce in our cornea, in order for it to correctly carry out its functions. The groups, as referred to corneal curvature, that we consider to be dangerous can be observed in Figure 23-5. As from the vision quality point of view, in particular under low illumination conditions, we begin to face problems when the final K's are found to be under 33 D, and we obviously consider it a high risk situation when the final K's are found to be under 31. In this last situation, patients frequently present a decrease in maximal corrected visual acuity. If this is not found under the standard conditions that can be present in our examination office, it can be found in their normal life.

To summarize, the relationship between maximal ablation depth, the lens we are sculpting on the cornea real diameter, and its relationship with pupillary diameter, as well as the final corneal curvature, are probably the most important parameters we must take into account to decide whether or not a patient is an optimal candidate for corneal refractive ablational surgery. I could not finish this chapter without insisting on two aspects I deem to be fundamental:

1. The presently available measurement methods. Despite the fact that we consider them to be most advanced, they present clear limitations that prevent us to accurately and repeatedly study them, while this limitation is extended to our patients' cases.
2. I would only like to indicate the lack of real knowledge of the optical and refractive aspects of a cornea after being operated. Why those patients to whom we have carried out an 18 D correction on the cornea, whose final corneal curvatures are extremely low, whose corneal thickness is very distant than what it was originally, have an excellent visual quality, despite the disagreement between the real optical zone where we have carried out the 18 D correction and the pupillary diameter, while on other patients under similar conditions, and even if a much slighter change has been induced, still present important symptoms and a decreased visual capacity, in particular under low illumination conditions?

New technology evaluating corneal contour as well as artificial intelligence will probably help us in understanding how important corneal asphericity is, how we can change it without altering visual conditions, etc.

The real fact is that there is still an important need to carry out work and research, in order to be able to truly understand what is really taking place after surgery in the amazing optical system called the eye.

Results of LASIK for the Treatment of Myopia at 1 Year from the University of Crete and the Vardinoyannion Eye Institute of Crete

IOANNIS G. PALLIKARIS, MD, DIMITRIOS S. SIGANOS, MD, THEKLA G. PAPADAKI, MD, VIKENTIA I. KATSANEVAKI, MD, KYRIAKI EVANGELATOU, MD

TABLE 1

Grouping and Number of Eyes

Group	Preoperative Myopia Sph Eq (D)	No. of Eyes (N=2170)
A	5 to 10	745
B	>10 to <16	1185
C	>16	240

TABLE 2

1-Year Results

Group	± 0.50 D (No. of Eyes%)	± 1.0 D (No. of Eyes%)	± 2.0 D (No. of Eyes%)
A	560 (75.1%)	610 (82.2%)	722 (96.9%)
B	450 (37.9%)	780 (65.8%)	988 (83.3%)
C	30 (12.5%)	88 (36.6%)	180 (75%)

SECTION 6

COMPLICATIONS

Chapter 24

LASIK COMPLICATIONS AND THEIR MANAGEMENT

Ioannis G. Pallikaris, MD, Dimitrios S. Siganos, MD, Vikentia I. Katsanevaki, MD

Compared with photorefractive keratectomy (PRK), LASIK is a more complex technique that demands a skilled surgeon. Based on 7 years experience with this procedure, I will present some of the most common LASIK, or laser in situ keratomileusis, complications as well as their management.

In this chapter, the complications of LASIK are divided into those related to the use of the microkeratome and those resulting from the use of the excimer laser. I use this classification for simplicity reasons alone.

Complications from both categories can occur in the same patient. I must emphasize that, apart from changes in shape and form of the cornea that may influence the optical system, there are also changes related to the corneal structure and properties as a refractive medium. Certain patients with satisfactory topography, manifest refraction, and slit lamp examination complain of poor vision. This is mostly related to light distortion at the interface that unfortunately cannot be detected from the common examination.

KERATOME-RELATED COMPLICATIONS

Apart from the surgeon's learning curve of LASIK, the operation can still be complicated since the flap making depends on a very sophisticated instrument—the microkeratome. Trained and reliable personnel must be responsible for its assembly

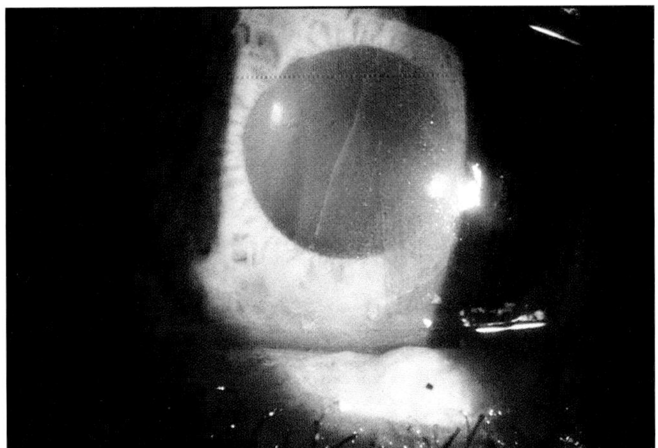

Figure 24-1.
Intermittent advancement of the keratome.

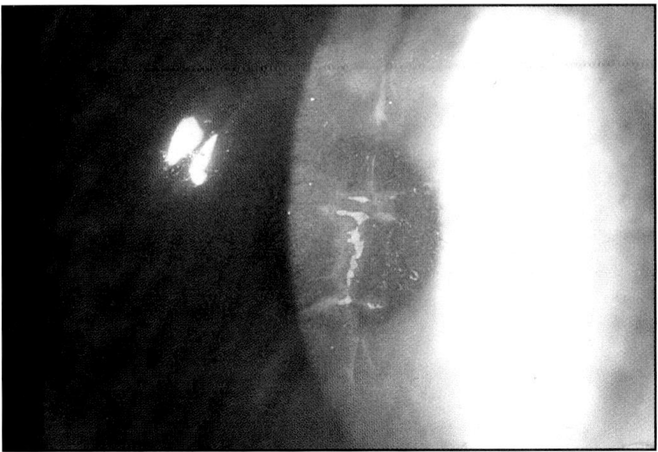

Figure 24-2.
Scar formation.

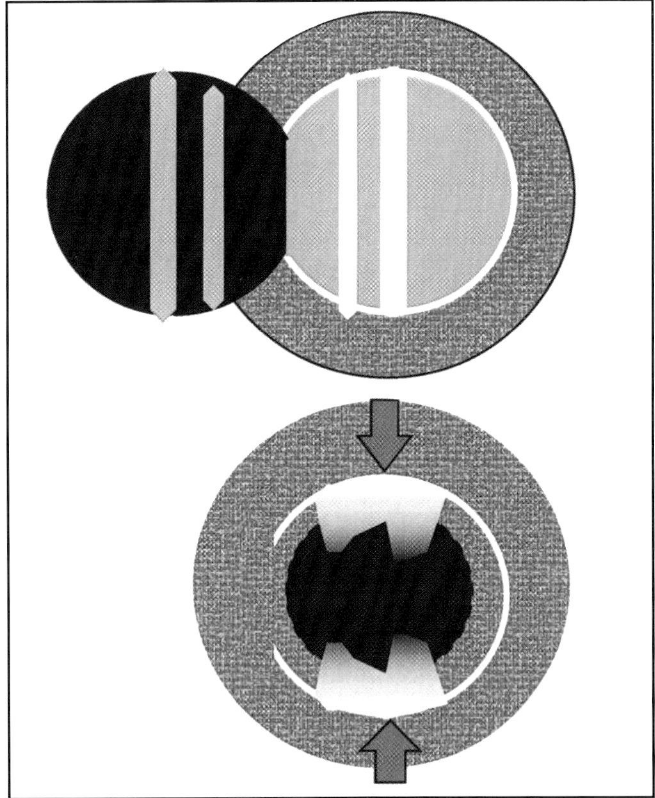

Figure 24-3.
Irregular cap thickness: Vertical direction of thinner part, very often multiple parallel lines consisting only of stromal tissue, irregular cap edges respectively to the thinner areas. Cause: Intermittent advancement of the blade (gear problems).
Early: Intrastromal epithelial ingrowth (occasional stromal melting). Late: Scar formation.

and maintenance. The microkeratome should be cleaned with a sterile hard brush and properly assembled before use. Dirty gears will result in intermittent advancement of the blade producing a flap of irregular thickness (Figures 24-1 through 24-4).

The quality of the blade is crucial for the results; with the Chiron microkeratome, a new blade must be used for each eye. A poor quality blade will result in a flap that is thinner than expected, with irregular borders and/or thickness (Figures 24-5a through 24-8). Regarding Figure 24-8, keep in mind the following points:

1—In case of PRK over PTK, after transepithelial removal of the initial 40 µm, add 1 D for every 20 µm removed to the final PRK correction (ie, to a patient with 5 D of residual myopia, in case of 60 µm of PTK prior to PRK, the attempted correction should be 4 D.)

2—In case of PRK over PTK with the use of a smoothing agent or masking material and epithelial debridement, add 1 to 2 D to the final PRK correction.

Ideally, flap thickness must range between 130 and 170 µm. Thicker flaps may not leave enough residual corneal stroma for the correction, while thinner flaps are difficult to manipulate on repositioning (Figures 24-9a through 24-9d).

A poor quality blade can leave metal particles in the stroma (Figure 24-10). These can be detected under the flap at slit lamp examination postoperatively. Metal particles must be removed immediately as they can induce scar formation.

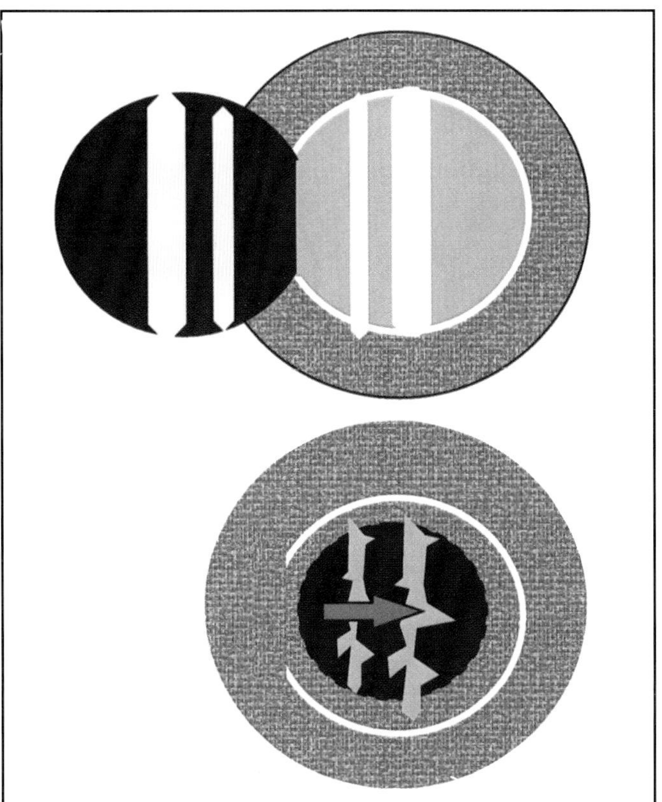

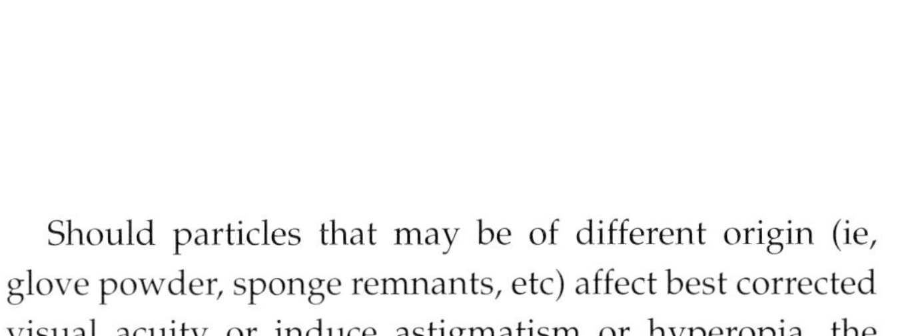

Figure 24-4.
Irregular cap thickness: Vertical direction of thinner part, multiple parallel lines consisting of epithelium only. Cause: Intermittent advancement of the blade, along with low IOP (gear and suction problems). Early: Intrastromal epithelial ingrowth (occasionally due to stromal melting). Late: Scar formation.

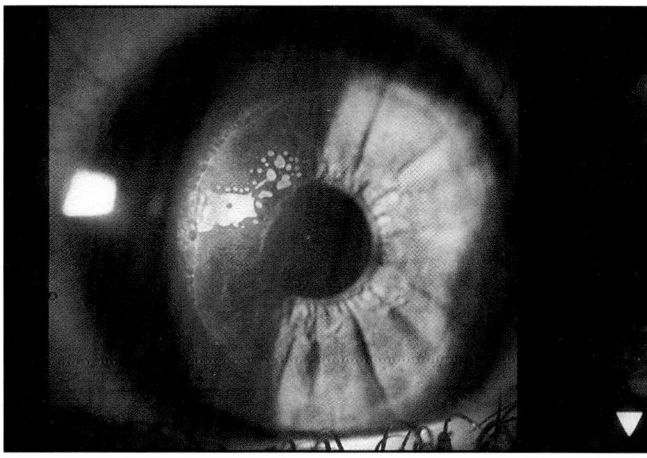

Figure 24-5a.
Corneal scar and intrastromal island.

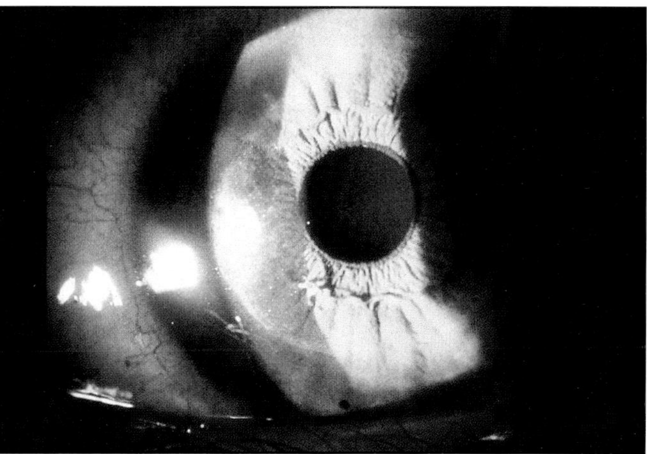

Figure 24-5b.
Corneal scar.

Should particles that may be of different origin (ie, glove powder, sponge remnants, etc) affect best corrected visual acuity or induce astigmatism or hyperopia, the stroma must be cleaned (Figures 24-11 through 24-13g).

The intraoperative IOP measurement should never be overlooked. Inadequate IOP (less than 65 mmHg) can result in a small or total cap with/or irregular cap thickness (Figures 24-2, 24-4, 24-14 through 24-17). Whatever the reason, irregular cap thickness will result in intrastromal epithelial ingrowth and eventually in corneal scarring.

OPTICAL COMPLICATIONS

The optical result of the photoablation can be evaluated with regard to three main factors that can be detected on the patient's postoperative topographic map.

1. The diameter of the central ablation (S)—This is defined as the size (in millimeters) of the area including 1.5 D of steepening, from the flattest value of refractive power, on an autoscaled topography map. Small-sized central ablation can induce glare or "ghosting" around headlights, especially at night. There are three sizes of central ablation that are discriminated. Size S1 refers to a central ablation larger than 5 mm (Figure 24-18). These patients are not expected to experience any glare or halos. Size S2 (Figure 24-19) refers to a central ablation measuring 3 to 5 mm and size S3 (Figure 24-20) refers to a central

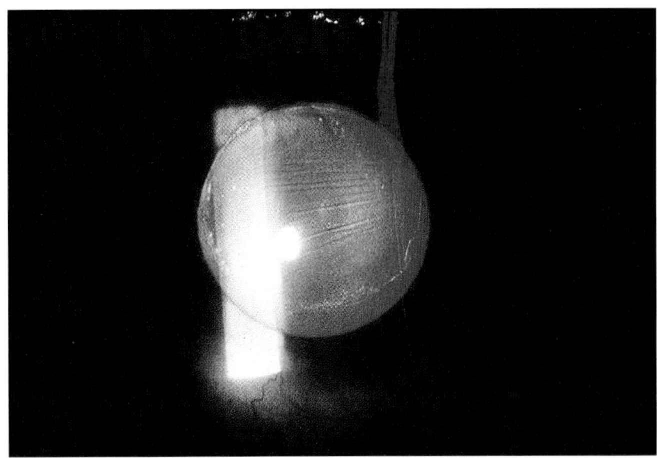

Figure 24-6a.
Irregular borders. Striae of the flap.

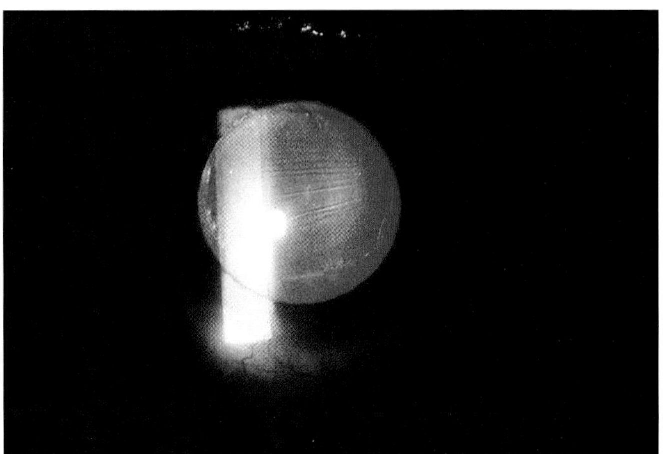

Figure 24-6b.
Irregular borders. Striae of the flap.

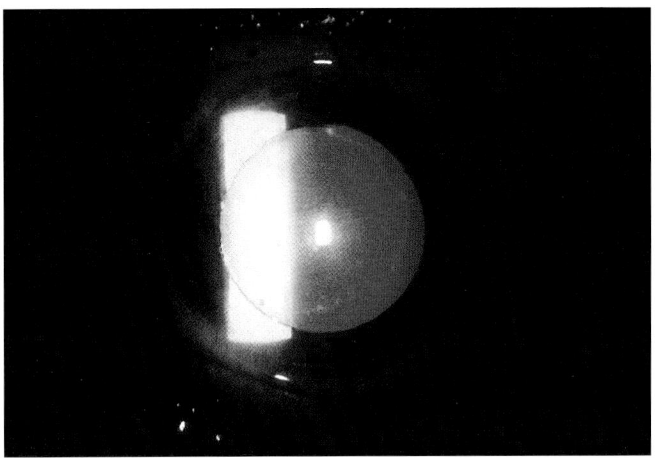

Figure 24-6c.
Irregular borders. Striae of the flap.

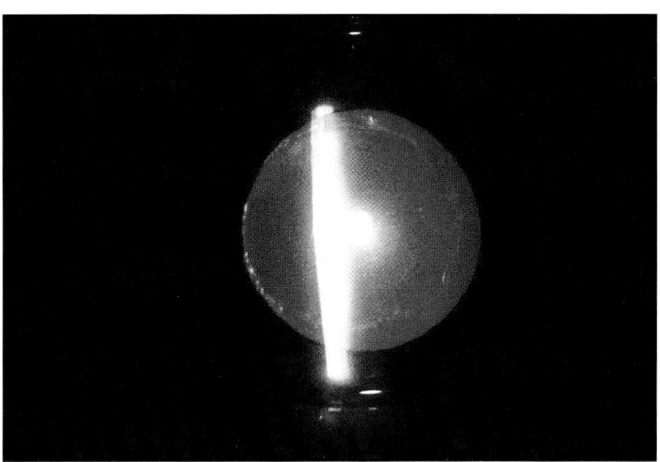

Figure 24-6d.
Irregular borders. Striae of the flap.

ablation that is smaller than 3 mm.

2. Ablation pattern (P)—Asymmetrical ablation patterns (Figures 24-21 through 24-23) can result in an irregular astigmatism and, in extreme cases, the patient complains of multiple images due to corneal prismatic effects. Ideally, the corneal refractive power should normally be increasing from the center to the periphery of the ablated zone. This means that in each meridian, symmetrical points from the center of the ablation should have the same refractive power and thus be represented with the same color on an autoscaled topographic map. Considering A as the smaller and B as the greater distance (in millimeters) between the flattest (deep blue) and the mean refractive power (middle green) area on the autoscaled topographic map, we define R as the ratio of A:B. In order to assess the extent of the irregularly ablated pattern, and to resolve it for a better visual outcome, we classify irregularity into three patterns in respect to R. P1 (see Figure 24-21) refers to ablation patterns where R is greater than 1/3. This case is within normal range and the patient may not suffer from subjective symptoms. On the other hand, in cases classified as P2 (R between 1/3 and 1/5) and P3 (R less than 1/5), severe complications exist and need to be treated (see Figures 24-22 and 24-23, respectively).
3. Centration of the ablation—In case the ablation center does not correspond to the center of the map, this

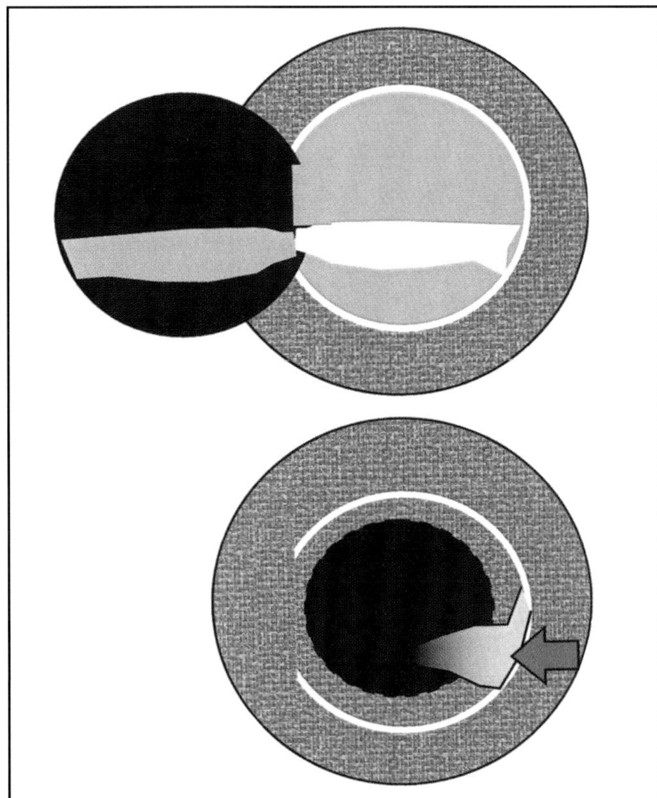

Figure 24-7.
Irregular cap thickness: Horizontal direction of thinner part (thinner part consists of epithelial and stromal tissue). Cause: Blade cutting edge irregularities.
Early: Intrastromal epithelial ingrowth, very often cornea melting. Late: Scar formation.

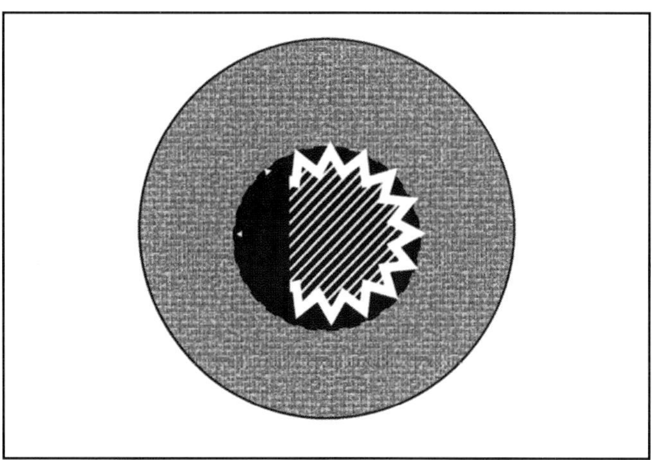

Figure 24-8.
Small cap or flap: size < 5 mm. Thickness: < 100 μm. Eccentric flap or cap borders within the 5-mm central optical zone.
Abnormal border with epithelial ingrowth or scar and central striae. (A) Best corrected visual acuity loss of two or more lines. (A1) Smooth anterior corneal surface (no irregular astigmatism) = transepithelial PTK, 60 μm in depth and 8 mm in diameter, centered at the pupil center, plus PRK for residual refractive error (7-mm tapered transition zone recommended). (A2) Irregular corneal surface (with irregular astigmatism) = epithelial debridement (using beaver, not brush) and PTK with smoothing agent (depth of the ablation will be optically estimated from the quality of the surface), plus PRK for residual refractive error (7-mm tapered transition zone recommended).
(B) Loss of best corrected visual acuity of one line or less. (B1) Intense glare and halos = transepithelial PTK 50 μm in depth with a 7-mm zone, plus PRK. (In case of myopic refraction up to 3 D, additional 30 μm PTK in 7-mm zone.) (B2) Minimal glare = secondary LASIK (second cut) for residual refractive error with flap thicker than 160 μm and wide ablation zone.

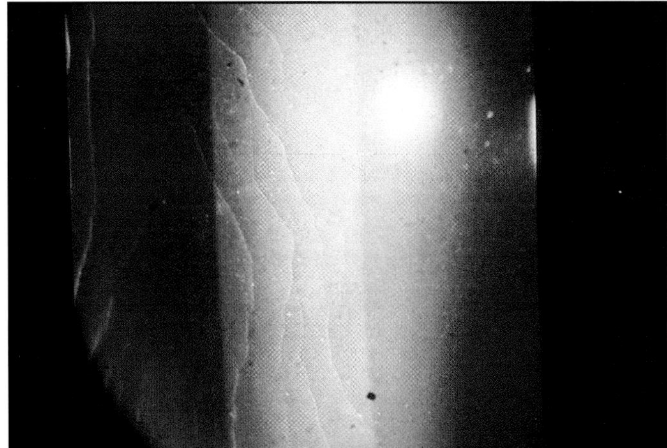

Figure 24-9a.
Thin flap with striae and regular borders.

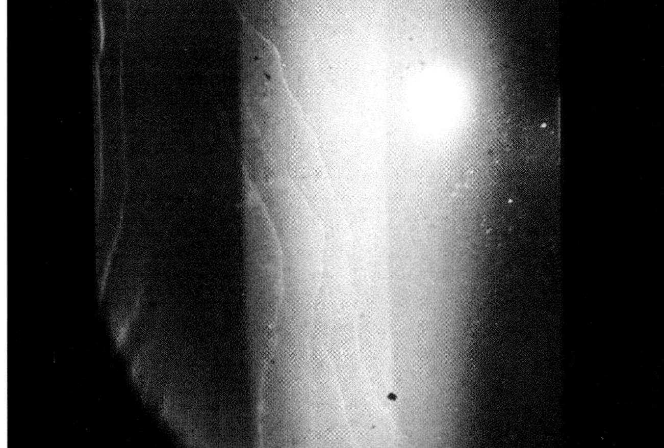

Figure 24-9b.
Thin flap with striae and regular borders.

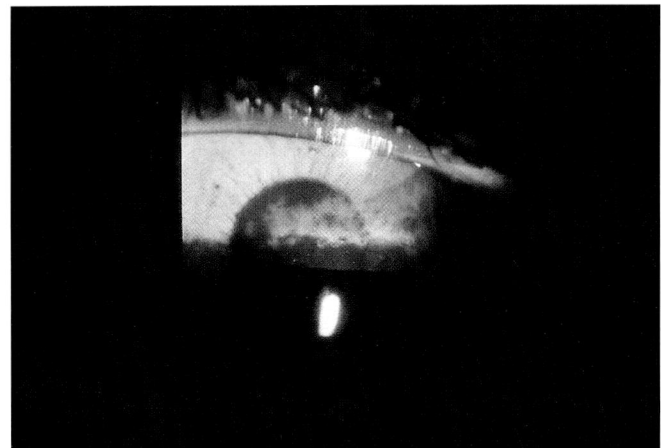

Figure 24-9c.
Thin flap with striae and regular borders.

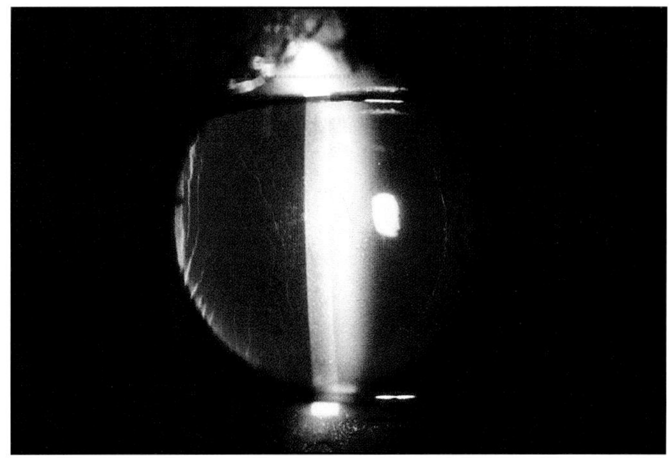

Figure 24-9d.
Thin flap with striae and regular borders.

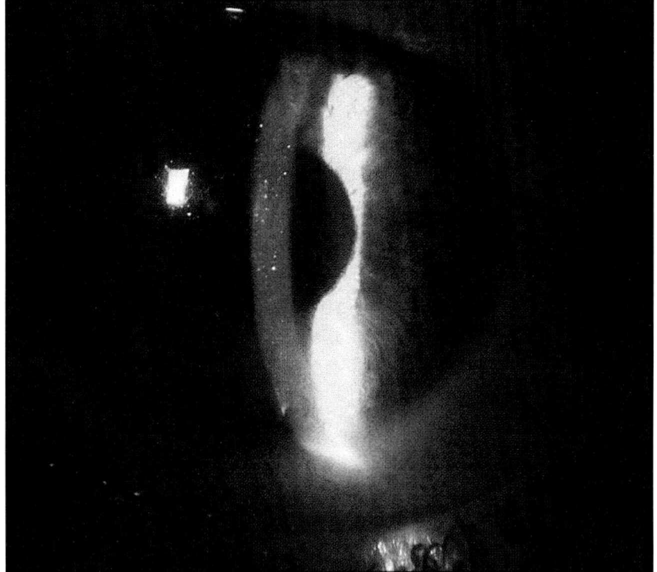

Figure 24-10.
Metal particles under the flap.

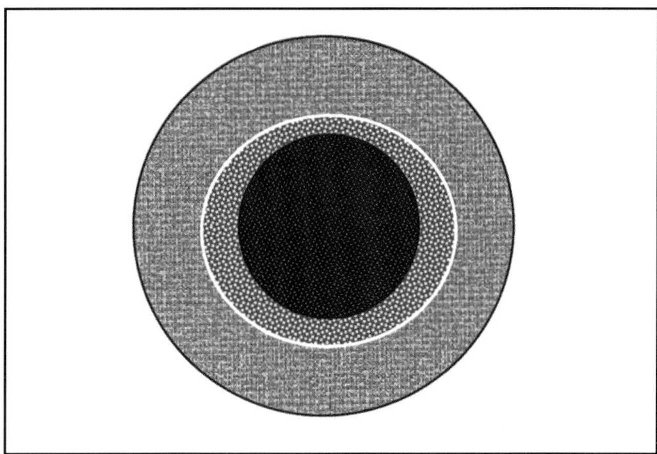

Figure 24-11.
Fine interface remnants. (1) Smooth corneal surface, no striae, no best corrected visual acuity loss at 1 month = wait. (2) Loss of best corrected visual acuity greater than or equal to one line, or no loss of best corrected visual acuity but induced cylinder greater than 1 D = immediate cleaning. (3) Metal particles = immediate cleaning.

ablation is considered to be eccentric (E). This is a severe complication that needs to be treated since it induces multifocality of the optical zone that could result into blurred images, glare, ghost images, poor visual acuity, or poor contrast sensitivity. Eccentricity is evaluated on an autoscaled topographic map where ideally the flattest (deep blue) area must include the center of the map. For treatment purposes, eccentricity is classified as E1 if the center of the map is situated within the area of the mean refractive power (middle green) and E2 if elsewhere (Figures 24-23 and 24-24). Both categories have subdivisions regarding the 3-mm optical zone. Subcategory A is defined as that having one quadrant of the 3-mm zone out of the green encircled area; subcategory B is defined as that having more than one quadrant of the

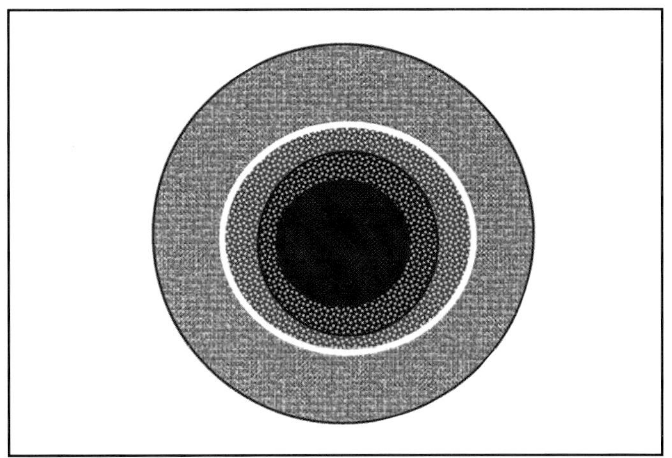

Figure 24-12.
Peripheral interface remnants or particles. (1) Not affecting best corrected visual acuity or inducing irregular astigmatism, no hyperopic shift = wait. (2) Not affecting best corrected visual acuity or inducing astigmatism, hyperopic shift (hyperopic effect due to the elevation of the periphery of the flap) = remove. (3) Affecting best corrected visual acuity or inducing irregular astigmatism = remove. (4) Metal particles = remove.

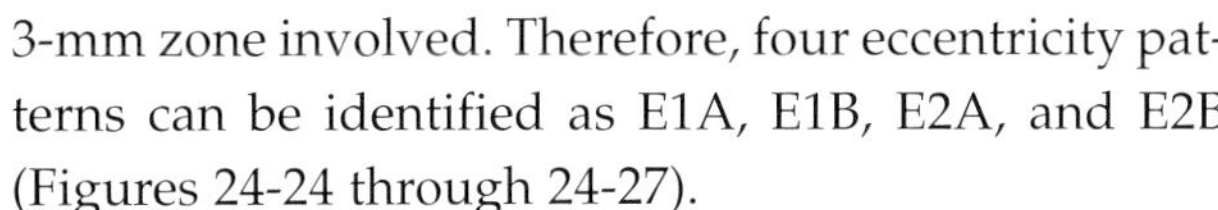

3-mm zone involved. Therefore, four eccentricity patterns can be identified as E1A, E1B, E2A, and E2B (Figures 24-24 through 24-27).

In fact, the topographic map of a complicated case reveals a combination of the above regarding the size, pattern, and centration of ablation. The treatment aims to restore a normal topographic map either by enlargement of the central ablated area using arcuate cuts (in milder cases) or with supplemental ablation which can be diagonal or masked.

Diagonal ablation is that centered at a distance equal to the smaller radius of the initial ablation, on an imaginary line passing from the center of the cornea to the center of the initial ablation (ie, 3 mm away from the center of the map, diagonally placed to the previous ablation of 6-mm zone). Diagonal ablation applies to cases with small-sized (S3) ablation combined with mild (P1), moderate (P2), or severe (P3) irregularity pattern and moderate (E1B or E2A) eccentricity (cases S3P1E1B, S3P2E2A, and S3P3E2A) See Tables 24-1 and 24-2.

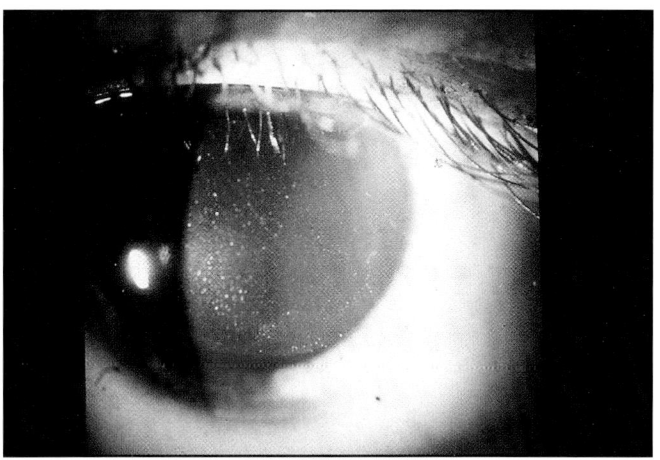

Figure 24-13a.
Fine interface remnants.

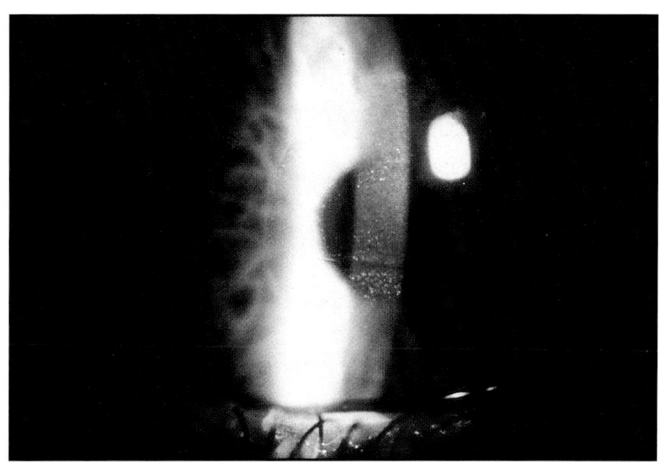

Figure 24-13b.
Fine interface remnants.

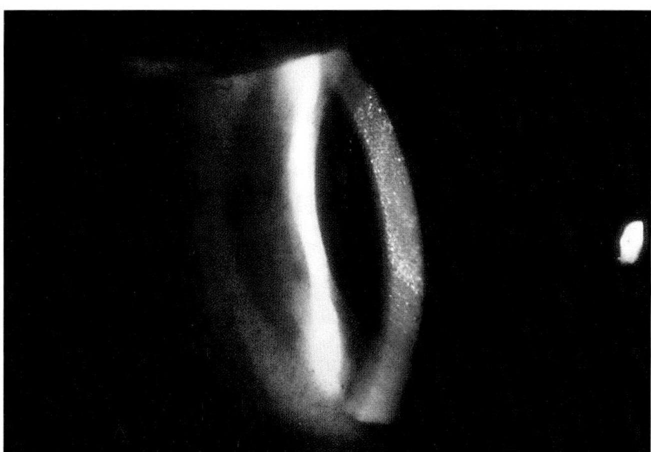

Figure 24-13c.
Peripheral remnants.

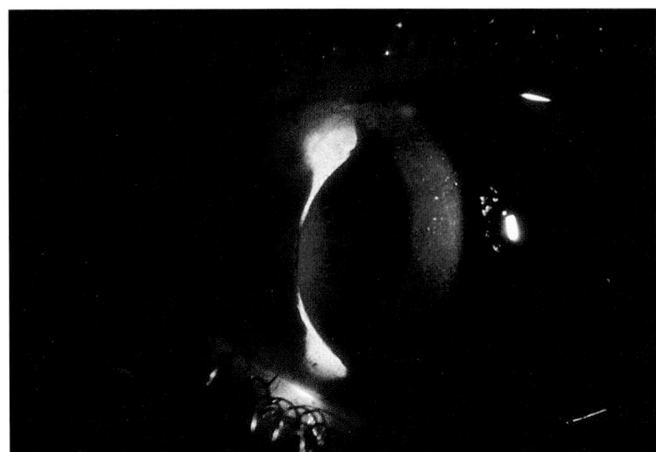

Figure 24-13d.
Peripheral remnants.

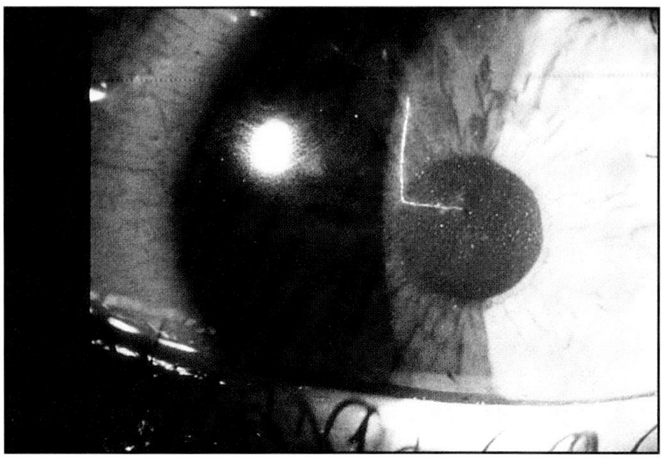

Figure 24-13e.
Sponge remnants.

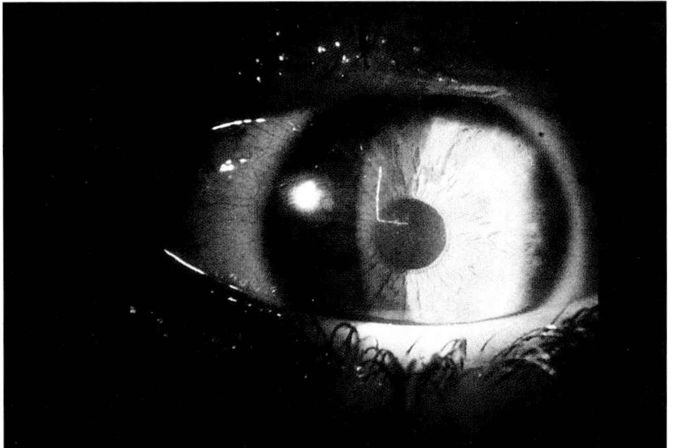

Figure 24-13f.
Sponge remnants.

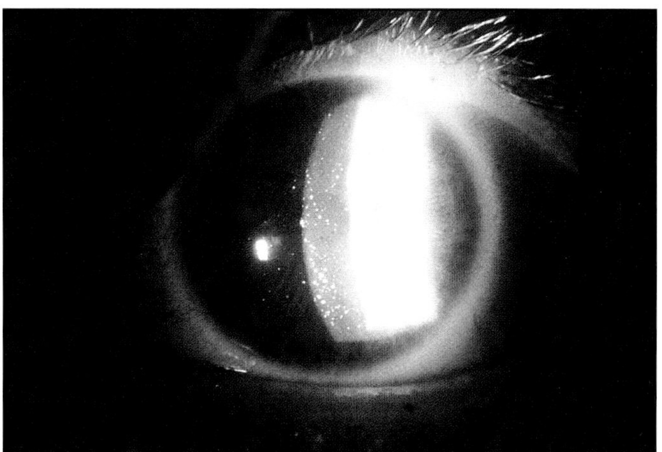

Figure 24-13g.
Glove powder under the flap.

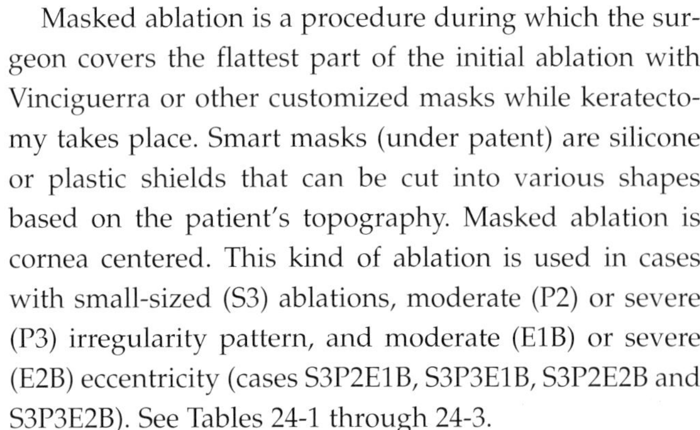

Masked ablation is a procedure during which the surgeon covers the flattest part of the initial ablation with Vinciguerra or other customized masks while keratectomy takes place. Smart masks (under patent) are silicone or plastic shields that can be cut into various shapes based on the patient's topography. Masked ablation is cornea centered. This kind of ablation is used in cases with small-sized (S3) ablations, moderate (P2) or severe (P3) irregularity pattern, and moderate (E1B) or severe (E2B) eccentricity (cases S3P2E1B, S3P3E1B, S3P2E2B and S3P3E2B). See Tables 24-1 through 24-3.

In every case, the amount of supplemental ablation should be the difference of the refractive power of the center of the ablation minus the refractive power of the flattest part of the cornea (ie, the center of the initial ablation). This is performed on a wide optical zone.

Attempted correction = Pc_1- Pc_2

(Pc_1=refractive power of the center of the ablation, Pc_2=refractive power of the center of the initial ablation)

This attempted correction applies even for patients who could in this way be overcorrected, since our major concern is to homogenize the optical zone. Any hyperopic shift could be corrected in a second approach. The residual corneal stroma must be at least 250-µm thick in order to prevent a possible corneal ectasia. During supplementary ablation, polishing with instillation of natural tears eye drops is recommended, so as to smooth the ablated surface.

Eccentric ablation E1A can be treated with an arcuate cut 70° long in every case of S or P. The smaller the opti-

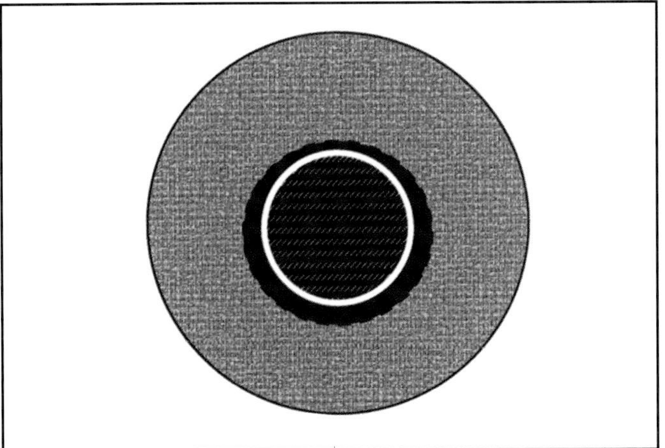

Figure 24-14.
Small flap or cap: 5 mm < size <7 mm. Thickness: >100 μm, well-centered, faint striae.
(1) No best corrected visual acuity loss, no induced astigmatism = wait. (2) Best corrected visual acuity loss or induced irregular astigmatism = early (within 1 month) repositioning and cleaning of the flap or cap. In case of a total cap, do not remove the cap, leave a small epithelial hinge, preferably where the cap is better fitted to the stroma, to prevent cap loss.

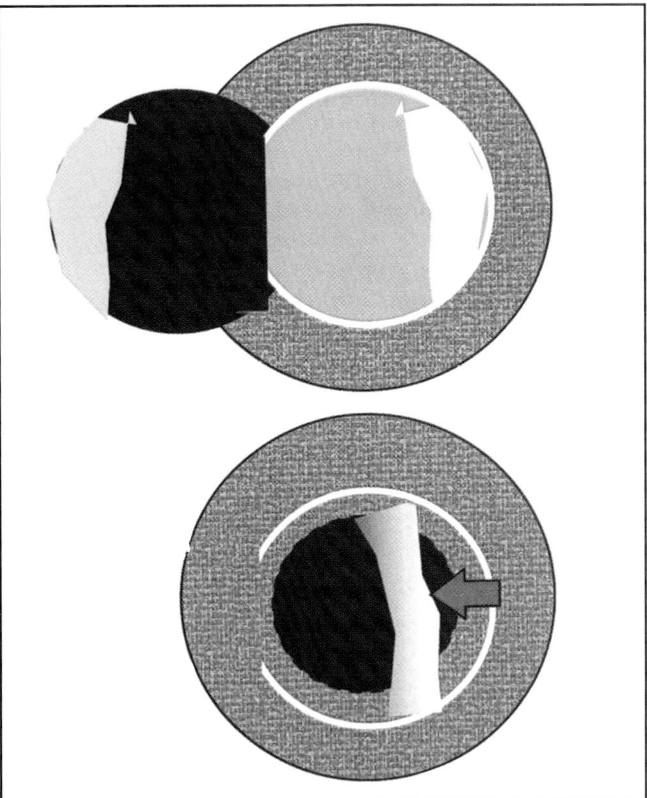

Figure 24-15.
Irregular cap thickness: Vertical direction of thinner part located at the temporal edge of the flap consisting only of epithelium. Cause: Inadequate suction, low IOP.
Early: Intrastromal epithelial ingrowth. Late: Scar formation.

cal zone, the more effective the cut (Table 24-4). In cases of more profound eccentricity (E1B or E2A), a longer arcuate cut (90°) is recommended (cases S1P2E1B, S1P3E1B, S2P1E1B, S2P2E1B, S2P3E1B, and S2P2E2A). See Tables 24-1 and 24-2.

Ablation-related complications constitute a problem for both the patient and the surgeon. Each complicated case is a unique entity in terms of objective signs as well as subjective symptoms and should be treated as such. An inappropriate keratectomy may result in a disabled patient whose treatment will require penetrating or lamellar keratoplasty. The abovementioned guidelines for the management of complicated eyes offer satisfactory results. Patients treated with arcuate cuts could obtain a homogeneous optical zone and thus a very good visual outcome. In more severe cases requiring supplemental ablation, the optical quality of the optical zone cannot always be uniform. This could be treated by using a biomaterial with certain properties that could serve as a special mold for the ablation. This biomaterial should be in liquid form when applied to the cornea where it will solidify within seconds. The preferred inner surface of a hard contact lens would be adjusted on the upper surface of the material while in liquid form. Ablation rate of this mask (when solid) is the same as that of the cornea. In this way, its surface is reproduced on the surface of the

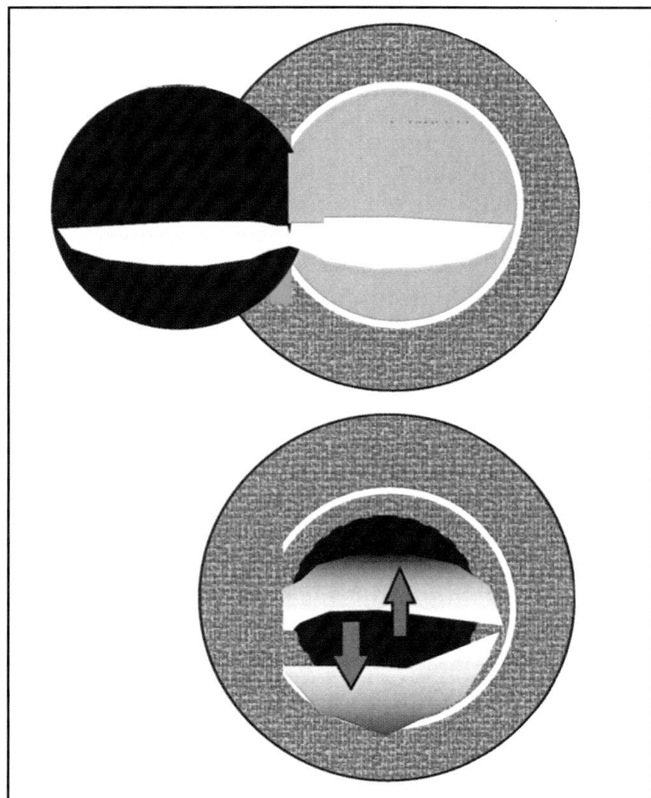

Figure 24-16.
Irregular cap thickness: Horizontal direction of thinner part or half cut flap (thinner part consists of epithelium only). Cause: Low IOP by inadequate suction.
Early: Intrastromal epithelial ingrowth. Late: Scar formation.

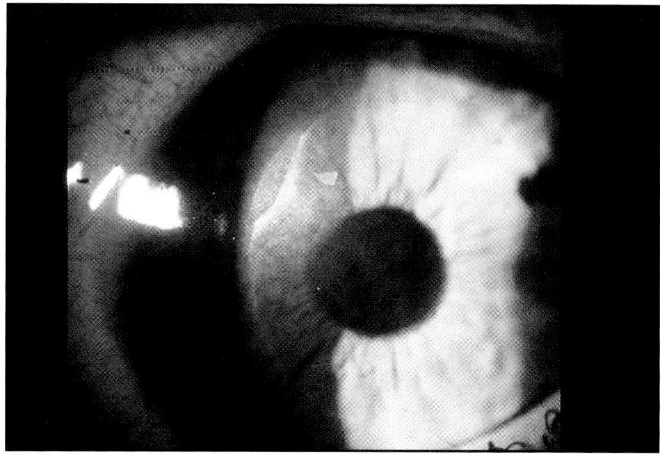

Figure 24-17.
Scar formation.

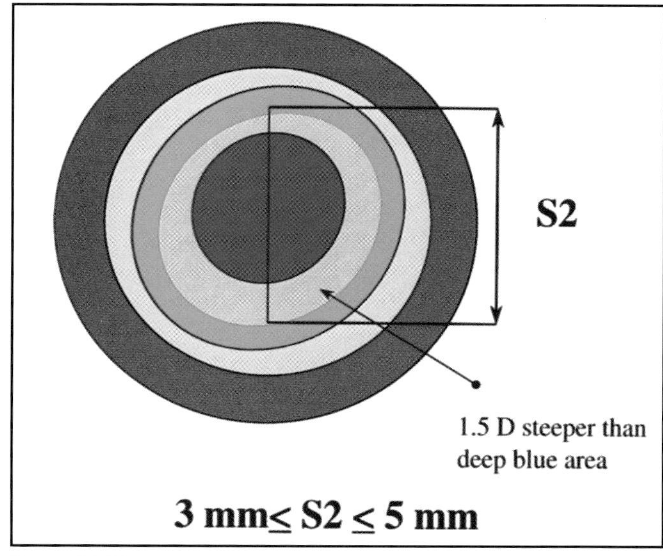

Figure 24-19.
Size S2.

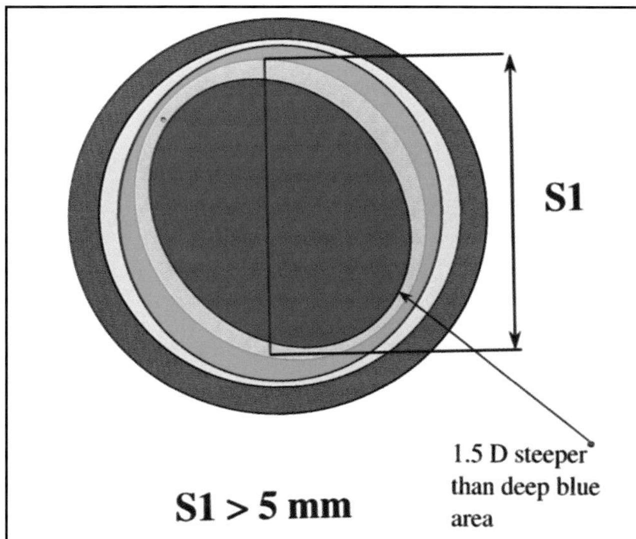

Figure 24-18.
Size S1.

cornea when ablated, leaving a perfectly smooth surface with the desired contour (under patent).

Case Example

Figures 24-28a and 24-28b are examples of a 24-year-old patient who underwent LASIK for the correction of -14.5 sph -2.25 cyl x 40. Nineteen months after the initial operation, the patient's refraction was -5.75 sph -4.75 cyl x 165. She underwent retreatment with a diagonal ablation. Attempted correction was -6 D with an optical zone of 6 mm. The center of the diagonal ablation was 2 mm up from the center of the pupil on the decentration axis. A second cut was performed at retreatment.

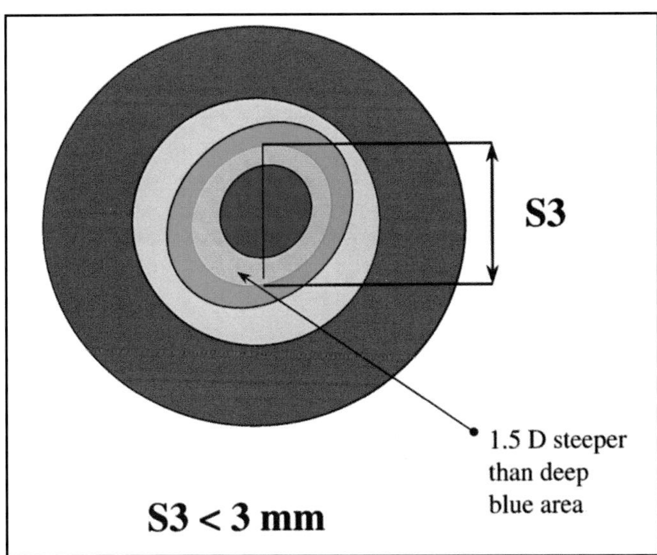

Figure 24-20.
Size S3.

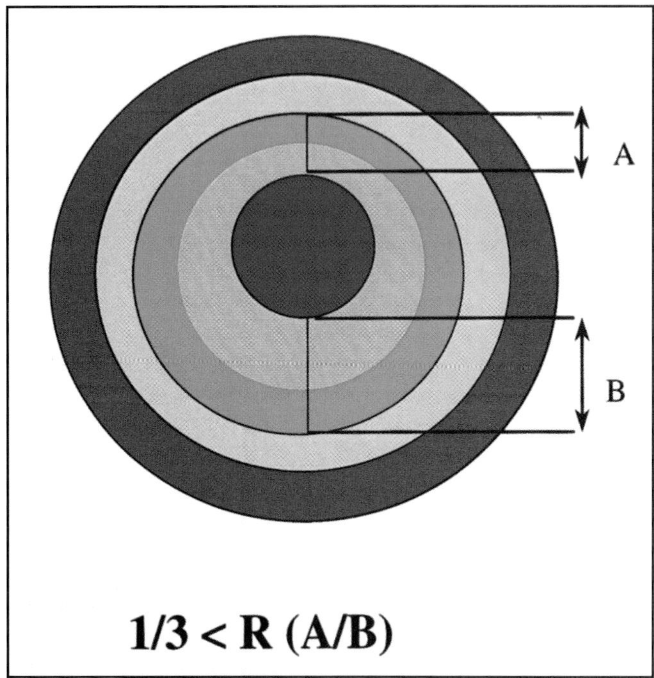

Figure 24-21.
Ablation pattern P1.

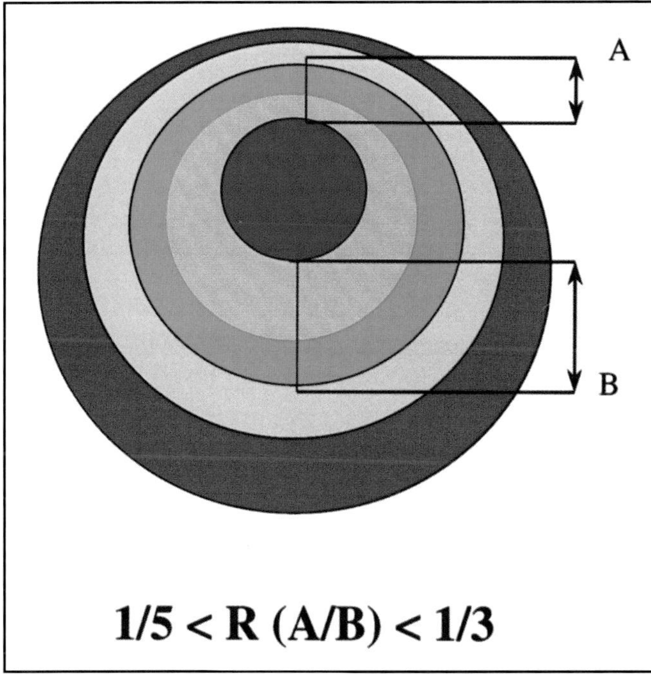

Figure 24-22.
Ablation pattern P2.

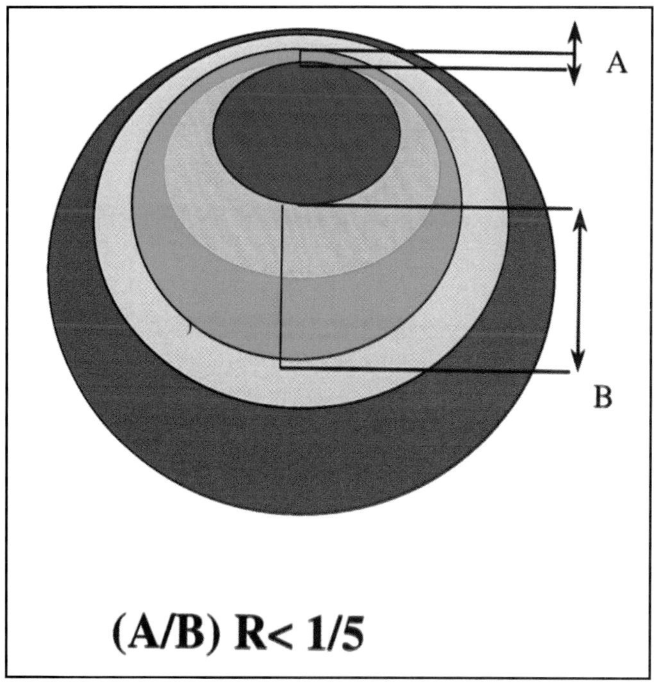

Figure 24-23.
Ablation pattern P3.

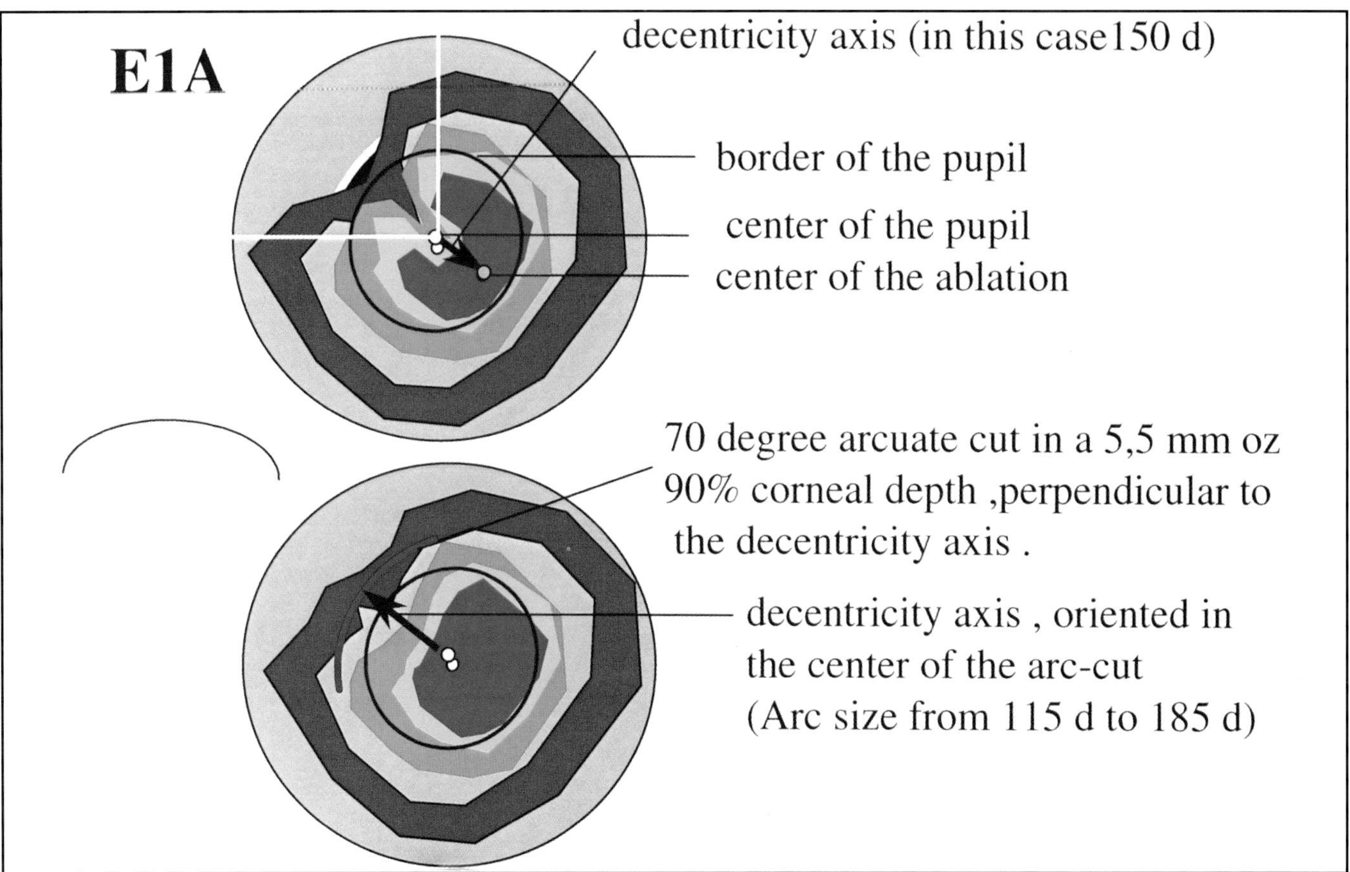
E1A
decentricity axis (in this case150 d)
border of the pupil
center of the pupil
center of the ablation
70 degree arcuate cut in a 5,5 mm oz
90% corneal depth ,perpendicular to
the decentricity axis .
decentricity axis , oriented in
the center of the arc-cut
(Arc size from 115 d to 185 d)

Figure 24-24.
E1A.

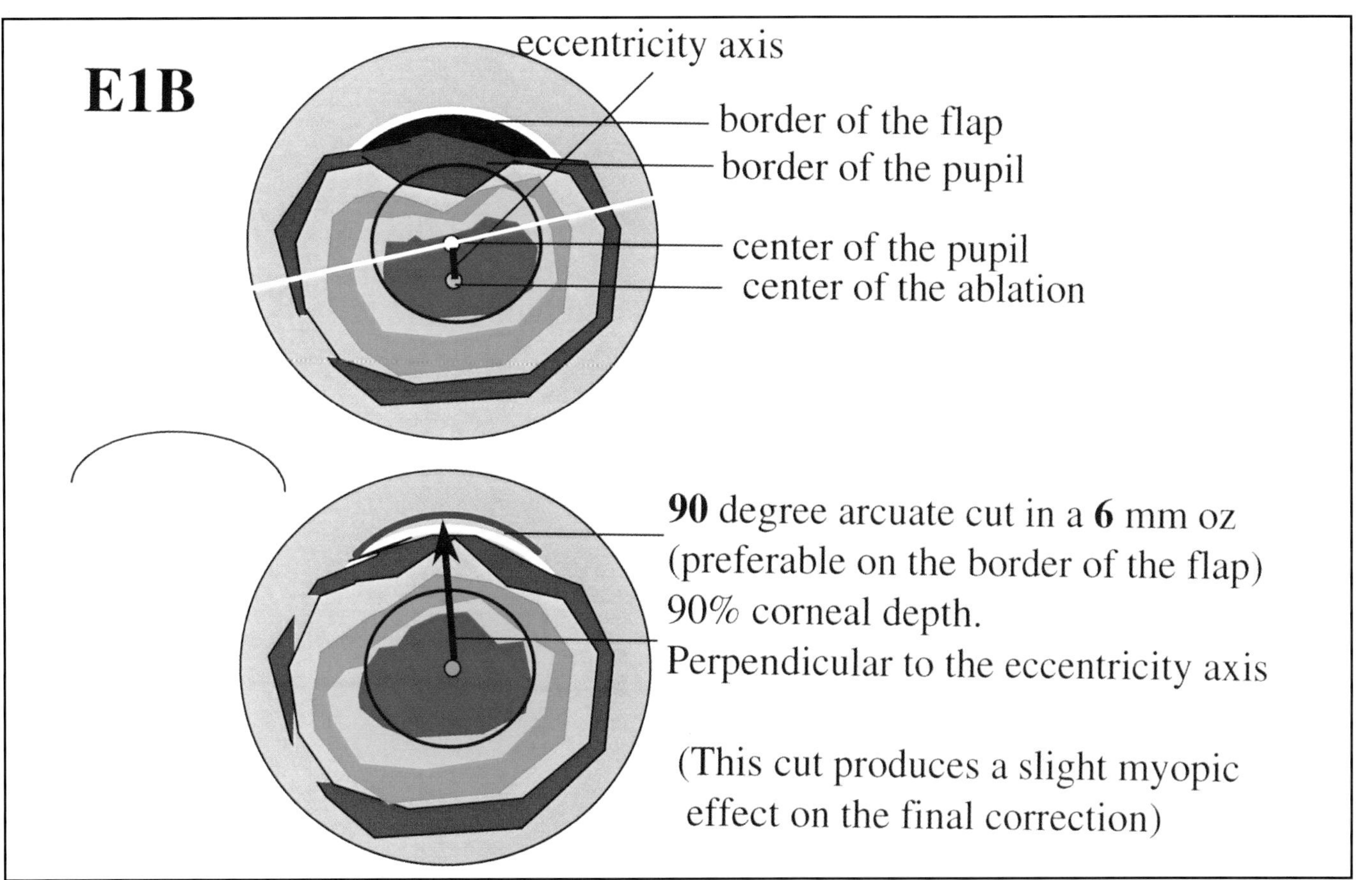
E1B
eccentricity axis
border of the flap
border of the pupil
center of the pupil
center of the ablation
90 degree arcuate cut in a 6 mm oz
(preferable on the border of the flap)
90% corneal depth.
Perpendicular to the eccentricity axis
(This cut produces a slight myopic
effect on the final correction)

Figure 24-25.
E1B.

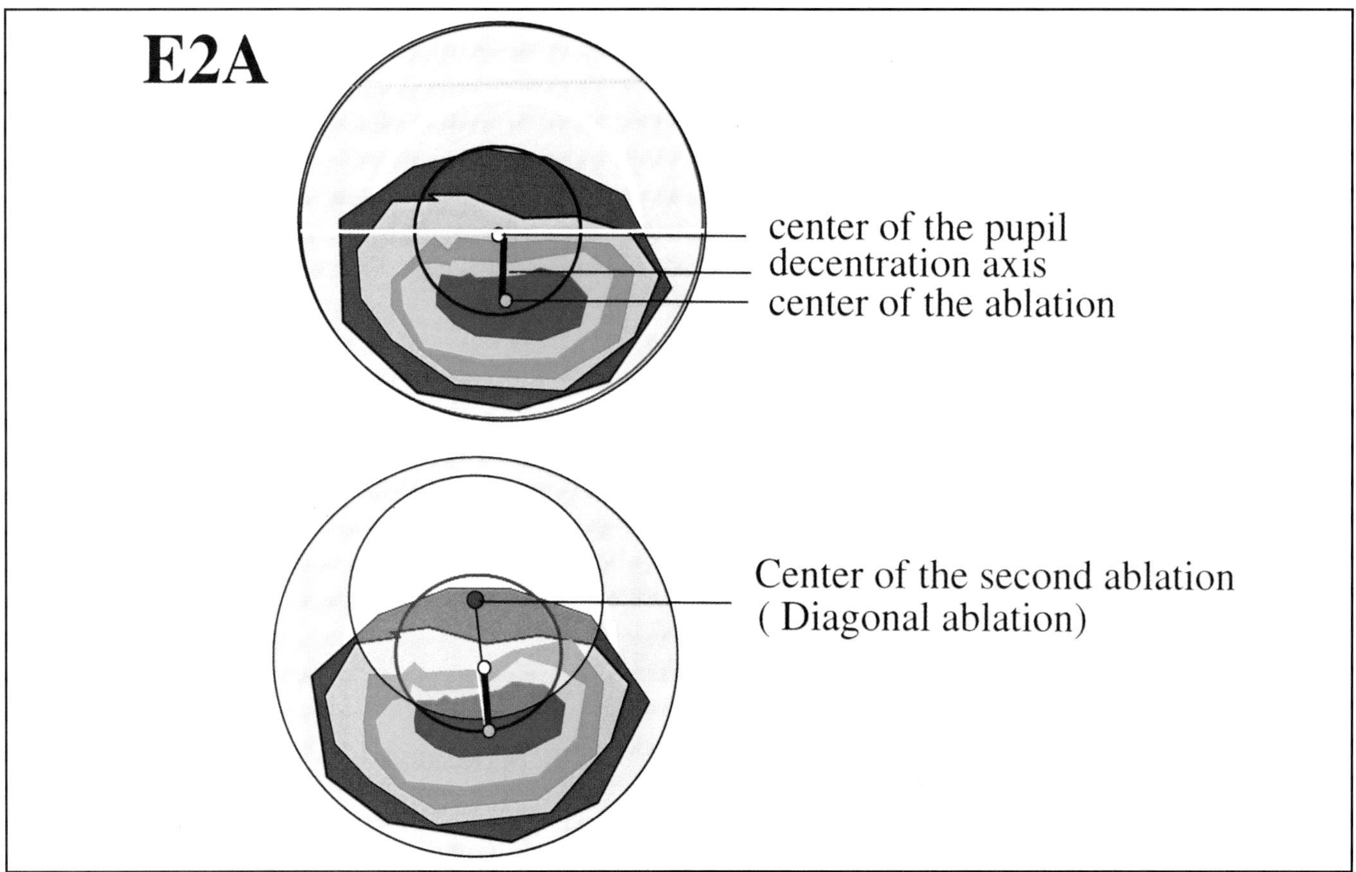

Figure 24-26.
E2A.

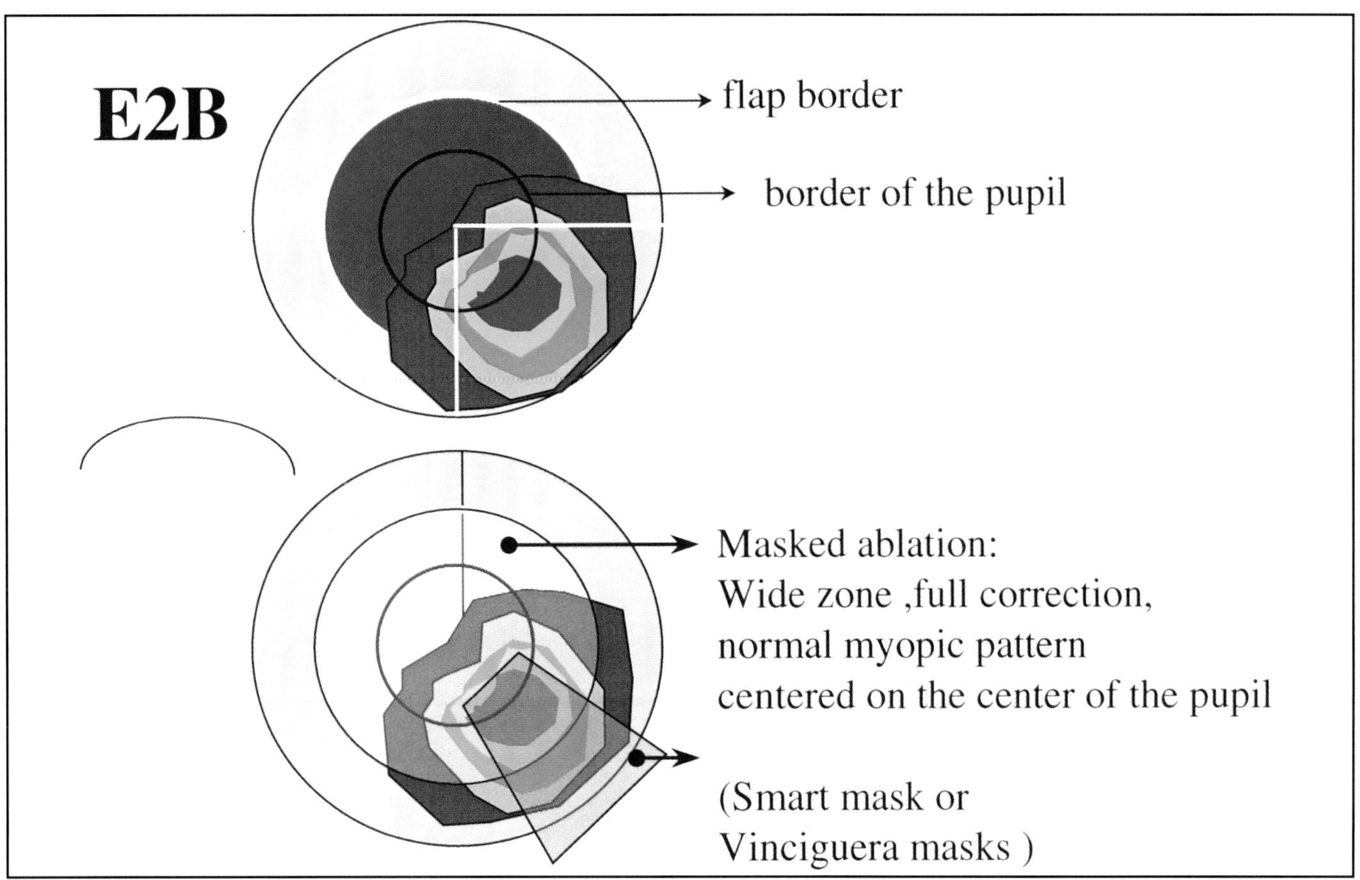

Figure 24-27.
E2B.

TABLE 24-1

E1B Management

	P1	P2	P3
S1	X	ARC 90°, OZ 7 mm	ARC 90°, OZ 6.5 mm
S2	ARC 90°, OZ 7 mm	ARC 90°, OZ 6.5 mm	ARC 90°, OZ 6 mm
S3	Diagonal ablation	Cornea centered-50% PRK (wide-sized zone), topography centered masking +50% PTK	Cornea-centered PRK (wide-sized zone) 3-mm topography centered masking

ARC=arcuate cut, OZ=optical zone.

TABLE 24-2

E2A Management

	P1	P2	P3
S1	X	X	X
S2	X	ARC 90°, OZ 6.5 mm	Cornea centered 30% PTK, +70% diagonal PRK
S3	Wide zone cornea centered PRK 100%	Wide zone diagonal PRK 100%	Wide zone, cornea centered 50% PTK, +50% OZ 5 mm, diagonal PRK

ARC=arcuate cut, OZ=optical zone.

TABLE 24-3

E2B Management

	P1	P2	P3
S1	X	X	X
S2	X	X	Cornea centered 100% PRK, 75% masking of the eccentric ablation area
S3	X	Cornea centered 100% PRK, 50% masking of the eccentric ablation area	Cornea centered 100% PRK, 75% masking of the eccentric ablation area

TABLE 24-4

E1A Management

	P1	P2	P3
S1	X	X	ARC 70°, OZ 8 mm
S2	X	ARC 70°, OZ 8 mm	ARC 70°, OZ 7 mm
S3	ARC 70°, OZ 8 mm	ARC 70°, OZ 7 mm	ARC 70°, OZ 7 mm

ARC=arcuate cut, OZ=optical zone.

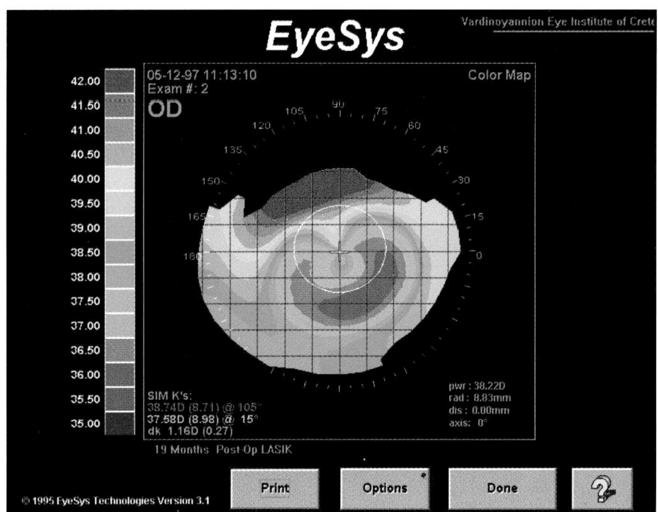

Figure 24-28a.
Topography of the patient 19 months after the initial treatment, preoperatively to retreatment.

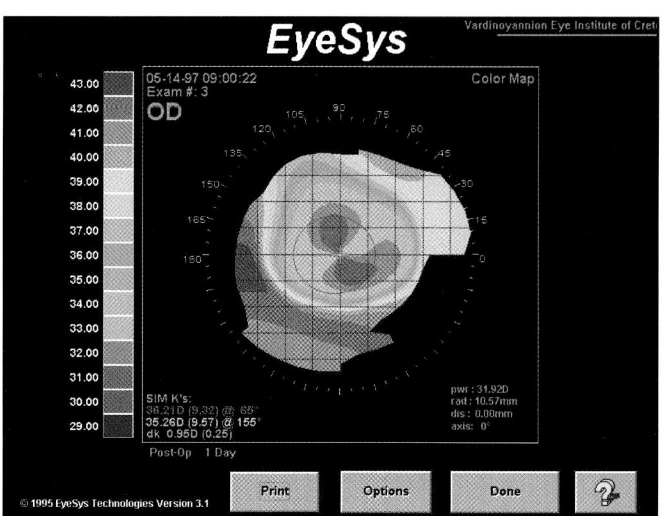

Figure 24-28b.
One day postoperatively to retreatment.

THE PALM TECHNIQUE: PHOTO-ABLATED LENTICULAR MODULATOR

IOANNIS G. PALLIKARIS, MD, SOPHIA I. PANAGOPOULOU, MD, VIKENTIA I. KATSANEVAKI, MD

A new two-component gel mold was developed in our institute to be used as a masking agent in photorefractive keratectomy (PRK) or phototherapeutic keratectomy (PTK). In a patented process, two solid components are dissolved to form an aqueous, homogeneous material. The solid-to-gel transition is determined by measuring the viscosity of the new material's aqueous solution as a function of temperature, using the viscobalance method of viscometry. The ablation rate of this mold was determined using an ArF excimer laser (200 mJ/cm^2/pulse at 5 Hz) and recording the number of pulses required to ablate a predetermined thickness gel film.

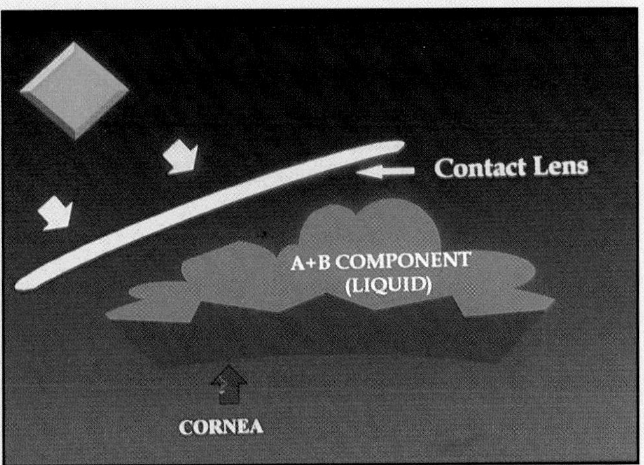

Figure 1.
Schematic diagram of the new two-component gel material (phakos). The material is applied to the irregular cornea in a liquid form and covered by a hard contact lens.

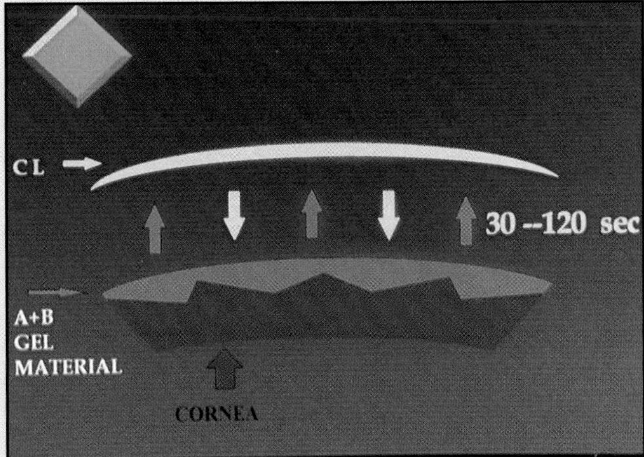

Figure 2a.
The material solidifies, and the hard contact lens is removed. The material that covers the cornea has now solidified, and the shape of the cornea is that of the posterior surface of the hard contact lens—a regular surface.

The material is maintained in solution at temperatures over 45°C. Below this temperature it solidifies. The temperature of the cornea at the moment the material is applied peaks at 39°C for 1.5 seconds and requires 2 more seconds to fall to its normal 35°C temperature. By altering the proportion of the components in the material, the ablation rate and the solid-to-gel transition time can be adjusted. By increasing the concentration of one of the two components, the ablation rate can be adjusted; by increasing the concentration of the other component, the solid-to-gel transition time can be adjusted from several minutes to 15 seconds, and the transition temperature can be adjusted from 35°C to 45°C (Figures 1 through 2b).

Transmission electron microscopy (TEM) was used to study the thermal effect of the material at the time of its application on epithelium-denuded rabbit corneas, as well as on those corneas after healing of the epithelium. Matching of the ablation rate and reproduction of a desired surface were studied by optical and scanning electron microscopy (SEM). TEM showed no thermal effect on the rabbit corneas, either immediately or following epithelialization, when

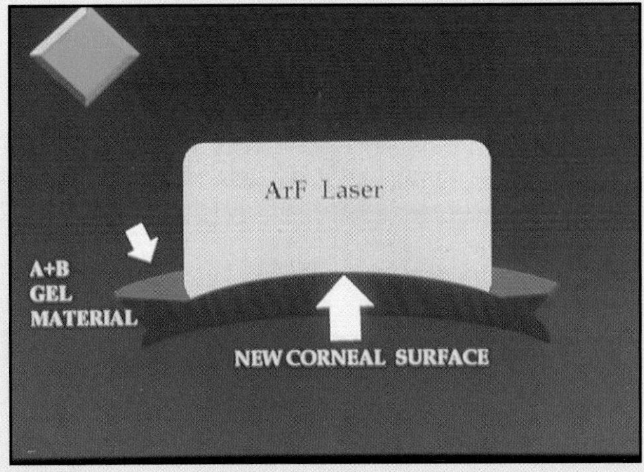

Figure 2b.
The excimer laser can now be applied on the new regular surface, treating any irregularities of the cornea.

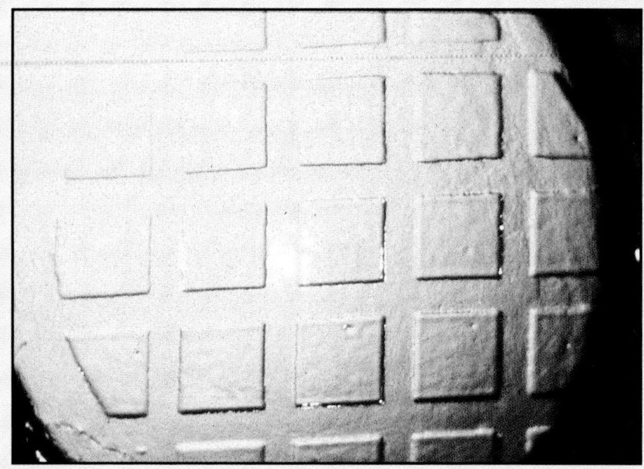

Figure 3.
Microphotography of a porcine cornea ablated through a grid using excimer laser.

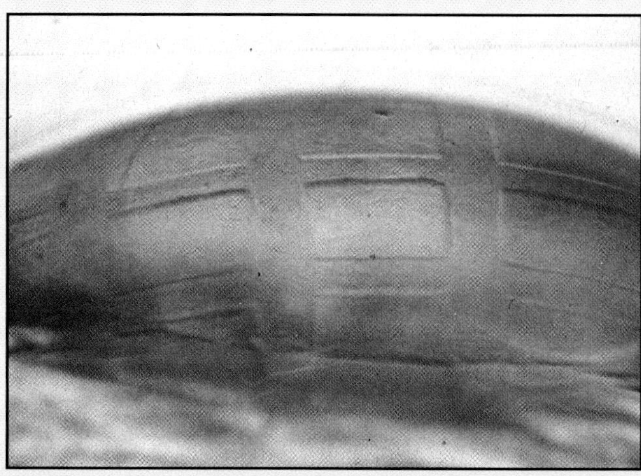

Figure 4.
Microphotography of a porcine cornea that is already ablated through a grid and then is covered with material shaped from a hard contact lens as in Figure 2a.

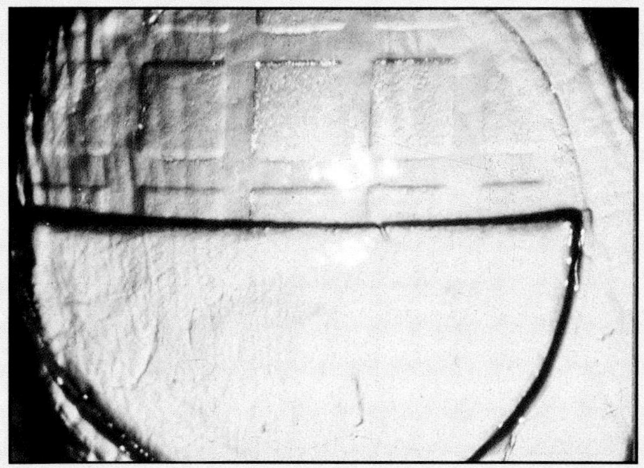

Figure 5.
Only the lower half of the area is irradiated through the gel material.

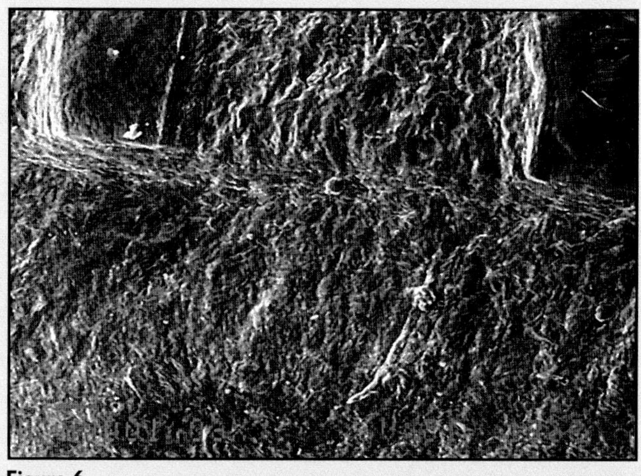

Figure 6.
Detail of Figure 5 in SEM at the interface of nude (without material) ablation (up) and through material ablation (down).

compared with controls. Optical microscopy, microphotography (Figures 3 through 5), corneal topography, and SEM (Figure 6) all revealed an excellent surface quality following excimer laser keratectomy. Owing to its adjustable properties, the new material seems to be very promising as an aid in both excimer laser PRK and PTK.

Long-term studies on a rabbit model reveal excellent results of the healing process and a very smooth corneal surface. Running clinical protocols on partially sighted human eyes are very promising. This technique may be the ultimate approach to making very high quality optical elements.

A New Technique for the Excimer Laser Correction of Decentration After PRK and LASIK

PAOLO VINCIGUERRA, MD, GUIDO MARIA NIZZOLA, MD, PIETRO AIRAGHI, MD,
ANDREA ASCARI, MD, FRANCESCO NIZZOLA, MD, MARCO AZZOLINI, MD

INTRODUCTION

Among the serious complications of photorefractive keratectomy (PRK) and laser in situ keratomileusis (LASIK), decentration occurs often. It causes visual acuity loss and glare and halos, disturbing the patient especially when driving at night.

Visual impairment is proportional to the decentration width and to the high correction. In these cases (Nizzola and Vinciguerra observations), corneal meridians modify their shape from sphere to parabolic. The corneal meridian connecting the pupillary center with the treatment center shows the biggest error. In fact, on this meridian lies a continuous transition from maximum dioptric power to minimum.

Oblique meridians present parabolic shape, too, but the dioptric gradient progressively decreases as the distance from the maximum error meridian increases. The only round arc-shaped meridian is perpendicular to the axis of decentration and obviously only this meridian allows a good focus.

The well-known Sturm conoid presents meridians with infinite, different but regular curvature radius; on the contrary, the "Nizzola-Vinciguerra" conoid, arising from a decentered treatment, is anarchic with different parabolic meridians.

TECHNIQUE

On this theoretical basis, Nizzola and Vinciguerra compared a well-centered treatment with a 1-mm decentered treatment, quantifying point by point the ablation error. To do this, lines were marked (isopters) that connect all the points with the same error.

By these profiles, it was possible to project a series of metallic diaphragms used successively during retreatments, starting with the biggest aperture and ending with the smallest one. These diaphragms must be well centered and located on the axis of decentration, so we put the diaphragms in a properly designed suction mask. This mask is not suitable for LASIK, so Vinciguerra utilizes the diaphragms alone with the help of a marking point on the cornea.

In all cases, a final PTK is mandatory to smooth the surface with a topography and refractive evaluation.

RESULTS

The asymmetric ablation obtained by this technique is complementary to the asymmetric ablation resulting from decentered treatment. Treatment and retreatment together create a well-centered ablation, the optical zone widens, and ablation is deeper, but the final refraction is the refraction desired during the first treatment. To do this is very important to correlate the exact algorithm according to the entity of decentration.

Chapter 25

LASIK COMPLICATIONS

Donald C. Fiander, MD, FRCSC

Any discussion of surgical complications must be prefaced by the acknowledgment that as physicians it is our responsibility to serve our patients; our responsibility to understand the details of any given procedure so that we may fulfill our Hippocratic oath to "first do no harm." The primary goal of refractive surgery is to reduce dependence on contact lenses and glasses while minimizing potential morbidity related to the surgical procedure. Complications, however uncommon, are always a management challenge that may result in permanent sequelae for the patient. As surgeons we must strive to eliminate potential problems.

LASIK, or laser in situ keratomileusis, is an advanced technique of lamellar refractive surgery that embraces the mechanical creation of a corneal flap for access to the stroma and the subsequent photoablation of corneal tissue for the correction of myopic, astigmatic, or hyperopic refractive errors. Complications that may arise during the surgery can be related to any of the successive stages in this procedure.[1-4] The observed complications and their prevention can be categorized with reference to the preoperative patient assessment, the use of the microkeratome and related instruments, the excimer laser ablation, and postoperative factors.

TABLE 25-1

MICROKERATOME COMPLICATIONS

- Inability to seat suction ring
- Inadequate suction
- Chemosis
- Incomplete keratome pass
- Free cap
- Irregular cap/flap
- Keratome fails to advance
- Perforation of anterior chamber

PREOPERATIVE ASSESSMENT

Although the principal deciding factor from the patient's perspective for any elective surgical procedure remains the desire of the individual to undergo the particular surgical intervention, successful outcomes are to some degree dependent on the patient's personal needs, goals, and expectations. It should always be remembered that it is the satisfaction of the patient that will ultimately determine if a given procedure is a success, regardless of our view as surgeons whether the outcome was satisfactory or not.

One of the most important aspects of any presurgical assessment must be the evaluation of the potential patient's psychological make-up and motivations for surgery. A person who will not accept the fact that reading glasses may become required post-surgery, a person who will not accept anything but 20/20 uncorrected acuity, or a person who appears unwilling to accept the realities of what refractive surgery can do should not undergo a procedure. Simply because a patient expresses a desire for a particular procedure should not be the deciding factor of that procedure's execution; the surgeon must make the final decision to actually perform the operation. If your better judgment suggests "Beware!", then by all means do not operate. The dissatisfied surgical patient can do more harm to your practice and reputation than can be offset by the generated surgical fee. As always, prevention is preferable to problem solving.

Having concluded the patient has reasonable expectations and goals, the prime consideration becomes the documentation of a stable and accurate refraction. Contact lens wearers, especially those using rigid lenses, must refrain from contact lens wear before their testing to ensure that the refraction is stable. Corneal topographic evidence that there is no sign of keratoconus, corneal warpage, or other causes of irregular astigmatism must be documented.

It may appear obvious, but a history of previous corneal disease such as keratoconus or herpes simplex keratitis should be considered a contraindication to LASIK or other refractive surgery.

KERATOME CONSIDERATIONS

The keratome and suction ring are sophisticated, highly engineered instruments that deserve a great deal of care and respect as the surgical outcome is closely related to their performance. The instruments must be kept meticulously clean from all debris that might impede the proper passage of the keratome head through the track. In addition to the standard checks of blade movement, plate position, and motor function, it is also strongly recommended to run the keratome head on the track prior to suction ring placement on the eye. This ensures the proper function of the instrument but does not relieve the surgeon of the responsibility for verifying that the track is free of cilia or other debris once the keratome is ready to be engaged. One should also verify that the aperture on the bottom of the ring is patent by placing a finger over the opening and depressing the suction switch before attempting to position the ring on the eye (Table 25-1).

Developments since the first ALK cases were performed have facilitated LASIK surgery. Today the non-adjustable suction ring designed specifically for LASIK makes the positioning of the ring much easier than with the larger adjustable ring provided with the original Automated Corneal Shaper. Current stopper designs are easier to manipulate than the earlier versions. Their use will help minimize the incidence of free caps when starting to perform LASIK.

Since the performance of the LASIK procedure

depends on the ability to place the suction ring on the eye and make the keratome pass to create a corneal flap, the anatomy of the prospective patient must be assessed. Failure to do so may result in failure to obtain satisfactory suction and thus cause the formation of an incomplete or irregular flap and compromise the surgical outcome. How deep is the orbit? What is the lid fissure width? If the orbit is deeply set and/or the lid fissure narrow, placement of the suction ring may be impossible. Attempts to seat the ring may abrade the corneal epithelium. Does the patient tend to squeeze his or her lids when tonometry is performed? Conjunctival chemosis may also interfere with suction. Any of the above may jeopardize the successful completion of the procedure. Even the experienced surgeon may have difficulty when the orbital configuration is suboptimal. If placement of the ring appears difficult, LASIK should not be attempted by the beginning LASIK surgeon.

In the situation of a deep orbit where the lid fissure is narrow, suction ring positioning may be easier if a small wire speculum is used rather than the one supplied with the Automated Corneal Shaper. In fact, we generally prefer to use the same wire speculum that we use for cataract surgery. There are some patients, however, where even this will not allow for the suction ring to be placed. The only available options in such cases are to either perform a lateral cathotomy or the preferred and less invasive maneuver of placing the suction ring directly on the globe without a lid speculum. This works well but it is even more important to be aware of the position of the cilia and the presence of any upper or lower eyelid skin protruding over the suction ring edges, particularly at the track for the keratome gears. Only rarely will these techniques not be successful in permitting completion of the procedure.

Chemosis tends to develop more frequently in the second eye of bilateral cases and when the patient squeezes lids excessively. To obtain satisfactory suction when the conjunctiva is chemotic is difficult. Gently massage the swollen conjunctiva with a Merocel sponge from anterior to posterior. Often this will permit adequate suction to be achieved. A second option is to wait approximately 30 to 45 minutes and try again. If that fails the safest course of action is to reschedule for 1 to 7 days later. Sedating the patient with Valium or another benzodiazepine agent may be of benefit to reduce the tendency to squeeze the lids, but it is essential that patients not be oversedated because patient cooperation during the photoablation is important.

In mechanical ALK, the suction ring position will determine not only the position of the corneal flap but also the location of the central tissue excision. With LASIK, however, centration of the flap and the ablation are independent. The hinge of the flap must not be ablated with the central stroma or else a double ablation will occur at the nasal portion of the flap. This would result in irregular astigmatism and effects similar to a primarily decentered ablation zone. Since the flap itself does not contribute to the eventual refractive correction it need not be centered on the optical zone itself. Decentering the flap nasally will generally prevent the excimer beam from impinging on the flap and still permits large optical zones from 6.5 to 7.5 mm at the outer edge of the ablation. It is wise in general to protect the nasal edge of the flap with a spatula or a moistened Merocel sponge.

Despite adequate suction and correct ring position, the ultimate size of the flap may be less than intended. In most instances this does not create any difficulty and the case may readily proceed. If the hinge occurs at or temporal to the pupil center, there is no option—the case must be aborted. To reposition the flap and attempt a second pass at that juncture would invite a severely disturbed, damaged, and perhaps amputated flap. If the hinge location is beyond the pupil center and preferably at or beyond the nasal edge of the pupil, the only modification in technique may be the reduction of the size of the maximum ablation zone.

If the flap size proves inadequate to complete the case, simply reposition the flap and reschedule the patient for 1 or 2 months later.

From the original work of Barraquer with the cryolathe to the development of current non-freeze keratome technology, keratomileusis was performed as a free cap procedure. Since the concept of the corneal flap was introduced by Pallikaris in 1991[1] it has become the standard of care in myopic keratomileusis. You may argue that a free corneal cap is not a true complication but it is not the optimal situation today, with the possible exception of hyperopic LASIK where a large centrally located ablation zone is necessary.

Complication or not, the surgeon must be able to properly manage a corneal cap. Anticipation of potential problems generally assists their solutions and that is certainly the case here. Consider this as you first position the patient at the microscope. Marking the cornea with a pararadial line temporally will enable proper reorientation of a free cap later. The cap should be gently removed from the keratome head and placed on the ALK spoon with the epithelial surface adherent to the spoon rather than in a fluid containing antidessication chamber which may allow the corneal marks to wash off. After the laser ablation, a single drop of BSS should be placed directly on the center of the corneal bed. The cap, which has been kept relatively dry, can be positioned. The surface tension of the fluid assists the deposition of the cap on the stromal bed. A non-toothed tying forceps is also useful to remove the cap from the spoon. At that point the orientation lines are used to realign the cap. It is generally recommended to wait 3 to 5 minutes from reapplication before removing the lid speculum. Unless there is a corneal abrasion, there is no indication for either a bandage contact lens or a patch.

An irregular or incomplete cut may result when suction is lost during passage of the keratome. Careful attention to detail may avert this. If you suspect suction has been lost due to globe movement or notice a hissing noise, stop and reverify the IOP. Use the Barraquer tonometer; lift up on the suction ring handle gently. When an irregular cap results there is no option but to abort the case. The cap must be repositioned accurately. Use a patch or bandage contact lens. Second interventions should be deferred for 1 to 2 months. Depending upon the size and location of the cap, the two options are to reattempt LASIK or to perform transepithelial PRK. In the case of a small, thin, irregular cap, significant irregular astigmatism may persist after reattempted LASIK. For that reason, transepithelial ablation may be the preferred course of action for these patients.

Debris in the keratome gears or track may on occasion prevent the advance of the keratome. An incorrectly connected power cord may also cause failure. If debris can be observed, gently remove it. Sometimes reversing the keratome minimally will allow the head to advance and complete the case. If these maneuvers are not successful, release suction and very gently disengage the keratome head. Once again, this problem can most often be addressed by meticulous attention to detail with the handling of the keratome and testing keratome passage in the suction ring before starting surgery.

Anterior chamber perforation is certainly the most dramatic surgical misadventure to arise from attempted keratomileusis procedures. The anecdotal reports presented at past meetings have indicated the cause as failure to ascertain that the proper plate was secured in position. Diligence on the part of the surgeon to **always** check that either plate #160 or #130 is correctly seated is essential to the prevention of this complication. Management obviously means discontinuing the refractive procedure. It may only be necessary to suture the corneal perforation, but if more severe damage has occurred, possible lens removal, iris suturing, and even anterior vitrectomy may be required.

LASER CONSIDERATIONS

No factor is of greater importance in achieving the desired outcome of excellent uncorrected visual acuity without disturbing secondary effects than accurate centration of the excimer laser beam (see Table 25-1). All of the preceding considerations lead to this brief period when the actual refractive component of the surgery takes place. Our greatest ally in this endeavor is the cooperative patient, well prepared for surgery because of our methodical explanation of the stages of the procedure, what is expected of the patient, and our calming assurance during the surgery, which is often more help than sedative medication. Although appropriate sedation also aids in the relief of anxiety, you must be careful not to overmedicate as an uncooperative patient may be unable to respond correctly to instructions during the surgery.

An additional point that became obvious when I began using both the Nidek EC-5000 and the VisX Star systems after several years working with the Summit ExciMed and later OmniMed lasers is that the fixation devices on all these units are different. It is necessary to be intimately familiar with the various targeting devices on any laser you may be using to be better able to explain to the patient what to look at during the procedure. The fixation target disappears on the Summit laser as the excimer is being armed before the ablation commences, for example. If the patient is not informed that "the flashing green light will disappear when the laser is ready," the patient may become unnecessarily anxious. Everything that can be done to help enlist the patient's cooperation will reward the surgeon in the end.

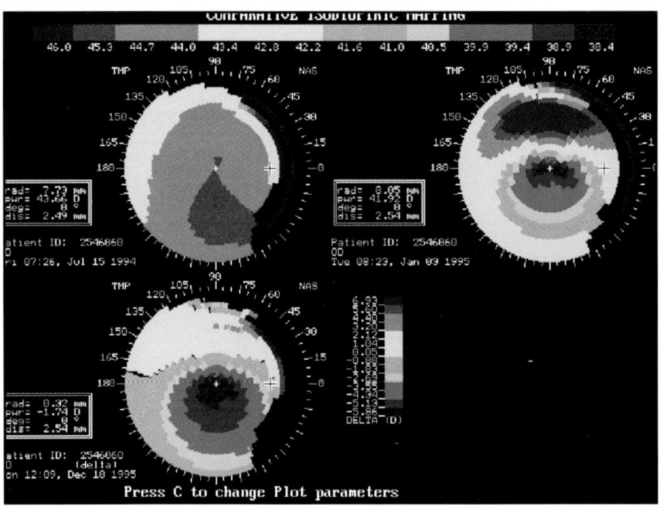

Figure 25-1.
Decentered ablation.

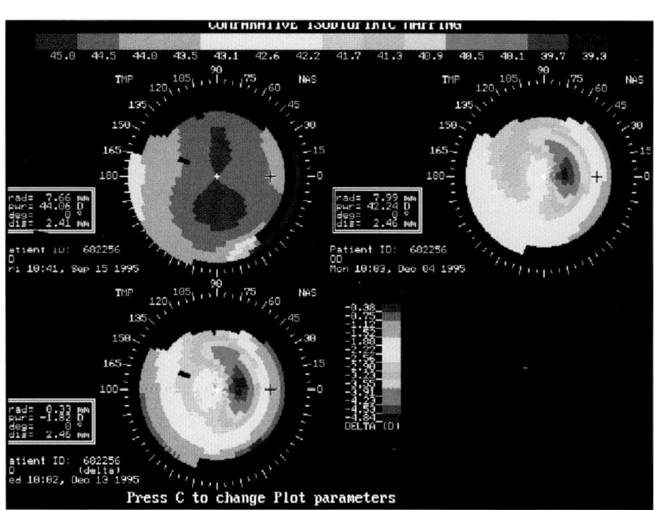

Figure 25-2.
Central island post-LASIK.

Throughout the case but especially prior to the ablation, be certain that the patient is positioned with the iris perpendicular to the beam of the laser. If a patient appears to be fixated and centration seems to be adequate based on your observation through the microscope, but the head is either hyperextended or flexed, the following ablation will occur eccentrically and either an inferior or superior decentration will result.

Before starting the actual ablation, it is advisable to remind the patient of the type of sound generated by the laser as well as the odor of the gas mixture often observed during ablations. Announce "I will be starting the laser on the count of three: one, two, three." Remind the patient to keep looking at the fixation target even though it will be somewhat blurred after the elevation of the flap than before the keratome passage. Always monitor the progress through the microscope and stop ablating immediately if fixation wanders. The first few seconds are critical for achieving good centration. Never be lulled into the attitude that the procedure will be over soon and everything will be all right. Recenter and commence the ablation again if necessary. If you observe fluid accumulating in the gutter at the flap hinge, aspirate it with a sponge to avoid the fluid acting as a mask over the nasal aspect of the ablation zone.

The consequences of decentered ablations range from regular and irregular astigmatism to symptoms of glare, ghosting of images, and diplopia. As noted in our series, significant decentrations are uncommon in experienced hands (Figure 25-1 and Table 25-2). Offsetting a subsequent ablation can help, but may be somewhat difficult to perform. Recently Dr. Pallikaris reported that peripheral arcuate incisions were useful in alleviating symptoms from significant ablation decentrations.[5]

TABLE 25-2

Postoperative Complications

- Infection
- Interface debris
- Epithelial ingrowth
- Central islands
- Folds
- Melt
- Haze
- Undercorrection
- Overcorrection
- Irregular astigmatism

Central islands (Figure 25-2) were first reported when surface PRK was performed using ablation zones of 6.0 mm or greater. Although initial cases were noted with VisX and Technolas lasers, they were also observed with Summit lasers. Although it still remains somewhat unclear as to the etiology of central islands, they can occur with LASIK but in most cases as with

TABLE 25-3

Excimer Laser Complications

- Decentered ablation
- Improper focus of targeting device
- Ablation of nasal edge flap
- Astigmatism: regular/irregular
- Undercorrection
- Overcorrection

TABLE 25-4

Change in Best Corrected Visual Acuity (N=715)

12	1.70%	Gained ≥	+3 lines
33	4.90%	Gained ≥	+2 lines
672	93.90%	No change ±	1 line
8	1.10%	Lost	2 lines*
0		Lost >	2 lines

*No eye worse than 20/40.

TABLE 25-5

Complications

	No.	%
Free cap	12/1045	1.1
Interface deposits	23/1045	2.2
Removal deposits	3/1045	0.3
Epithelial ingrowth	23/1045	2.2
Removal epithelium	5/1045	0.5
Folds	2/1045	0.2
Steps in bed	1/1045	0.1
Melt	1/1045	0.1
Incomplete flap	4/1045	0.3
Haze	2/1045	0.2
Decentered ablation	5/1045	0.5
Induced astigmatism	6/1045	0.6
Irregular astigmatism*	6/1045	0.6

*4 flap induced, 2 decentered ablation.

PRK, topographically observed islands usually resolve and usually are not a concern. Current software approaches with larger size ablation zones have largely eliminated this concern. Nonetheless, should a visually significant island occur, elevating the flap and retreating centrally will solve this problem.

POSTOPERATIVE FACTORS

As with all surgery, possible complications from LASIK do not end when the flap has been repositioned after a successful, well-centered ablation. This merely signals the onset of a new stage in the surgical process (Tables 25-2 and 25-3). With all refractive procedures, loss of best corrected visual acuity has been used as one of the benchmarks for assessing safety of a given procedure. Reports of from 5% to 15% loss of two or more lines of best corrected acuity in PRK eyes have generated justifiable concern about the effects of haze and scarring in that procedure. Observations on our series of 715 eyes followed for more than 3 months revealed that only eight eyes (1.1%) suffered a two line loss of visual acuity and none of these eyes was worse than 20/40. No one had more than a two line loss (Table 25-4). This certainly attests to the safety of the procedure.

One of the concerns once expressed about lamellar surgery in general was that if an infection developed beneath the flap without the barrier effect of the corneal epithelium, devastating corneal destruction could ensue. All our patients are treated with routine antibiotic coverage in the initial postoperative period and receive either Tobrex, gentamicin, or Ciloxan drops four to six times daily for 5 to 7 days. We have not to date observed any infections. This experience does not parallel our experience with PRK with a large central epithelial defect that requires several days to heal. In fact, as our observations (Table 25-5) seem to bear out, the incidence of infection following LASIK is exceedingly low, probably in part

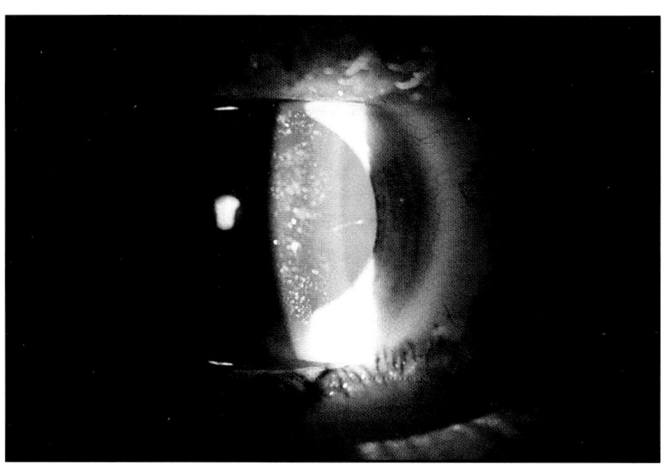

Figure 25-3.
Interface debris.

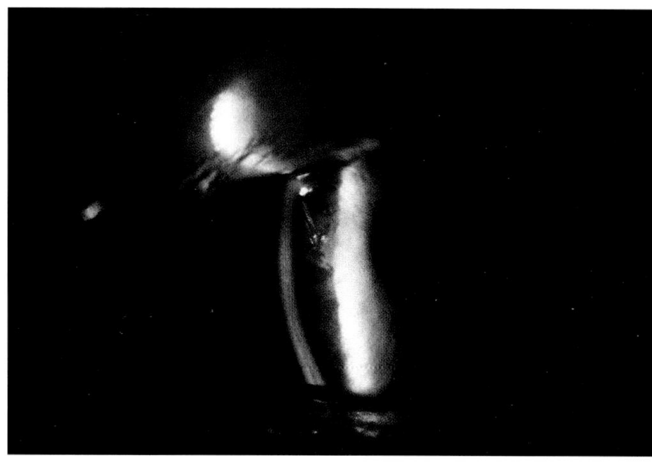

Figure 25-4.
Epithelial ingrowth at interface 2 months post-LASIK.

because the lamellar flap retains most of the corneal epithelial barrier function undisturbed with only a small circular defect at the site of the keratome passage, which is usually totally re-epithelialized at the first postoperative visit less than 24 hours after surgery. I believe that it is wise, however, to caution patients about exposure to possible infection and instruct them to avoid exposure to swimming pools, hot tubs, or other situations where there is a risk of exposure to pathogens.

In ALK for hyperopia, a thick, heavy cap or flap was generated by the surgery increasing the tendency for flap dislocation over observations in myopic cases. Since flap thickness for both myopic and hyperopic LASIK is generally either 130 or 160 µm, this should no longer be a concern. It is important to test the flap adherence prior to removing the lid speculum. Noting that striae extend readily into the flap when the peripheral cornea is depressed with an instrument is a good sign that the flap is stable. One additional step is useful to avoid an unwelcome surprise on the first postoperative visit—have the patient wait 15 to 20 minutes following surgery before discharge and examine the cornea at the slit lamp. A flap that is not positioned properly should prompt an immediate return to the surgical suite for repositioning.

Slit lamp observation has the added benefit of permiting the immediate recognition of interface particles and debris, permitting their removal at once (Figure 25-3). Striae in the flap, indicating that it has not been smoothed over the corneal bed sufficiently, is also an indication to elevate and reposition. Management at this stage becomes part of the primary procedure, precluding the need for a later reoperation, and eliminating potential complications.

Epithelial ingrowth can be minimized by limiting tissue manipulation and avoiding touching the lamellar bed with instruments that have been in contact with the corneal epithelium. Although it may be possible to introduce epithelial cells into the lamellar interface, the post-ablation routine of irrigation beneath the flap should remove this source. Most cases of ingrowth probably result from situations where flap-bed adherence is suboptimal, such as with a poorly aligned free cap, a flap with an abrasion at its edge, and resulting local corneal edema.

Epithelial ingrowth can be recognized by the occurrence of small nests of cells in the interface or the appearance of a translucent sheet which tends to radiate from the edge of the flap centrally (Figure 25-4). Frequently epithelial ingrowth does not progress and, therefore, does not necessarily indicate reoperation. If vision is compromised and/or the ingrowth is progressive, the flap must be lifted and the epithelium removed. Once the flap is elevated, the epithelium can usually be wiped away with a sponge or spatula. Extra care must be taken when replacing the flap to prevent recurrence of the ingrowth.

When there has been excessive tissue manipulation and/or marked epithelial ingrowth local melting rarely occurs at the flap edge. Residual epithelium should be removed to prevent further progression.

TABLE 25-6

ASTIGMATISM (N=715)

	No.	%
Induced cyl>1.25 D	16/715	2.2
Induced cyl>1.5 D	6/715	0.6
Induced cyl≥2.0 D	4/715	0.5

The integrity of central Bowman's membrane is not disrupted with LASIK. The healing haze so typical of surface PRK does not occur following LASIK. Presumably the healing response observed in PRK is dependent upon the interactions following ablation of Bowman's. In fact it is not uncommon to note a faint haze type response at the edge of the corneal flap in LASIK patients where the keratome passed through Bowman's layer. Rarely, LASIK patients may exhibit a ground glass type haze appearing centrally but this does not appear the same as the typical healing response of PRK. It tends to occur in patients who have had a free cap and probably results from the additional manipulation required in those patients to correctly replace the cap on the bed.

COMPLICATION INCIDENCE

The preceding discussion has focused on the spectrum of possible complications with LASIK, methods of prevention, and management considerations. How frequently are problems encountered? Several authors have published reports outlining the incidence of complications with LASIK.[4-10] To provide a concise perspective on this issue, I will review the past 3 years' experience with LASIK. As referred to earlier, my colleague Dr. Fouad Tayfour and I have been performing LASIK since November 1993. Our complication data which was recently presented will be summarized here.[11] To date we have tabulated data on 1045 eyes. There was follow-up greater than 3 months in 715 eyes to permit assessment of visual outcomes (Table 25-6).

As mentioned earlier the data regarding change in best corrected visual acuity is presented in Table 25-4. In more than 1000 eyes we did not experience any cases of flap/cap loss, infection, or perforated globes. The incidence of other surgical complications is tabulated (see Table 25-2).

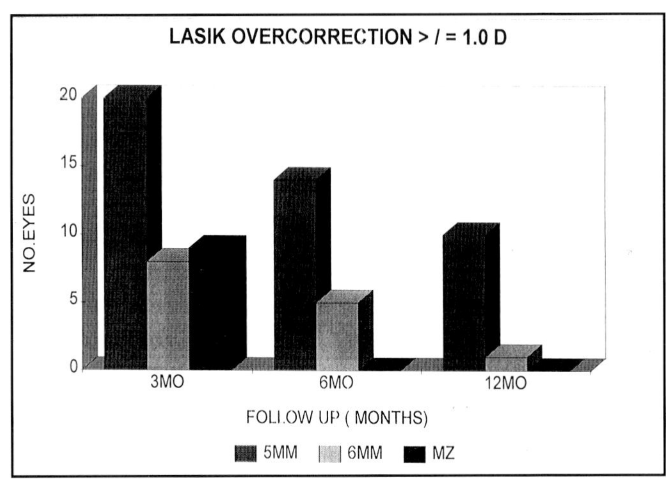

Figure 25-5.
Overcorrection by more than 1.0 D following LASIK.

There was a tendency in the initial cases performed with a 5.0-mm ablation zone to note overcorrections postsurgery. Subsequent modification of nomograms and additional software refinements permitted 6.0 mm and multiple zone ablations. The problem of overcorrection has been largely eliminated (Figure 25-5). The number of eyes with a postoperative spherical equivalent greater than 2.0 D for each of the 5.0 mm, 6.0 mm, and multizone groups are shown in Figure 25-2 for follow-up of 3, 6, and 12 months.

SUMMARY

LASIK has been demonstrated to be an elegant, effective method for the correction of refractive errors. Although the potential for significant morbidity from complications exists, the experience of surgeons performing LASIK has indicated that incidence of complications is minimal. Furthermore, in my personal experience, the overall morbidity from LASIK is substantially less than noted with surface PRK. LASIK does necessitate a level of skill beyond what is required to perform PRK. With appropriate training and attention to detail this procedure can be performed safely with minimal adverse effects.

REFERENCES

1. Pallikaris IG, Papatzanaki ME, Siganos DS, Tsilimbaris MK. A corneal flap technique for laser in situ keratomileusis. *Arch Ophthalmol*. 1991;145:1699-1702.

2. Pallikaris IG, Papatzanaki ME, Stathi E, Frenschock O, Georgiadis A. Laser in situ keratomileusis. *Lasers Surg Med*. 1990;10:463-468.

3. Buratto L, Ferrari M, Rama P. Excimer laser intrastromal keratomileusis. *Am J Ophthalmol*. 1992;113:291-295.

4. Fiander DC, Tayfour F. Excimer laser in situ keratmileusis in 124 myopic eyes. *J Refract Surg*. 1995;11:S234-238.

5. Pallikaris IG, Siganos DS, Detorakis ET, Papadaki TG, Astirakakis NI. Enhancement of PRK or LASIK ablated zone using arcuate corneal cuts. Presented at ISRS Mid Summer Symposium, Minneapolis, Minn, July 1996.

6. Pallikaris IG, Siganos DS. Excimer laser in situ keratomileusis and photorefractive keratectomy for correction of high myopia. *J Refract Corneal Surg*. 1994;10:498-510.

7. Helmy SA, Salah A, Badawy TT, Sidky AN. Photorefractive keratectomy and laser in situ keratmileusis for myopia between 6.00 and 10.00 diopters. *J Refract Surg*. 1996;12:417-421.

8. Guell JL, Muller A. Laser in situ keratomileusis (LASIK) for myopia from -7 to -18 diopters. *J Refract Surg*. 1996;12:222-228.

9. Maldonado Bas A, Onnis R. Excimer laser in situ keratomileusis for myopia. *J Refract Surg*. 1995;11:S229-233.

10. Knorz MC, Liermann A, Seiberth V, Steiner H, Wiesinger B. Laser in situ keratomileusis to correct myopia of - 6.00 to -29.00 diopters. *J Refract Surg*. 1996;12:575-584.

11. Fiander DC, Tayfour F. LASIK—complications in the first 1000 cases. Presented at ISRS Pre AAO Meeting, Chicago, Ill, October 1996.

Treatment of Eccentric Ablation

GUILLERMO AVALOS, MD

The treatment of ablations requires the aid of elevation topography and the capacity of the laser to decenter the beam and send it to the zone to be treated. To achieve these two purposes, I have found it very useful to use the PAR System Topographer and the Apollo excimer laser (International Ophthalmic Technologies).

The PAR System Topographer has surgery simulation software with which, in complicated cases (eg, eccentric ablations), before realizing the treatment, we know the result that we will obtain once realized, and to modify it according to the image that we desire to obtain.

In the topography, the depth of the ablation is measured in microns and we use a grid to determine the millimeters of the decentration. With this data, we pass the information from the Topographer to the laser in order to execute the desired program once the various alternatives have been analyzed.

EXAMPLES

Case 1: Left Eye

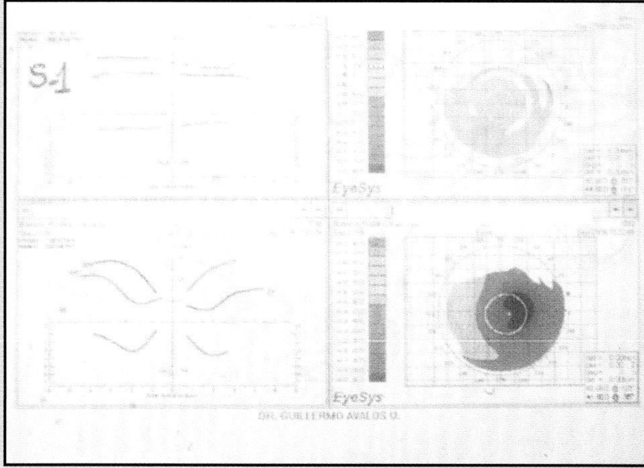

Figure 1.
Patient 3 months postoperatively after LASIK. Visual acuity 20/50, best corrected visual acuity 20/25, -2.00 -1.00 x 175°.

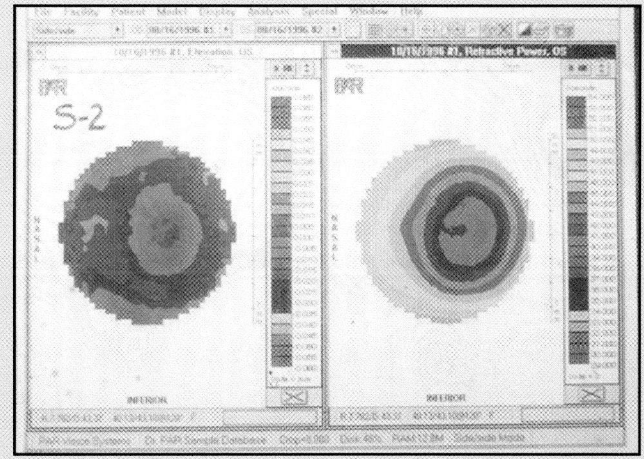

Figure 2.
PAR topography, where decentration and irregular ablation are demonstrated.

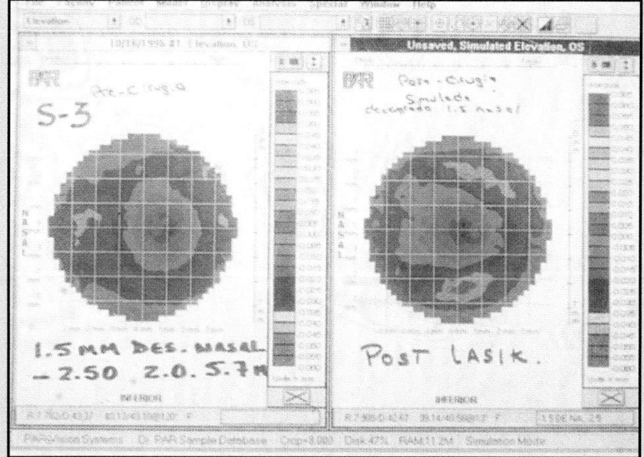

Figure 3.
The decentration is measured from the visual axis and the difference of ablation is measured in microns between the zone already treated and the visual axis. In this case, programming a nasal decentration of 1.5 mm and an ablation zone of 5.7 mm with 31 μm of depth. On the right side topography, the result of the treatment is appreciated, achieving an adequate centration and improvement of vision to 20/25.

Case 2: Left Eye

Patient with previous KMIS and with a very significant decentration of the second cut. Preoperative refraction of the KMIS -16.00 D and postoperative KMIS -9.00 D with best corrected visual acuity 20/60.

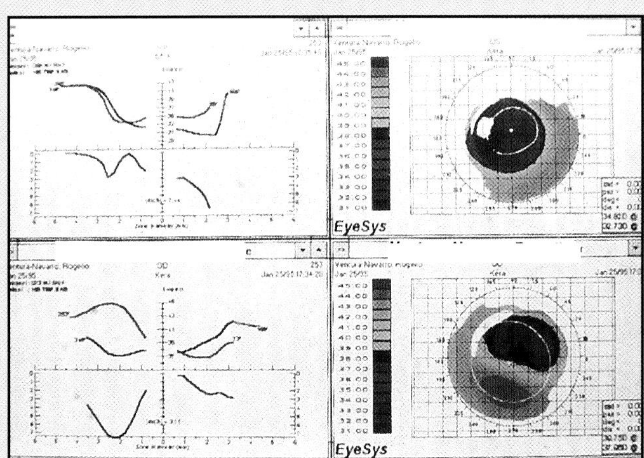

Figure 4.
EyeSys topography demonstrating the decentration.

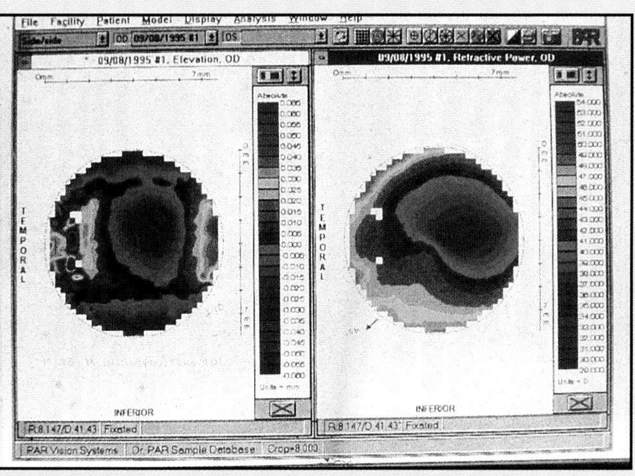

Figure 5.
PAR System topography demonstrating a difference of the level of 25 μm with decentration of 1 mm to 45° axis was programmed.

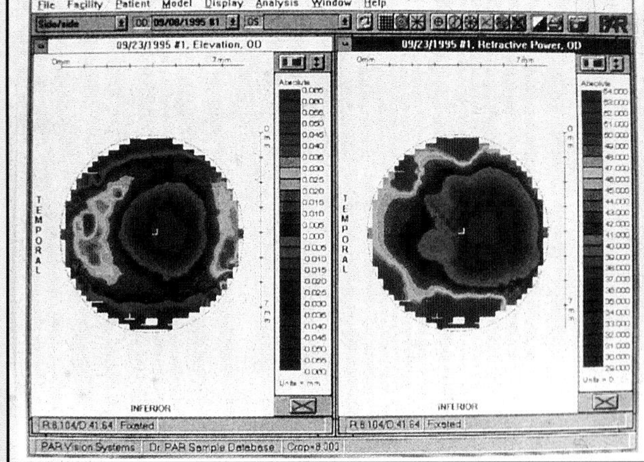

Figure 6.
Postoperative topography demonstrating good centration and uniform ablation. Postoperative visual acuity 20/30.

Case 3: Right Eye

Patient with previous RK of 16 months' evolution.

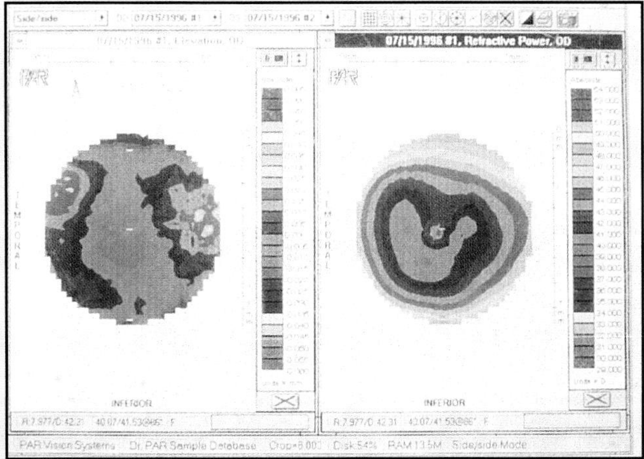

Figure 7.
Pre-LASIK topography. Demonstrates eccentricity of the central area of the cornea with a central elevation zone. Visual acuity 20/60, refraction -1.00 -2.00 x 90°, best corrected visual acuity 20/25.

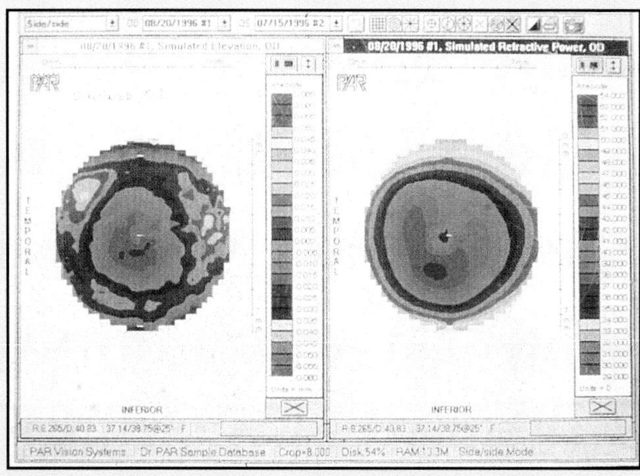

Figure 8.
Simulation of ablation. Note that the central zone most elevated still persisted.

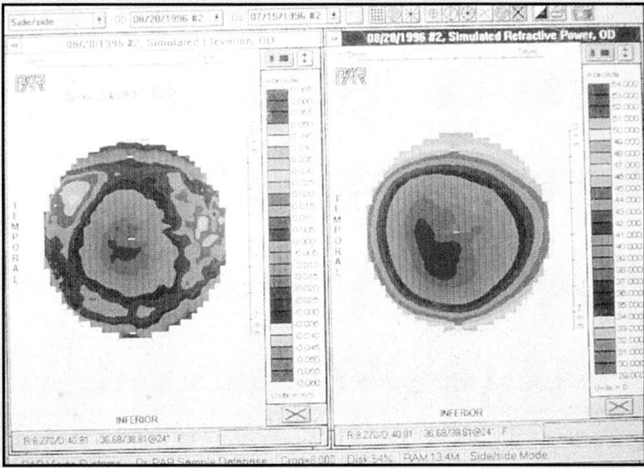

Figure 9.
Simulation. A uniform ablation with disappearance of the central zone most elevated was observed. This program is chosen.

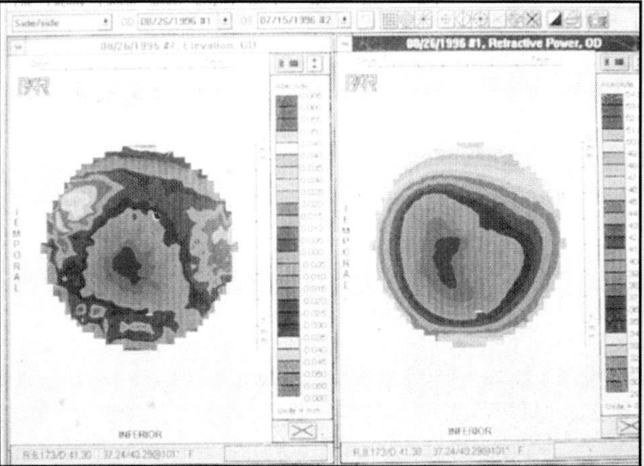

Figure 10.
Postoperative. The similitude of the simulation program with the postoperative result is observed. Postoperative visual acuity 20/20.

Chapter 26

A NEW OPTICAL EFFECT OF ARCUATE KERATOTOMY

Ioannis G. Pallikaris, MD, Dimitrios S. Siganos, MD

INTRODUCTION

Eccentric ablation following photorefractive keratectomy (PRK) or laser in situ keratomileusis (LASIK) is reported in different series to range from 1% to 9%.[1-4] Decentrations producing significant visual and refractive symptoms, such as glare, asymmetric halos, due to a prismatic effect especially during night, and diplopia, are only those exceeding 1 mm from the pupil center.[1-5] Excimer laser systems utilizing mask techniques, such as hand-held rotating or erodible masks, or using smaller ablation zones are more liable to result in eccentric ablations.[6] All the above techniques increase the rate of decentrations by more than 1 mm to 5% to 9%.[6] Incorporation of tracking systems in the excimer laser units probably reduces the incidence of eccentricity. In any case, a huge number of eyes have been treated with first- and second-generation laser systems and the percentage of patients requiring retreatment for correction of decentration may also be large.

Retreatment of decentrations by means of a second PRK was suggested by Seiler et al.[6] He tried eccentric reablation by the identical distance to the center of the pupil but opposite to the initial PRK. The attempted refractive change should amount to the local undercorrection at the center of the pupil as deduced from the corneal map. The epithelium inside the area of the second ablation is removed with the excimer laser.

Where decentration was associated with significant amounts of undercorrection,

TABLE 26-1

GRADING OF SUBJECTIVE SYMPTOMS

Grade	Characteristics
+3	Continuous
+2	Only after constant work
+1	Sporadically noticed
--	Absent

we have tried retreatment using a larger ablation zone after evaluating the topography thoroughly and including the primary ablation in the new area (unpublished data). A possible source is excimer laser beam inhomogeneity or incomplete removal of the corneal epithelium.

Before proceeding to more radical and invasive procedures, such as a corneal transplantation, which is known to carry certain hazards,[7] and based on manipulation of the elastic properties of the cornea, we tested an approach of placement of one or more arcuate cuts on the cornea to enhance the ablation zone by shifting it toward the cut by fractions of a millimeter.

INDICATIONS

Any patient who has undergone excimer laser correction of his or her ametropia, either by LASIK or PRK, and has a small (less than 4.5 mm) or decentered ablation zone (usually more than 1 mm) causing visual symptoms.

PREOPERATIVE EXAMINATION

Arcuate cuts based on computer-assisted topography were performed on 10 eyes of 10 patients who had undergone LASIK (seven eyes) and PRK (three eyes). All eyes had loss of best spectacle corrected visual acuity and complained of subjective symptoms, such as night glare and halos, uniocular or binocular diplopia, and symptoms of asthenopia. Preoperatively, both eyes are examined for uncorrected and best spectacle corrected visual acuity and manifest refraction. Corneal topography is performed and the ablation zone diameter, its amount of decentration from the vertex normal, and the pupil center, as well as the axis of decentration, are determined.

Subjective symptoms are recorded in each case. Subjective symptoms considered are glare, halos, uniocular or binocular diplopia, and asthenopia. We use a grading we suggested in our published study: If the symptom is continuous, then it is given a 3+; if after only constant work, a 2+; if sporadically noticed a 1+; and if absent a "-" sign (Table 26-1).

The patient should be properly informed about the nature of the procedure and a written informed consent is obtained. It is important that the patient understands that it is a technique to be tried before we resort to more invasive procedures.

DETERMINATION OF THE AXIS OF DECENTRATION

The axis of decentration from the pupil center is determined on the topographer by moving the cursor to the center of the eccentric ablated area. Among others, the data obtained from the point the cursor is placed are distance from the pupil center, distance from the vertex normal, and the axis.

DETERMINATION OF THE ABLATION ZONE DIAMETER

Actually two diameters are to be determined: a horizontal and a vertical one, or, in case the ablation zone is ovoid, as in astigmatic corrections, the longest and shortest ones. This is also performed by placing the cursor at the borders of each diameter and deriving its value by calculating the data on the distance from the vertex normal.

SURGICAL PLAN

Decentered Ablation Zone

The arcuate cut to be performed is one having an arc of 90°, centered along the same axis but 180° opposite to the direction of decentration. For example, if the decentration lies toward the 90°, an arc should be placed between 225° and 315° (ie, centered equally around the 270° axis).

To Widen a Small but Well-Centered Ablation Zone

If merely the enhancement of an otherwise centered but small ablation zone is intended, then two mirror-image cuts, each 70° arc, 90% depth, at 7-mm zone, centered along the axis of the smallest diameter of the ablation zone are performed. The ablation zone in such eyes is smaller than 4 mm in at least one diameter.

THE PROCEDURE

Anesthesia

Proparacaine hydrochloride 0.5 % or any other topical anesthetic drops may be used, one drop every 5 minutes for a total of three drops. The patient lies down and the eye area is wiped with povidone-iodine 9%. The eye is covered with a steri-drape and a Barraquer's wire speculum is introduced. The patient is asked to fixate to the light of the microscope while the fellow eye is covered. Covering the fellow eye facilitates fixation by the operating eye. A 5.5-mm ring marker is centered over the pupil and pressed to mark its impression. The probe of an ultrasonic corneal pachymeter is used to take several readings on the 5.5-mm ring impression in the region of the planned cut. The 90% of the smallest depth is selected for the cut.

Although the cut can be preformed by any diamond knife capable of producing arcuate cuts, we use the arcutome (Duckworth & Kent, Herts, England), a device that was designed in our clinic (Figure 26-1). The plugs determining the cut ends are applied to the corresponding degrees on the outer ring cone of the device and the proper (5.5 mm) inner ring is fit within the outer cone. The plug determining the cut depth is introduced in the microdiamond knife. The arcutome with these predetermined cut specifications is applied and centered over the pupil and its incorporated suction is turned on. The microdiamond knife is then inserted in its corresponding inner ring slot. The knife moves between the plugs determining the arc's boundaries performing the arcuate cut, which is then washed with BSS.

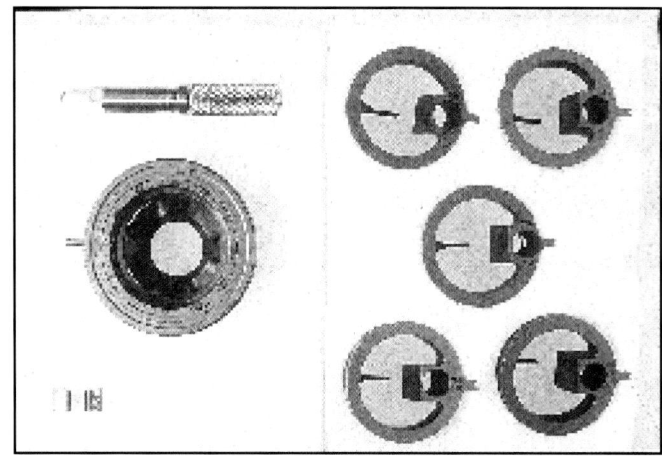

Figure 26-1.
The arcutome (Duckworth & Kent).

In case an enhancement of a small but centered ablation zone is intended, the corresponding 7-mm inner ring is inserted, and four plugs marking the beginning and the end of the two cuts to be performed are preset in the arcutome.

One drop of cyclopentolate 1% and tobramycin 0.3 %-dexamethasone drops are immediately applied to the eye after the operation and a bandage soft contact lens is fit. The wire speculum and steri-drape are removed. The whole operation is performed under a surgical microscope or the microscope of the excimer laser unit.

POSTOPERATIVE THERAPY AND FOLLOW-UP

One drop of Tobradex four times daily is prescribed for 15 days, and is then discontinued. Patients are seen the next 1 or 2 days until epithelialization of the cut is negative to fluorescein dying. Once epithelialization is complete, the therapeutic contact lens is removed. Patients are asked to return at 1 month, or to report earlier should they feel something they would consider unusual.

Corneal topographies are taken at the first or the second day, as well as at 1 and 3 months. During these visits, eyes are examined at the slit lamp and their uncorrected and best corrected visual acuities and manifest refraction are determined. The size of the ablation zone and amount of decentration from the vertex normal and the pupil center, as well as the axis of decentration, are determined in the same manner as preoperatively. We

TABLE 26-2

PREOPERATIVE AND 6-MONTH POSTOPERATIVE SUBJECTIVE SYMPTOMS DATA

Case Number	Subjective Symptoms									
	Glare		*Halos*		*Uniocular Diplopia*		*Binocular Diplopia*		*Asthenopia*	
	Preop	*Postop*	*Preop*	*Postop*	*Preop*	*Postop*	*Preop*	*Postop*	*Preop*	*Postop*
1	+	-	+	-	+++	+	-	-	+++	+
2	+	-	+	-	++	-	++	-	+++	-
3	+	-	+++	+	-	-	-	-	-	-
4	+	-	++	+	+	-	++	-	++	-
5	++	+	++	+	+++	++	-	-	+++	++
6	+	-	+	-	-	-	-	-	++	-
7	++	+	++	+	++	-	-	-	++	-
8	+	+	+	-	-	-	-	-	+++	-
9	++	-	++	+	++	-	+	-	+++	-
10	++	-	++	-	-	-	-	-	-	-

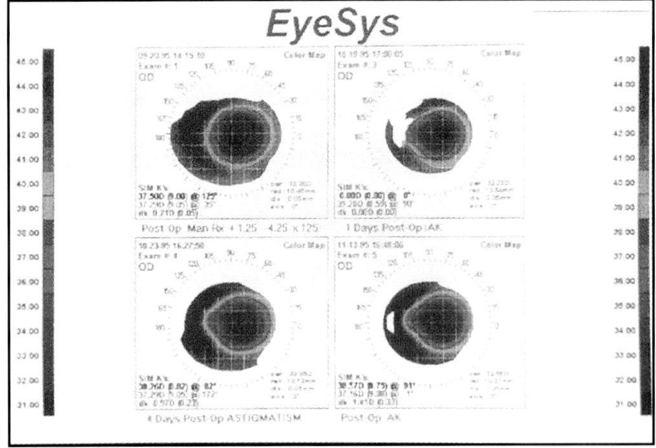

Figure 26-2.

Pre- and postoperative corneal topographies. There is an obvious shift of the ablation zone.

defined enhancement as "the increase in size of the ablation zone radius closer to the cut." Subjective symptoms are recorded in each case. The patient is asked to report any improvement or deterioration of his or her subjective symptoms or the appearance of new symptoms; the patient's responses are recorded.

RESULTS

In our cohort, clinical trial study, 10 eyes of 10 patients who had undergone LASIK (seven eyes) and PRK (three eyes) underwent arcuate keratotomy based on corneal topography.

All operations were uneventful. In all patients the cut healed between 2 to 4 days. Until contact lens removal, all patients felt a mild discomfort and lacrimation. In all eyes the ablation zone was preoperatively decentered from the vertex normal by 1.9 to 2.4 mm.

During the first postoperative visit, there was a topographic shift of the ablation zone by 0.2 to 0.8 mm toward the side of the cut in all eyes, followed by moderate to marked improvement in the uncorrected and best corrected visual acuities and asthenopic and subjective symptoms. The shift did not actually involve the entire ablation zone. A "nipple shift" (ie, a small central part) was seen protruding from the decentered ablation zone toward the arcuate cut. While topography remained stable thereafter, minimal alterations were seen in the uncorrected and best corrected visual acuities during the next

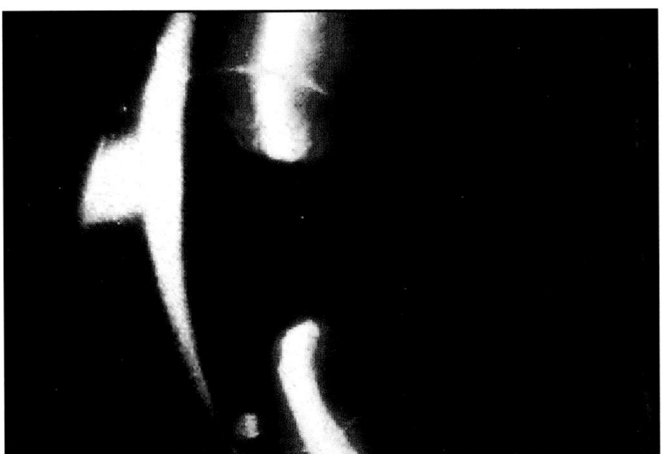

Figure 26-3.
Two arcuate corneal cuts produced by the arcutome.

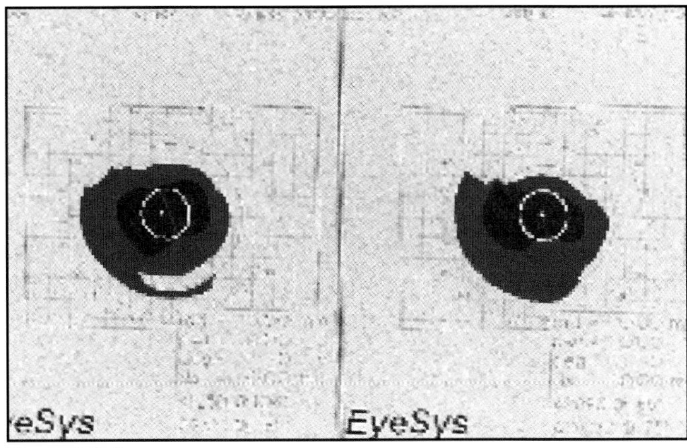

Figure 26-4.
Enhancement effect produced by two cuts where the aim was to enlarge the small ablation zone.

two visits, at 1 and 3 months.

Amelioration of patient subjective symptoms is seen in Table 26-2. Figure 26-2 shows the pre- and postoperative corneal topographies. Figure 26-3 shows two arcuate corneal cuts. Figure 26-4 shows the enhancement effect produced by two cuts where the target was to enlarge the small ablation zone.

COMMENTS

Arcuate keratotomy is considered an effective method for treating astigmatism.[8] In at least one PRK study, arcuate cuts were used to treat induced regular astigmatism of 1.5 D to 2.5 D in three eyes following PRK.[9] However, in these cases, the cuts are done peripheral to the ablation. Asymmetric arcuate cuts have also been used by other authors for topographically asymmetrical astigmatism using special software.[8]

The cuts should not be performed at a zone smaller than 5.5 mm in order to avoid inducing a glare effect by the cut itself. The suggested depth is 90%—although a 95% depth may have a more significant effect—however, increasing the rate of possible perforation into the anterior chamber. The shift occurring following the cut did not actually involve the entire ablation zone.

One should always have in mind that in our case, the aim of the procedure is not to correct astigmatism, but to shift the excimer laser ablated eccentric zone toward an arcuate cut placed away and opposite to the ablation zone.

Amelioration of asthenopia and diplopia symptoms could be achieved with this method. In some cases, there was no noticeable difference between pre- and postoperative uncorrected or best corrected visual acuity. However, the subjective symptoms patients endured after having their initial refractive procedure, whether LASIK or PRK, were relieved.

Our preliminary results showed that the technique might prove safe and effective, and an alternative to selective excimer laser retreatment in decentered ablations. It might be tried before resolving to more invasive procedures, such as penetrating keratoplasty.

REFERENCES

1. Webber SK, McGhee NJ, Bryce IG. Decentration of photorefractive ablation zones after excimer laser surgery for myopia. *J Cataract Refract Surg*. 1993;22:299-303.
2. Cavanaugh TB, Durrie DS, Riedel SM, et al. Topographical analysis of the centration of excimer laser photorefractive keratectomy. *J Cataract Refract Surg*. 1993;19:136-143.
3. Cantera E, Cantera I, Olivieri L. Corneal topographic analysis of photorefractive keratectomy in 165 myopic eyes. *Refract Corneal Surg*. 1993;9(2):S19-S22.
4. Wilson SE, Klyce SD, McDonald MB, et al. Changes in corneal topography after excimer laser photorefractive keratectomy for myopia. *Ophthalmology*. 1991;98:1338-1347.
5. Seiler T. Photorefractive keratectomy. European experience. In: Thompson FB, McDonnel PJ, eds. *Color Atlas/Text of Excimer Laser Surgery. The Cornea*. New York, NY: Igaku-Shoin Medical Publishers; 1993:53-62.
6. Seiler T, Schmidt-Petersen H, Wollensak J. Complications after myopic PRK primarily with the Summit Laser. In: Salz JJ, McDonnell PJ, McDonald MB, eds. *Corneal Laser Surgery*. St. Louis, Mo: CV Mosby; 1995:131-142.
7. Paton D. The principal problems of penetrating keratoplasty: graft

failure and astigmatism. In: *Symposium on Medical and Surgical Diseases of the Cornea. Trans New Orleans Academy of Ophthalmology.* St. Louis, Mo: CV Mosby; 1980:248.

8. Pallikaris IG, Xirafis ME, Naoumidis LP, Siganos DS. Arcuate transverse keratotomy with a mechanical arcutome based on videokeratography. *Refract Corneal Surg.* 1996;12(2):S296-S299.

9. Salz JJ, Maguen E, Nesburn AB, et al. A two year experience with excimer laser photorefractive keratectomy. *Ophthalmology.* 1993:90;873-882.

Related Readings

Cavanaugh TB, Durrie DS, Riedel SM, et al. Centration of excimer laser photorefractive keratectomy relative to the pupil. *J Cataract Refract Surg.* 1993;19:144-148.

Doane JF, Cavanaugh TB, Durrie DS, Hassanein KM. Relation of visual symptoms to topographic ablation zone decentration after excimer laser PRK. *Ophthalmology.* 1995;92(1):42-47.

Englanoff, Kolahdouz-Isfahani AH, Moreira H, et al. In situ collagen gel mold as an aid in excimer superficial keratectomy. *Ophthalmology.* 1992;99(8):1201-1208.

Klyce SD, Smolek MK. Corneal topography of excimer laser photorefractive keratectomy. *J Cataract Refract Surg.* 1993;19:122-130.

Lin DTC, Sutton HF, Berman M. Corneal topography following excimer laser photorefractive keratectomy for myopia. *J Cataract Refract Surg.* 1993;19:149-154.

Pallikaris IG, Siganos DS. LASIK complications management. In: Talamo JH, Krueger RR, eds. *The Excimer Manual.* Boston, Mass: Little, Brown and Co; 1997:227-243.

Schwartz-Goldstein BH, Hersh PS. The Summit photorefractive keratectomy study group. Corneal topography of phase III excimer laser photorefractive keratectomy; optical zone centration analysis. *Ophthalmology.* 1995;92:951-962.

Chapter 27

REOPERATION FOLLOWING LASIK

Tarek Salah, MD, FRCS

One important criterion for judging the utility of a method of refractive surgery is adjustability, the ability to repeatedly alter the refractive correction in order to adapt to changing conditions, such as surgical under- or overcorrection, increasing myopia with increasing axial length of the globe, and physiological aging with presbyopia. Adjustability is a major advantage of spectacles and contact lenses for the correction of ametropia; patients accept the idea of changing their optical correction periodically. A fully adjustable technique of refractive surgery is an elusive goal because repeated surgery involves risk and morbidity for patients and the results are not accurately predictable. Most patients seem to expect that one operation will permanently eliminate their refractive error, and therefore, explaining the need for repeated surgery requires considerable patient education. Repeated surgery has become an accepted part of contemporary refractive keratotomy. For example, Werblin and Stafford[1] did one to seven repeated keratotomies on 66 of 203 (33%) eyes and Waring and colleagues[2] reported repeated keratotomies on 241 of 546 eyes (39%).

ADJUSTABILITY OF LAMELLAR REFRACTIVE PROCEDURES

Surgeons also seek adjustability in lamellar refractive procedures. Table 27-1

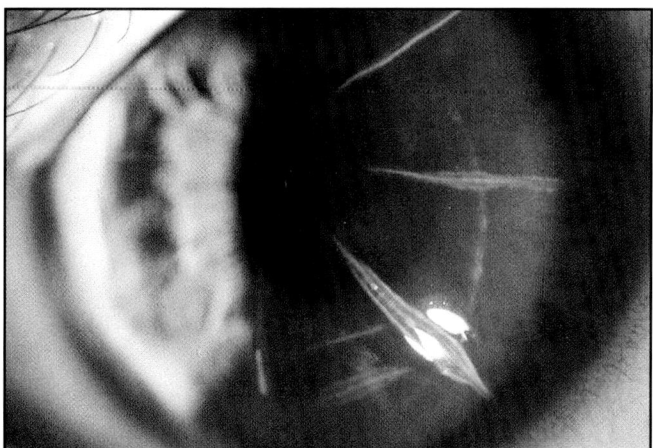

Figure 27-1.
Tissue "melting" and fusiform gaping at the intersection of the RK incisions with the edge of the LASIK flap.

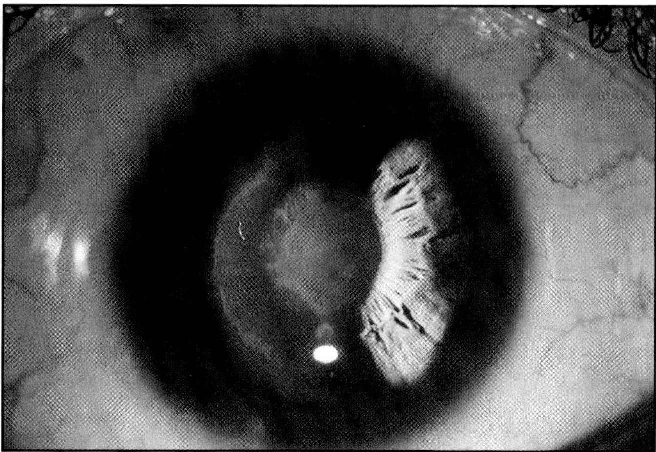

Figure 27-2.
Central scarring after PRK which is done to treat residual myopia following LASIK. The edge of the flap is evident.

shows the possible procedures used to treat residual myopia after different lamellar refractive techniques.

Adjustment of keratomileusis performed on the back of the disc (cryolathe, planar non-freeze, and excimer laser on the disc) is impractical because of the limited amount of tissue that can be removed from the disc in a second operation. Perforation is a possibility or it might be so thin that scarring occurs or it might be thin enough to be difficult to handle intraoperatively and create irregular astigmatism, thus requiring homoplastic donor lenticle for repeated keratomileusis on the disc.[3,4] Otherwise, a second different procedure is usually needed to correct the residual amount of myopia or astigmatism.

The advent of keratomileusis in situ (KMIS),[5,6] in which the refractive cut is made in the thicker stromal bed, has opened the possibility of adjustable keratomileusis because the corneal disc or flap can be easily lifted from the bed since its major adhesion is around the edges where the epithelium contacts the stroma and there is minimal healing within the stromal lamellar interface. Attempting to do repeated KMIS with the microkeratome is difficult, due to the fact that it is hard to center the microkeratome in the same position as the initial keratectomy and because it is usually difficult to create an accurate thin excision with the microkeratome, especially when trying to reoperate for small correction of -3.00 D or less; the microkeratome is simply too inaccurate and imprecise and results in overcorrection or irregular cut causing irregular astigmatism.

Laser in situ keratomileusis[7] (LASIK) is potentially repeatable and adjustable in an accurate and practical manner because the lamellar bed can be opened easily, the hinged flap can be folded back and then easily repositioned, the laser can be centered around the pupil with the guidance of helium-neon laser alignment beams, and small accurate correction can be created with the laser.

OPTIONS FOR TREATING UNDERCORRECTED LASIK

Table 27-1 shows the different possible surgical interventions that can be utilized to treat residual myopia following LASIK. These fall into the following types:

1. Incisional keratotomy. Radial keratotomy (RK) and astigmatic keratotomy (AK) were the main available procedures for treatment of undercorrection after cryolathe or KMIS.[8,9] The drawbacks of such an approach are unpredictable outcome, possibility of inducing irregular astigmatism, the occurrence of a fusiform gaping, tissue melting,[4] epithelial inclusions at the site of the intersection of the radial incision and the edge of the flap (Figure 27-1), possibility of a hyperopic shift, and limitation in correcting high degrees of residual myopia of -3.00 D or more.
2. Photorefractive keratectomy (PRK) or photoastigmatic refractive keratectomy (PARK). PRK or PARK are possible options in treating undercorrected LASIK cases. Like incisional keratotomies they have their drawbacks. LASIK has the advantage of preserving

Bowman's layer, an advantage that is lost when PRK is performed following LASIK with the subsequent possibility of inducing various degrees of corneal haze, scarring, and regression (Figure 27-2). PRK is followed by a painful recovery period, delayed visual rehabilitation, and it is inappropriate to treat high degrees of residual myopia.

3. Repeated laser in situ ablation. One of the main advantages of LASIK[10] is that postoperative modification of the refractive outcome is still possible using reablation of the bed after simple dissection and elevation of the flap. This makes the procedure somewhat adjustable.

We have been using the last technique since early 1994 for treating residual myopia following LASIK in more than 90 eyes. We will now discuss the various aspects of this approach regarding the timing, the surgical technique, the results, and advantages.

Timing (When to Do It?)

There is no rule-of-thumb to determine the ideal timing for reoperation after LASIK. Theoretically, there are two factors that may play a role in choosing the right time: first is the stability of refraction, and second is the corneal wound healing and the adhesions between the flap and the stromal bed. It is theoretically ideal to postpone the second intervention until a significant stability has been reached, but before the healing process hinders the ease of dissecting and elevating the flap from its bed. There have been few reports on stability; some[11,12] have shown that following LASIK, there is a trend toward regression of the surgical effect which was maximized between 1 and 3 months after surgery. This is followed by little change in the refraction with considerable stability after 6 months. Where the healing factor is concerned, theoretically, it is easier to dissect the flap earlier than later. We have noticed that the flap can be easily peeled from its interface and elevated up to 9 months postoperatively. After 1 year, when the adhesion is between the flap and the bed, the procedure is somewhat more difficult but is still possible; we have been able to elevate the flap as late as 24 months after the initial LASIK procedure. Accordingly, it is preferable to wait for 3 to 6 months postoperatively when considerable stability in refraction has been reached and the strength of wound healing will permit easier dissection and elevation of the flap.

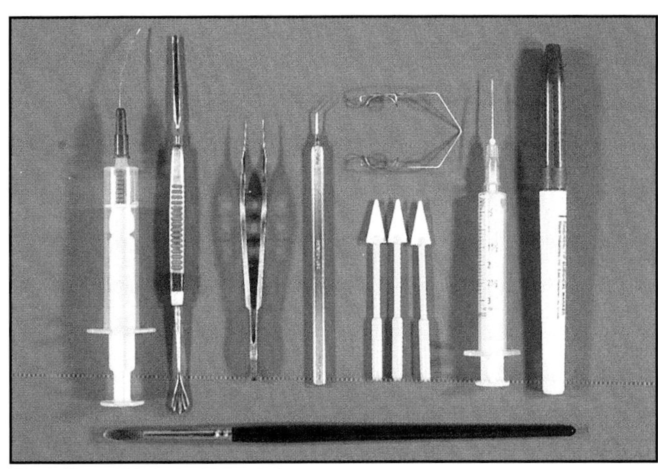

Figure 27-3.
Instruments used for repeated excimer laser in situ ablation.

Surgical Technique (How to Do It?)

The technique of repeated laser in situ ablation is done as an outpatient procedure in the excimer laser suite under topical anesthesia. Preoperatively, a full description of the procedure is given to the patient and instructions of the importance in maintaining fixation throughout the procedure need to be emphasized especially during elevating the flap and applying the laser.

INSTRUMENTS

The instruments used in this technique are shown in Figure 27-3. They include a wire lid speculum, an irrigating cannula, a 23-gauge needle inked with methylene blue, a surgical marking pen, a dry sponge or Weck-cels, a Sinskey hook, an iris spatula, a fine-toothed forceps, and a red sable brush.

SURGICAL STEPS

Figures 27-4a through 27-4f demonstrate the surgical steps for repeated laser in situ ablation. Before surgery, the edge of the previous flap is marked with a surgical marking pen at the slit lamp microscope to enable the surgeon to identify the edge of the flap intraoperatively. Topical pilocarpine 2% is instilled 30 and 15 minutes before surgery; the entire procedure is performed under topical anesthesia with 0.5% benoxinate.

The patient is placed beneath the laser, prepped with povidone-iodine, and draped in a sterile fashion with an adhesive drape securing the eyelashes to the eyelid. A wire lid speculum is inserted and the conjunctival cul-de-sac is irrigated with BSS and carefully dried. A vertical reference

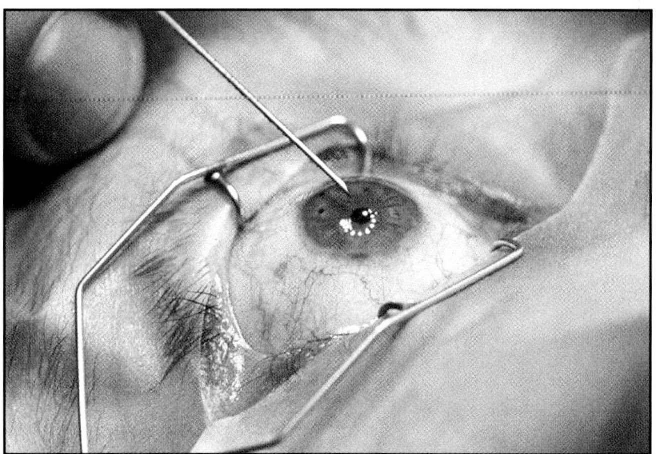

Figure 27-4a.
Demonstration of the steps in repeated excimer laser in situ ablation. The eyelashes are sequestered beneath an adhesive drape. Two spot marks were done to mark the edge of the flap. A vertical reference mark is made with a 23-gauge needle.

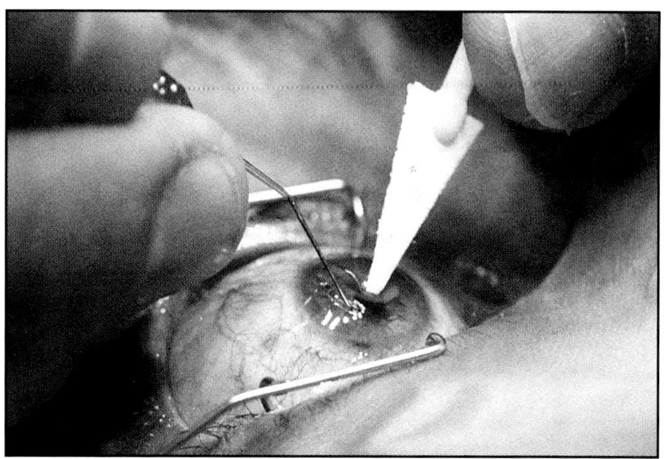

Figure 27-4b.
The central cornea is depressed with a dry Weck-cel to accentuate the location of the edge of the flap and a Sinskey hook is used to break into the interface.

TABLE 27-1

Repeated Surgeries for Treating Undercorrection Following Lamellar Refractive Procedures

Cryolathe Keratomileusis	In Situ Keratomileusis	PRK	Excimer Keratomileusis on Disc (Buratto's Technique)	LASIK
• Repeat keratomileusis • RK • AK • PRK or PARK • ALK • LASIK	• Repeat in situ keratomileusis • Repeat in situ keratectomy (with a microkeratome) • RK and AK • PRK or PARK • LASIK • Repeated in situ laser ablation	• Repeat PRK • Scraping of epithelium • RK or AK • LASIK	• RK and AK • PRK or PARK • LASIK	• RK or AK • PRK or PARK • Repeat LASIK • Repeat laser in situ ablation

mark is made with a 23-gauge needle inked with methylene blue tangent with the pupil at 9:00 and extending vertically to the limbus for orientation of the flap during repositioning (Figure 27-4a). The surgeon depresses the central cornea with a dry microsponge to accentuate the location of the edge of all around the flap and uses a Sinskey IOL hook to break into the interface and stroma at the marked or accentuated edge of the flap (Figure 27-4b).

The edge of the flap is teased up with a fine-toothed forceps and the flap is gently peeled from the stromal bed toward the nasally located hinge. This is sometimes assisted by introducing a flat spatula, and gently advanced in the previous lamellar interface with an outward sweeping movement to separate the flap from the bed and to break all adhesions, especially if reoperation is done after a longer period of time has passed since the

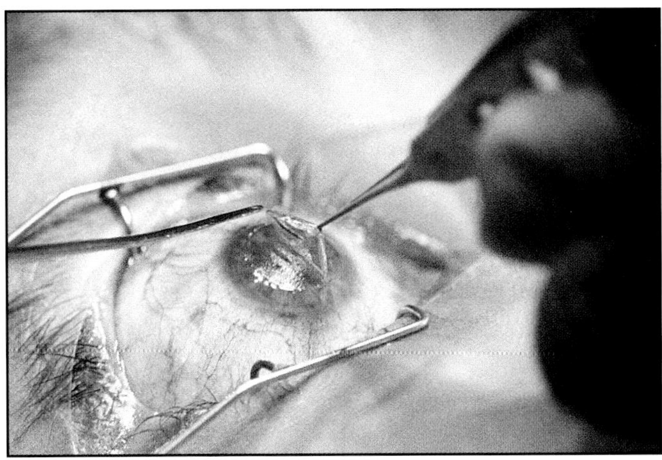

Figure 27-4c.
The edge of the flap is teased up with a fine-toothed forceps and the flap is peeled off gently from the stromal bed assisted by a flat spatula to break any adhesions present.

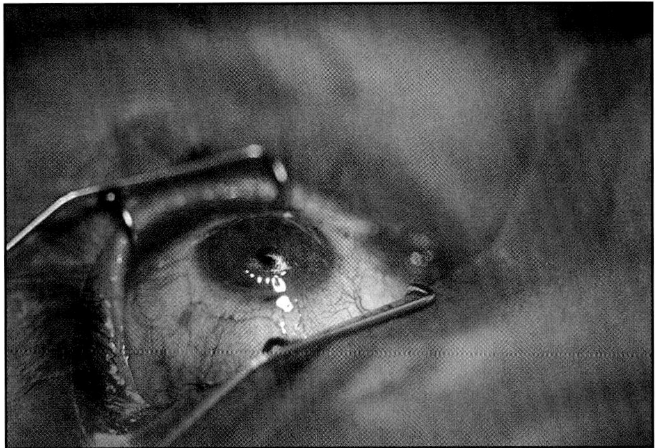

Figure 27-4d
Laser ablation is done to the previous stromal bed after focusing and centering the helium-neon laser beams.

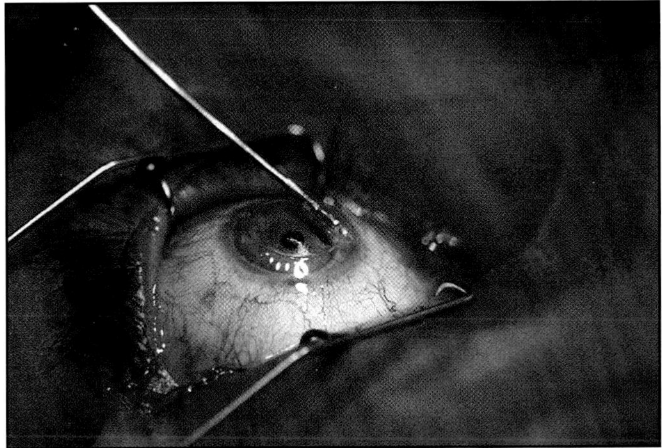

Figure 27-4e.
The stromal surface of the flap is flooded with BSS and the flap is flipped with a blunt irrigating cannula back into place matching the reference mark.

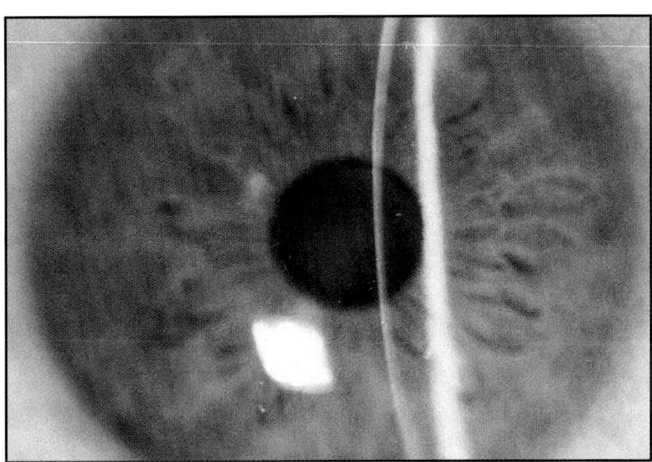

Figure 27-4f.
Eye 6 months after repeated excimer laser in situ ablation shows the margin of the flap and the clear central cornea.

initial LASIK procedure (Figure 27-4c). The previous ablation site and the concentric laser marks in the bed are revealed. Laser ablation to treat the residual myopia or astigmatism is then completed in the stromal bed centered around the center of the entrance pupil (Figure 27-4d). After the laser ablation, BSS is placed on the stromal surface of the flap and the flap is folded back to its normal anatomical position with a blunt irrigating cannula so that the reference marks are aligned (Figure 27-4e). The edge of the flap is dried with a microsponge and the surface is dried with humidified air which passed through a millipore filter from a distance of 6 inches. One drop of tobramycin is applied and the eye is inspected 30 minutes after the procedure to ensure approximation of the flap. The patient is then discharged without patching the eye, and topical antibiotic and steroids are prescribed for 5 to 7 days.

Results

The first 20 consecutive eyes of 12 patients (nine males and three females) who received initial LASIK that resulted in an undercorrection were followed by repeated excimer laser in situ ablation procedure (Table 27-2). Patients were selected for repeated surgery because both the patient and the surgeon judged that visual function with residual myopia was unacceptable. Repeated excimer laser in situ ablation was done 3 to 18 months (mean: 7 months) after the initial surgery and was fol-

TABLE 27-2

Results of 20 Eyes Before and After Repeated Excimer Laser In Situ Ablation

Patient No.	Baseline			After Initial LASIK			After Retreatment		
	VAsc	*Sph Eq (D)*	*VAcc*	*VAsc*	*Sph Eq (D)*	*VAcc*	*VAsc*	*Sph Eq (D)*	*VAcc*
1. Rt	20/200	-3.25	20/22	20/40	-1.00	20/25	20/25	-0.25	20/22
Lt	20/200	-3.50	20/20	20/30	-1.25 -0.25 x 25	20/22	20/20	-0.25	20/20
2. Rt	20/400	-5.00 -0.50 x 90	20/30	20/40	-1.00 -0.50 x 10	20/30	20/25	+0.50 -0.50 x 80	20/25
Lt	20/400	-7.00 -1.75 x 150	20/100	20/40	-3.50	20/30	20/25	Plano -1.00 x 10	20/25
3. Rt	20/400	-5.00 -0.50 x 10	20/20	20/40	-1.25 -0.50 x 40	20/20	20/20	Plano	20/20
Lt	20/400	-5.00 -1.00 x 180	20/20	20/40	-1.37 -0.25 x 180	20/20	20/25	Plano -0.75 x 170	20/20
4. Rt	20/800	-10.00 -1.75 x 30	20/40	20/160	-2.75 -1.00 x 40	20/40	20/40	Plano -0.75 x 40	20/40
Lt	20/800	-11.00 -1.25 x 160	20/40	20/250	-3.25 -0.75 x 160	20/40	20/70	+1.00	20/40
5. Lt	20/400	-5.00 -0.50 x 30	20/20	20/70	-1.50	20/20	20/20	Plano	20/20
6. Rt	20/800	-11.50	20/25	20/70	-1.25	20/25	20/25	Plano	20/25
7. Rt	20/800	-18.50 -1.50 x 25	20/30	20/400	-5.00 -1.00 x 20	20/40	20/40	-0.50 -1.00 x 20	20/30
8. Rt	20/800	-18.50 -1.00 x 40	20/70	20/100	-3.00 -1.50 x 10	20/50	20/50	-0.50 -0.50 x 75	20/40
Lt	20/800	-19.25 -1.00 x 160	20/50	20/160	-4.50 -1.75 x 160	20/40	20/50	-0.50 -1.00 x 25	20/40
9. Rt	20/250	-5.00 -0.75 x 008	20/20	20/100	-2.00 -0.25 x 25	20/22	20/20	+0.25 -0.25 x 40	20/20
Lt	20/250	-5.50 -0.25 x 150	20/20	20/100	-2.00 -0.50 x 145	20/20	20/30	+0.50 -0.50 x 125	20/25
10. Rt	20/400	-6.50 -0.50 x 30	20/25	20/50	-1.75 -0.50 x 35	20/25	20/30	+0.25 -0.25 x 35	20/25
Lt	20/400	-6.25 -0.50 x 95	20/25	20/50	-1.50 -0.50 x 95	20/25	20/25	+0.25 -0.50 x 125	20/22
11. Rt	20/400	-3.50	20/20	20/70	-1.75	20/20	20/20	Plano	20/20
Lt	20/400	-3.50 -0.50 x 40	20/20	20/50	-1.00 -0.75 x 20	20/20	20/20	+0.50	20/20
12. Rt	20/800	-7.50 -1.50 x 20	20/30	20/100	-2.75 -1.50 x 005	20/30	20/30	-0.75 -0.50 x 20	20/25

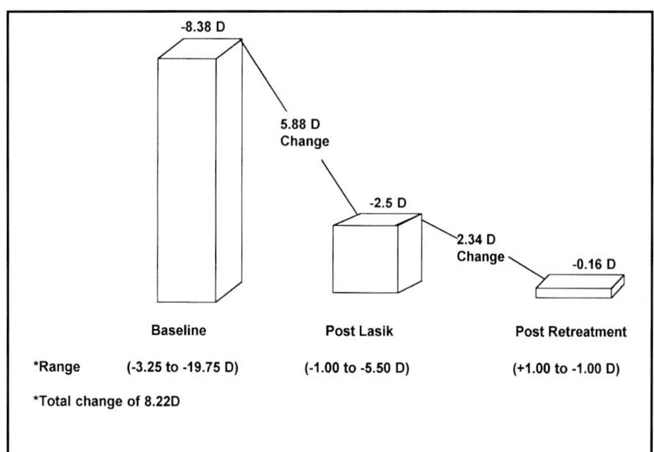

Figure 27-5.
Mean spherical equivalent (20 eyes) before and after LASIK retreatment.

lowed up for 6 to 18 months (mean: 12 months) after the retreatment procedure.

The mean baseline spherical equivalent refraction before the initial LASIK procedure was -8.38 D (range: -3.25 D to -19.75 D) with a mean refractive cylinder of -0.73 D (range: plano to -1.75 D). The mean spherical equivalent refraction before the repeated excimer laser in situ ablation was -2.50 D (range: -1.00 D to -5.50 D). The repeated laser in situ ablation was done using the Summit OmniMed excimer laser; the initial LASIK was done according to the Salah-LASIK nomogram which has been described in detail elsewhere.[11] It is a modification of the original Ruiz KMIS nomogram for myopia. For the repeated ablation, the same nomogram was used based on the spherical equivalent of the manifest refraction.

At 1 year after repeated laser in situ ablation (Figure

27-5), the mean spherical equivalent of the manifest refraction was -0.16 D (range: +1.00 D to -1.00 D), 15 eyes (75%) had refraction between ± 0.50 D, 20 eyes (100%) had refraction between ± 1.00 D. The refractive cylinder remained essentially unchanged by the repeated excimer laser in situ ablation, the mean cylinder was -0.40 D (range: plano to -1.00 D) (Figure 27-6). At 1 year after the retreatment procedure, the uncorrected visual acuity was 20/20 or better in 6 eyes (30%), 20/25 or better in 12 eyes (60%), 20/40 or better in 17 eyes (85%), and 20/50 or better in 20 eyes (100%).

Videokeratography after the retreatment procedure showed greater flattening in the central ablated zone and the center of the ablation was within 1.00 mm of the center of the pupil image in all eyes (Figures 27-7a through 27-7d).

No serious intra- or postoperative complications were observed in this group of eyes. Only one eye of one patient lost one line of best corrected visual acuity because of implanted epithelial cells at the interface (Figure 27-8). His unaided visual acuity was 20/30, and best spectacle corrected visual acuity was 20/25 with a manifest refraction of +0.50 -050 x 125. The patient's other retreated eye had an unaided visual acuity of 20/20 with manifest refraction of +0.25 -0.25 x 40. The patient was satisfied with the result and no attempt was needed to remove the epithelial cells.

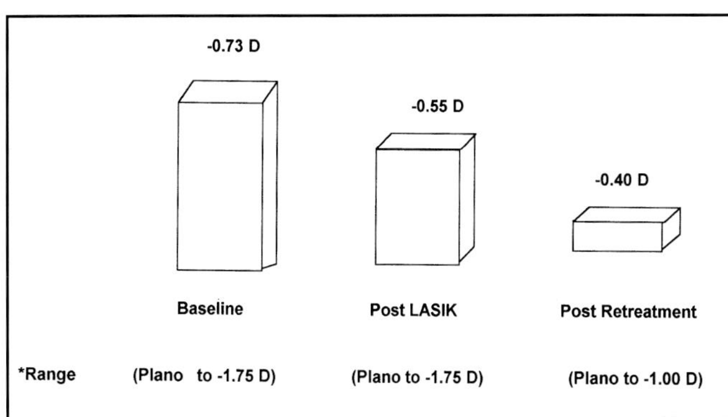

Figure 27-6.
Mean refractive cylinder (20 eyes) before and after LASIK retreatment.

Advantages (Why to Do It?)

Our experience and this report demonstrate the feasibility of repeating an excimer laser in situ ablation after elevating the flap manually to treat residual myopia after a previous LASIK procedure. We think that this approach is superior to incisional keratotomy or PRK because of the following advantages:

- The surgical technique is a straightforward, quick procedure and less complicated than the original LASIK procedure that required a microkeratome section.
- Recovery of useful vision is rapid within 24 to 48 hours with minimal postoperative pain when compared to PRK.
- Repeated excimer laser in situ ablation avoids destabilizing the cornea with a possible hyperopic shift that occurs after refractive keratotomy[13] and avoids subepithelial stromal haze as occurs after PRK.[14,15]
- Because there is minimal stromal corneal wound healing in the lamellar interface,[16] the repeated surgery does not restart wound healing that can affect the outcome, as may occur after repeated PRK,[17] but rather acts more like a direct adjustment of the refraction, as demonstrated in this reported series.
- Corneal topography[18] can remain as regular after the repeated excimer laser in situ ablation as it was after the initial LASIK.
- The refractive correction with the excimer laser is a spherocylindrical one, which can correct a wide range of myopia and myopic astigmatism as well; the laser can be centered over the pupil with the laser alignment beams.
- The procedure is considerably safe, effective, and more predictable; all 20 eyes reported here had a refractive outcome within ± 1.00 D and only one eye lost only one line of best corrected visual acuity.
- Theoretically, the procedure can be used to treat overcorrection if excimer lasers can be configured to effectively treat hyperopia and the diameter of the required ablation falls within the diameter of the resected flap.
- This technique of repeated laser ablation in the old stromal bed after elevating the previous flap is preferred to performing another LASIK with the microkeratome because:

1. There is no need to use the microkeratome with its hazards.
2. It is difficult to center the new flap with the previous one.
3. There is a high possibility of dissecting another plane and creating a double interface.

- The same technique can effectively be used to treat residual myopia after ALK and induced central

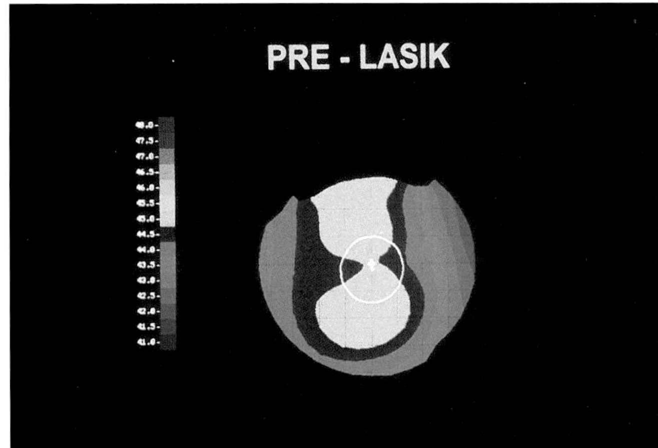

Figure 27-7a.
Sequential videokeratographs of the right eye of one patient. At baseline a bowtie pattern is present demonstrating with-the-rule astigmatism. At the 3-mm diameter zone, the corneal power is 42.5 x 95 / 41.50 x 05.

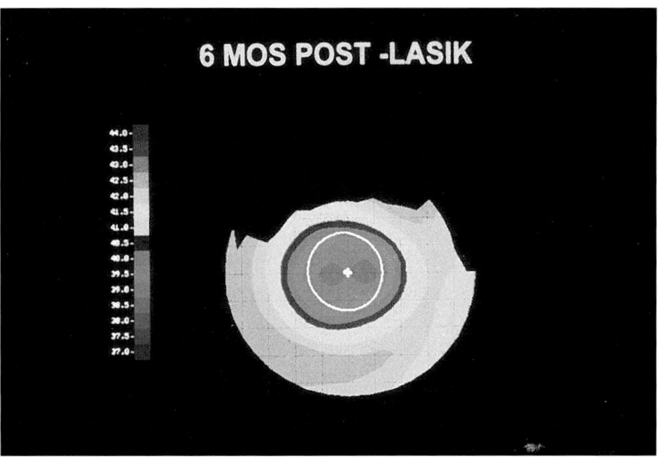

Figure 27-7b.
Six months after the initial LASIK procedure a well-centered round central flat zone is present, measures approximately 5.00 mm in diameter, and exhibits a small bowtie pattern centrally. The average central power is approximately 39.5 D.

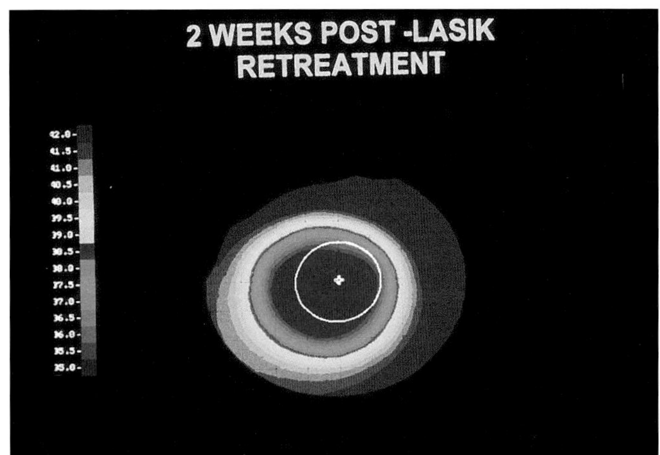

Figure 27-7c.
Two weeks after repeated excimer laser in situ ablation, the central zone is still round and is flatter (average power of 35.0 D) and more uniform.

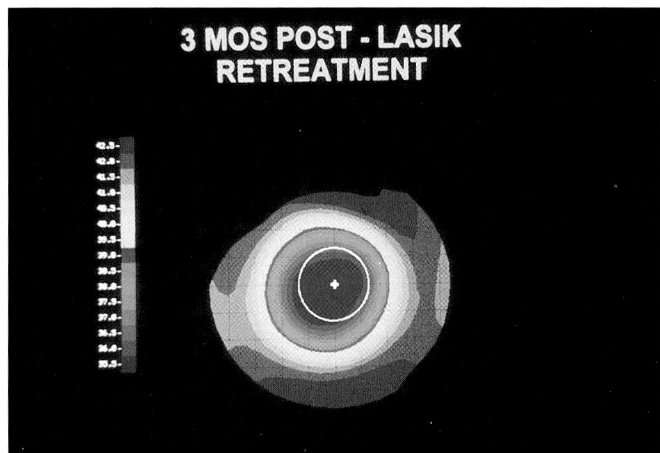

Figure 27-7d.
Three months after the repeated surgery the round uniform central flat zone is still present with more tapered edges and an average central power of 35.5 D. (The scale contains colored-coded steps that are in 0.50 D increments. The scale is normalized so an individual color does not represent the same power on each keratograph.)

islands or implanted epithelial cells at the interface following LASIK.

Despite the abovementioned advantages, we would like to draw your attention to the following:

- The procedure involves repeated surgery with its attendant risks, morbidity, and inconvenience. Among these risks is the possibility of implanting epithelial cells in the interface so great care should be taken while breaking though the interface, remove any tags of epithelium at the edge of the bed, and clean the stromal bed by irrigation and brushing before flipping the flap back to its position.
- Preoperatively, the corneal thickness should be accurately measured, and following the reablation the residual thickness of the stromal bed should not be less than 250 µm or corneal ectasia may occur.

CENTRAL ISLAND

A central island is a topographic abnormality that has been reported following excimer laser ablation of the cornea. It is defined[14] as a central or paracentral steepening of at least 1 D to 3 D in height, a diameter of at least 1 to 3 mm, measured at least 1 month postoperatively, and associated with clinical symptoms of ghosting of images, blurring, and qualitative visual changes. There are four main theories explaining its cause:

1. Focal central epithelial hyperplasia.
2. The vortex plume theory.
3. Degradation of laser optics.
4. The acoustic shockwave theory.

Central islands have been primarily reported following PRK[19]; their occurrence following LASIK has not been reported. I have seen central islands in two eyes following LASIK; both eyes were treated with the VisX 20/20 excimer laser.

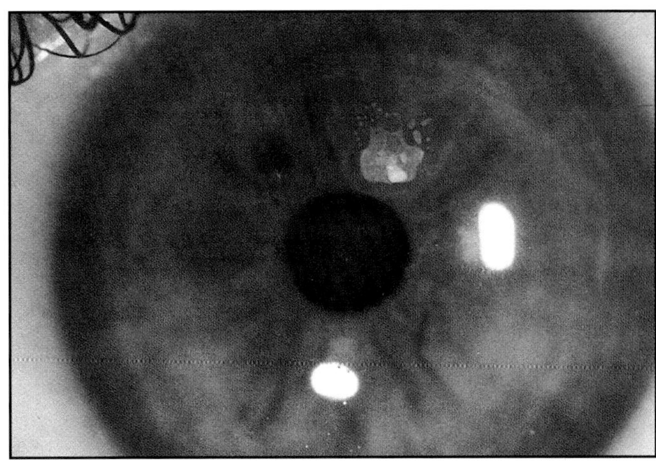

Figure 27-8.
Implanted epithelial cells at the interface following repeated laser in situ ablation.

Case Report: Treatment of Central Islands Following LASIK

A 34-year-old man received LASIK to correct his myopic astigmatism in July 1995. Preoperatively, his unaided visual acuity was counting fingers at 5 m, and with a manifest refraction of -10.25 -4.50 x 170 he could see 20/30. Corneal topography using the EyeSys topography unit machine showed regular bowtie topographical patterns and 4.5 D with-the-rule myopic astigmatism (Figure 27-9a). LASIK was done on the left eye using the VisX 20/20 excimer laser which has a laser pulse rate of 6 Hz. The operative parameters were

- Refraction, -10.50 DS -4.50 D cyl x 170.
- Treatment zone of 6.00 mm.
- 752 total pulses.
- Total ablation depth of 123 µm.

Four days post-LASIK the patient complained of ghost images, shadowing, and something blocking his central vision. Unaided visual acuity was 20/70; slit lamp biomicroscopy examination showed a clear centered flap with a clear interface. Corneal topography was done and it showed a significant well-defined central island of 3 mm in diameter approximately 5.5 D in height (Figure 27-9b). The decision to follow the patient at 1, 3, and 6 months was made hoping that the central island might disappear or decrease. At 1 month, the topographic picture remained the same; his unaided visual acuity was 20/50, manifest refraction was +0.75 -1.50 x 90, and the symptoms persisted even with spectacles.

After 9 months, the central island measured 3.0 mm in diameter and 4.0 D in height. The patient was still complaining of ghost images; his manifest refraction was +0.75 -1.00 x 130, and the decision to treat the central island was made. Treatment was done under topical anesthesia. Preparation of the eye and marking of the cornea was done as usual. The flap was manually elevated as previously described for retreatment of residual myopia following LASIK, the previous stromal bed was exposed, then the Nidek excimer laser was used to ablate the central island using the PRK program with the following parameters:

- Diameter of 3 mm.
- Transition zone of 0.5 mm.
- Refraction of 3.5 D.

These parameters were chosen according to the diameter and height of the central island as demonstrated by corneal topography done preoperatively (Figure 27-9c). The preoperative refraction was not put into consideration.

Postoperatively, unaided visual acuity in the left eye was 20/40, refraction remained the same +0.75-1.00 x 140, best spectacle corrected visual acuity was 20/30, and corneal topography showed a central area of homogenous flattening of 6 mm in diameter. The central island almost resolved and the patient symptoms of ghost images and shadowing disappeared (Figure 27-9d).

In conclusion, we think that the presence of an anterior corneal flap is a great step forward in lamellar refractive surgery, since it leaves the door open for another enhancement procedure, in which the flap can be elevated and another laser ablation could be done to treat under- or overcorrections and central islands following LASIK. For the higher degrees of myopia, LASIK can be

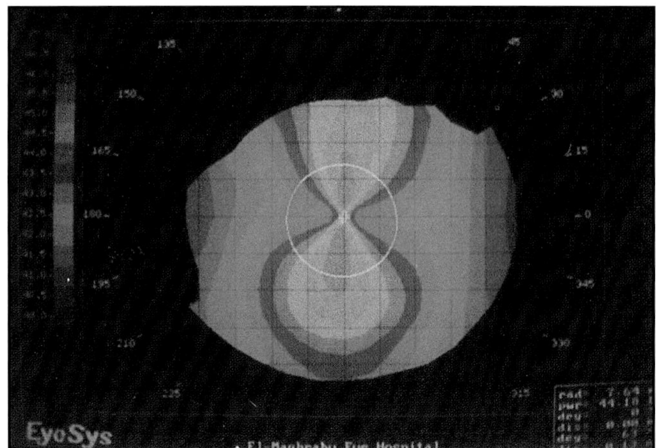

Figure 27-9a.
Sequential videokeratographs of the left eye of one patient who developed central island following LASIK. At baseline a bowtie topographic pattern is present demonstrating a 4.5 D with-the-rule astigmatism.

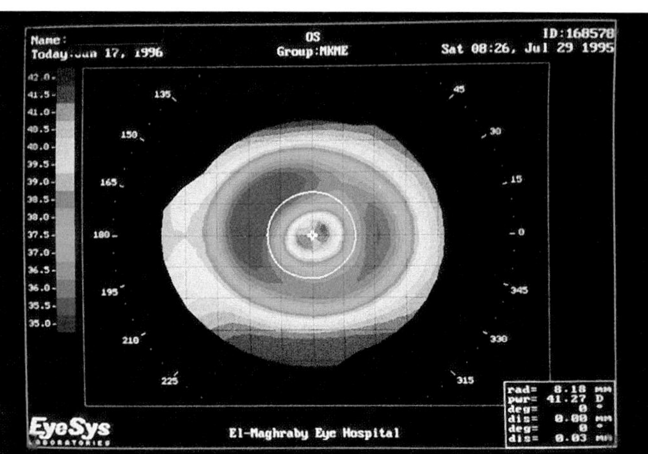

Figure 27-9b.
Corneal topography 4 days post-LASIK shows a well-centered oval ablated zone with a well-defined central island of 3 mm in diameter and approximately 5.5 D in height.

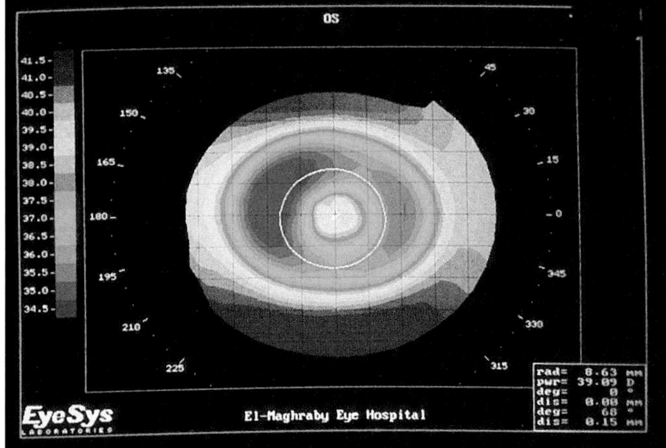

Figure 27-9c.
Nine months following LASIK shows the central island of 3.00 mm in diameter and about 4.0 D in height.

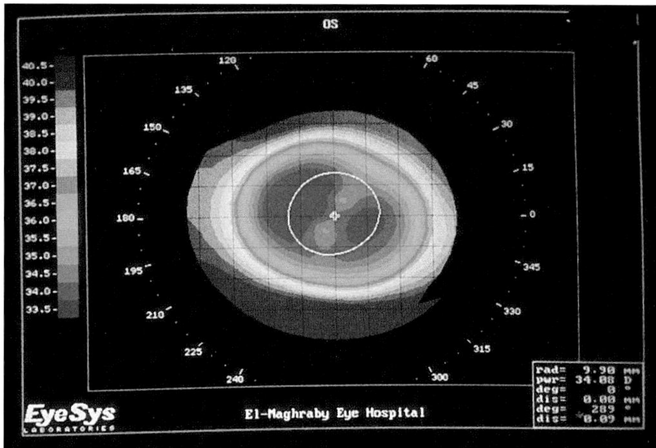

Figure 27-9d.
Corneal topography 1 month after treatment of the central island demonstrates a central area of homogeneous flattening of 6 mm in diameter and exhibits a small bowtie pattern centrally.

staged and results titrated in order to avoid overcorrection.

References

1. Werblin TP, Stafford GM. The Casebeer system for predictable keratorefractive surgery: one year evaluation of 205 consecutive eyes. *Ophthalmology*. 1993;100:1095-1102.
2. Waring GO, Allen R, Verg JC, Casebeer JC, et al. A prospective multicenter study of refractive keratotomy for myopia and astigmatism. *Ophthalmology*. 1994;101(suppl):90.
3. Price FW. Keratomileusis. In: Thompson KP, Waring GO III, eds. *Ophthalmology Clinics of North America. Contemporary Refractive Surgery*. Philadelphia, Pa: WB Saunders Co; 1992:673-681.
4. Barraquer J. *Cirugia refractive de la cornea*. Bogota, Columbia; Instituto Barraquer de America; 1989.
5. Arenas-Archilla E, Sanchez-Thorin J, Naranzo-Uribe J, Hernandez-Lozano A. Myopic keratomileusis in situ: a preliminary report. *J Cataract Refract Surg*. 1991;17:424-435.
6. Rozakis GW, ed. *Refractive Lamellar Keratoplasty*. Thorofare, NJ: SLACK Inc; 1994:112.
7. Pallikaris IG, Siganos DS. Excimer laser in situ keratomileusis (LASIK) versus photorefractive keratectomy for the correction of high myopia. *J Refract Corneal Surg*. 1994;10:1-13.
8. Binder PS, Charlton KH. Surgical procedures performed after refractive surgery. *J Refract Corneal Surg*. 1992;8:61-74.
9. Bores LD. Side effects and complications of refractive surgery. In: Bores L, ed. *Refractive Eye Surgery*. Blackwell Scientific Publications; 1993:500-554.
10. Salah T, Waring GO, El-Maghraby A. Excimer laser keratomileusis, Part I. In: Salz JJ, ed. *Corneal Laser Surgery*. St. Louis, Mo: Mosby-Year Book, Inc; 1995:187-194.

11. Salah T, Waring GO, El-Maghraby A, et al. Excimer laser keratomileusis under a corneal flap for myopia of 2 to 20 diopters. *Am J Ophthalmol*. 1996;121:143-155.

12. Guell JL, Muller A. Laser in situ keratomileusis (LASIK) for myopia from -7 to -18 diopters. *J Refract Surg*. 1996;12:222-228.

13. Waring GO, Lynn MJ, McDonell PJ. The PERK study group results of the prospective evaluation of radial keratotomy (PERK) study 10 years after surgery. *Arch Ophthalmol*. 1994;112:1298-1308.

14. Maguen E, Machat JJ. Complications of photorefractive keratectomy, primarily with the Visx excimer laser. In: Salz JJ, ed. *Corneal Laser Surgery*. St. Louis, Mo: Mosby-Year Book; 1995:143-158.

15. Epstein D, Fagerholm P, Hamberg-Nystrom H, Tengroth B. Twenty-four month follow up of excimer laser photorefractive keratectomy for myopia. *Ophthalmology*. 1994;101:1558-1563.

16. Tester JV, Rodriguez MM, Villasenor RA, Schanzlin DJ. Keratophakia and keratomileusis: histopathologic, ultrastructural and experimental studies. *Ophthalmology*. 1984;91:793-805.

17. Seiler T, Ders CM, Pham T. Repeated excimer laser treatment after photorefractive keratectomy. *Arch Ophthalmol*. 1992;110:1230-1233.

18. Lin DTC. Corneal topographic analysis after excimer photorefractive keratectomy. *Ophthalmology*. 1994;101:1432-1439.

19. Parker PJ, Klyce SD, Ryan BL, et al. Central topographic islands following photorefractive keratectomy. *Invest Ophthalmol Vis Sci*. 1993;34(suppl):803.

SECTION 7

EVALUATION OF LASIK OPTICS

Chapter 28

ADVANCED VISUAL FUNCTION TESTING IN LASIK

Brian S. Boxer Wachler, MD, David W. Evans, PhD, Ronald R. Krueger, MD, MSE

BACKGROUND

Each keratorefractive procedure has advantages and disadvantages. Laser in situ keratomileusis (LASIK) delivers faster visual rehabilitation and largely obviates the need for steroids compared to surface photorefractive keratectomy (PRK). In exchange for these benefits, LASIK invokes a unique set of risks. The ultimate measure of a refractive procedure is its effect on visual function. Visual acuity was first developed by Snellen in 1865 to aid practitioners in refracting and prescribing spectacles.[1] As diagnostic and treatment modalities for ocular diseases developed, visual acuity was modified and integrated beyond the area of refraction and into assessment of disease states. In ocular disease, contrast sensitivity has shown to be more sensitive in detecting changes in vision than visual acuity.[2-4] A similar relationship has recently been observed in PRK.[5] In LASIK, there have been no published studies reporting both visual acuity and contrast sensitivity results. As contrast sensitivity testing is recognized in refractive surgery to be an important diagnostic tool, the results of such testing will likely be forthcoming.

VISION LOSS IN LASIK

Both visual acuity and contrast sensitivity are important safety tools for detecting

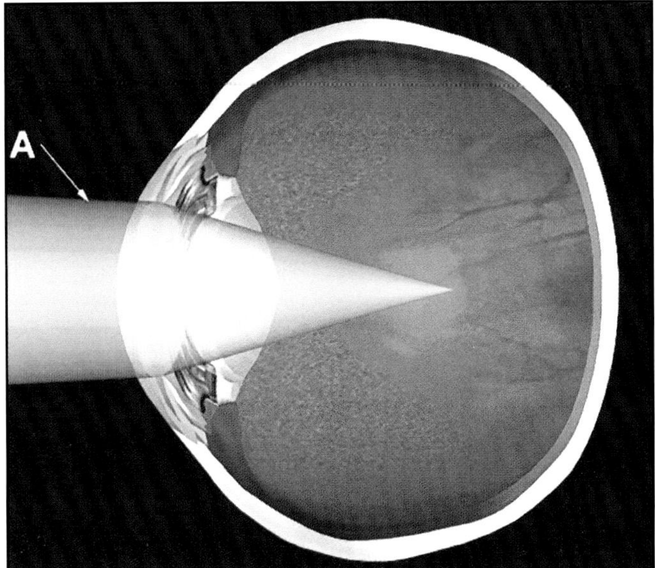

Figure 28-1.
The myopic eye. Light rays A focus anterior to the fovea.

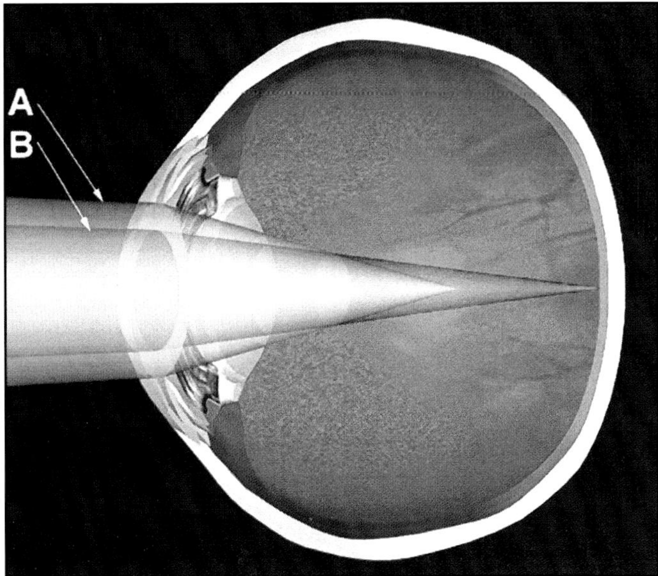

Figure 28-2.
Post-LASIK negative clearance. Light rays A pass through unablated cornea and focus anterior to rays B which travel through the optical zone and focus on the fovea. This situation creates halos and reduced vision which can occur at night when the pupil naturally dilates.

visual consequences of LASIK complications. Vision loss may result from mechanical (flap), medical, and optical etiologies.

Mechanical etiologies are flap related and result in irregular astigmatism:

- Missing flap.
- Perforated flap.
- Repair of free flap.
- Incomplete flap.
- Slipped flap.

Medical etiologies are visually obstructive and may result in opacity or haze:

- Central epithelial ingrowth.
- Stromal haze.
- Infection.
- Interface debris.

Optical etiologies are refractive disorders and may result in spheric or aspheric aberrations:

- Negative clearance (pupil larger than optical zone).
- Decentered ablation.
- Steep central island.
- Irregular astigmatism.

CLEARANCE

Halos and visual loss at night may result from negative clearance, a condition where the pupil naturally dilates larger than the optical zone.[6] Halos may occur following PRK[7-10] and LASIK.[11] One study reported 29% of patients experience halos and were treated with ablation zones that ranged from 4.5 to 6.0 mm.[12] An illustration of optical ray tracing of a myopic eye is illustrated in Figure 28-1. Figure 28-2 demonstrates the spherical aberration caused by the situation of negative clearance when the pupil is larger than the optical zone. The mechanism for this phenomenon has been described for PRK,[13] and applies to LASIK as well. Such aberration would be expected to reduce contrast sensitivity.[14,15] In PRK, we have shown that ablation diameter correlated with contrast sensitivity, not visual acuity.[5] To avoid such aberrations, positive clearance is desired where the optical zone is equal to or larger than the pupil (Figure 28-3).

To quantify the degree of negative clearance, accurate measurement of the pupil under dim (mesopic) conditions is required. Using the comparison method (Rosenbaum card) is not as accurate as infrared pupillometry.[16] Although topography units can capture and

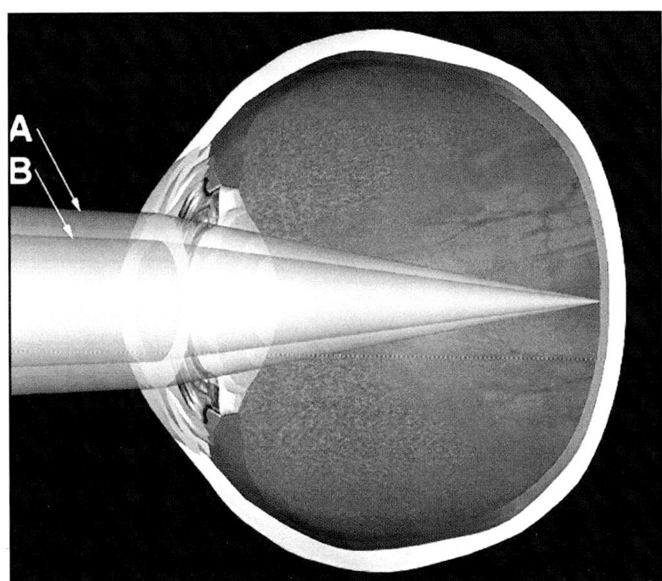

Figure 28-3.
Post-LASIK positive clearance. A larger optical zone allows light rays A and B to pass through the optical zone and focus on the fovea, thereby avoiding halos and decreased vision from aberrations.

measure the image of the pupil, the luminance of the Placido rings yields pupils that are smaller than measured in the dark-adapted state.[17] Infrared pupillometers can accurately measure pupils in darkness which may aid in determining negative clearance.[18] If pupil diameters are accurately measured preoperatively, patients at risk of halos may be appropriately counseled or directed toward another procedure. Alternatively, preoperative pupil measurements may guide the surgeon to use a larger ablation diameter pending laser capability. As the success of treating halos by enlarging the optical zone is not universal,[19,20] it does not seem prudent to disregard the opportunity to prevent halos.

If clearance is positive, patients will not likely complain of halos but may still report glare even in the absence of corneal haze. Veiling glare results from forward light scatter from corneal haze.[21] With a clear visual axis, glare may result from off-axis light rays that pass between the pupil and optical zone and enter the eye.[22] These light rays fall peripheral to the fovea and can result in night vision disturbances, but would not be expected to reduce visual function. Since the fovea is spared, central visual function should not be affected.

MASKING SPHERICAL ABERRATIONS

After LASIK, there is potential spherical aberration from the junction between the ablated and non-ablated cornea. The iris determines whether such aberration exists in the eye's optical system. Any condition that causes a small pupil may potentially mask deleterious optical disorders. We have performed contrast sensitivity and visual acuity testing in post-PRK patients with a peripheral glare source and noted improved visual function since the glare source resulted in smaller pupils (unpublished data).

Glare sources are not the only mechanism that induce pupillary miosis in vision testing. The test condition itself may be the cause. During visual acuity testing, bright ambient room lights will affect the pupil. A similar potential bias exists in contrast sensitivity testing. Some contrast sensitivity devices are externally illuminated. If these charts are used with high illumination, pupils will be small. Dim illumination will elicit large pupils. Internally illuminated light boxes can be used with the room lights completely out. It is important to be aware of possible light-related factors that may mask corneal aberrations during vision testing. An attempt to minimize such luminance-based artifacts will increase the sensitivity of vision testing.

EXPLANATION OF CONTRAST SENSITIVITY

Over the past decade, improvements in refractive surgery techniques have greatly reduced the number of patients who have lost lines of best corrected visual acuity. But even as surgical techniques improve, it has become obvious that better methodology is needed to accurately define surgery outcome. Contrast sensitivity testing was first developed in the mid-1950s by an RCA television engineer, Otto Schade,[23] who developed a vision testing technology to make the television screen image compatible with the human visual system. He measured individual sensitivity to varying size bar patterns at different contrast levels and incorporated this information into television screen designs. This technolo-

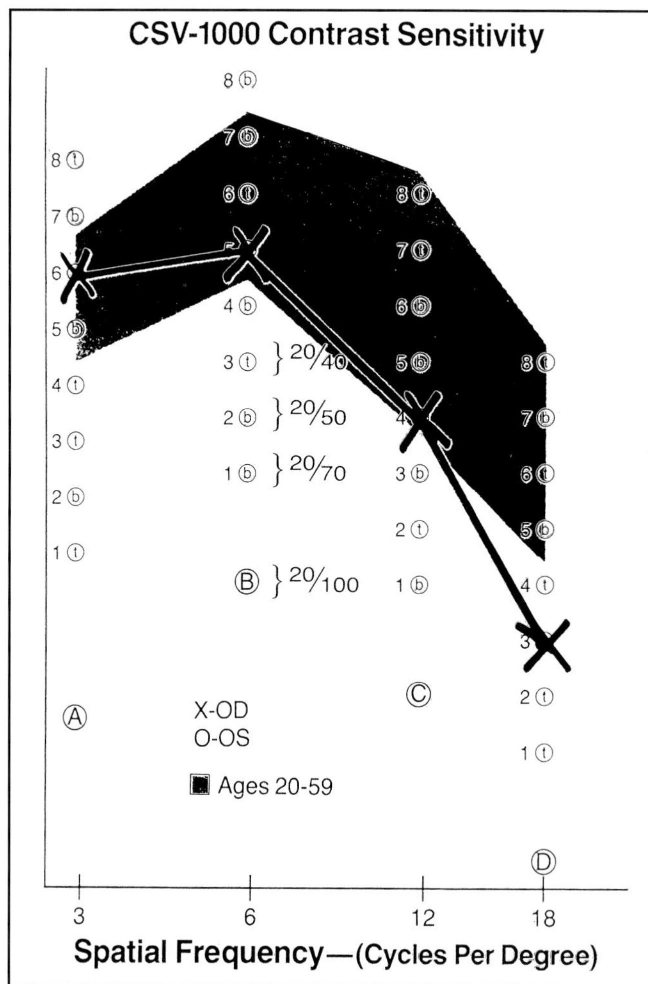

Figure 28-4.

Traditionally, contrast sensitivity results were plotted on separate graph paper which proved difficult for clinicians to use in practice.

gy was further developed by Campbell and Green who studied the effects of optical blur on contrast.[24] Since that time, contrast sensitivity has come into clinical use, primarily as a tool to evaluate and document cataract vision loss.[25]

A simple means to understand contrast sensitivity is to consider it as an improved measure of central vision just as automated threshold visual field perimetry is more sophisticated than Goldmann visual field testing. Similar to threshold visual field testing, contrast sensitivity also determines a threshold, but only in the central field of vision. In visual field testing, the threshold level is that at which the patient can no longer detect the spot of light. In contrast sensitivity testing, a bar pattern is presented to the patient and the contrast level is reduced until the patient can no longer detect this pattern. This contrast level is the patient's contrast sensitivity threshold. Just as in perimetry where different size spots can be used for different test purposes, in contrast sensitivity different size bar patterns (spatial frequencies) can be used to test different aspects of vision. However, unlike perimetry, in which only one size test spot is used within a given test, in contrast sensitivity four or five different size bar patterns (spatial frequencies) are used within the same test.

One aspect of visual field perimetry that has made it useful to clinicians is the normalized reference values. Clinicians do not speak of a patient's visual field sensitivity in terms of the lux or illuminance level that a patient requires to detect each spot of light. Instead, software is used to compare the patient threshold scores to a normalized score for a given age group. The resultant comparison is expressed in terms of a logarithmic difference between the patient and the normalized score in units of dB (1 dB = 1/10 of a log unit). Clinicians describe a patient's peripheral vision in terms of the dB loss at each location.

To better evaluate surgical outcome, contrast sensitivity testing has been suggested as an adjunct to visual acuity. Research has shown that contrast sensitivity is a better predictor of real-world visual performance than visual acuity, such as for nighttime driver performance and pilot target detection.[26,27] For refractive surgery, recent data also shows that patient satisfaction following surgery is associated with contrast sensitivity.[28] For patients such as professional and Olympic athletes who are uniquely dependent on visual performance, contrast sensitivity is of key importance. In such fields, contrast sensitivity has virtually replaced acuity as the primary measure of visual capability in the field of sports vision testing.

Figure 28-5 shows the CSV-1000 contrast sensitivity test and internally luminated light box. There are four rows of different spatial frequencies: 3, 6, 12, and 18 cycles per degree. Within each row, there are paired circles, one above another. Alternating light and dark bars exist in only one circle in the pair. The contrast between these bars systematically decreases toward the right side of the chart, which corresponds to higher contrast sensitivity. The patient is instructed to identify whether the bars are in the top circle, bottom circle, or neither. The last correct identification is taken as the contrast sensitivity.

Although contrast sensitivity is an important measure, it has not experienced the prolific use that visual acuity has. Historically, contrast sensitivity was used by researchers, not clinicians. The results were plotted as curves on special graph paper (Figure 28-4). Such representation is difficult for a clinician to use in practice. Additionally, the contrast sensitivity values were absolute. It seems that clinicians appreciate notations that incorporate a relative standard which both visual acuity and threshold visual perimetry do. Two of the authors (BSBW, RRK) have developed a similar notation to aid in interpreting contrast sensitivity scores.[29] Just as in field testing, contrast sensitivity is measured on a logarithmic scale. This new contrast sensitivity notation establishes a ratio between the average logarithmic threshold value for the population and the individual logarithmic threshold score. If the patient score is equal to the average score, then the contrast sensitivity value is expressed as 1.0. If the patient score falls below the average, then the score is expressed as a ratio less than 1.0. If the patient scores above the average, then the score is expressed as a ratio greater than 1.0. Such normalized ratios may be applied to any contrast sensitivity testing medium. Figure 28-6 shows the Normalized CSV-1000E from VectorVision (Dayton, Ohio) and Figure 28-7 shows the Normalized F.A.C.T. chart from Stereo Optical (Chicago, Ill) as examples.

There have been no published studies reporting the results of contrast sensitivity in LASIK. In PRK, reports have shown that best corrected vision as measured by contrast sensitivity falls following PRK,[30-32] but other studies have shown no loss in contrast sensitivity.[33,34] The lack of consensus may reflect the different luminance levels of contrast sensitivity devices used which would affect pupil size. In normal eyes, luminance-induced changes in pupil diameter significantly affect both visual acuity and contrast sensitivity.[35] In order to determine the changes in visual function and quality of vision in LASIK, long-term studies utilizing contrast sensitivity in a controlled environment are needed.

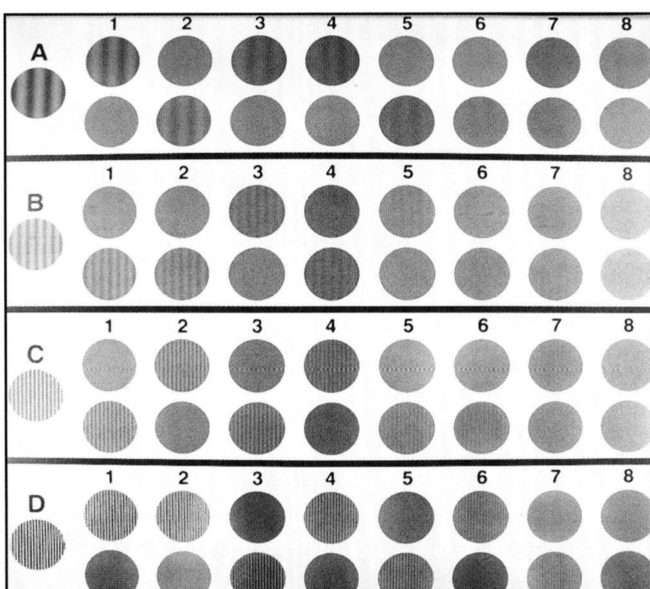

Figure 28-5.
The CSV-1000E Contrast Sensitivity chart. Patients are to identify whether the vertical bars are in the top or bottom circle.

ROLE OF CONTRAST SENSITIVITY

A common complaint from highly myopic patients concerns the quality of vision through spectacles. Even with 20/20 acuity, patients indicate that the vision is not crisp. The cause of these complaints is thought to be image distortion and miniaturization induced by the high spectacle power. These patients typically achieve good acuity with spectacles, but the contrast sensitivity falls below or in the lower portion of the normal range. When patients wear contact lenses, they subjectively comment that the vision has improved, even though acuity has not changed. Similar comments are associated with LASIK patients. This clinical situation is where contrast sensitivity can play a very valuable role, ie, a change in vision is too subtle to be measured by standard acuity, but both the clinician and patient suspect that the vision has changed. Contrast sensitivity testing provides an objective measure of this change.

Here we present two case reports of highly myopic patients who underwent LASIK. These individual reports are not presented as conclusive evidence regarding the impact of LASIK on contrast sensitivity and the quality of patient vision. Rather, these reports are presented to help in educating the refractive surgeon concerning the value of monitoring visual function with measures other than visual acuity to objectively assess subtle changes in vision that are important for patient care. The results for only one eye will be described for each patient.

Patient 1 is a 40-year-old male with entering refractive state and visual acuity as follows for the right eye: -8.75 -1.00 x 40 (20/20-1).

Contrast sensitivity was measured at four spatial fre-

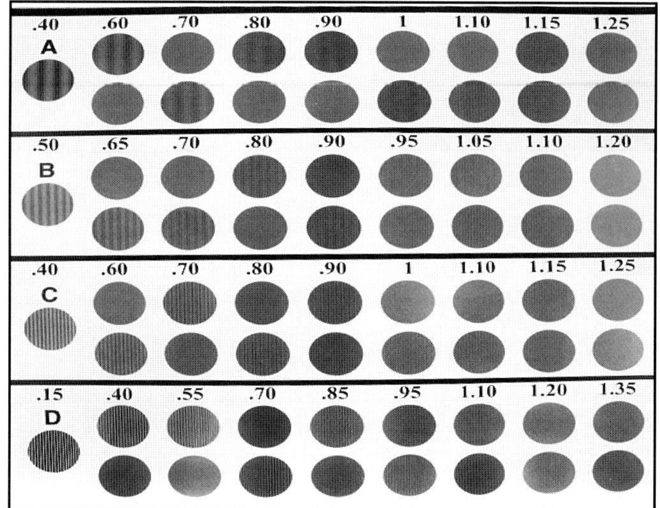

Figure 28-6.
The Normalized CSV-1000E chart. Normalized ratios indicate to the clinician the patient's performance relative to a normal population. Results can be notated directly in the patient's chart for each spatial frequency.

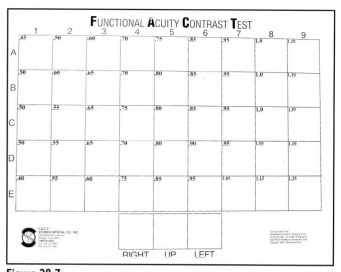

Figure 28-7.
The Normalized F.A.C.T. chart. All contrast sensitivity testing media can incorporate the normalized notation.

quencies (3, 6, 12, and 18 cycles per degree) under standardized illumination using the CSV-1000 contrast testing instrument. For purposes of our explanation, these spatial frequencies will be referred to as A, B, C, and D, respectively. These letters correspond to the row on the test instrument (see Figure 28-5) for each spatial frequency. The results are expressed in normalized ratios where numbers greater than 1.0 correspond to percent contrast sensitivity above the population average and numbers below 1.0 represent percent of the average contrast sensitivity below the population average.

Preoperative contrast sensitivity is shown below.

A	B	C	D
1.15	.95	1.0	.70

The patient underwent LASIK on December 20, 1996 and returned for contrast sensitivity examination 1 month later. The patient status is shown below.

-1.75 -0.50 X 75 (20/20)

A	B	C	D
1	1.05	.90	.85

This patient has retained very good contrast sensitivity. The patient returned 2 months later for re-examination. The refractive state, visual acuity, and contrast sensitivity are shown below.

-2.00 -0.50 X 90 (20/16 + 2)

A	B	C	D
1	1.05	1.25	.95

The patient now demonstrates an improvement in contrast sensitivity from the baseline pretreatment condition, particularly in Rows C and D. (Rows C and D test the higher spatial frequencies and are most important for refractive surgery evaluation.) The patient improved from an original score on C and D of 1.0 and .70 (100% of normal and 30% below normal) to 1.25 and .95 (25% above normal and 5% below normal), respectively. This improvement provides a good indication that this patient has better functional vision following LASIK, than he had through his spectacles.

Patient 2 is a 39-year-old female with the entering visual acuity, refractive state, and contrast sensitivity as follows for the right eye:

8.75 -2.50 x 18 (20/20)

A	B	C	D
.90	.90	.70	.40

This high myope displays contrast sensitivity well below the normal value for her age group, even though standard acuity is 20/20. She is 30% and 60% below normal for C and D, respectively, the most important rows for refractive surgery evaluation.

She underwent LASIK on January 10, 1997 and returned for contrast sensitivity evaluation 1 month later. Her examination showed the following.

-0.50 -0.75 x 80 (20/50)

A	B	C	D
.90	.90	.60	.40

Her contrast sensitivity has fallen a little on Row C and

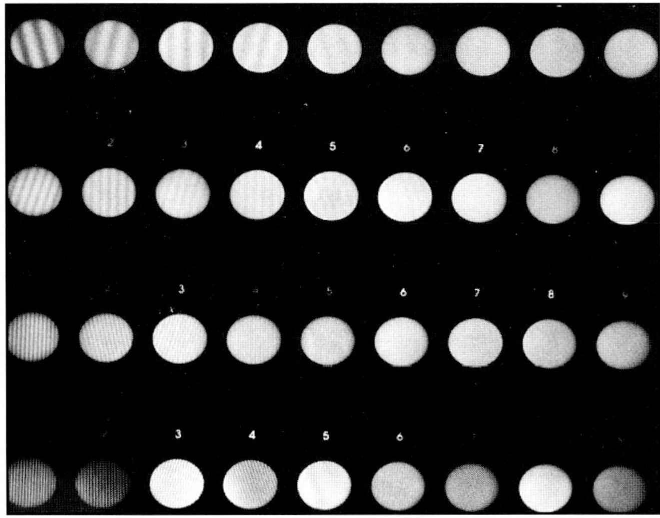

Figure 28-8.
The Horizon chart. By blocking out light that is not used to illuminate the contrast gratings, ambient room luminance is minimized. This allows maximum natural pupil dilation for contrast sensitivity testing and provides for increased sensitivity to optical aberrations caused by negative clearance.

remains low for Row D. Note that acuity has also dropped to 20/50. Unlike before surgery, now her visual acuity and contrast sensitivity provide similar information. Both are depressed.

Her examination 2 months later showed the following.

-0.50 -0.50 X 80 (20/25)

A	B	C	D
.90	.90	.90	.85

Three months after surgery, the patient's contrast sensitivity has improved. On Rows C and D the patient improved from a preoperative level of .70 and .40 to .90 and .85, respectively. Just as in the preoperative condition, contrast sensitivity and visual acuity provide different information. Visual acuity dropped to 20/25, but the contrast sensitivity measure of functional vision shows that the vision has improved to a level similar to average for the patient's age group.

Diagnostic testing is essential for properly evaluating patients in refractive surgery. One of the most important factors to understand and control is the pupil diameter. A small pupil during vision testing will mask the aberrations of the junction between central optical zone and unablated cornea. As the most common cause for induced miosis during vision testing is ambient luminance, attention to chart designs is important. The Horizon contrast sensitivity chart (VectorVision, Dayton, Ohio) attempts to maximize the natural pupil diameter by blocking out all chart light that is not being used to retro-luminate the contrast sensitivity patches (Figure 28-8). In a study of normal untreated eyes, we found that the Horizon chart had largest pupil diameters compared to the CSV-1000E and the visual acuity chart. As a result, the Horizon chart had lower contrast sensitivity than the CSV-1000E.[35]

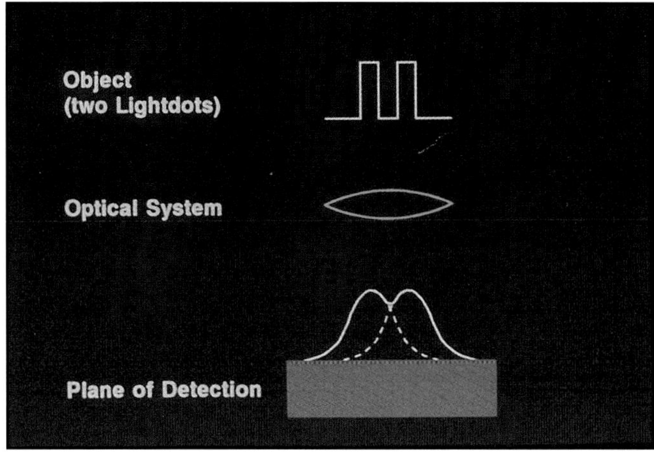

Figure 28-9.
Elements of ray tracing analysis. Two points in space are projected through the anterior optical system of the eye and are represented as a sinusoidal wave at the image plane.

EXPLANATION OF RAY TRACING ANALYSIS IN VISUAL FUNCTION TESTING

An objective method to assess visual function has been developed for the Technomed C-Scan videokeratography unit. This module uses ray-tracing analysis and the pupil diameter to determine the potential corneal visual acuity from the videokeratography map. The ray tracing module of the C-Scan accomplishes this by graphically displaying the image quality of two points from the object plane as they are projected through the videokeratography map (optical system) onto the best fit image plane as shown in Figure 28-9. Since visual acuity is defined as the ability to separate two isolated points, it is possible to objectively determine the best visual acuity from the ray tracing analysis of the corneal maps.

The corneal map, however, is not the only component necessary to determine visual acuity. The resolving power of the cornea also depends on the anterior cham-

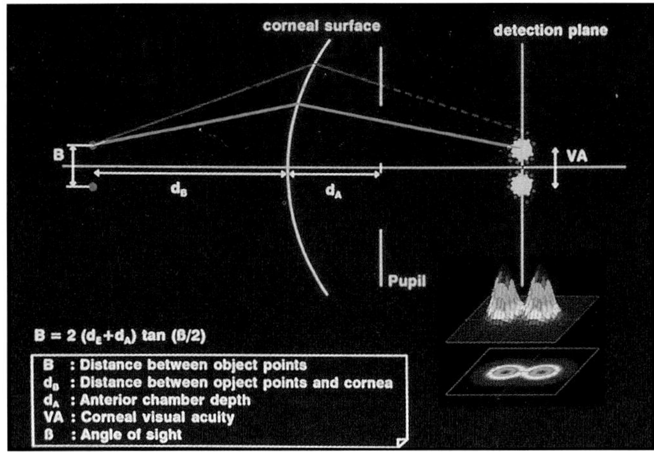

Figure 28-10.
Factors that influence ray tracing. Based on the topographic map, the ray tracing module projects light through the cornea and determines the image plane that provides the highest degree of two-point focus of all projected light rays. The pupil serves as a sentry for light rays entering the eye which may dramatically affect the results of ray tracing. Changing the anterior chamber depth results in a small refractive change compared to the cornea and axial length.[36]

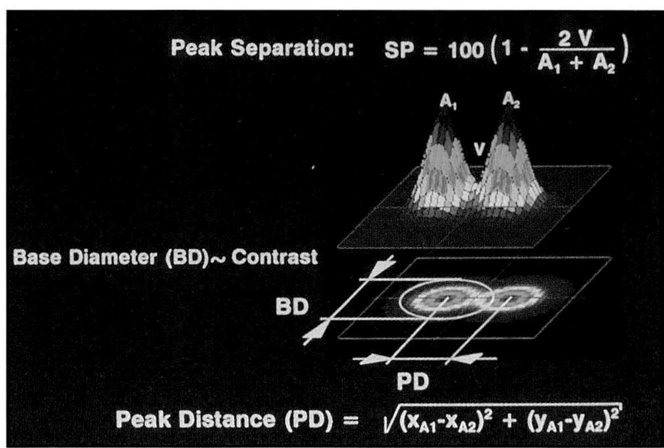

Figure 28-11.
Determinants of two-point resolution. At the image plane, the quality of the sinusoidal curves are determined based on peak distortion, peak distance, and minimum resolvable (not shown). The contrast between the peak and base of the curve is a function of the base diameter, where large base diameters lead to peripheral distortion spikes that rise from the plane of the base and decrease the two-point resolution. Figure 28-12f illustrates this phenomenon.

ber depth and pupil size. Hence, ray tracing analysis requires information about the corneal shape, pupil size, and anterior chamber depth in order to determine potential corneal visual acuity as demonstrated in Figure 28-10. Of these three parameters, anterior chamber depth probably has the least effect in ray tracing. A previous study has shown that variability of chamber depths may result in a maximum 2 D change compared a potential 26 D and 16 D change from variability of axial lengths and anterior corneal curvatures, respectively.[36]

To understand this further, the imaged points on the detection plane are represented by two intensity peaks which must be spatially resolved in order to discriminate them as separate and individual. The peak distortion, peak distance, and minimum resolvable percentage are three parameters defined to help us understand when these two peaks are spatially resolved (Figure 28-11). The minimum resolvable percentage (or peak separation) is the most useful parameter, and spatial resolution (visual acuity) is best determined when this value equals 100%. Potential corneal visual acuity can therefore be determined by ray tracing two isolated spots through the videokeratography map, anterior chamber depth, and entrance pupil onto a detection plane which determines the spatial distance necessary to discriminate these spots as separate.

The ray tracing display assumes an anterior chamber depth of 3.0 mm (which may be adjusted), and calculates the pupil size by the captured image of the pupil during videokeratography. This pupil, which is measured under the luminance of the videokeratography rings (25.5 cd/m^2), is automatically integrated into the ray tracing analysis with the videokeratography map to determine potential corneal visual acuity. The pupil may be manually adjusted as well. Since two point discrimination (visual acuity) is linear (one dimensional) discrimination, potential corneal visual acuity is automatically calculated along the flat axis of corneal astigmatism on the videokeratography map. A 90° shift function can be implemented to calculate the potential corneal visual acuity along the steep axis of astigmatism as well. This gives a two-dimensional assessment of potential corneal visual acuity which correlates better with the two-dimensionality of the videokeratography map.

ROLE OF RAY TRACING ANALYSIS IN VISUAL FUNCTION TESTING

In laser keratorefractive surgery (PRK and LASIK), regularity and uniformity of corneal shape are impera-

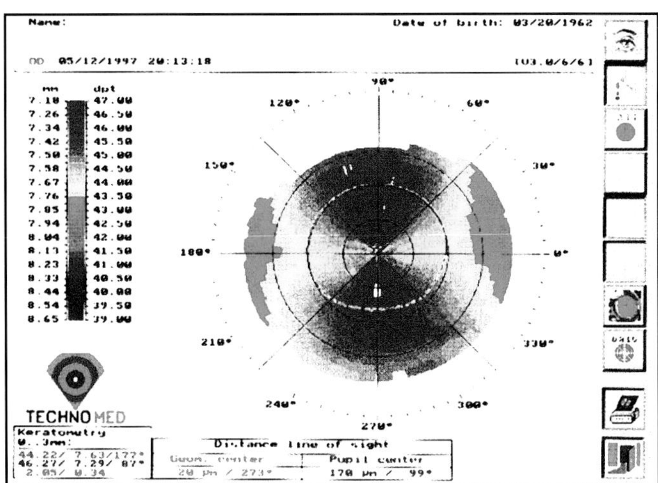

Figure 28-12a.
A case report (Figures 28-12a through 28-12f) illustrating the postoperative aberrations following PRK. The preoperative cornea.

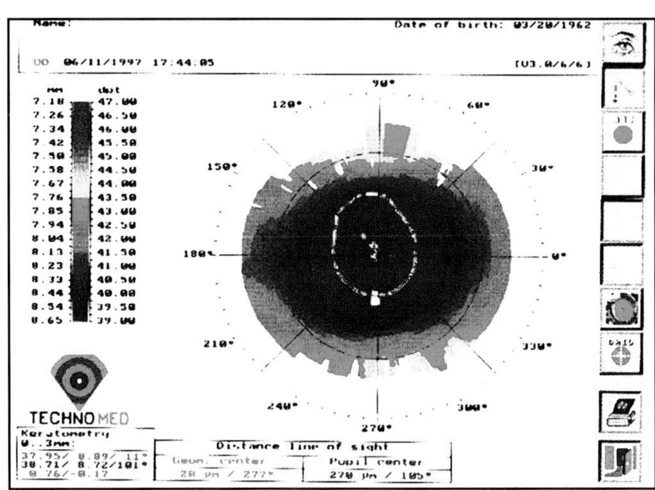

Figure 28-12b.
The postoperative cornea shows uniform central flattening.

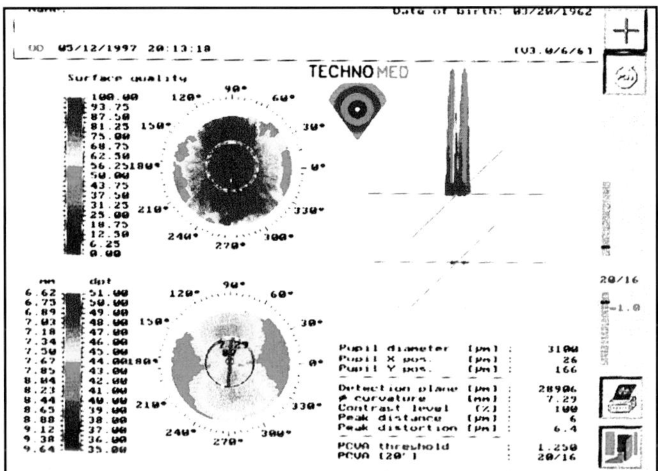

Figure 28-12c.
Ray tracing analysis of the preoperative cornea with a 3.0-mm pupil indicates potential corneal visual acuity of 20/16.

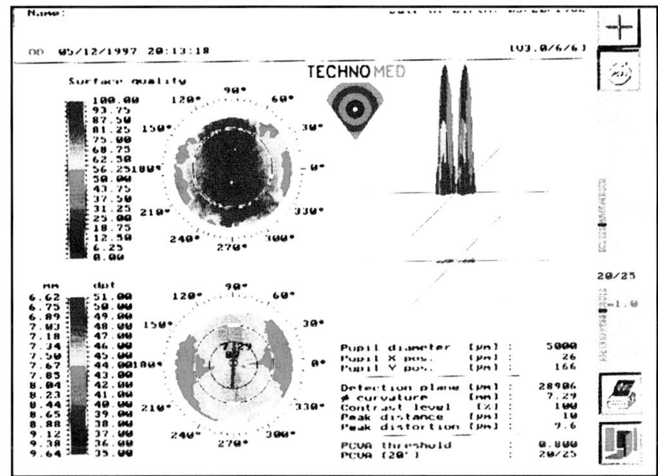

Figure 28-12d.
Ray tracing analysis of same cornea with a 5.0-mm pupil yields a potential corneal visual acuity of 20/25.

tive in order to achieve a good visual outcome. Corneal shape that is grossly irregular results in visual loss. Even subtle irregularities determined by videokeratography can result in visual loss and visual function complaints. Rarely, however, does a well-performed procedure that is topographically well-centered, uniform, and symmetric result in visual loss under standard testing conditions. Subtle complaints, however, can be elicited regarding night driving vision even in the best of patients. The diagnostic power of ray tracing analysis in LASIK and PRK can be illustrated in association with nighttime vision in the following example.

A 35-year-old white male underwent excimer laser PRK for compound myopic astigmatism (optical zone 5.5 x 7.5 mm) with an excellent visual outcome in his right eye. His preoperative refraction and vision was -9.25 +2.25 x 100° (20/20++), and 1 month postoperatively he was +0.75 +0.75 x 150° (20/16++) spectacle corrected and (20/16++) uncorrected. In moderate light, his pupil size was 3.0 mm, but this increased to 5.0 mm in dim light. Although very happy with the procedure, he did note that his vision was cloudy at night.

Pre- and postoperative corneal topography with the Technomed C-Scan shows a 46 D steep astigmatic cornea (Figure 28-12a) reshaped to a well-centered 39 D cornea with negligible astigmatism (Figure 28-12b). Ray tracing analysis reveals that with a 3.0-mm pupil, his preoperative potential corneal visual acuity is 20/16

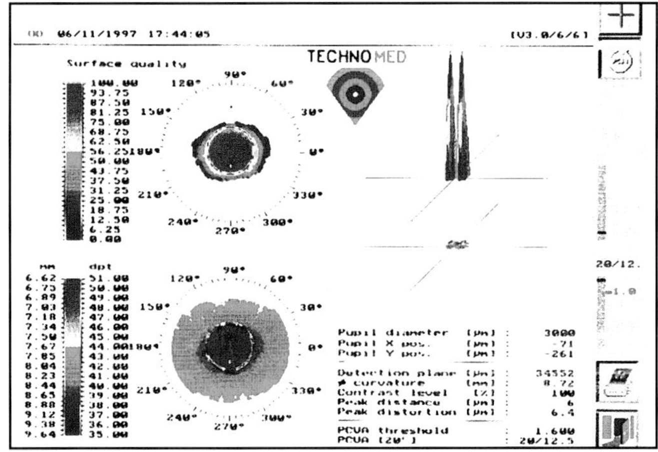

Figure 28-12e.
Ray tracing analysis of postoperative cornea with a 3.0-mm pupil produces 20/12.5 potential corneal visual acuity with a small pupil.

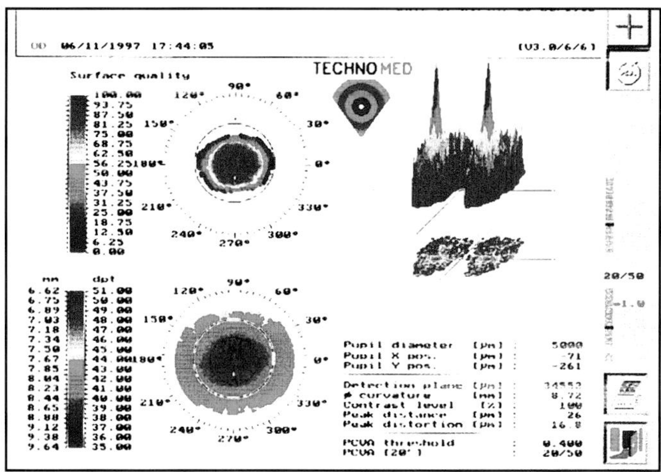

Figure 28-12f.
Ray tracing analysis of postoperative cornea gives 20/50 with a larger pupil. The pupil is beyond the functional optical zone which creates detrimental aberrations. Notice the surface quality map (upper left) where the pupil (red circle) is outside the 100% quality. This accounts for the peripheral distortion spikes that rise from the base of the sinusoidal wave (right).

(Figure 28-12c) and with a 5.0-mm pupil is 20/25 (Figure 28-12d). However, his postoperative potential corneal visual acuity increases to 20/12.5 with a 3.0-mm pupil (Figure 28-12e) but decreases to 20/50 (Figure 28-12f) with a 5.0-mm pupil. This is due to peripheral aberrations of his now oblate cornea which can only be observed at night when his pupil naturally dilates to expose unablated cornea.

This example illustrates that even with an excellent outcome in correcting moderately high myopic astigmatism, peripheral corneal aberrations can impact nighttime vision when the pupil is largest. This effect can be well illustrated and explained with ray tracing analysis using the Technomed C-Scan.

CONCLUSION

In conclusion, it is incumbent upon practitioners to understand basic principles of vision testing, such as contrast sensitivity, and have an appreciation for the mechanisms behind optical aberrations that arise from refractive surgical procedures. This chapter provides the knowledge to assist practitioners in caring for their patients. Understanding these concepts will increase one's ability to pre- and postoperatively assess patients. Additionally, such information will allow one to critically evaluate the results of refractive surgery in order to advance the capability of oneself and the field toward the ultimate outcome—complete patient satisfaction.

Dr. Evans has a financial interest in VectorVision, Inc.

REFERENCES

1. Donders FC. On the anomalies of accommodation and refraction of the eye. London, England: The New Sydenham Society; 1864:96-107.
2. Pomerance GN, Evans DW. Test-retest reliability of the CSV-1000E contrast test and its relationship to glaucoma therapy. *Invest Ophthalmol Vis Sci.* 1994;35:3357-3361.
3. Sekuler R, Owsley C, Berenberg R. Contrast sensitivity during evoked visual impairment in multiple sclerosis. *Ophthl Physio Opt.* 1986;6:228-232.
4. Wolkstein R, Atkin A, Bodis-Wollner R. Contrast sensitivity in retinal disease. *Ophthalmology.* 1980;87:1140-1149.
5. Boxer Wachler BS, Krueger RR, Durrie DS, Assil KK. The role of clearance and optical zones in contrast sensitivity: significance in refractive surgery. *J Cataract Refract Surg.* In review.
6. Boxer Wachler BS, Krueger RR, Durrie DS, Assil KK. Variability of pupil size in contrast sensitivity testing: significance in refractive surgery. *J Refract Surg.* In review.
7. Anschutz T. Pupil size, ablation diameter, and halo incidence after photorefractive keratectomy. Symposium on Cataract, IOL, and Refractive Surgery Best Paper of Session. 1995:1-4.
8. Shah SI, Hersh PS. Photorefractive keratectomy for myopia with a 6-mm beam diameter. *J Refract Surg.* 1996;12:341-346.

9. O'Brart DPS. Lohmann CP, Fitzke FW et al. Disturbances in night vision after excimer laser photorefractive keratectomy. *Eye.* 1994;8:46-51.

10. Schallhorn SC, Blanton CL, Kaupp SE, et al. Preliminary results of photorefractive keratectomy in active-duty United States Navy personnel. *Ophthalmology.* 1996;103:5-22.

11. Knorz MC, Liermann A, Seiberth V, Steiner H et al. Laser in situ keratomileusis to correct myopia of -6.00 to -29.00 diopters. *J Refract Surg.* 1996;12:575-584.

12. Perez-Santonja JJ, Belot J, Claramonte P, et al. Laser in situ keratomileusis to correct high myopia. *J Cataract Refract Surg.* 1997;23:372 386.

13. Roberts CW, Koester CJ. Optical zone diameters for photorefractive corneal surgery. *Invest Ophthalmol Vis Sci.* 1993;34:2275-2281.

14. Baron WS, Munnerlyn C. Predicting visual performance following excimer photorefractive keratectomy. *Refract Corneal Surg.* 1992;8:355-362.

15. Ludwig K, Schaffer P, Gross H, et al. Mathematical simulation of retinal image contrast after photorefractive keratectomy with a diaphragm mask. *J Refract Surg.* 1996;12:248-253.

16. Boxer Wachler BS, Krueger RR. Agreement and repeatability of infrared pupillometry and the comparison method. *Ophthalmology.* In review.

17. Boxer Wachler BS, Krueger RR. Agreement and repeatability of pupillometry using videokeratography and infrared devices. *Ophthalmology.* In review.

18. Loewenfeld IE. Methods of pupil testing. In: Loewenfeld IE, Lowenstein O, eds. *The Pupil: Anatomy, Physiology, and Clinical Applications.* Iowa City, Iowa: Iowa State University Press; 1993:828-899.

19. Egginik FAGJ, Beekhuis WH, Trokel SL, den Boon M. Enlargement of the photorefractive keratectomy optical zone. *J Cataract Refract Surg.* 1996;22:1159-1164.

20. Lafond G. Treatment of halos after photorefractive keratetomy. *J Refract Surg.* 1997;13:83-88.

21. Van Den Berg TJTP. Importance of pathological intraocular light scatter for visual disability. *Doc Ophthalmol.* 1986;61:327-333.

22. Uozato H, Guyton DL. Centering corneal surgical procedures. *Am J Ophthalmol.* 1987;103:264-275.

23. Schade OH. Optical and photoelectric analog of the eye. *J Opt Soc Am.* 1956;46:721-739.

24. Campbell FW, Green DG. Optical and retinal factors affecting visual resolution. *J Physiol.* 1965;181:576-593.

25. Kock D, Lui J. Survey of the clinical use of glare and contrast testing. *J Cataract Refract Surg.* 1990;6:707-711.

26. Evans D, Ginsburg A. Contrast sensitivity predicts age-related differences in highway sign discriminability. *Human Factors.* 1985;27:637-642.

27. Ginsburg A, Evans D, Sekuler R, Harp S. Contrast sensitivity predicts pilots' performance in aircraft simulators. *Am J Opt Physiol Opt.* 1982;59.

28. Boxer Wachler BS, Frankel RA, Krueger RR, Durrie DS, Assil KK. Contrast sensitivity and patient satisfaction following photorefractive keratectomy and radial keratotomy. *Invest Ophthalmol Vis Sci.* 1996;37:3:S19.

29. Boxer Wachler BS, Krueger RR. Normalized contrast sensitivity: a new notation for mainstream contrast sensitivity testing in refractive surgery. *Invest Ophthalmol Vis Sci.* 1997;38:530.

30. Ficker LA, Bates AK, Steele ADMcG, Lyons CJ et al. Excimer laser photorefractive keratectomy for myopia: 12 month follow-up. *Eye.* 1993;7:617-624.

31. Shimizu K, Amano S, Tanaka S. Photorefractive keratectomy for myopia: one-year follow-up in 97 eyes. *J Refract Corneal Surg.* 1994;10(suppl):S178-S187.

32. Dutt S, Steinert RF, Raizman MB, Puliafito CA. One-year results of excimer laser photorefractive keratectomy for low to moderate myopia. *Arch Ophthalmol.* 1994;112:1427-1436.

33. Heitzmann J, Binder PS, Kassar BS, Nordan LT. The correction of high myopia using the excimer laser. *Arch Ophthalmol.* 1993;111:1627-1634.

34. Sher NA, Barak M, Daya S, DeMarch J, et al. Excimer laser photorefractive keratectomy in high myopia. *Arch Ophthalmol.* 1992;110:935-943.

35. Boxer Wachler BS, Krueger RR. The effect of luminance-induced pupil changes on contrast sensitivity. *Invest Ophthalmol Vis Sci.* In review.

36. Klonos GG, Pallikaris J, Fitzke FW. A computer model for predicting image quality after photorefractive keratectomy. *J Refract Surg.* 1996;12:S280-S284

Chapter 29

A NEW CORNEAL ANALYSIS AFTER EXCIMER LASER ABLATION: DIGITIZED RETROILLUMINATION

Paolo Vinciguerra, MD,
Marco Azzolini, MD, Paola Radice, MD

A comprehensive examination of the ablated surface is becoming more important for the refractive surgeon, as the patients' requests and the competition among surgeons increase, because it allows the surgeon to understand how the ablation characteristics influence the functional outcome and helps to explain the reasons of any cases of visual acuity impairment not explained by the simple slit lamp examination (eg, transparent corneas). Videokeratography is an important aid; its development is inseparably bound to the refractive surgery. However, videokeratography can only examine the cornea at its surface so it is not always able to identify the cause of visual acuity loss. The observation of a visual impairment in the presence of a transparent cornea and a regular topography calls for deeper investigation, especially after laser in situ keratomileusis (LASIK).[1]

These assumptions prompted us to develop a system for the examination of the ablation beyond the surface and to identify the problems of the ablated area even under the epithelium and within the stroma. We identified it with digitized retroillumination (DR). A retroillumination image is an image of the cornea obtained by illuminating the ocular fundus and using the light reflected by the fundus to "lighten" the cornea from the inside of the eye, if the other dioptric means are transparent.[2] The images obtained in this way offer a representation of the optic qualities of the cornea. These depend on tissue opacities and superficial irregularities, but also on refraction index (RI) dishomogeneities within the corneal thickness due to a different RI between two adjacent layers or to the formation of an

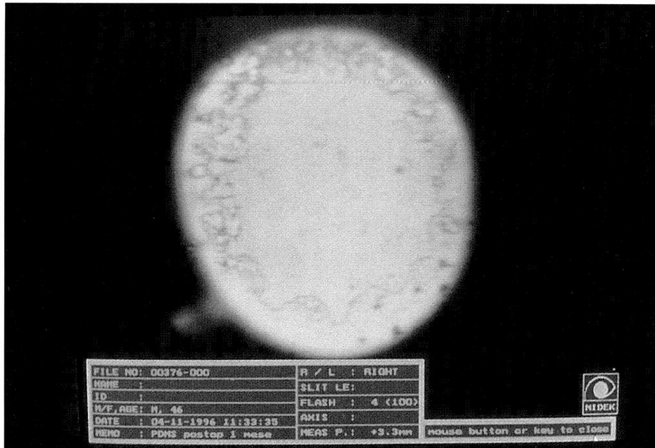

Figure 29-1.
DR image of cortical lens opacities in a vitrectomized eye (male, 46 years old).

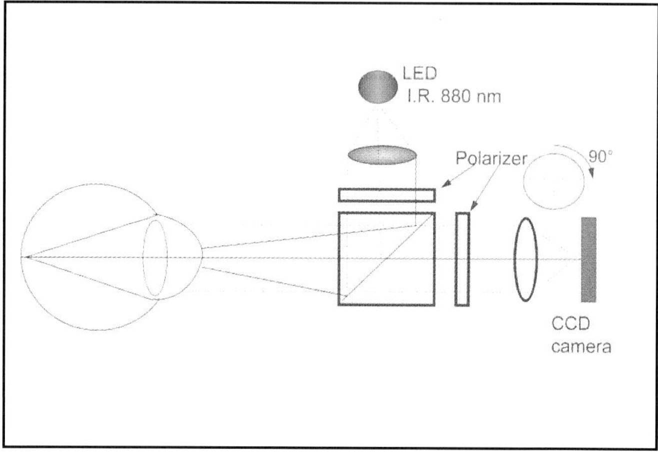

Figure 29-2.
A schematic representation of the photography system we use (see text for details). Note the 90° angle between the polarizers.

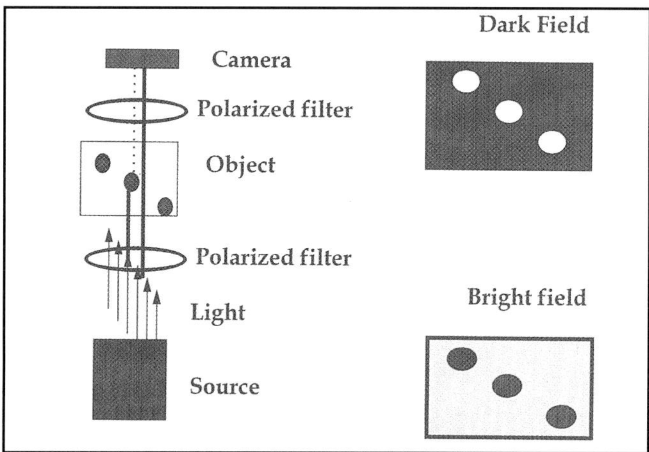

Figure 29-3.
A schematic representation of the dark field and bright field illumination. In the former the diffracted light areas appear clear, with the bright field illumination they appear dark.

interstice between the flap and the stroma that cause light diffraction.

DR has been used in the past mainly to detect morphological changes of the crystalline lens in vivo, often in association with densitometric analysis systems that measured the progression of the lens opacities (Figure 29-1).[3-5] To extend its applications to the field of refractive surgery, we use a modified Nidek Eas-1000 Anterior Eye Segment Analysis System (Nidek Co Ltd, Gamagory, Japan) to obtain these images. The photography system used is shown in Figure 29-2. It includes an infrared light (wavelength = 880 nm) LED used for the illumination, a CCD camera to obtain the images and also for alignment and focusing using a television screen, two polarized light boards in which polarized light axis at right angles for floodlighting side and projecting side are arranged. When examining the eye, a retroillumination image appearing on the monitor screen is observed under infrared light. A focusing operation for this image is performed on the screen; when the appropriate focus on the cornea (to obtain a perfect focusing on the cornea, we modified the image acquiring technique, considered for the crystalline) is attained, the image is frozen on the screen, stored on a database and if necessary printed out and analyzed with an appropriate analysis software (eg, the measurement of opaque areas in the pupillary zone documented in the retroillumination image is possible). During the focusing and alignment steps it is very important to try different positions in order to reach the best vision possible of the areas of interest; this is especially true for eyes with localized defects which greatly impair the function but difficult to be detected.

The light, emitted by the infrared LED, passes through the first polarizer and illuminates the eye. The reflected light is captured by the CCD camera after the second passage through a polarizer placed orthogonally with respect to the first one. In this way, in case of no diffraction of light by the eye tissues, no light should reach the camera, the eye appearing completely dark; only the diffracted light should appear on the image ("dark field illumination," see Figure 29-3); nevertheless the tonality of the light is automatically inverted by the instrument so that the diffracted light is shown as dark on the image ("bright field illumination," see Figure 29-

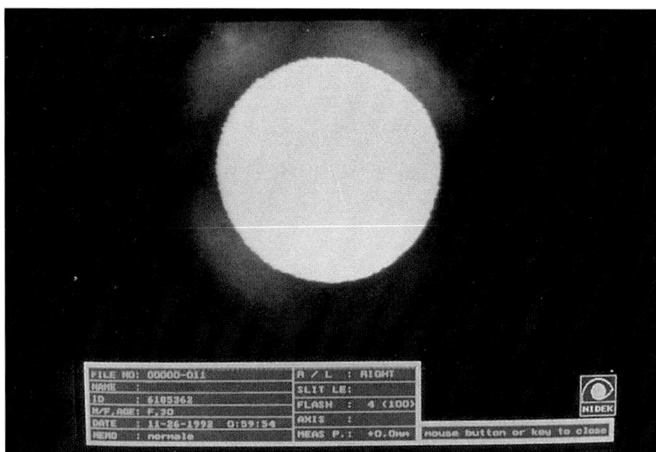

Figure 29-4.
A DR image of a normal cornea (female, 34 years old).

3). Figure 29-4 shows a DR image of a normal cornea in bright field illumination with the instrument we use.

As the diffraction of light is caused by the difference of RIs among the means crossed, not only the corneal opacities, but even more the surface irregularities and the intrastromal dishomogeneities appear to be influent on the amount of diffracted light. This is of great importance for the study of the interface of the LASIK, where, if the ablated surface and the inner flap layer are not perfectly congruent, diffraction phenomena occur.

In this way the DR gets the importance of an interferential analysis system that defines the quality of the light transmission of the cornea, not only in relation to surface opacities or irregularities, but also to subepithelial and stromal dishomogeneities that impair the light transmission quality and, in the final analysis, the patient's visual acuity.

At first, we applied the DR to the study of surface refractive surgery, in particular to PRK and PTK. Our first clinical use was the evaluation of the clinical importance of scars and opacities to be treated by PTK. It is common experience that the influence on vision of a scar not only depends on its density, but also on the superficial irregularity it creates. By DR we noticed that the subepithelial irregularities and the different RI with respect to the stromal one are important too. For example, a very dense but thin scar is seen brighter than a less dense but thicker and multilayered one at the DR (Figure 29-5), due to the greater light diffraction, resulting from the sum of the single diffractions between the consecutive layers. This means that a not very dense but multilayered scar greatly influences the visual function. A very dense but with regular edges intrastromal scar causes a lower diffraction of light than a less dense but more irregular one, so that in the DR image it appears less dark. In this way we were able to detect the more impairing the visual acuity scars, even in the presence of a low opacity at the slit lamp examination and to decide their treatment by PTK.

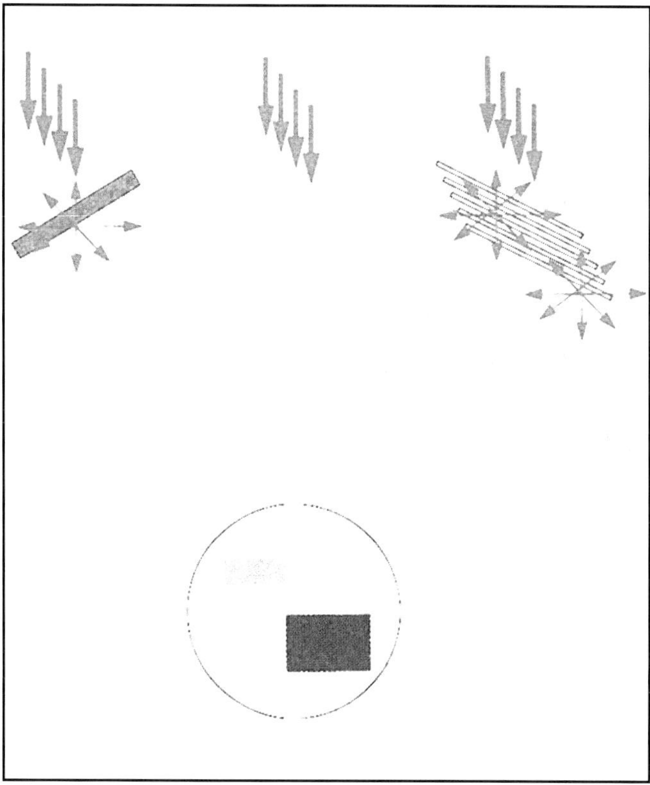

Figure 29-5.
The lower part shows the DR image representation of the scars drawn in the upper scheme. Notice how the left scar, denser but monolayered, appears clearer in the DR image than the right, which is less dense but multilayered.

Then we tried to use the DR to detect the causes of visual impairment after PRK not recognized by videokeratography (regular topographic flattening) and clinical observation (no corneal haze). The DR,

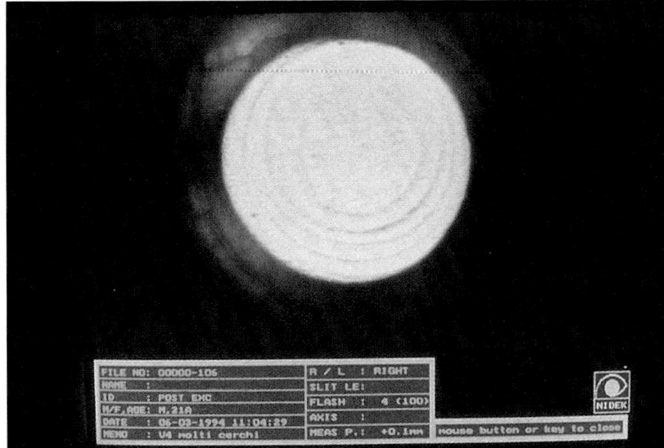

Figure 29-6.
DR image of a multizone PRK (four optical zones) for a correction of -16 D. At the topography, the ablation appeared regular and centered, but the patient complained of halos and glare. After this examination, we retreated the patient with a simple PTK smoothing, obtaining the regression of the symptoms without refractive change.

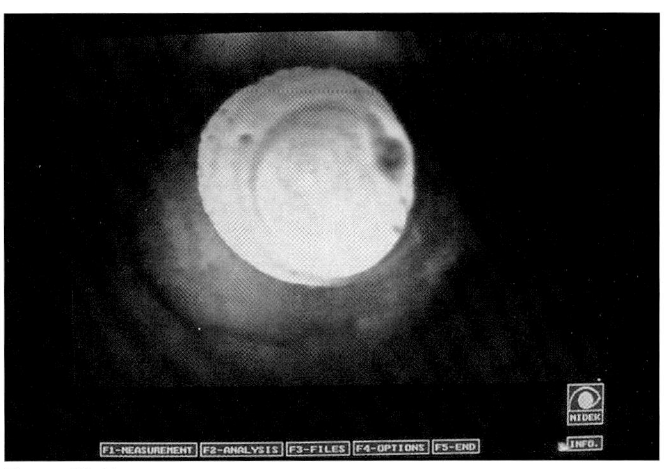

Figure 29-7.
DR image of a -2.5 D PRK with a loss of fixation during the treatment, clearly visible on the upper temporal part of the cornea. We immediately corrected this aspect at the end of PRK and obtained a regular ablated surface, with no visual acuity loss in the postoperative. The dark mass visible in the upper right part of the cornea is conjunctival secrete.

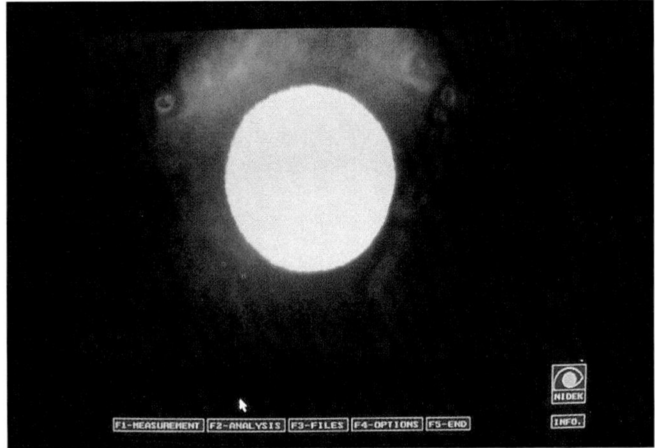

Figure 29-8.
DR image of a V0 immediately postoperative cornea, with the LASIK reversed flap visible on the right side. Note the extremely smooth ablated surface with slight edges and the regularity of the cut surface.

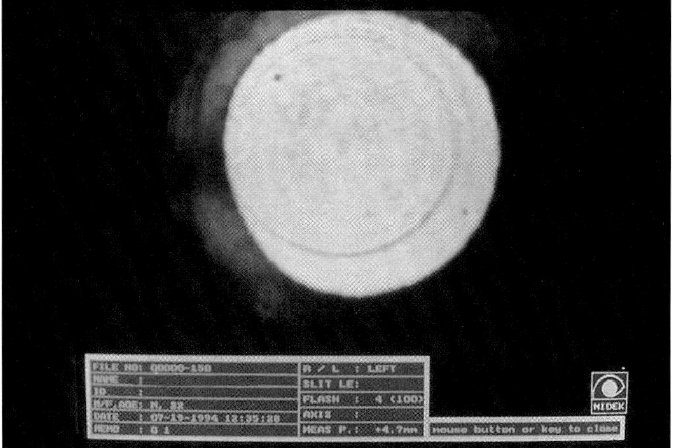

Figure 29-9.
A V1 post-PRK eye with stromal irregularities of the ablated surface and an evident but not too sharp edge.

focused under the corneal epithelium, was able to offer an image of the ablation. In this way we were able to confirm the importance of the ablation regularity on the visual outcome of PRK.

In fact, DR reveals, with or without the epithelium, all the ablation irregularities not clear at a topographic or slit lamp exam, such as the edges of a multizone treatment (Figure 29-6), the results of fixation losses (Figure 29-7), and so on. We have developed an ablated surface homogeneity scale (called Vinciguerra scale/V-scale) based on the dishomogeneities observed in the immediate postoperative retroillumination image (V0=undetectable, V1=mild, V2=severe), samples of which are shown in Figures 29-8 through 29-10. To demonstrate a correlation between the ablated surface homogeneity and the postoperative results, we treated 40 eyes by PRK with a Nidek EC-5000 excimer laser (mean spherical equivalent: -7.03 ± 2.4 D) and evaluated the corneal surface at the end of the PRK. In this way the eyes divided in three groups: V0 = 9 eyes, V1 = 16 eyes, and V2 = 15 eyes. After 12 months we measured corneal haze and the refractive outcome, obtaining the

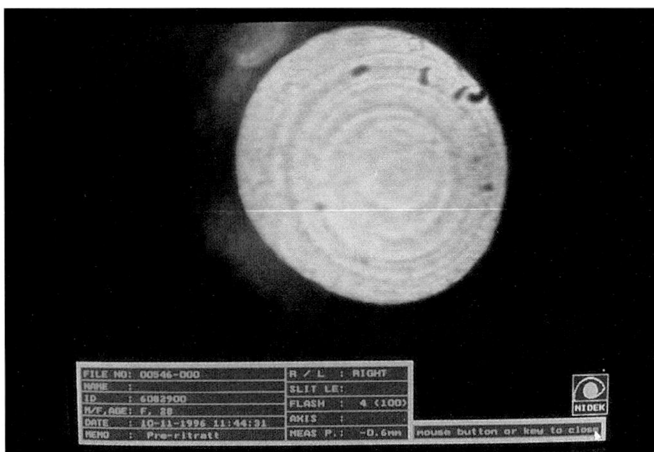

Figure 29-10.
DR image of a V2 cornea, with an irregular ablation surface and many fixation losses, resulting in this case in a strong regression.

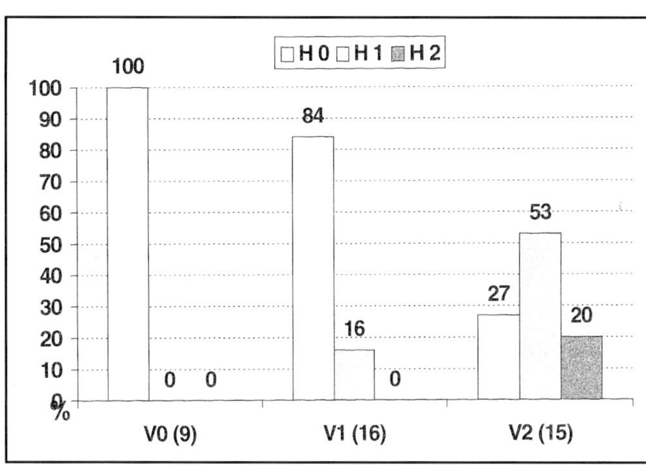

Figure 29-11.
Percentages of corneal haze 0, 1, and 2 in the three groups of V-scale after 1 year from the PRK. Haze 0=transparent cornea or barely detectable opacity, haze 1=mild opacity noticeable by various angles of the slit lamp, haze 2=opacity evident with the direct illumination.

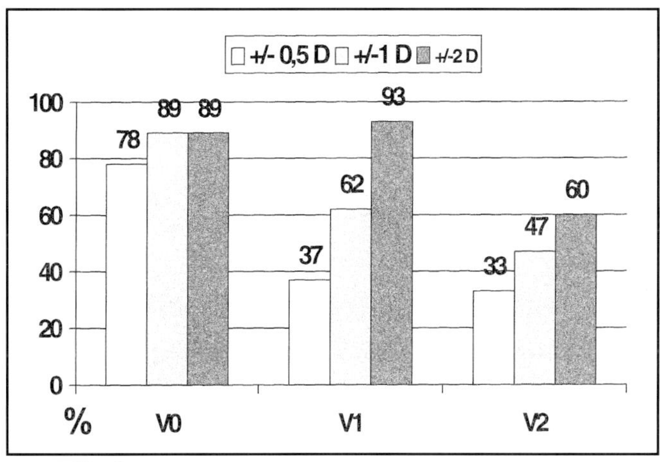

Figure 29-12.
Percentages of eyes with a 12-month refractive outcome within 0.5, 1, and 2 D from the plano in the three V-groups.

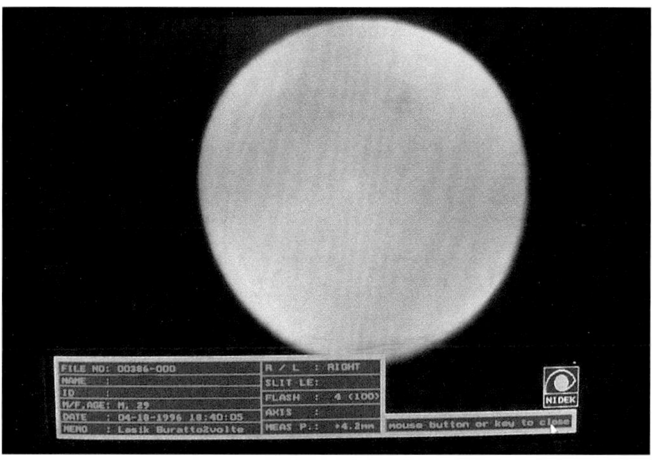

Figure 29-13.
DR image of LASIK with no interface problems but a slight one in the upper mid-periphery not affecting the vision.

results shown in Figures 29-11 and 29-12. The patients with a postoperative grade of V0 had a sharply lower incidence of haze and a better refractive outcome with respect to the plano, confirming the influence of the ablation regularity on the results of the PRK.

Actually, we use DR daily for the intraoperative, immediate postoperative, and late postoperative evaluation of the ablation quality obtained with PRK. In particular, after PRK the DR distinguishes the ablation irregularities (and the decenterings as well) impairing the visual acuity immediately after the treatment, and not after at least 1 week as with videokeratography, and to correct them with a final smoothing (PTK), if necessary. Our PRK technique now provides a DR control at the end of the ablation, an evaluation of the V-scale of the ablated surface, and a smoothing of the V1 and V2 eyes to bring them to a V0 grade. In this way we were able to increase our outcomes with PRK.

The same principles are true for the examination of eyes having undergone LASIK, as the DR, having been properly focused and aligned, can study the diffraction of light at the interface level. At this level, if any incon-

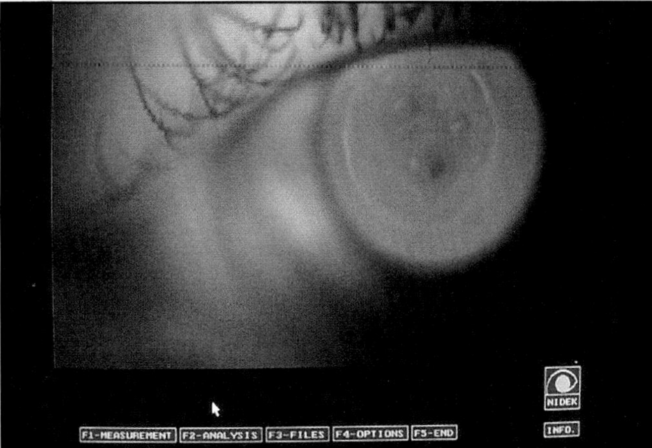

Figure 29-14.
DR image of a postoperative case treated by LASIK for -8 D with an optical zone of 5.5 mm with a bad transition zone. At this level, interface causes light diffraction impairing the patient's visual acuity. Fourteen months after LASIK visual acuity was 20/50 with spectacle correction of -1.25 D; after retreatment it reached 20/25 with -0.50/100°.

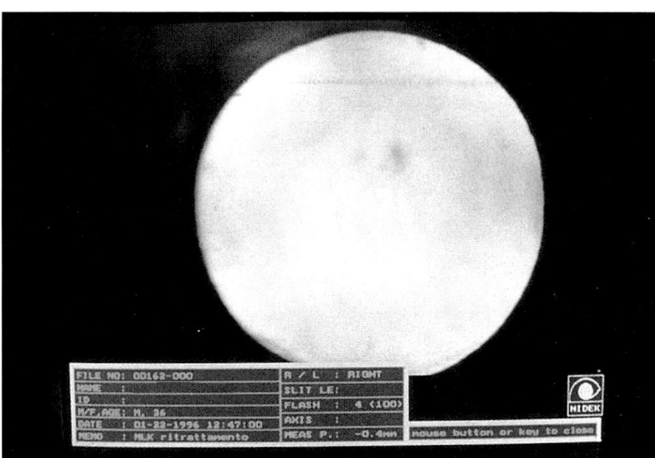

Figure 29-15.
DR image of a 3-month post-LASIK case with central irregularities of the ablated surface.

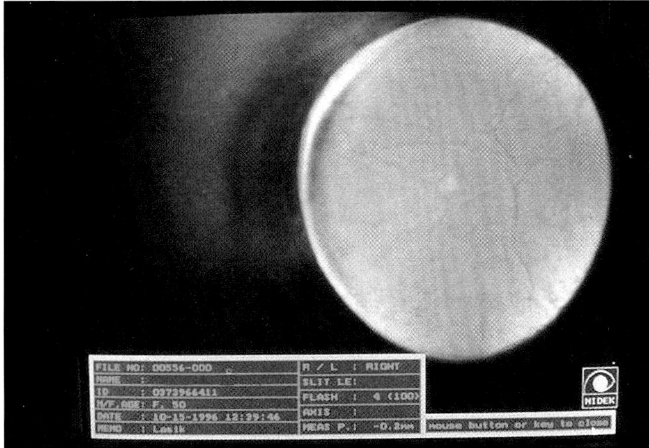

Figure 29-16.
Lines of tension observed at the interface level after 40 days from LASIK. In presence of a good videokeratography and a transparent cornea, these lines caused a visual acuity impairment of three lines.

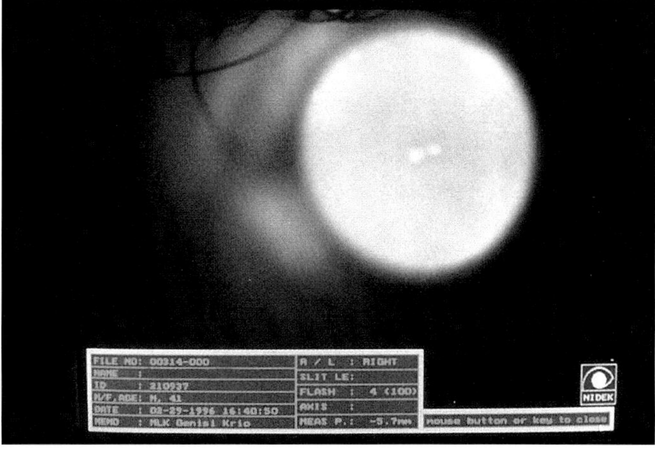

Figure 29-17.
DR image of a post-LASIK cornea with central stromal hypertrophy.

gruence between the stromal and the inner flap layers has occurred, there is a RI variation inducing a loss of light transmission. This is a very interesting characteristic for the surgeon, for so far no other diagnostic means has been able to give a representation of the LASIK interface in such detail.

In Figure 29-13, LASIK with no interface problems is shown; in this case we had a good postoperative visual acuity and a good videokeratography, too. But DR is very useful mainly to examine LASIK eyes with a functional loss in presence of a good videokeratography and a "normal" slit lamp aspect. Until now we have observed 19 cases with these characteristics, and in all of them DR allowed us to identify the cause of the visual impairment with an incongruence between the ablated stroma and the inner flap layer. In fact, it is very important for the surgeon to build a regular ablated surface with no sharp edges, so that the flap, when replaced, can follow it. Otherwise, a undesired interstice remains, creating light distortion.

The most frequent reason for such an interface problem is a bad ablation surface with no transition zone.

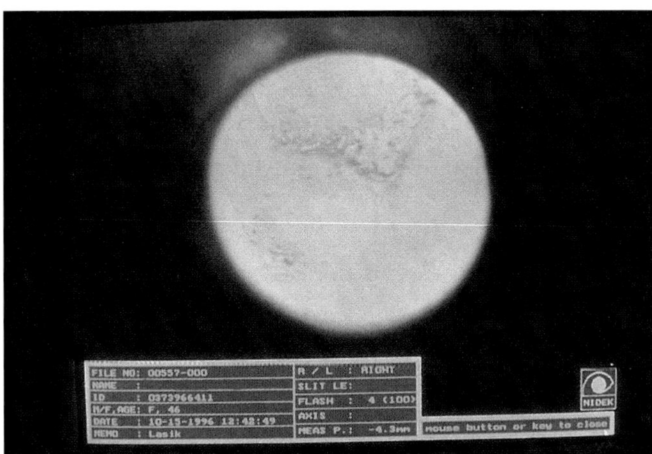

Figure 29-18.
Epithelial regrowth under the LASIK flap.

Figure 29-14 shows a DR image of an 8-month postoperative LASIK for a correction of -7 D, with an optical zone of 5 mm and bad transition. Figure 29-15 shows a 3-month postoperative LASIK with central irregularities of the ablated surface that, at slit lamp examination, were not visible but caused a 0.3 visual acuity loss after the treatment.

During the replacement of the flap after the ablation it is important to avoid distortions or tractions that could bring to the formations, at the level of the inner flap surface, of lines of tension like the ones shown in Figure 29-16.

Less frequent reasons of visual acuity impairment after LASIK are stromal hypertrophy at the interface (Figure 29-17) and an epithelial regrowth with epithelium filtered under the flap (Figure 29-18).

In all 19 eyes, once the reason for the visual acuity loss was detected by DR, we were able to correct it by reintervention. For the future, our goal will be to use DR, as we already do for PRK, immediately at the end of the ablation, before the flap replacement, to examine the ablated surface and eventually correct it.

With this objective, we think that utilizing DR could increase LASIK results and safety.

References

1. Pallikaris IG, Papatzanaki ME, Siganos DS, Tsilimbaris MK. A corneal flap technique for laser in situ keratomileusis. Human studies. *Arch Ophthalmol.* 1991;109:1699-1702.

2. Sasaky K, Sakamoto Y, Shibata T, Emori Y. The multi-purpose camera: a new anterior eye segment analysis system. *Ophthalmic Res.* 1990;22(suppl):3-8.

3. Sasaky K, Sakamoto Y, Shibata T, et al. New camera for crystalline lens photography. *J Ophthal Opt Soc.* 1985;6:40-44.

4. Weale R. The Oqual: a new device for measuring the optical quality of the anterior segment of the human eye. *Exp Eye Res.* 1992;55:507-510.

5. Lindstrom B, Philipson B. Microdensitometer system for microradiography. *Histochemie.* 1969;17:187-193.

Chapter 30

TOPOGRAPHY IN LASIK

Carlos E. Martínez, MD, MS, Stephen D. Klyce, PhD,
George O. Waring III, MD, FACS, FRCOphth,
Mohammad Akef El-Maghraby, MD

INTRODUCTION

The cornea is the major refracting element of the eye and the shape of its anterior surface determines the quality of the retinal image. Thus, keratorefractive surgery can result in emmetropia by producing small changes in central corneal curvature, but small postoperative deviations from the ideal topography can result in devastating consequences for the patient undergoing refractive surgery. For example, irregular astigmatism, central islands, and multifocality introduced by keratorefractive surgery can lead to patient complaints of blurred vision, halos, starburst, decreased contrast sensitivity, and disabling problems with night driving. Hence, the specific aim of refractive surgery should be to maximize visual acuity while achieving a corneal shape that minimizes any optical aberrations that can cause a decrease in contrast sensitivity or degrade the retinal image.[1]

Videokeratography was developed in order to quantitatively as well as qualitatively evaluate the specific corneal topographic changes that may result in these problems after keratorefractive surgery.[2] With the demonstration by Trokel[3] that the 193-nm excimer laser could sculpt corneal tissue, videokeratography continued to play an active role in the fine-tuning of the surgical results and in the evaluation of this new refractive technique.

Today, excimer laser photorefractive keratectomy (PRK) has been shown to provide good accuracy and predictability in tissue removal.[4] Clinically, PRK has been shown to be effective in the correction of myopia from 1.50 D to 6.00 D.[1,5-7] However, for higher corrections, PRK can result in halos, glare, difficulty with night vision, and decreased contrast sensitivity even when emmetropia, 20/20 vision, and apparently clear corneas are achieved.[8-17] Furthermore, patients who undergo PRK can experience unpredictable amounts of regression, have long periods of rehabilitation, and in some instances develop corneal haze, particularly those with higher corrections.[18,19]

More recently, several authors have proposed using laser ablation of the stromal bed under a corneal flap in order to produce the same changes in corneal curvature as PRK for patients with higher degrees of myopia. In 1989, Peyman et al[20] used an infrared (2.9 μm) erbium:YAG laser to ablate the stroma of rabbits under a lamellar flap. In 1990, Pallikaris[18,21] introduced LASIK. In 1992, Buratto[22] used excimer laser ablation of the corneal lenticle rather than the stromal bed (in situ). Clinical[18,23-25] as well as experimental reports[4,24] suggest that refractive stability could be achieved earlier with LASIK than PRK, providing faster visual rehabilitation.

Nevertheless, all of these refractive procedures, including those that utilize the excimer laser,[1,22,26,27] can produce irregular astigmatism which may result in decreased vision or alternatively 20/20 vision with visual distortion, in the absence of slit lamp findings.[17,28,29] The relationship between these visual disturbances and irregular astigmatism can go undetected without videokeratography.[30] Furthermore, this technology has been used to evaluate multifocality,[31] decentration,[18,19,32,33] fluctuating vision,[17,34] and regression,[18,35,36] which can occur after refractive surgery and may go undetected with other clinical diagnostic modalities.[30,35,37-39]

Videokeratography can provide the refractive surgeon with the information needed to ensure the highest quality result, to understand the optical performance of the postoperative cornea, and to compare new surgical techniques.[1,8,9,28,35] A thorough understanding of videokeratography is therefore of fundamental importance to all refractive corneal surgeons. Nevertheless, there is little topographic information available in the literature on some of the more recently developed procedures, particularly LASIK. In this chapter, we will review the advantages, limitations, and fundamentals of videokeratography as well as introduce global descriptors of corneal topography found in the literature. This information will then be used to characterize the corneal topography after LASIK.

ADVANTAGES OF VIDEOKERATOGRAPHY IN THE TOPOGRAPHIC ANALYSIS OF THE CORNEA

Computer-assisted corneal topography,[2] or videokeratography, offers a variety of advantages over other ways of examining corneal topography, including keratometry and photokeratoscopy.[40] The keratometer or ophthalmometer, first described by Helmholtz,[41] measures the radius of curvature of the anterior corneal surface using four reflected points, each 1.5 to 2.0 mm (depending on corneal power and keratometer) from the corneal apex. The radius of curvature for two orthogonal meridians are then converted into dioptric powers using the standard keratometric index. This instrument is capable of measuring the power of a regular surface with an accuracy of better than 0.25 D. However, it does not give any information about the corneal shape within or outside this 3.0- to 4.0-mm diameter zone. In addition, it assumes that the cornea has a spherocylindrical surface with orthogonal flattest and steepest meridians. In many abnormal corneas (postoperative and diseased), the flattest and steepest meridians are not orthogonal. In addition, keratometry is unable to quantitate irregular astigmatism or asymmetric regular astigmatism. Photokeratoscopes, on the other hand, provide information about a larger portion of the cornea, but do not provide good coverage of the central cornea, missing as much as a 3-mm central diameter. In addition, photokeratoscopes can provide only a subjective, qualitative impression of corneal topography.

Videokeratography can provide accurate keratometry readings in the paracentral cornea with sensitivities comparable to keratometry after surgery.[40] It also gives important information about the peripheral cornea, and quantitative indexes that measure irregular astigmatism and correlate this to potential visual acuity.[40,42] Furthermore, videokeratography is not as affected by tilt and off-axis misalignment as the Placido disk keratoscope.[43]

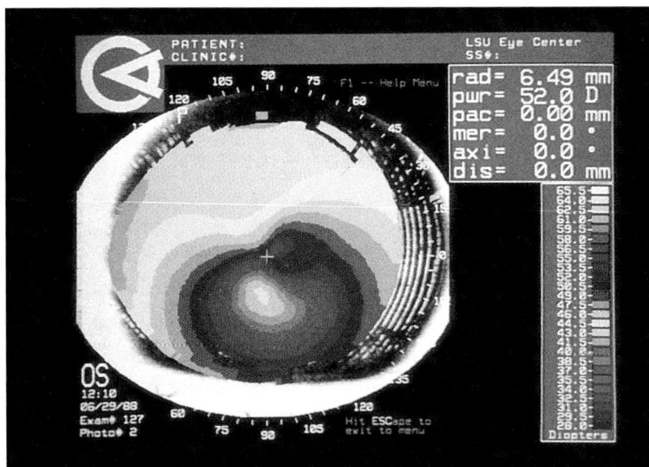

Figure 30-1.
Videokeratography of the left eye of a patient with keratoconus.

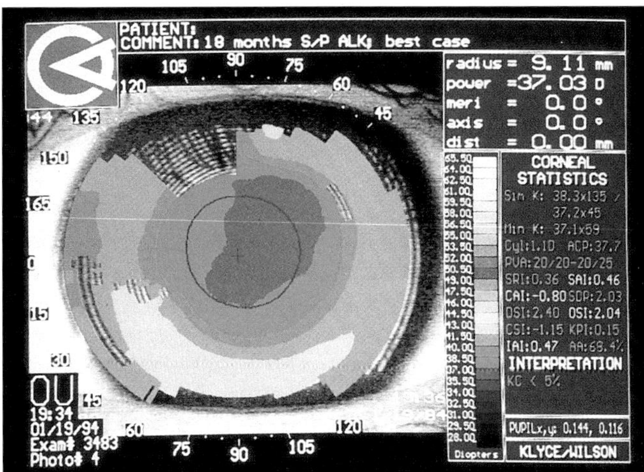

Figure 30-2.
Videokeratography of the left eye 18 months after ALK.

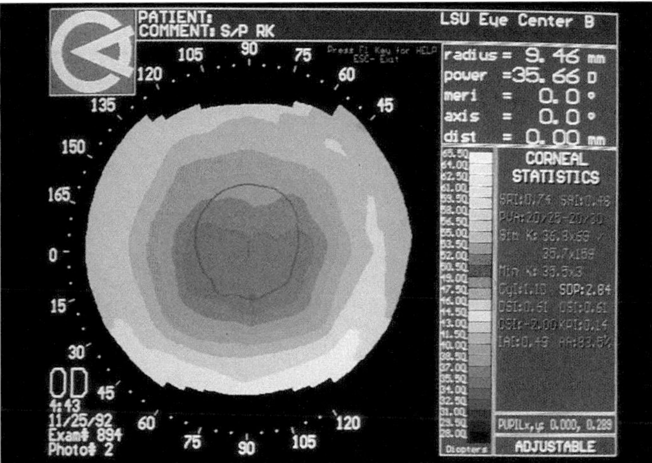

Figure 30-3.
Videokeratography of the right eye 18 months after RK.

VIDEOKERATOGRAPHY DURING THE PREOPERATIVE EVALUATION

Corneal topographic analysis is invaluable in the preoperative evaluation of all corneal refractive surgery patients.[35] Videokeratography should always be done prior to refractive corneal surgery in order to detect contact lens-induced corneal warpage and corneal ectasias such as keratoconus. If these go undetected, they may lead to complications such as inadequate correction or exacerbation of the preexisting disease. In the case of keratoconus (Figure 30-1), patients undergoing LASIK, ALK (Figure 30-2), or RK (Figure 30-3) could experience perforation of the globe. This is particularly important when one considers that corneal topographical abnormalities such as keratoconus are more frequent (6% or more) in the population interested in refractive surgery.[35] It is also important to remember that contact lens warpage can look like keratoconus,[44] necessitating repeat examinations in the absence of contact lens wear to differentiate these two conditions.

FUNDAMENTALS AND LIMITATIONS OF VIDEOKERATOGRAPHY

A basic understanding of the methodology behind videokeratography is needed in order to facilitate its interpretation as well as its limitations. A detailed description of its specific methods has been published.[2,45] The Topographic Modeling System, TMS-1, manufactured by Computed Anatomy, Inc (New York, NY), was used in our analysis. Briefly, it uses a 25- or 30-ring cone videokeratoscope to produce high resolution, graphic representations of corneal topography.[2] The size of the analyzed cornea varies with the cone type and corneal curvature, with the diameter of the keratoscopic mires being larger for flatter corneas.[45] However, for most corneas, the 30-ring cone can provide detailed information from the entire cornea from the visual axis to the periphery of the cornea.

On each ring, 256 points are sampled and the resolution is less than 0.25 D.[37] The analysis assumes central fixation as well as a constant distance from the photoker-

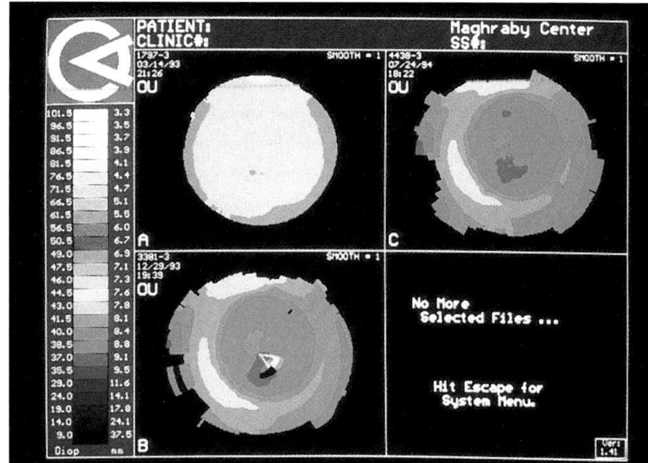

Figure 30-4.
Improperly aligned and focused exam producing an artifact that resembles a central island.

atoscope to the image of the innermost ring in order to calculate the corneal curvature. Errors in corneal surface powers are generally smallest centrally and greatest peripherally.[46,47] Color-coded contour maps of the corneal surface power distribution are generated to facilitate interpretation.[45] Tear film abnormalities and debris can result in poor quality or interrupted mires and misleading results. In addition, off-centered videokeratographic and analysis performed when the photokeratoscope is not focused can be misleading, unless compensation algorithms are employed. Figure 30-4 shows an improperly aligned and focused exam producing a minor central irregular artifact that resembles a "central island."

Videokeratographs can be displayed using normalized (self-adapting) or absolute (fixed) scales. In the absolute scale, each color always represents a fixed dioptric power.[39,45] In addition, powers found in normal corneas (40 D to 44 D) are depicted in greens and yellows, while steeper than normal powers are represented with reds and whites, and flatter than normal powers with blues and black.[39,45] With the normalized scale, the range of powers in a given exam is calculated and the scale is then adjusted to fit this range. Thus, in the normalized scale, power-color associations are not fixed from cornea to cornea. In this type of scale, each cornea can have a different color to power association. This type of scale may also emphasize changes that are not clinically relevant.[39] The Wilson/Klyce scale[39] is a fixed scale with powers ranging from 28 to 65.5 at intervals of 1.5 D which is recommended for routine clinical exams with the TMS-1 and other videokeratoscopes with similar sensitivity and resolution. All LASIK videokeratographs in this chapter will use this scale.

Global Descriptors of Corneal Topography

Global quantitative descriptors of corneal shape have been developed to facilitate evaluation of changes in topography, to explain the current visual results, to improve optical outcomes, and to project potential visual acuity from topography.[8,42,48-51] In particular, these global descriptors include the Klyce/Wilson indexes,[42] the Holladay diagnostic summary,[52] point spread function,[53] fourier analysis,[54,55] spherical aberration,[8,9,50,51] and coma.[8,50,51]

THE EL-MAGHRABY LASIK SERIES

In this section, we will report a comprehensive analysis of the corneal topography of the LASIK procedure in a series performed at the El-Maghraby Eye Hospital and El-Maghraby Eye Center in Jeddah, Saudi Arabia. This study consisted of 26 sighted and partially sighted eyes treated for 2.7 D to 9.0 D of myopia with a mean follow-up time of 5.2 months (2.9 to 8.4 months). The specific aim of the analyses performed was to address the following issues: centration of the treated area relative to the pupil center; the size, power, and prevalence of central islands; potential quantitative topographic correlates to vision; and treatment stability. Qualitative as well as quantitative (Klyce/Wilson indexes) changes in the post-LASIK cornea were obtained from videokeratographs. Calculated quantitative indexes are described in Tables 30-1 and 30-2. Many of these are presently provided on the TMS-1 (see Table 30-1).

In our analysis of the El-Maghraby LASIK series, TMS-1 videokeratographs were collected at each site but not every TMS for each exam period was available for every patient. Where preoperative data were not available for an eye, none of the exams for the eye could be used in the case of correlations derived from changes from preoperative levels. Corneal topography was evaluated with custom software for the preoperative exams plus all postoperative visits as available from the 26 eyes in the study. The custom software required the operator to indicate the exam to be processed, to interactively indicate on the TMS video

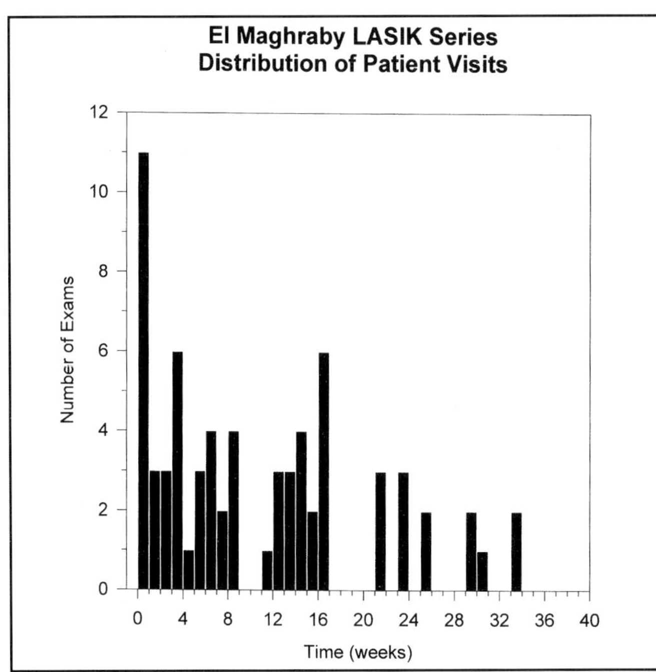

Figure 30-5.
El-Maghraby LASIK series distribution of patient visits.

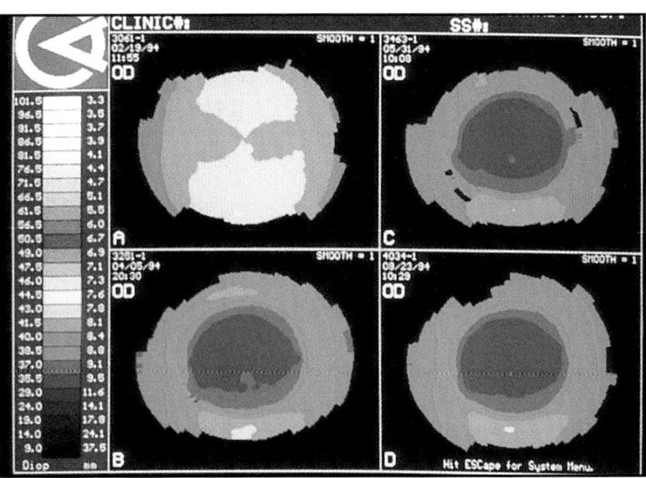

Figure 30-6.
Videokeratography of left eye preoperatively (upper left) and 2 (lower left), 3 (upper right), and 6 months (lower right) after LASIK. Note the prolate (steeper centrally than peripherally) shape of the preoperative cornea and the oblate (flatter centrally than peripherally) configuration of the post-LASIK cornea.

the size and position of the patient's pupil, and subsequently the position of the ablation. The program then calculated the statistics shown in Tables 30-1 and 30-2.

Patients underwent LASIK using the Chiron microkeratome and the ablation was performed with the VisX Model 20/20 B excimer laser, as described.[56] The follow-up visit schedule for this cohort was variable (Figure 30-5). Because of this, for some analyses all follow-up data were employed collectively, while for other analyses data were collected in three time intervals: less than 1 month, 1 to 4 months, and more than 4 months.

Qualitative Impressions

After LASIK, the cornea changes from a prolate (steeper centrally than peripherally) (Figure 30-6, upper left) to an oblate (flatter centrally than peripherally) configuration (Figure 30-6, lower left). As expected, this is not unique to LASIK and has been noted with other refractive procedures.[1] Nevertheless, the aspherical, prolate shape of the normal preoperative cornea is designed to reduce the amount of spherical aberration and the postoperative cornea may result in increased spherical aberration.

Holladay[57] has previously measured the asphericity of the normal cornea (-0.26) indicating that it flattens by about 7% in its radius of curvature compared to a sphere at a distance of 5 mm from the center.[52] His measurements of the post-LASIK cornea found that asphericity ranges from +0.01 to +2.00 depending on the size of ablation zone and diameter of the flap and indicating that the post-LASIK cornea steepens as we move to the periphery.[57] A sphere would have asphericity of zero. Once again, this change in curvature from the pre- to postoperative cornea would be expected to correlate with an increase in spherical aberration.

In general, the topography appeared to change little after the first postoperative visit (see Figure 30-6) in contrast to both RK and PRK. In six eyes, the postoperative topography showed features that might signal the presence of a central island (Figure 30-7) or peninsula (Figure 30-8). However, the preoperative topographies showed astigmatism and other shape anomalies that could have confounded the issues in some cases. In order to accurately determine the presence or absence of these defects, difference maps were analyzed and only four (15%) were determined to contain significant central islands (see Figure 30-7). Three of these four eyes with significant central islands also had the preexisting bowtie pattern of corneal cylinder. Islands in patients with preexisting corneal cylinder have been seen previously in the VisX phase III eyes (SD Klyce, unpublished data).

Regression

Clinical,[18,23-25] as well as experimental, reports[4,24] sug-

TABLE 30-1

Definitions and Sample Applications of the TMS-1 Indexes

Term	Definition	Application
Sim K[42,68]	Simulated Keratometry—Greatest power from an average of rings 6-8 along every meridian and power and axis orthogonal to the highest power.	Higher values are often associated with keratoconus, penetrating keratoplasty (PK), and the occasional steep normal. Lower values- myopic refractive surgical corrections and the rare flat normal.
Min K	Minimum Keratometry Value—Lowest power observed from an average of rings 6-8 along every corneal meridian.	Non-orthogonality most often occurs with keratoconus, PK, trauma, and may be present after cataract surgery as well.
ACP[69]	Average Corneal Power—The ACP is an area-corrected average of the corneal power ahead of the entrance pupil. Used here to measure topographic stability.	Equal to the keratometric spherical equivalent except for decentered refractive surgical procedures and when ablation zone is smaller than entrance pupil.
SRI[42,68]	Surface Regulatory Index—A measure of local fluctuations in central corneal power.	Correlates to potential visual acuity. High SRI values are found with dry eyes, contact lens wear, trauma, and after PK.
SAI[42,68]	Surface Asymmetry Index—The difference in corneal powers at every ring (180°apart) over the entire corneal surface.	High in keratoconus, PK, decentered refractive surgical procedures, trauma, and warpage. Good spectacle correction often not achieved for high SAI.
PVA[42,68]	Potential Visual Acuity—Given as the range of best spectacle corrected Snellen visual acuity that might be expected from a functionally normal eye with the topographical characteristics of the analyzed cornea. Evaluation should consider that tear film breakup can influence PVA (and SRI).	Prolonged gazing at a fixation target by a patient without blinking can produce tear film breakup, transiently reduced vision, and abnormal values of PVA and SRI. With proper blinking, abnormal values of PVA are associated with true irregular corneal astigmatism observed with keratoconjunctivitis sicca, contact lens warpage, lamellar keratoplasty, and herpes keratitis.
KPI[70]	Keratoconus Prediction Index—Numerical estimator of the presence of a keratoconus pattern in corneal topography.	Has a range of 0 (no keratoconus-like patterns) to 1 (100% keratoconus-like features).
IAI[70]	Irregular Astigmatism Index—An area-compensated average summation of inter-ring power variations along every meridian for the entire corneal surface.	Increases as local irregular astigmatism increases. IAI is high in corneal transplants shortly after surgery; persistence heralds suboptimal best spectacle corrected vision.
SDP[71]	Standard Deviation of Corneal Power—The SDP is calculated from the distribution of all cornea powers in a videokeratograph.	SDP is often high for keratoconus corneas, transplants, and trauma—all situations in which there is a wide range of powers occurring in the measured topography.
CVP	Coefficient of Variation of Corneal Power—Calculated from SDP.	This measure should correlate with the sharpness of the power distribution.
Pupil Data	Pupil_x_ctr, pupil_y_ctr, and pupil_radius are measured interactively by manually matching the diameter and position of a circle superimposed on the video image of the patient's eye.	Used to measure decentration of the ablation with respect to the entrance pupil.

TABLE 30-2

Other Topographic Statistics

Term		
Ablation Data	Ablation_x_ctr and ablation_y_ctr are measured interactively by manually adjusting the position of a 5-mm diameter circle superimposed on the color-coded contour map using the Maguire/Waring scale (32.0 D start with 1.0 D intervals).	Data regarding the ablation characteristics is collected from a 4-mm diameter circle centered on ablation_x_ctr and ablation_y_ctr.
Centration Data	This reports the distance between and direction to the estimated center of the ablation from the estimated center of the pupil.	Decentration_amount and decentration_direction are calculated from: **decentration_amount** =sqrt(sqr(pupil_x_ctr - ablation_x_ctr) + sqr(pupil_y_ctr - ablation_y_ctr)) **decentration_direction** =Radians2Degrees * arctan((ablation_y_ctr - pupil_y_ctr) / (ablation_x_ctr - pupil_x_ctr)).
CIP	Central Island Power (cip, in diopters) calculated from a 4-mm diameter centered on the ablation center. Within the analyzed area, the most frequently occurring power is found and this is taken to represent the base plane of the ablation. Any power value that is found to lie over 1 D, more or less, from the most frequent power (mfp) is subtracted from the mfp and the absolute value of this difference multiplied by the corneal surface area it represents (area compensation) is summed.	The final sum is divided by the total area included in the summation to provide the average power of elevation/depressions in a given cornea. The ± 1 D window is sensitive enough to detect anomalies well below clinical significance. Additionally, this method treats elevations and depressions equally, as each might be expected to have the same visual consequence, if it can be shown that such consequences do indeed occur.
CIA	Central Island Area (cia, in mm) is calculated during the collection of the cip data above. It becomes the denominator for the area compensation of the cip.	Used to calculate EDM.
EDM	The Elevation/Depression Magnitude (edm, diopter * mm^2) is the integral of the elevation/depression data expressed as the product of the average power (cip) and the elevation/depression area (cia).	Used to measure central island or central depression size.

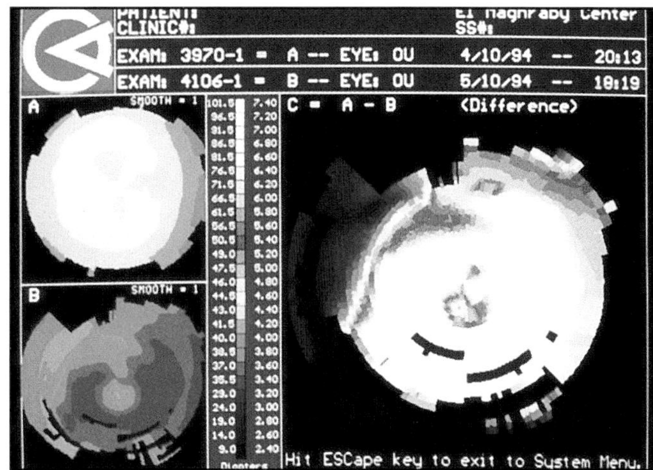

Figure 30-7.
Videokeratographic images showing the preoperative cornea (upper left), postoperative (1 month) cornea (lower left), and the differential map (right). On the postoperative topography, notice the presence of an area within the treated area suggestive of a central island. The differential map (right) shows the presence of a significant elevation within the treated area of the postoperative cornea.

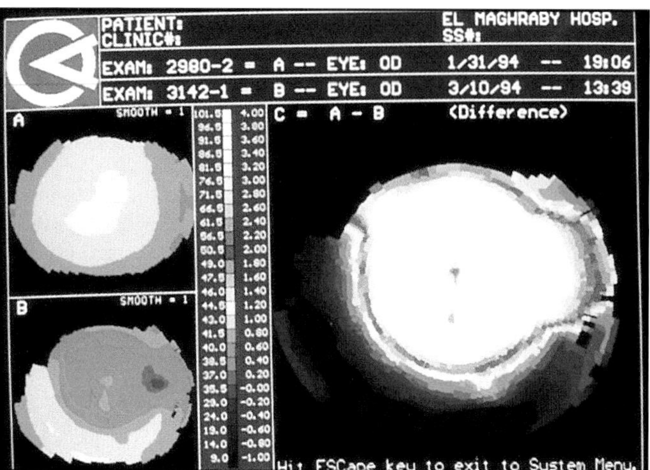

Figure 30-8.
Postoperative topography (B, lower left) of right eye shows features that might signal the presence of a peninsula. A differential map is shown on the right which shows no significant difference in elevations within the treated area when compared to the preoperative cornea.

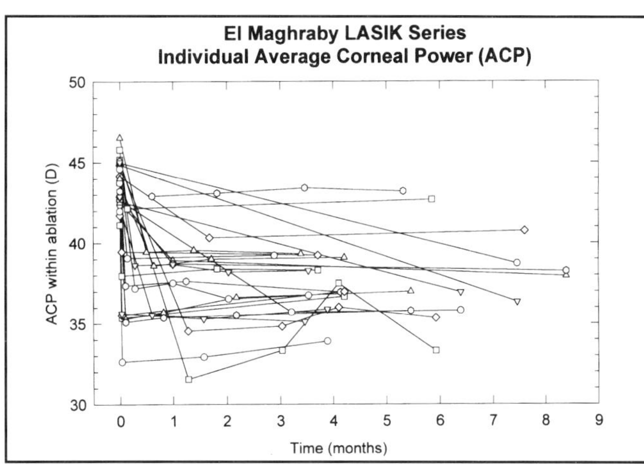

Figure 30-9.
Individual data for the ACP obtained from the 4-mm diameter measuring circle centered on the apparent treated area. Stability as represented by the ACP was excellent. The apparent negative slopes occur for corneas that lacked short-term postoperative follow-up.

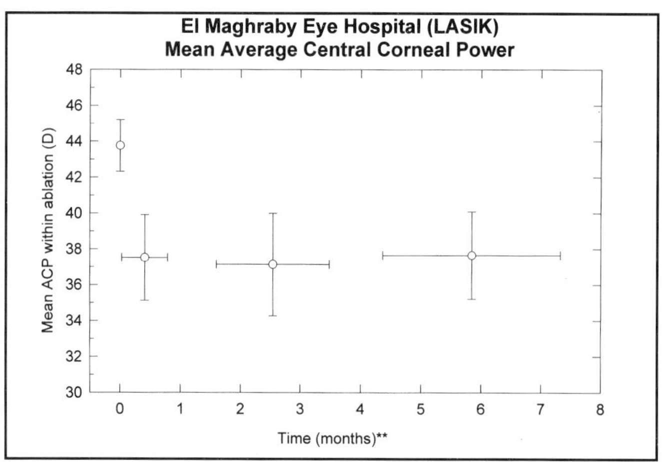

Figure 30-10.
Mean ACP as a function of time. There was no statistically significant difference in the values for the postoperative follow-up period.

gest that refractive stability could be achieved earlier with LASIK than PRK, providing faster visual rehabilitation. In order to test this hypothesis, we evaluated topographic stability using the average central corneal power (ACP) (see Table 30-1) within the treated area. In Figure 30-9 we present the individual data for the ACP obtained from a 4-mm diameter measuring circle centered on the apparent treated area. For this study cohort stability was excellent; the apparent negative slopes seen in the figure occur for corneas that lacked short-term postoperative follow-up. Figure 30-10 presents the means of ACP within the treated area for the preoperative exams and the three averaged time intervals. No statistically significant difference was noted among the three time averages. To look at possible regression more closely, in Figure 30-11 we present the difference between the intended correction and the ACP within the treated area. Note the curious trend for corneas that appear to initially be over- or undercorrected to drift with time toward the intended correction. This is in agreement with the clinical findings

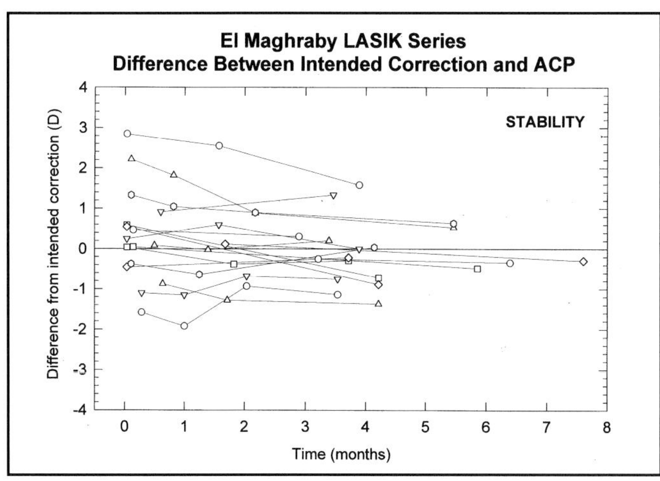

Figure 30-11.
The difference between the intended correction and the ACP within the treated area. Note the curious trend for corneas that appear to initially be over- or undercorrected to drift with time toward the intended correction.

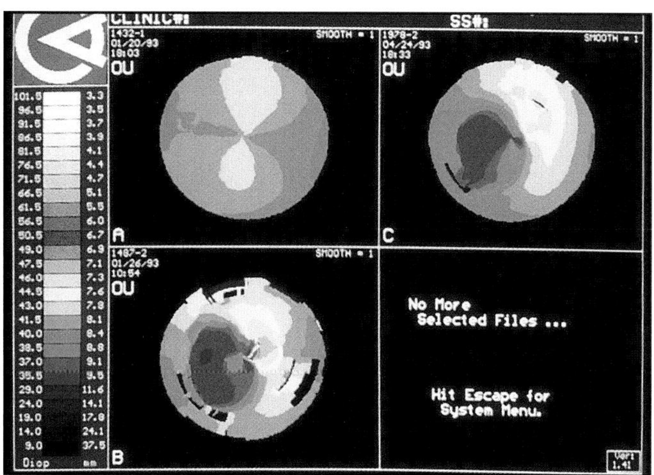

Figure 30-12.
Videokeratograph of the left eye after ALK, 1 and 3 months after surgery showing marked decentration. The patient experienced glare and ghost images.

of other authors in that LASIK patients have earlier stabilization of their vision and refraction[18,23-25] and consistent with keratometric measurements after LASIK published by Salah.[56]

Comparing ACP in post-PRK corneas using the same excimer laser utilized for this study, we found the difference in the stability pattern between LASIK and PRK to be striking.[32,36] In the PRK cornea, there was an early reduction in the effect of treatment which continued to decrease and resulted in stabilization by 6 months.[32] In some cases, stabilization has been reported to take even longer.[18,25] Stabilization with LASIK appears to take a few weeks. It is believed that, after PRK, regression occurs as a result of communication between the epithelium and underlying keratocytes when the intervening Bowman's layer is removed.[4] It is possible that this communication results in keratocyte activation and new collagen formation or that it results in epithelial hyperplasia which fills in some of the defect.[4,58] Solomon[24] has implicated cytokine levels such as epithelial growth factor in this rapid stabilization. He showed that the wound healing in LASIK is very rapid and blunted whereas PRK has a prolonged response which lasts 4 to 6 months and may be responsible for the regression found in PRK. There is no a priori reason to suppose that LASIK corneas would regress after 6 months since even after PRK, wound healing has tapered by this time. However, in the absence of additional follow-up, long-term topographical stability for the LASIK procedure cannot be proven.

Centration

The issues of centration and size of the optical zone were first noted in the development of epikeratophakia,[59,60] but affect all keratorefractive procedures. Decentration may be difficult to detect without topographical analysis[35,37] and yet it is easily detected, but not quantified, by simple inspection of color-coded maps (Figure 30-12).[35,37] Decentration of the optical zone may increase glare,[28,33,61] induce astigmatism, produce ghost images, and reduce contrast sensitivity,[33] and/or Snellen visual acuity[33] particularly when the central zone of uniform power is restricted to a small portion of the corneal surface.[28]

Therefore, it is important to measure decentration, defined as the direction and magnitude of the vector from the center of the entrance pupil to the center of the treated area. Decentration of the treated zones can be measured manually by aligning a computer-generated mask within the TMS-1 video image, and storing the displacements and diameter (in the case of the pupil) in a permanent computer record for each exam. This procedure can be repeated for all available exams of an individual cornea (minimum N=3) and the data averaged for each cornea. The grand average can then be calculated for all treated corneas.

Figure 30-13 (left) illustrates the decentration results for the cohort, with each point representing the average centration for a given eye. All decentrations were less

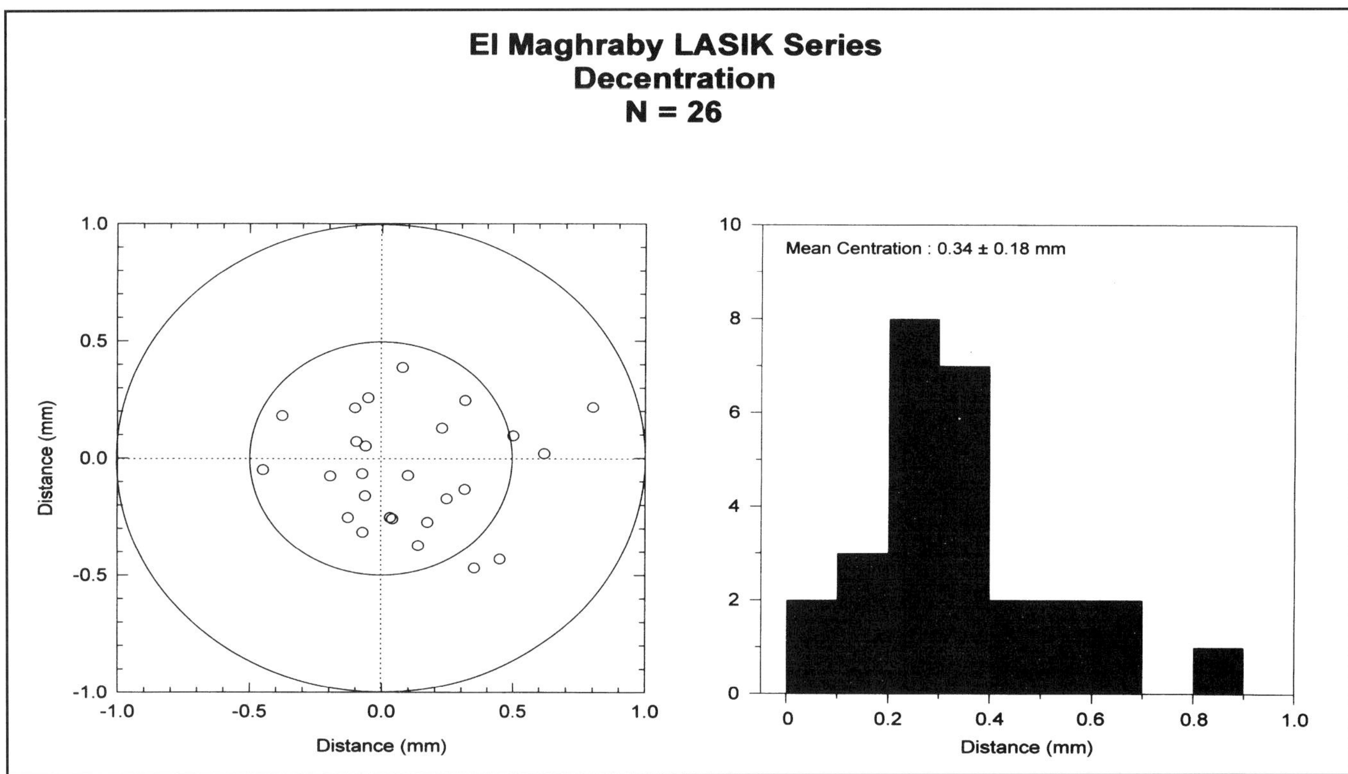

Figure 30-13.
Decentration results for the cohort, with each point representing the average centration for a given eye. All decentrations were less than 1 mm, while 80% were less than 0.5 mm (left). Frequency distribution of decentration. The distribution is not gaussian with a mode near 0.25 mm. The average amount of decentration for this group was 0.34 ± 0.21 mm (mean ± standard deviation). There was no significant systematic error in centration. This result indicates the absence of alignment error with the laser used (right).

than 1 mm, while 80% were less than 0.5 mm, values which are comparable to the better PRK results in the literature.[32,36,62,63] This would also be expected to be better than centration during ALK.[25,64] The frequency distribution of this data is shown in Figure 30-13 (right). The distribution is not gaussian with a mode near 0.25 mm. The average amount of decentration for this group was 0.34 ± 0.21 mm (mean ± standard deviation [SD]). Similar to PRK,[32] there was no significant systematic error in centration; the horizontal offset was +0.10 ± 0.29 mm while the vertical offset was -0.06 ± 0.23 mm. This result indicates the absence of alignment error with the laser used.

Clinically, surgical technique and misalignment of the laser can also result in decentration. In order to minimize decentration, careful attention is needed and the ablation should be centered on the center of the entrance pupil, not the visual axis.[61] In addition, the natural pupil should be used because medications used to constrict or dilate the pupil can sometimes shift its center.[61] Decentration is also expected to be greater when the ablation is performed in situ (on the stromal bed) rather than on the back of the lenticle.[64] This is because the eye can move during in situ ablation. An eye movement tracking device such as that present in the Autonomous Technologies Corp Laser Ladar Tracking System may prove to be useful if its response time is fast enough.

Irregular Astigmatism Measurement

Irregular astigmatism can be defined as any optical distortion that cannot be corrected with spherocylindrical optics (spectacles), a useful functional definition when evaluating keratorefractive surgery. Some authors have suggested that patients who undergo LASIK have a substantial risk of loss of best spectacle corrected visual acuity apparently due to irregular astigmatism.[26] Brint et al reported that 21% of patients who underwent LASIK had irregular astigmatism.[64] However, Salah et al reported only one case of clinically significant irregular astigmatism resulting in the loss of two or more lines of best spectacle corrected visual acuity in the El-Maghraby LASIK

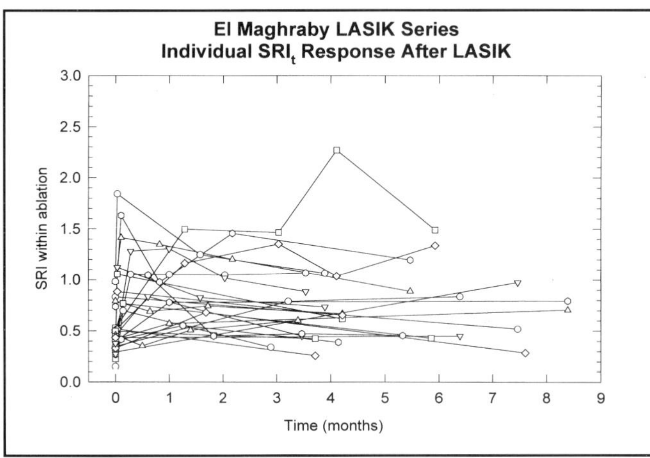

Figure 30-14.
Individual responses of SRI_t to LASIK. In general, SRI_t was increased in the first postoperative exam, but decreased with time. However, there were a few examples of steadily increasing SRI_t. Since SRI is specifically designed to correlate to potential visual acuity,[42] such a finding is a concern.

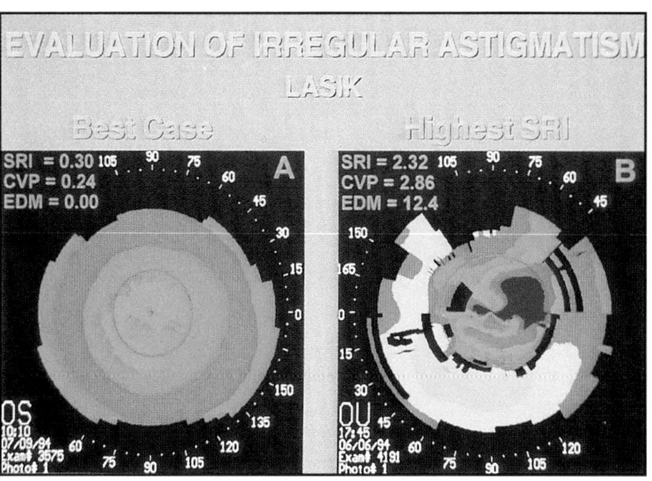

Figure 30-15.
Videokeratograph of the postoperative cornea with the lowest values for SRI, CVP, and EDM (left). Videokeratograph of the postoperative cornea with the highest surface regularity index (right).

series.[56] In general, all refractive procedures may cause irregular astigmatism[26] which may result in decreased vision or cause visual distortion, decreased contrast sensitivity, and symptoms such as monocular diplopia, halos, starburst, and problems with night vision.[28] Any irregular astigmatism introduced by this elective procedure would be a concern.

Several attempts to quantitate irregular astigmatism and predict visual acuity from corneal topography have been made. Holladay has developed a corneal uniformity index (CUI) which is a measure of the uniformity of the central 3-mm of the cornea. He has found that LASIK corneas have CUI that range from 50% to 90%.[57]

We have developed topographic descriptors to evaluate irregular astigmatism, mainly the Surface Regularity Index (SRI), the Coefficient of Variation of Power (CVP), and the Elevation/Depression Magnitude (EDM) (see Table 30-1), that would be expected to correlate with visual acuity. The SRI and EDM measure high and low frequency surface distortions, respectively, while CVP measures the amount of dispersion in the corneal power. CVP should correlate to the collective sharpness of the power distribution. The lower the CVP, the narrower will be the distribution of powers within the area of consideration. EDM is another measure of irregular astigmatism and also a measure of central islands and will be discussed later.

SRI and CVP were calculated for two different corneal areas. To correlate with vision, SRI_p and CVP_p were calculated from the area of the cornea ahead of the entrance pupil ${}_p$. To evaluate the quality of the refractive procedure, SRI_t and CVP_t were measured for a corneal area 4-mm in diameter and centered on the apparent treatment optical zone, t.

The individual responses of SRI_t to LASIK are shown in Figure 30-14. Videokeratographs for the best and worst SRI values are shown in Figure 30-15. In general, SRI_t was increased in the first postoperative exam, but decreased with time. However, there were a few examples of steadily increasing SRI_t. Since SRI is specifically designed to correlate to potential visual acuity,[42] such a finding is a concern. Averages of SRI_t for the preoperative and three postoperative periods are shown in Figure 30-16. There is a statistically significant elevation of SRI_t postoperative for all time periods ($P \leq 0.01$ to $P \leq 0.0001$). Our SRI changes with treatment showed that the theoretical potential visual acuity changed from 20/20 to 20/25 preoperatively to 20/25 to 20/30 at an average of 6 months, a loss of one Snellen line. This is consistent with Holladay's finding[57] on distortion maps that even at 6 months postoperatively there were concentric wrinkles near the 3-mm pupil when treatments were performed using single pass single zone lasers. His topographically predicted visual acuities ranged from 20/16 to 20/30, but there was no mention of attempted correction.[57] While there is a trend toward a diminution (improvement) of the surface regularity within the treated area, SRI_t, a

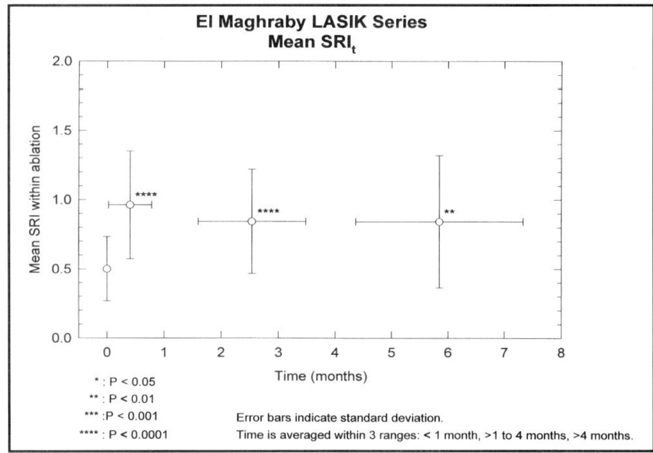

Figure 30-16.
Averages of SRI$_t$ for the preoperative and three postoperative periods. There is a statistically significant elevation of SRI$_t$ postoperative for all time periods ($P \leq 0.01$ to $P \leq 0.0001$).

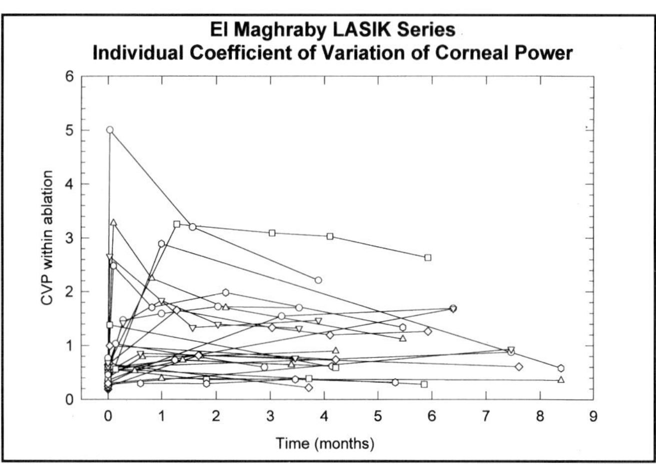

Figure 30-17.
Coefficient of variation of corneal power within the treatment zone for individual corneas. For most corneas, there was a substantial increase in CVP$_t$.

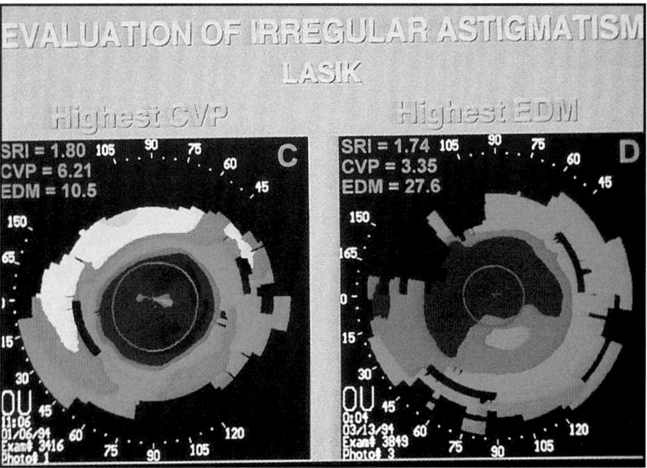

Figure 30-18.
Videokeratograph of the postoperative cornea with the highest CVP (left). Videokeratograph of the postoperative cornea with the highest EDM (right).

longer follow-up is needed for appropriate evaluation.

Clinically, the outcome of this procedure is most affected by the success or failure of the microkeratome cut. The best and most predictable results are obtained when a smooth cut is achieved. Other possible ways to decrease the amount of irregular astigmatism include:

- Not allowing the flap to dehydrate in order to prevent wrinkling of the flap.
- Rinsing the flap-cornea interface prior to replacing the flap in order to prevent deposits under the flap.
- Making sure the flap is well adhered to the stromal bed in order to prevent intrastromal epithelial ingrowth.
- Flattening wrinkles and performing videokeratography immediately after the procedure to detect any wrinkling of the flap.

Gimbel et al[23] found that 10% of eyes had mild wrinkling near the flap edges. In their study, however, they did not extend centrally and did not affect visual acuity.[23] Contrast sensitivity was not measured, but may be affected.

The coefficient of variation of corneal power within the treatment zone for individual corneas is shown in Figure 30-17. The videokeratograph for the cornea with the lowest CVP is shown in Figure 30-15 (left) whereas that with the highest CVP is shown in Figure 30-18 (left). For most corneas, there was a substantial increase in CVP$_t$ and a more extended follow-up may be necessary to determine where this determinant of irregular astigmatism stabilizes. In Figure 30-19 the averages and standard errors for CVP$_t$ with time are plotted. CVP$_t$ remains elevated at all postoperative periods ($P < 0.0001$), although there is a clear trend toward a diminution with time.

Central Islands

Since the very first reports of central islands (a local contiguous area of elevated power sometimes several diopters higher than the surround and 2 mm or more in diameter) within an otherwise homogeneous ablation with the PRK procedure (see Figure 30-7), investigators have tried to quantitate these and to formulate causes and cures.[1,65,66] This is because they can lead to decreased

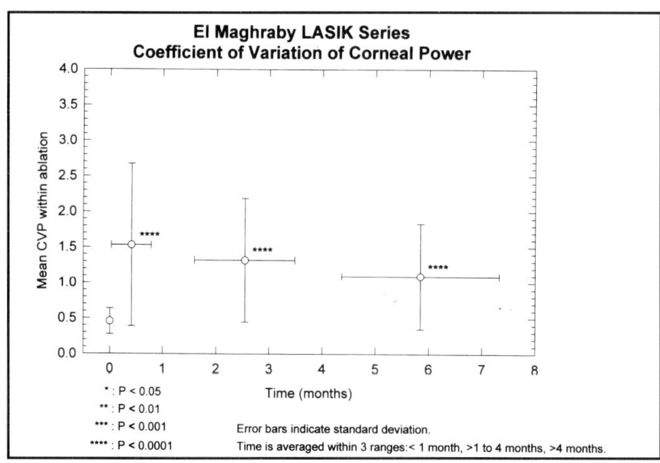

Figure 30-19.

Averages and standard errors for CVP_t with time are plotted. CVP_t remains elevated at all postoperative periods ($P < 0.0001$), although there is a clear trend toward a diminution with time.

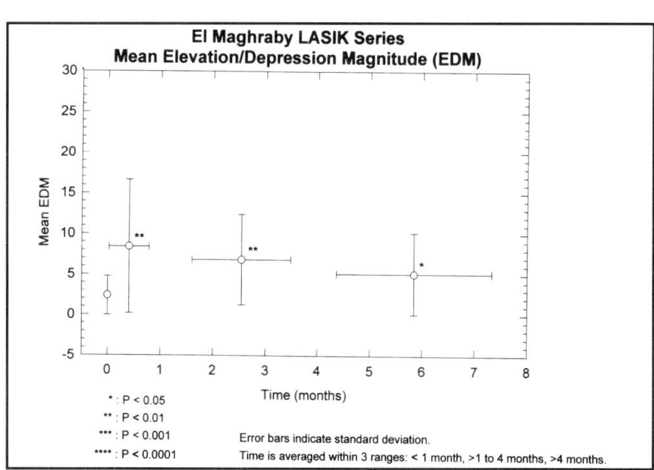

Figure 30-20.

EDM for the three postoperative periods. Immediately postoperatively there is a 3.5-fold increase in EDM ($P < 0.01$). This value decreases subsequently and at the third postoperative interval is only twice the preoperative value ($P < 0.05$).

vision, monocular diplopia, and decreased contrast sensitivity. Clinically they can also create apparent over- and undercorrections. Initially, it was believed that their appearance was confined to the VisX PRK laser patients, but there is now anecdotal information appearing that suggest the presence of similar features within the treated zone of the Summit excimer laser and procedures performed with the Chiron Automated Lamellar Keratectomy device. There may be multiple causes and/or there may be causes that are unrelated to the specific modality used to achieve corneal flattening, such as intraoperative variables or postoperative regimen.

Improperly aligned and focused exams can cause a minor central irregular artifact that resembles a central island under unusual circumstances (see Figure 30-4). It has also been pointed out that central islands stand out in topographical maps because with the absolute scale they appear yellow or orange on a blue background. It is also true that the converse feature, a central depression, might tend to be obscured on the color maps because a deeper blue would not stand out on a lighter blue background. Theoretically, if a central island can cause reduced contrast sensitivity or monocular diplopia, a central depression should cause a similar difficulty. Clearly from these considerations, there is a need for objective evaluation of such features. One such method would be to evaluate difference or change maps of an ablation pre- and postoperatively (see Figures 30-7 and 30-8). However, without further analysis, this method is left to subjective grading of island size and power.

It was felt that a more objective grading scheme would be one in which a feature was clearly above the noise of the topographic measuring system, but clearly well below something that would degrade vision. In fact, a good test of such a metric would be its occasional occurrence in normal 20/20 or better preoperative eyes. To this end, we have derived an algorithm described below to calculate the size and power of low frequency "bumps" and "pits" within corneal topography, calling this index or topographic metric the EDM (see Table 30-1).

There was a range of responses that the EDM achieved among the individual corneas with some extremely small values throughout the postoperative period, some examples of steadily increasing values, as well as some that match the trend for an early postoperative increase followed by a decrease, as shown by the average EDM for this group of eyes in Figure 30-20. The videokeratograph for the postoperative cornea with the lowest EDM is shown in Figure 30-15 (left) whereas that of the highest EDM is shown in Figure 30-18 (right). The EDM for the three postoperative periods was elevated by comparison to preoperative values ($P < 0.05$ to $P < 0.01$). This overall trend to a decrease in EDM but a persistently elevated EDM at 6 months is in agreement with Seiler's[66] work where he found that after LASIK, 24% of patients had central islands at 1 month and 8% at 6 months. However, as noted above, EDM and central islands can take longer than the average 6 months follow-up to return to preop-

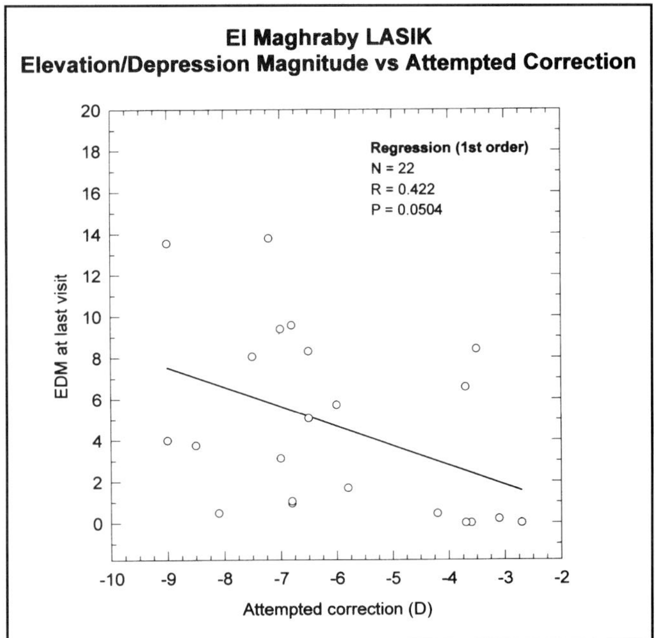

Figure 30-21.
The correlation between the EDM and the attempted correction tended to be weak. At the last follow-up period, linear regression showed R = 0.422 with P = 0.0504.

erative values after PRK, which suggests that a longer follow-up time is necessary. There is a trend for EDM at the last visit to be related to the amount of the attempted correction (Figure 30-21); the correlation coefficient was 0.422 with P = 0.0504 by linear regression. This is also in agreement with Seiler's observation that in cases of high corrections, the central islands increased in height.[66]

Central islands have been theorized to occur secondary to unequal ablation over areas of unequal stromal hydration or areas of external hydration such as tear build-up.[1,67] Therefore, it is possible that not drying the stromal bed before ablation during LASIK procedures may lead to an increased incidence of islands and an increased EDM. The corneal surface should also be dried before lifting the flap. Likewise, deposits under the flap or intrastromal particles included during the procedure may increase this coefficient. Intrastromal epithelial ingrowth secondary to a poorly adherent flap may also increase the EDM.

Predictors of Visual Acuity After LASIK

The SRI is a sensitive tool with which to follow high frequency irregularity on the corneal surface. CVP should correlate to the collective sharpness of the power distribution. The lower the CVP, the narrower the distribution of powers will be within the area of consideration. In this section we examine visual acuity to search for correlations to topographic (EDM, SRI, CVP, ACP, decentration) and clinical (attempted correction) data.

This study contained six partially sighted eyes preoperatively. In addition, preoperative visual acuity was unavailable for two additional eyes whose acuity remained worse than 20/20 at the last postoperative visit. Two of the six patients had lost a line of vision at their last postoperative visit; the origin of this visual loss is confounded by their ocular pathology. Of some note, all of the remaining eyes that had 20/20 or better vision preoperatively had 20/20 or better best corrected vision at their last postoperative visit.

As noted above, the centration of this procedure was excellent, comparable to the best reports for excimer PRK for myopia. No statistically significant correlation (R = 0.03; P = 0.78) was found between visual acuity with correction and decentration (Figure 30-22A). In this sample of patients there was also no statistically significant correlation found between patient age and the visual acuity with correction achieved. The sample size was far too small to expect a correlation between visual acuity results and age.

However, a statistically significant correlation was found between all measures of irregular astigmatism and the best corrected visual acuity. This contrasts with several reports that show that irregular astigmatism is mild and does not affect the spectacle corrected visual acuity after LASIK.[18] There was a statistically significant, although somewhat weak, correlation (R = 0.43; P < 0.0001) between the SRI for the pupil (SRI_p) and the best corrected visual acuity as shown in Figure 30-22B which plots all postoperative data. As SRI was specifically designed to correlate well with visual acuity, this correlation is not surprising. However, it does corroborate Brint's assertion that loss of early best corrected visual acuity is probably related to irregular astigmatism and wound healing.[64]

There was also a statistically significant correlation (R = 0.46; P < 0.0001) between the coefficient of variation of corneal powers within the apparent entrance pupil and visual acuity with correction as shown in Figure 30-22C which plots all postoperative data. Reduced acuity in PRK for myopia with high CVP_p has also been shown (Klyce et al, unpublished data).

However, the strongest correlate to visual acuity with

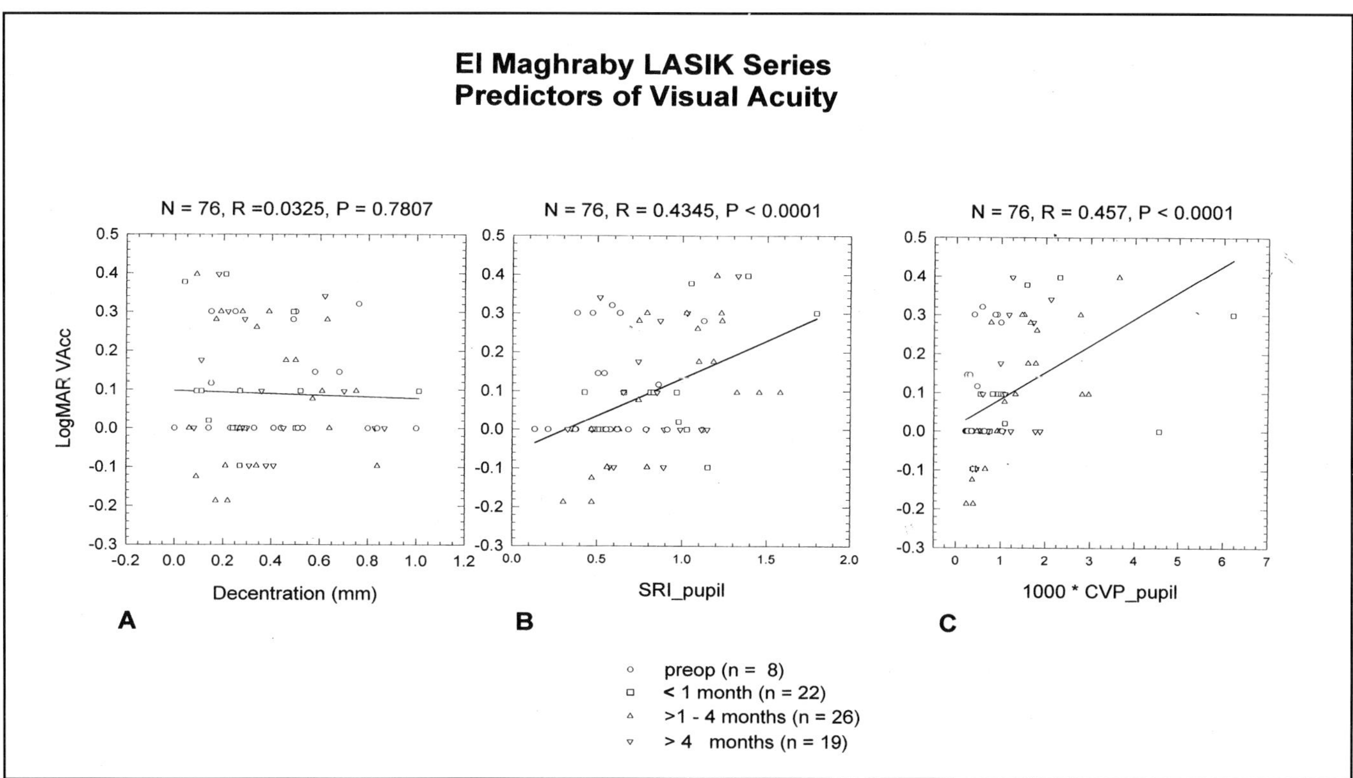

Figure 30-22.

Plots of the LogMAR of the visual acuity vs the postoperative decentration, SRI, and CVP data. (A) Decentration—No statistically significant correlation ($R = 0.03$; $P = 0.78$) was found between visual acuity with correction and decentration. (B) SRI—There was a statistically significant although weak correlation ($R = 0.43$; $P < 0.0001$) between the surface regularity index for the pupil (SRI_p) and the best corrected visual acuity. (C) There was also a statistically significant correlation ($R = 0.46$; $P < 0.0001$) between the coefficient of variation of corneal powers within the apparent entrance pupil and visual acuity with correction. In general these correlations would be expected to be strongest for the early postoperative periods.

correction in the LASIK study was EDM. As Figure 30-23A shows there is a statistically significant correlation ($R = 0.62$; $P < 0.0001$) between the EDM and best corrected visual acuity. EDM, SRI, and CVP are not independent parameters; they are each measures of irregular astigmatism, but as we shall see below, EDM may be the most sensitive to the type of irregular astigmatism that correlates best with reduced acuity after LASIK.

There was a statistically significant correlation ($R = 0.39$; $P = 0.001$) found between attempted correction and visual acuity with correction when assessed with all individuals from all time points (Figure 30-23B). This could easily be explained since we showed that the change in EDM was at least partly determined by the attempted correction. The average corneal power within the apparent entrance pupil will also correlate directly with the attempted correction given that preoperative ACP_p had a narrow range. It is, therefore, not surprising that there is a statistically significant correlation ($R = 0.32$; $P = 0.0051$) between ACP_p and visual acuity with correction as shown in Figure 30-23C which plots all postoperative data.

SUMMARY AND CONCLUSION

In this chapter we have reviewed some of the fundamentals of videokeratography, discussed the advantages of videokeratography over other methods of evaluating corneal topography, and discussed global descriptors of corneal topography found in the literature. We also describe a topographic analysis of the postoperative LASIK cornea. The topographic analysis described here is a most rigorous objective analysis of refractive surgical procedures. In the past, it has been applied to study the results of excimer PRK for myopia using the VisX laser; the conclusions from that analysis, where the visual results of nearly all patients were excellent, argued

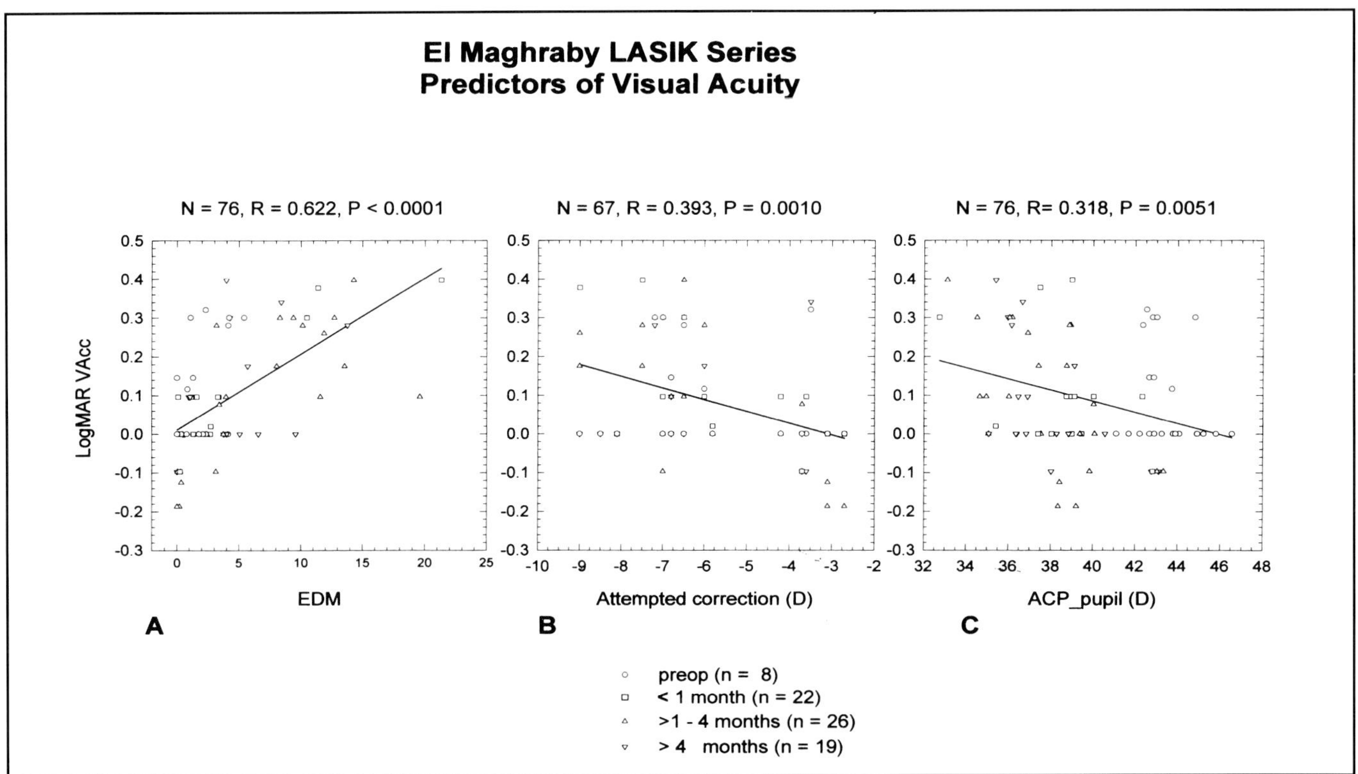

Figure 30-23.
Plots of the LogMAR of the best corrected visual acuity vs the postoperative EDM, attempted correction, and ACP data. (A) A statistically significant correlation ($R = 0.62$; $P < 0.0001$) between the EDM and best corrected visual acuity is shown. (B) A statistically significant correlation ($R = 0.39$; $P = 0.001$) was also found between attempted correction and visual acuity with correction when assessed with all individuals from all time points. (C) In addition, there was also a statistically significant although weak correlation ($R = 0.32$; $P = 0.0051$) between ACP_p and visual acuity with correction. Once again, these correlations would be expected to be strongest for the early postoperative periods.

toward the safety and efficacy of the excimer laser area ablation technique as embodied by the VisX 20/20 laser system.[32,36] In this chapter, we report the first comprehensive analysis of the corneal topography of LASIK. The issues that have received the most attention and could be of concern to the success of the procedure (centration, stability, and irregular astigmatism) have been carefully measured in this study and have been carefully correlated with vision.

Treatment stability within this group after LASIK was remarkable, with no statistically significant variations occurring from the first postoperative exam throughout the average 6-month postoperative follow-up. In addition there was a trend toward emmetropia rather than to the original refractive error in the months after LASIK. This contrasts with first-generation excimer laser PRK, where stability is not achieved generally until the sixth postoperative month and regression is common.[18] Centration of the treated area compares favorably with the best published reports for centration accuracy in PRK.

An elevation/depression detection algorithm was devised to objectively assess islands and depressions in topography—the EDM. EDM was significantly increased in all postoperative periods; it was found that some elevations/depressions were transient and diminished with time, others increased with time, and some remained relatively constant. These findings are in contrast to PRK corneas with islands; PRK central islands diminish with time and are essentially absent by 18 months postoperative.

Analysis of the SRI changes with treatment showed that the theoretical potential visual acuity changed from 20/20 to 20/25 preoperatively to 20/25 to 20/30 at an average of 6 months, a loss of one Snellen line. The correlations of best corrected visual acuity with ACP_p, SRI_p, CVP_p, EDM, and attempted correction were statistically significant. For best corrected Snellen acuity, a forward stepwise linear regression analysis showed that the EDM was most strongly correlated to visual acuity. When the variations in best corrected Snellen acuity due to EDM were eliminated, none of the other variables retained statistical significance. In this test, we show that EDM could be the most responsible for the correlation with acuity. Further follow-up is needed to see if this type of irregular astigmatism decreases to immeasurable levels with time as it does with PRK.

The visual results and the topographic analyses indicate the need for improving the uniformity of the treated zone obtained with the LASIK procedure. However, it is clear from some of the correlations of very sensitive objective topography measures that additional patients need to be enrolled and the follow-up time needs to be extended for a good assessment of the safety and efficacy of the procedure as well as for a good comparison to alternative refractive surgical procedures.

During excimer refractive surgery procedures, the wider the diameter of the ablation zone desired, the deeper the ablation would have to be done to achieve the same correction. Thus, for ablations being performed after a deep flap cut, or on a thin cornea, a smaller optical zone may be needed which can lead to halos, glare, and problems with night vision.[27,33] We suspect that thinner flaps may decrease the incidence of these complications but may increase the incidence of wrinkles and irregular astigmatism of the flap. We are presently looking at characterizing the aberration structure of the post-LASIK cornea and comparing this to the post-PRK cornea. In the future, this data could be used to describe the ideal corneal shape after refractive surgery for a given correction that would maximize uncorrected visual acuity while minimizing decreased contrast sensitivity.

Topographic analysis of the clinical trial presented in this chapter indicates good predictability, rapid achievement of good uncorrected visual acuity, and apparent long-term stability with few or no reports of haze over the entrance pupil. However, the early postoperative irregular astigmatism needs further evaluation to see that it resolves. Improvements of the microkeratome design are clearly needed to reduce complications.

References

1. Rabinowitz YS, Wilson SE, Klyce SD. *Atlas of Corneal Topography*. New York, NY: Igaku-Shoin Medical Publishers Inc; 1993.
2. Klyce SD. Computer-assisted corneal topography: high resolution graphical presentation and analysis of keratoscopy. *Invest Ophthalmol Vis Sci*. 1984;25:1426-1436.
3. Trokel SL, Srinivasan R, Braren BA. Excimer laser surgery of the cornea. Am J Ophthalmol. 1983;96:710-715.
4. Pallikaris IG, Papatzanaki ME, Stathi EZ, Frenschock O, Georgiadis A. Laser in situ keratomileusis. *Laser Surg Med*. 1990;10:463-468.
5. McDonald MB, Liu JC, Byrd TJ, et al. Central photorefractive keratectomy for myopia. *Ophthalmology*. 1991;98(9):1327-1337.
6. Seiler T, Wollensak J. Myopic photorefractive keratectomy with the excimer laser. One year follow-up. *Ophthalmology*. 1991;98(8):1156-1163.
7. Waring III GO, O'Connell MA, Maloney RK, et al. Photorefractive keratectomy for myopia using a 4.5-millimeter ablation zone. *J Refract Surg*. 1995;11(3):170-180.
8. Martinez CE, Applegate RA, Howland HC, et al. Photorefractive keratectomy and the monochromatic aberrations of the cornea. In Pre-AAO International Society of Refractive Surgery Meeting. Chicago, Ill, 1996.
9. Seiler T, Reckmann W, Maloney RK. Effective spherical aberration of the cornea as a quantitative descriptor in corneal topography. *J Cataract Refract Surg*. 1993;19(5):155-165.
10. Ficker LA, Bates AK, Steele ADMcG, et al. Excimer laser photorefractive keratectomy for myopia: 12 month follow-up. *Eye*. 1993;7:617-624.
11. Halliday BL. Refractive and visual results and patient satisfaction after excimer laser photorefractive keratectomy for myopia. *Br J Ophthalmol*. 1995;79(10):881-887.
12. Shimizu K, Amano S, Tanaka S. Photorefractive keratectomy for myopia: one-year follow-up in 97 eyes. *J Refract Corneal Surg*. 1994;10(suppl 2):S178-S187.
13. Hamberg-Nystrom H, Fagerholm P, Tengroth B, Epstein D. Photorefractive keratectomy for low myopia at 5 mm treatment diameter. A comparison of two excimer lasers. *Acta Ophthalmologica*. 1994;72(4):453-456.
14. Kim JH, Hahn TW, Lee YC, Joo CK, Sah WJ. Photorefractive keratectomy in 202 myopic eyes: one year results. *Refract Corneal Surg*. 1993;9(suppl 2):S11-S16.
15. Gartry DS, Kerr Muir MG, Marshall J. Photorefractive keratectomy with an argon fluoride excimer laser: a clinical study. *J Refract Corneal Surg*. 1991;7:420-435.
16. O'Brart DPS, Lohmann CP, Fitzke FW, et al. Night vision after excimer laser photorefractive keratectomy: haze and halos. *Eur J Ophthalmol*. 1994;4(1):43-51.
17. Maguire L. Keratorefractive surgery, success and the public health. *Am J Ophthalmol*. 1994;117(3):394-398.
18. Pallikaris IG, Siganos DS. Excimer laser in situ keratomileusis and photorefractive keratectomy for correction of high myopia. *J Refract Corneal Surg*. 1994;10(5):498-510.
19. Fiander DC, Tayfour F. Excimer laser in situ keratomileusis in 124 myopic eyes. *J Refract Surg*. 1995;11(suppl 3):S234-S238.
20. Peyman GA, Badaro RM, Khoobehi B. Corneal ablation in rabbits using infrared (2.9mm) erbium:YAG laser. *Ophthalmology*. 1989;96(8):1160-1169.
21. Pallikaris IG, Papatzanaki ME, Siganos DS, Tsilimbaris MK. A corneal flap technique for laser in situ keratomileusis. Human studies. *Arch Ophthalmol*. 1991;109(12):1699-1702.

22. Buratto L, Ferrari M, Rama P. Excimer laser intrastromal keratomileusis. *Am J Ophthalmol*. 1992;113:291-295.

23. Gimbel HV, Basti S, Kaye GB, Ferensowicz M. Experience during the learning curve of laser in situ keratomileusis. *J Cataract Refract Surg*. 1996;22:542-550.

24. Solomon K. The wound healing response following LASIK and PRK. In Pre-AAO International Society of Refractive Surgery Meeting. Chicago, Ill, 1996.

25. Kremer FB, Dufek M. Excimer laser in situ keratomileusis. *J Refract Surg*. 1995;11(suppl):S244-S247.

26. Kliger CH, Maloney RK. Excimer laser myopic keratomileusis at the Jules Stein Eye Institute. In: Salz J, McDonnell, McDonald M, eds. *Corneal Laser Surgery*. St. Louis, Mo: CV Mosby; 1995:196-200.

27. Bas AM, Onnis R. Excimer laser in situ keratomileusis for myopia. *J Refract Surg*. 1995;11(suppl):S229-S233.

28. Maguire LJ. Topographical principles in keratorefractive surgery. *Int Ophthalm Clin*. 1991;31:1-6.

29. Maguire LJ, Zabel RW, Parker P, Lindstrom RL. Topography and raytracing analysis of patients with excellent visual acuity 3 months after excimer laser photorefractive keratectomy for myopia. *Refract Corneal Surg*. 1991;7(2):122-128.

30. Maguire LJ, Klyce SD, Sawelson H, McDonald MB,, Kaufman HE. Visual distortion after myopic keratomileusis: computer analysis of keratoscopy photography. *Ophthalmic Surg*. 1987;18(5):352-356.

31. Maguire LJ, Bourne WM. A multifocal lens effect as a complication of radial keratotomy. *Refract Corneal Surg*. 1989;5(6):394-399.

32. Klyce SD, Smolek MK. Corneal topography of excimer laser photorefractive keratectomy. *J Cataract Refract Surg*. 1993;19(suppl):122-130.

33. Maloney RK. Corneal topography and optical zone location in photorefractive keratectomy. *Refract Corneal Surg*. 1990;6:363-371.

34. McDonnell PJ, McClusky DJ, Garbus JJ. Corneal topography and fluctuating visual acuity after radial keratotomy. *Ophthalmology*. 1989;96:665-670.

35. Wilson SE, Klyce SD. Screening for corneal topographic abnormalities before refractive surgery. *Ophthalmology*. 1994;(101):147-152.

36. Wilson SE, Klyce SD, McDonald MB, Liu JC, Kaufman HE. Changes in corneal topography after excimer laser photorefractive keratectomy for myopia. *Ophthalmology*. 1991;98(9):1338-1347.

37. Wilson SE, Klyce SD. Advances in the analysis of corneal topography. *Surv Ophthalmol*. 1991;35(4):269-277.

38. Wilson SE, Lin DT, Klyce SD. Corneal topography of keratoconus. *Cornea*. 1991;10(1):2-8.

39. Wilson SE, Klyce SD, Husseini ZM. Standarized color coded maps for corneal topography. *Ophthalmology*. 1993;100:1723-1727.

40. Martinez CE, Klyce SD. Corneal topography in cataract surgery. *Curr Opinion Ophthal*. 1996;7(1):30-38.

41. Helmholtz HV. *Hanndbuch der physiologicschen Optik*. Hamburg, Germany: Leopold Voss; 1909.

42. Wilson SE, Klyce SD. Quantitative descriptors of corneal topography. A clinical study. *Arch Ophthalmol*. 1991;109(3):349-353.

43. Rabinowitz YS, Wilson SE, Klyce SD. *Color Atlas of Cornel Topography*. New York, NY: Igaku-Shoin Medical Publishers; 1993.

44. Bond W. LASIK in keratoconus: A case history. In Pre-AAO International Society of Refractive Surgery Meeting. Chicago, Ill, 1996.

45. Maguire LJ, Singer DE, Klyce SD. Graphic presentation of computer-analyzed keratoscope photographs. *Arch Ophthalmol*. 1987;105(2):223-230.

46. Wang JW, Silva DE. Wave-front interpretation with Zernike polynomials. *Applied Optics*. 1980;19(9):1510-1519.

47. Wang J, Rice D, Klyce S. A new reconstruction algorithm for improvement of corneal topographical analysis. *Refract Corneal Surg*. 1989;5(6):379-387.

48. Hersh PS, Shah SI, Geiger D, Holladay JT, The Summit PRK Topography Study Group. Corneal optical irregularity after excimer laser photorefractive keratectomy. *J Cataract Refract Surg*. 1996;22(3):197-204.

49. Maloney RK, Bojan SJ, Waring III GO. Determination of corneal image properties from corneal topography. *Am J Ophthalmol*. 1993;115:30-41.

50. Applegate RA, Howland HC, Buettner J, et al. Corneal aberrations before and after radial keratotomy (RK) calculated from videokeratometric measurements. In: Vision Science and Its Applications Topical Meeting. Santa Fe, NM; 1994.

51. Applegate RA, Howland HC, Buettner J, et al. Changes in the aberration structure of the RK cornea from videokeratographic measurements. *Invest Ophthalmol Vis Sci*. 1994;35(suppl):1740.

52. Holladay JT. The Holladay diagnostic summary. In: Gills J, et al, eds. *Corneal Topography: The State of the Art*. Thorofare, NJ: SLACK Inc; 1995:309-323.

53. Greivenkamp JE, Schwiegerling J, Miller JM, Mellinger MD. Visual acuity modeling using optical raytracing of schematic eyes. *Am J Ophthalmol*. 1995;120(2):227-240.

54. Olsen T, Dam-Johansen M, Bek T, Hjortdal JO. Evaluating surgically induced astigmatism by Fourier analysis of corneal topography data. *J Cataract Refract Surg*. 1996;22(3):318-323.

55. Hjortdal JO, Erdmann L, Bek T. Fourier analysis of video-keratographic data. A tool for separation of spherical, regular astigmatic and irregular astigmatic corneal power components. *Ophthalmic Physiol Opt*. 1995;15(3):171-185.

56. Salah T, Waring III GO, Maghraby AE, Moadel K, Grimm SB. Excimer laser in situ keratomileusis under a corneal flap for myopia of 2 to 20 diopters. *Am J Ophthalmol*. 1996;121:143-155.

57. Holladay JT. Correlating visual performance with corneal topography following RK, PRK, and LASIK. In Pre-AAO International Society of Refractive Surgery Meeting. Chicago, Ill, 1996.

58. Taylor DM, L'Esperance FA, Del Pero RA, et al. Human excimer laser lamellar keratectomy: a clinical study. *Ophthalmology*. 1989;96:654-664.

59. Maguire LJ, Klyce SD, Singer DE. Corneal topography in myopic patients undergoing epikeratophakia. *Am J Ophthalmol*. 1987;103(3pt2):404-416.

60. Reidy JJ, MCDonald MB, Klyce SD. The corneal topography of epikeratophakia. *Refract Corneal Surg*. 1990;6(1):26-31.

61. Uozato H, Guyton DL. Centering corneal procedures. *Am J Ophthalmol*. 1987;103:264-275.

62. Cavanaugh TB, Durrie DS, Reidel SM, Hunkeler JD, Lesher MP. Topographical analysis of the centration of excimer laser photorefractive keratectomy. *J Cataract Refract Surg*. 1993;19(suppl):136-143.

63. Amano S, Tanaka S, Shimizu K. Topographical evaluation of centration of excimer laser myopic photorefractive keratectomy. *J Cataract Refract Surg*. 1994;20:616-619.

64. Brint SF, Ostrick DM, Fisher C, et al. Six-month results of the multicenter phase I study of excimer laser myopic keratomileusis. *J Cataract Refract Surg*. 1994;20(6):610-615.

65. Lin DTC, Sutton HF, Berman M. Corneal topography following excimer photorefractive keratectomy for myopia. *J Cataract Refract Surg*. 1993;19(suppl):149-154.

66. Seiler T. Central islands after LASIK. In Pre-AAO International Society of Refractive Surgery Meeting. Chicago, Ill, 1996.

67. Michalos P, Avila EN, Florakis GJ, Hersh PS. Do human tears absorb ultraviolet light? *CLAO J*. 1994;20(3):192-193.

68. Dingeldein SA, Klyce SD, Wilson SE. Quantitative descriptors of corneal shape derived from computer-assisted analysis of photokeratographs. *Refract Corneal Surg*. 1989;5(6):372-378.

69. Maeda N, Klyce SD, Smolek MK, McDonald MB. Disparity of keratometry readings and corneal power within the pupil after refractive surgery for myopia. *Cornea*. In press.

70. Maeda N, Klyce S, Smolek M, Thompson HW. Automated keratoconus screening with corneal topography analysis. *Invest Ophthalmol Vis Sci*. 1994;35:2749-2757.

71. Mafra CH, Dave AS, Pilai CT, Klyce SD, Wilson SE. Prospective study of corneal topographic changes produced by extracapsular cataract surgery. *Cornea*. 1996;15(2):196-203.

Chapter 31

AN ALTERNATIVE TOPOGRAPHY IN LASIK

Ioannis G. Pallikaris, MD, Petros V. Kapoulas, BSc,
Dimitrios S. Siganos, MD

INTRODUCTION

Computer-aided corneal topography has proven to be a powerful tool in the hands of ophthalmic surgeons in relation to diagnostic procedures and surgery planning, as well as postoperative evaluation of the surgical outcome. The technology related to such systems is rapidly evolving, mainly due to an increasing demand by the clinicians for more enhanced features and concrete diagnostic results, in their attempt to have a better grasp of the specifics of each clinical case. Here we present briefly a novel approach to corneal topography, namely the ORBSCAN Slit Scan Corneal Topography/Pachymetry System by ORBTEK Inc and its advantages in the area of evaluating the immediate outcome of a keratorefractive procedure. We assume that the reader is familiar with the use of corneal topography systems and interpretation of the offered examination data.

DESCRIPTION

In general, corneal topography systems project a light pattern on the eye's surface and employ image analysis software to derive the shape of its anterior surface. Most systems employ a Placido to project a number of concentric rings on the tear film, acquire an image of their reflected pattern, and derive the shape of the surface based

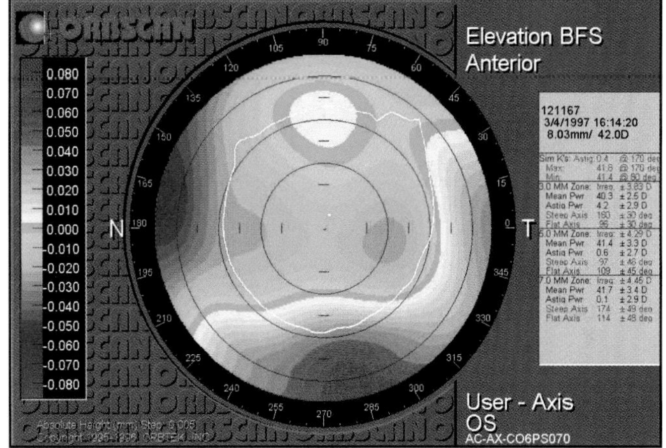

Figure 31-1.
Each given point on the cornea is presented as being on the surface of the best fit sphere, under it, or over it.

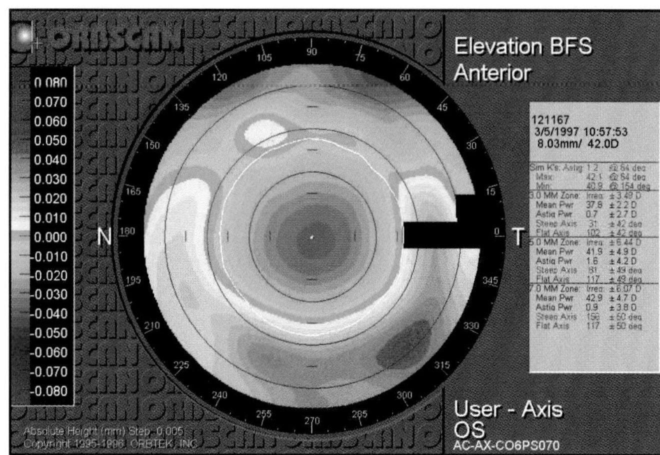

Figure 31-2.
Preoperative state of posterior surface.

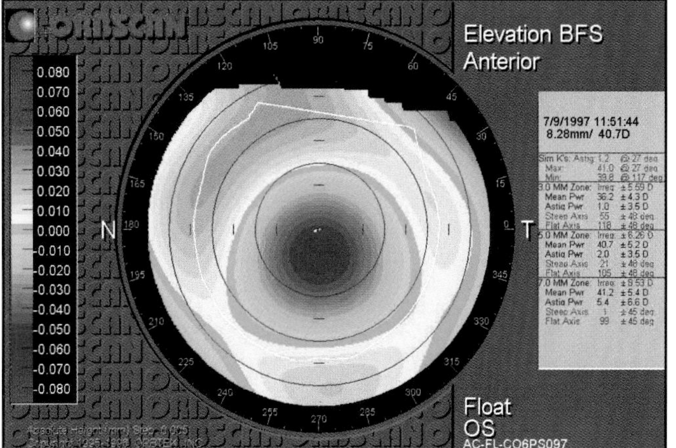

Figure 31-3.
Postoperative state of posterior surface.

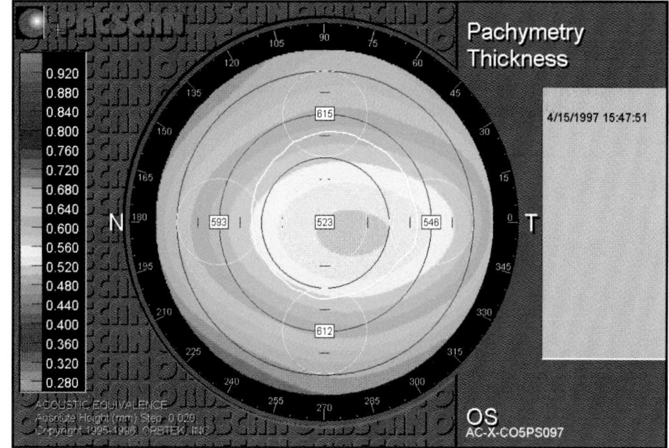

Figure 31-4.
An important feature is pachymetry.

on the distortion of that pattern. The ORBSCAN system projects a series of light slits, 20 from left to right and 20 from right to left, acquires an image for each projection, and uses edge detection to derive the curvature of the anterior and posterior surface of the cornea.

Corneal topography systems in general present the derived data in the form of color-coded topography maps, with each specific color depicting a corresponding level of refraction for a particular area of the cornea's surface. ORBSCAN calculates a "best fit sphere," which is the sphere whose surface contains the maximum of the cornea's surface. Each given point on the cornea is presented as being on the surface of the best fit sphere (ie, has the same curvature as the best fit sphere, represented by the color green), under it ("cold" colors, shades of blue to purple) or over it ("warm" colors, shades of yellow to red). An example is given in Figure 31-1. This way, a more realistic presentation of the changes of the elevation of the corneal surface is given.

The first and obvious advantage is that both surfaces of the cornea are examined, offering valuable diagnostic data. Particularly in relation to LASIK, the occasional severe thinning of the cornea may have dramatic effects on the posterior surface of it. With the use of this particular system, the corneal posterior surface ectasia effect, extremely important for LASIK, can be readily examined. An example is given in Figures 31-2 (preoperative state of the posterior surface) and 31-3 (postoperative state of the posterior surface). Other important features are pachymetry (Figure 31-4) and difference maps between pre- and postoperative pachymetry of a treated cornea, where the exact correction introduced is presented. A fine point is

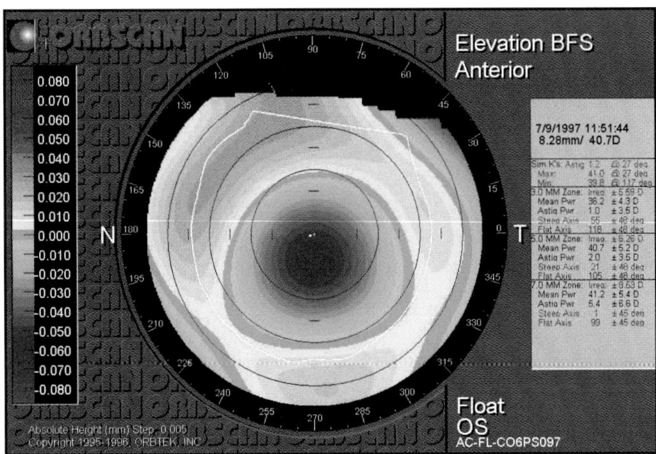

Figure 31-5.
The best fit sphere is floating.

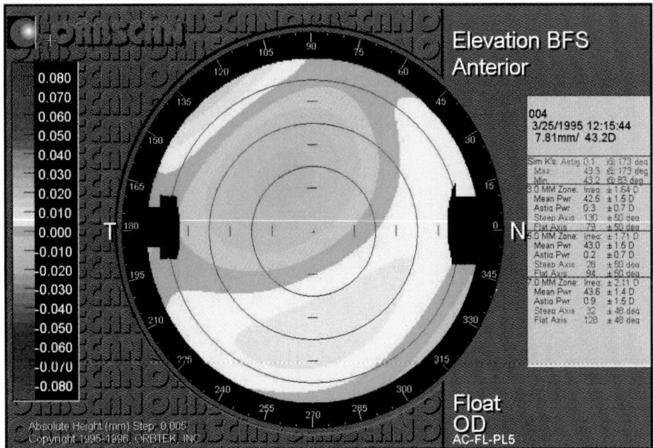

Figure 31-6.
The best fit sphere is axially aligned.

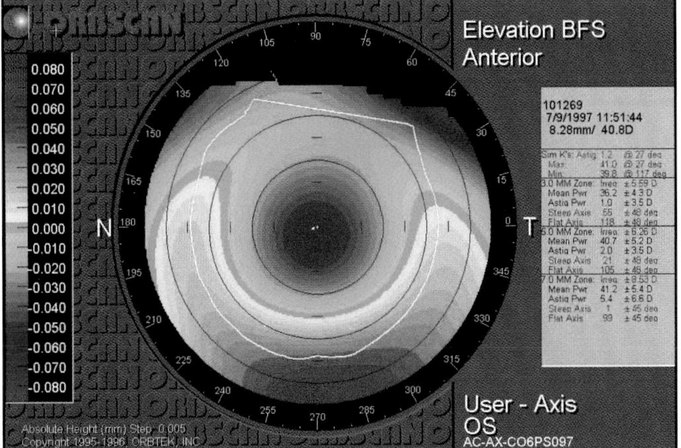

Figure 31-7.
The best fit sphere is floating.

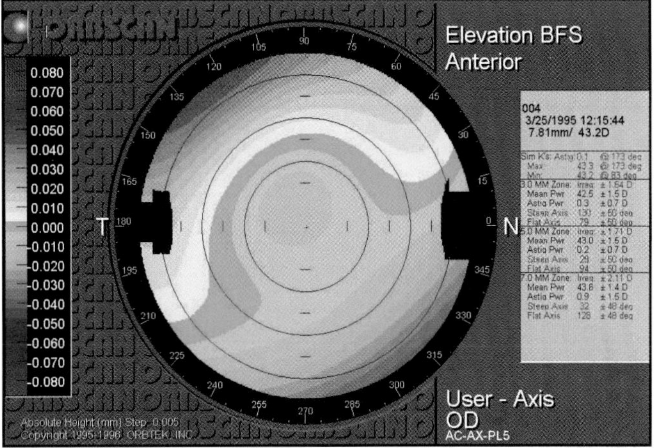

Figure 31-8.
The best fit sphere is axially aligned.

that the system does not rely on the existence of the tear film for the acquisition of the data, therefore, an examination may be performed immediately after surgery, when the epithelium is absent.

The most interesting feature of the system, revealed by the preliminary investigation of its use, is the ability to force the center apex of the best fit sphere onto an axis through the apex of the cornea. The ability to choose the size and placement of the sphere that fits on the corneal surface exists for examination of specific and/or extreme surface anomalies. If the chosen sphere has the same size as the best fit sphere, and its center apex is placed onto the optical axis, then a more detailed presentation of the region around the apex of the eye is available. This form is extremely useful for determining the exact location of the performed ablation. In Figure 31-5, the best fit sphere is floating, whereas in Figure 31-6, the same sphere is axially aligned. The latter case shows a better centered ablation than the one in the initial presentation. Systems that employ a Placido do not possess such an ability, due to their fixed centration of the projected pattern.

In Figures 31-7 and 31-8, an extreme case is presented, which clearly demonstrates the benefits of this feature. Examinations taken with Placido systems show essentially the same image of the corneal curvature as the one in Figure 31-7, where the best fit sphere is floating. The ablation seems to be extremely decentered. In Figure 31-8, the same best fit sphere is axially aligned. Here, there appears to be a good centration of ablation. We note that PRK was performed on this particular patient with an excellent postoperative visual acuity result, which clearly agrees with the examination data of Figure 31-8. It is therefore safe to conclude that proper use of this particular feature gives a more realistic presentation of the actual shape of the cornea while providing for better evaluation of the effect of photorefractive surgical procedures on the eye.

CONCLUSION

As a final comment, we want to stress the significance of such enhancements in computerized corneal topography. A clear perspective of the actual effect of surgical procedures on the eye brings the surgeon a step closer to proper planning of surgery and ideal treatment approach of each individual case.

SECTION 8

FINAL THOUGHTS

Chapter 32

FUTURE DEVELOPMENTS IN LASIK

George O. Waring III, MD, FACS, FRCOphth

INTRODUCTION

Telling the future is easy—it requires no data and only personal speculation. I will make some predictions about new developments in laser in situ keratomileusis (LASIK) based on what we know.

SELECTION OF PATIENTS

The most important feature in selecting patients will not change: the patient must have realistic expectations of the procedure based on honest communication from the surgeon and professional staff, regardless of portrayal of the procedure in advertising and the popular media.

As increasing experience is published in the peer-reviewed literature from LASIK surgeons around the world, it will be easier for the surgeon to help patients form realistic expectations because more information will be available on which objective predictions can be made in terms of refractive outcome, uncorrected visual acuity, quality of vision, topography, and complications.

Since there will inevitably be scatter in the results, as occurs in all human surgical procedures, patients must be aware that they may need spectacle correction after surgery for specific tasks (eg, night driving) or for reading if they are over age 40 and do not have residual myopia.

TREATMENT OF COMPOUND MYOPIC ASTIGMATISM AND HYPEROPIA

The future is now. Lasers that use expanding slit apertures and scanning beams can now correct compound myopic astigmatism and in the future, this capability will be a feature of all excimer lasers.

The challenge will remain to align the appropriate astigmatic meridian of the cornea with the laser beam with anatomic accuracy. This requires proper identification of the steep meridian on the patient's eye.

Ablation algorithms and contours to correct hyperopia require flattening a large circular zone of paracentral cornea with an inner diameter of approximately 4 mm and an outer diameter of 8 to 10 mm. Thus, the anterior corneal flap will have to be at least 9 to 10 mm in diameter to reveal enough stroma for the hyperopic ablation—a requirement that necessitates new designs of the microkeratome and the suction ring.

LASIK FOR PRESBYOPIA

Whether it is possible to ablate a cornea with intentionally designed multifocal contours that allow a presbyopic person to see sharply at distance and near is unknown. Experience with bifocal contact lenses and multifocal IOLs continues to improve, offering a prototype of how the cornea might be shaped for presbyopes. However, the degradation of image quality inherent with multifocal IOLs and contact lenses and with inadvertently created multifocal corneas after refractive surgery remains a serious drawback. Most patients are unwilling to tolerate slightly blurred vision with poor contrast for freedom from reading glasses.

A lamellar plano corneal flap can be raised to create a location for a multifocal or presbyopic intracorneal lens. However, such lenses are probably more easily placed in a simple lamellar pocket.

OPTIMAL CORNEAL CONTOURS AND OPTICS

The algorithms that control the dosing and distribution of laser energy to reshape the cornea must undergo continual improvement in order to create more physiological contours of the cornea that do not create optical aberrations, which the patient perceives as glare and halos or simply as loss of sharp vision. This requires gradual transition zones and large diameter ablations, probably at least 7 mm in diameter, so the edge of the ablation is outside the diameter of the entrance pupil.

Our current standard for correcting ametropia is glasses and contact lenses. Refractive surgery will have to be as good as those optical devices in terms of accuracy of correction and quality of vision if surgery is to become the treatment of choice for ametropia. But the real goal is to be able to shape the cornea or insert an IOL so that the patient has better vision than is achieved with spectacles and contact lenses. This creates a serious challenge for the LASIK community—laser engineers, optical engineers, manufacturers of microkeratomes, and ophthalmic surgeons. Flying spot lasers that use fractal mathematics to create algorithms that can ablate each cornea into a custom shape are now being developed.

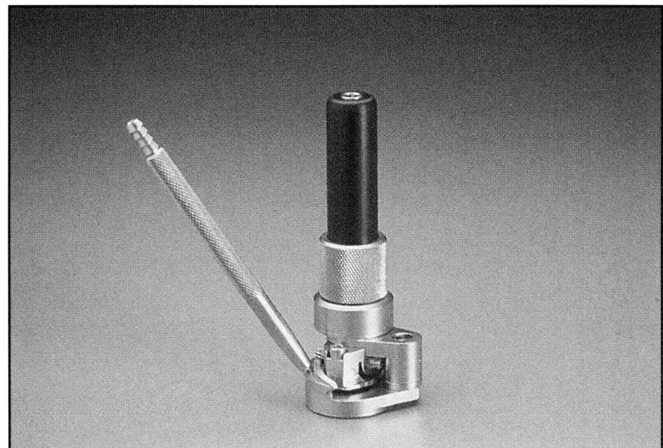

Figure 32-1.
The Hansatome.

MICROKERATOMES

The most widely used microkeratome currently is the Chiron Automated Corneal Shaper, which is a modified version of the original Barraquer microkeratome with a motorized advance. A new design, the Hansatome (Figure 32-1), is easier to assemble and use. A reliable, economical, totally disposable microkeratome would be ideal; because if it were manufactured with high quality control, all of the intensive daily maintenance, technician training, repairs, and adjustments would disappear.

A suction ring that would obviate conjunctival suction, the circumstance in which the conjunctiva occludes the aspiration hole without elevating the IOP, would increase the safety of the suction ring. A larger diameter suction ring to create a 9- to 10-mm diameter flap and allow for hyperopic correction is needed. Since only one diameter is required for LASIK, an adjustable suction ring is unnecessary. However, multiple diameters might allow the surgeon to operate on eyes with variably sized corneas. The suction ring should also allow for operating on eyes with unusually shaped anterior corneal curvatures, a need that may require some custom manufacturing. The size of the suction ring handle should be short enough to fit easily beneath the excimer laser.

New ways of fashioning a corneal flap may obviate the use of microkeratomes altogether. Waterjets and lasers hold forth this promise, but none has proven practical yet.

HANDLING OF THE CORNEAL FLAP

Although creating a corneal flap is reasonably automated and doing the ablation is somewhat robotic, replacing the flap is still a matter of surgical skill. Wet techniques, dry techniques, damp techniques, no-touch, painting it flat, the current variety of approaches are being replaced by a consensus technique that will allow firm adherence, absence of wrinkles and microwrinkles, elimination of epithelial ingrowth, and creation of a clean interface. Elements of this technique are:

- Keeping a clean, dry ocular surface.
- Folding the flap back dry immediately after ablation to decrease exposure time of the bed to foreign material.
- Floating the flap on a bed of BSS to relieve torsion and stress on the tissue and to align the fiduciary lines.
- Squeezing the fluid out of the interface to approximate the stromal tissue faces.
- Stretching the flap in all directions with gentle massage to eliminate wrinkles.
- Pushing the edge of the flap adjacent to the edge of the bed to minimize the peripheral scar and the chance of epithelial ingrowth.

EXCIMER LASER DESIGN

Detailed discussion of excimer laser design is carried out in many chapters of this text. Let us clearly state the future goal: the invention and clinical realization of an excimer laser that can do the following:

- Create corneal contours that obviate optical aberrations.
- Custom shape the cornea based on the individual's preoperative corneal shape.
- Modify corneal shape in a custom manner when an undesired shape occurs postoperatively or after corneal disease.
- Operate not just on corneal topography, but on the actual refractive system of the eye to create visual acuity better than that achieved with spectacles and contact lenses. Will this be done with ablatable masks, with a flying spot, with fractal mathematics, with fuzzy logic algorithms? The future will tell.

ADJUSTABLE LASIK

LASIK has one big advantage—it can correct a large range of myopia, astigmatism, and hyperopia; myopia from -1.00 D to -15.00 D with current technology, and maybe higher corrections in the future. The fact that a surgeon can lift the corneal flap years after surgery (or simply make another microkeratome pass) allows for adjustability of the LASIK procedure, as long as there is enough corneal tissue left (currently, 200 μm in the bed). One can conceive the following sequence of events: A patient with compound myopic astigmatism undergoes LASIK, but with a resultant undercorrection. A repeated LASIK leaves residual astigmatism. Yet another LASIK corrects the astigmatism, but induces hyperopia. Another repeated LASIK treats the hyperopia and renders the patient plano and happy. However, the natural progression of myopia produces more myopia, which is treated again by a LASIK enhancement. The patient remains stable and happy until the onset of presbyopia, when a hyperopic LASIK steepens the central cornea in one eye to induce myopia and give the patient monovision. Such adjustability is feasible, but current techniques require refinement to realize it.

THE CHALLENGE TO LASIK: PHAKIC IOLS

LASIK has two major disadvantages: it is not reversible and it creates an abnormally shaped cornea. Phakic IOLs share neither of these disadvantages and offer another major advantage to the ophthalmologist and the patient—the procedure is much cheaper; no need for expensive microkeratomes and excimer lasers, no need for special vision correction facilities, no need for extensive surgical training. Since most surgeons know how to implant an IOL, simple refinement of these techniques will allow the surgeon to implant a phakic IOL. The reduced cost to the surgeon should reduce the cost to the patient.

Currently, phakic IOLs are in the early stages of development and new designs, new surgical techniques, new optical refinements, and new materials will all be forthcoming. The contest between LASIK and phakic IOLs will be an interesting one that will carry refractive surgery into the 21st century.

Chapter 33

REFRACTIVE PROCEDURES: WHERE ARE THE BORDERS?

Ioannis G. Pallikaris, MD

Today, there are numerous operations available for the correction of refractive errors. Some of them, such as intracorneal rings or corneal inlays, are still developing and have not reached the stage of perfection of others. With all these operations, sometimes it is difficult to chose what is the best for the patient, as there is an overlap in the indications and the range of refractive error they correct.

In order to select the proper operation, patient expectations should be kept in mind. The patient's age and needs (not always expectations) are the two most crucial parameters in the decision-making process.

We will try an evaluation approach for these procedures, based on the following parameters:

- The range of refractive error that can be corrected.
- The rehabilitation time required for the patient to regain useful vision (ie, the stability of the refractive outcome).
- The current cost.
- The extra skills that may be required by the surgeon.
- Whether the operation affects the central zone of the cornea.
- Reversibility of the procedure.
- Predictability.

As some intraocular procedures, such as clear lensectomy and phakic IOLs, are also used in treating refractive errors, two more parameters should be also kept in mind, namely invasiveness and accommodation.

CORNEAL REFRACTIVE PROCEDURES

PRK

PRK, or photorefractive keratectomy, has proven in many studies to be safe and effective in treating myopia up to -6.0 D. Refinement of excimer lasers, perfection of optics, and incorporation of tracking systems have improved the results and may have widened the range of its application to -8.0 D or -10.0 D, or even more. It is a simple procedure and does not require special skills. Its predictability in the indicated range is relatively high, almost 90% ± 1.0 D. On the other hand, it is an operation that affects the central (optical) zone of the cornea, it is not reversible, and current cost is high. Since it is performed on the cornea, it does not affect the accommodation and is probably the refractive procedure of choice in young patients with this range of myopia. It is expensive due to the very high cost of the excimer laser system. What seems to be sometimes a problem is the rehabilitation time required for the patient to regain useful vision. Besides the 3 days on average required for epithelial healing, it tends to produce an initial overcorrection (ie, temporary hyperopia), which is very annoying especially to those near their 40s, who are unable to perform near work for a variable period of weeks to sometimes months.

RK

Although RK, or radial keratotomy, was the operation of choice for the range of myopia between 1.0 D to 5.0 D till the early 1990s, it is now being gradually replaced by PRK, despite its almost similar predictability with that of PRK and the very low cost of the procedure. It definitely requires special skills, especially mini-RK. Rehabilitation is rapid and is an operation that preserves accommodation.

In any case, RK is being revived by some surgeons as new instruments are constantly being developed, and it does not affect the optical zone of the cornea. On the other hand, it is not reversible.

LASIK

LASIK, or laser in situ keratomileusis, is considered by many surgeons to be the rising star in the arena of refractive procedures. It is an operation that can be used for the correction of moderate to high myopia, although many refractive surgeons use it routinely for the lower ranges of myopia, too. We believe that its application should be limited to the range of -6 D to -18 D. Below this range, PRK is simpler, predictable, and potentially less hazardous. Over this range, one must go very deep into the cornea, something that may affect the corneal biomechanics. It is an operation that has not yet reached the utmost level of refinement, mainly because of the microkeratome problems. The main advantage of LASIK over PRK or RK is that it offers immediate rehabilitation and rapid stability of refraction. Its predictability is moderate to high, and it will further improve with improvement of microkeratomes. On the other hand, it is a very expensive procedure because of the use of both the excimer laser and the microkeratome. Also, its learning curve may be long.

INTRAOCULAR PROCEDURES

Clear Lensectomy

From the refractive result point of view, it is the operation that offers the highest accuracy and a very rapid stability. Its accuracy is within ± 1 D in over 90% of cases using the majority of existing IOL calculating formulas. It can also be applied for any refractive error and it is an operation within the grasp of any cataract surgeon. The factors that limit its application are its invasive nature and permanent loss of accommodation. It is not reversible, and it has a one in 1000 risk of sight loss.

Implantable Contact Lenses

There are different types of phakic IOLs available today. Some of them have been tried extensively, while new types are still being evaluated. Irrespective of the type, it is an operation that can be handled by the average phaco surgeon. It deals with inserting an IOL in a phakic eye, meaning that it is potentially cataractogenic. It is expensive owing largely to the high cost of the phakic IOL. These do not seem to affect accommodation although there are injectable types that rest on the crystalline lens and may partially restrict accommodation. It

TABLE 33-1

Preferable Procedure for the Treatment of Myopia

AGE	0 D to 3 D	3.5 D to 6 D	6.5 D to 8 D	8 D to 12 D	12 D to 18 D	>18 D
>40	PRK, RK	PRK, RK, LASIK	LASIK, PRK	LASIK, CLE	CLE, LASIK	CLE
<35	PRK, RK	PRK, LASIK, RK	LASIK, PRK	LASIK, ICL	ICL, LASIK	ICL, CLE

is an operation that is preserved for medium to high refractive errors, especially in young patients, and its rehabilitation is very rapid.

CHOICE OF THE APPROPRIATE OPERATION

Based on the above, we can see that there is significant overlap in many procedures. For example, a patient having -18 D of myopia can be actually treated with three of the above procedures, namely LASIK, implantable contact lenses (ICLs), and clear lens extraction. Which, then, is the most appropriate?

We should go back to the age of the patient and his or her needs.

The age that could be considered as a borderline, although not strictly, is that of 40 years. The patient approaches the presbyopia age, which is going to tax his or her declining accommodation power. So accommodation is not an issue here. In such a case, all three operations can be performed. What is the next issue to be considered? This is the condition of the lens. Any nuclear sclerosis or presence of even minimal opacities in the lens periphery or the posterior subcapsular area is an indication for clear lens extraction. If these observations are absent, then a less invasive procedure is chosen. When we talk about invasiveness we mean intraocular procedures, thus the ICL is also ruled out. We are now left with LASIK. This is the operation to be performed.

Take another example—a patient who has the same refractive error, but is 25 years old. He or she will be able to use his or her accommodation for many years to come. We then rule out clear lens extraction, so as not to deprive the patient of accommodation. This patient is within the range of LASIK and ICL. The following factors should be taken into consideration: invasiveness and possible hazards. ICL is the only intraocular procedure of the two. But LASIK also carries potential hazards, such as irregular astigmatism formation and line loss of best spectacle corrected visual acuity. In our opinion, as 18 D is at the extreme range of indication for LASIK, then LASIK should be ruled out and ICL is the operation to be performed.

When there is an overlap of indications of two or more procedures, and knowing the advantages and disadvantages of each, the next most important parameters in selecting the appropriate procedure are the patient's age, lifestyle, and needs (ie, occupation).

Before making our final decision, we have to bear in mind the difference between vision accuracy and vision quality. For many professions, visual quality, without halo, glare, prismatic effect, interface striae and metamorphotic images, impaired binocular fusion, and low contrast sensitivity are more important than a 20/20 uncorrected visual acuity.

People with myopia working as watchmakers and computer users, who need to work for long periods with very accurate near vision, in the sense that their efficiency depends on detail, need to be slightly undercorrected by procedures that do not produce or have the minimum incidence of haze, decrease in contrast sensitivity, and more specific metamorphotic effect. In such patients, PRK is preferred over LASIK, if under 40 and with lower degrees of myopia, while clear lens extraction may be the most appropriate and preferred over LASIK in patients over 40 or with higher degrees of myopia.

Myopic truck drivers and pilots very often need night vision with high accuracy, so they could be slightly overcorrected with wider, very well-centered optical zones.

TABLE 33-2

PREFERABLE PROCEDURE FOR THE TREATMENT OF HYPEROPIA

		PRK	LTK	LASIK	Phakic IOL	CLE
<40	≤ 4	+	-	+	-	-
>40		++	+	+	-	+ (C)
<40	>4-8>	±	-	++	+	±
>40		±	-	+	-	+ (C)
<40	>8-12>	-	-	+	++	+
>40		-	-	-	-	++
<40	>12	-	-	-	++	+

TABLE 33-3

PREFERABLE PROCEDURE FOR THE TREATMENT OF ASTIGMATISM

Type	PRK	LTK	LASIK	AK	Wedge Resection
Hyperopic	+	+	++	+	-
Mixed	-	-	-	++	-
Myopic, ≤ 4	+	+ (>40 years)	+	+ RK	-
Myopic, >4-8	+	-	++	-	-
Myopic, >8	-	-	+	+	+

Small and eccentric ablations zones lead to glare, causing the biggest problem in this category.

Low vision patients, because of macular degeneration, should be slightly hyperopic; a preferable solution will be ICL or clear lens extraction with wide optics.

Based on this way of thinking, we present our nomogram of the preferred procedure for each case. This nomogram reflects our personal view, and overlaps may still be present. We have not included the ICR, as it is not clinically a widely applied procedure (Table 33-1).

On the same grounds, the operations available for hyperopia are the following: PRK, LTK, LASIK, phakic IOL, and corneal lens extraction. Based on the current "performance" of these operations we use the nomograms in Tables 33-2 and 33-3 in the selection of the appropriate procedure.

Refractive surgery is becoming an art more than a science. In many occasions, the good old adage stands more than ever. Do to your patient what you would have done to yourself. It is almost absolutely sure that you would choose the correct procedure.

Chapter 34

BEYOND LASIK

Ioannis G. Pallikaris, MD

Today, LASIK is, undoubtedly, one of the best techniques for the correction of refractive errors because it combines two important elements: accuracy of the laser cut, as well as better anatomical restoration of the cornea, since tissue removal takes place in the stroma. However, it is a surgical technique that requires high surgeon experience, and one that depends on microkeratome technology.

The next step in the development of LASIK, and in order to render it a procedure capable of correcting the whole range of refractive errors—however, as far as this is allowed and limited by the corneal thickness—is the development of the microkeratome. This will diminish or eliminate complications attributed today to the microkeratome. Even when we reach the ultimate point of microkeratome technology, LASIK will continue to present at least two important "limitations" regarding the best quality of the optical system of the eye. The first is the laser itself, and the patterns of different beam profiles that could be created by the existing technology. The second, and probably more important, is the fact that we are working at the corneal level, meaning that we are modifying only one optical element out of the refractive media constituting the optical system of the eye. LASIK, probably, in its ultimate form, could manage to correct refractive errors in the range of moderate to low myopia, moderate to low astigmatism, and moderate to low hyperopia. What it could not achieve is optimization of the optical system of the eye as a whole. In order to attain optimization, we may have to use one or a combination of procedures where the aim of any operation on the cornea, or wherever on the optical system, is the total correction of all optical aberrations of the optical system of the eye. This means that the laser beam or technique should be designed in such a way as to correct all chromatic, spherical, or other aberrations of the optical system; all phakic astigmatism; and all peripheral optical effects of the optical system of the cornea, as well as the non-planar construction of the retinal surface.

In the future, no matter whether the intervention is done by LASIK, PRK, ICL, etc, our efforts should be aimed not at merely optically correcting the refractive abnormalities of the eye, but at optimizing the visual performance of the optical system of the eye as a whole. New technology should be able to provide intervention, in improving the quality of vision in people who otherwise do not require spectacles, for people who may have an unaided vision of 20/20.

Manolis Manolas, PhD, and I, following a detailed and meticulous signal processing of visually evoked responses, came to the conclusion that the time required for organizing time of the eye signal to become a best visual image varies according to the quality of the optical system, regardless of whether quantitative visual acuity in those patients is 20/20 or better. The organizing time of the image is what the eye needs in order to correct any optical errors on a retinal or central nervous system level, so as to achieve the best visual image in the retina and thus in the brain. This simply means that there is a process of multiple reflexes either from the ciliary body (by accommodation), from the pupil (with its reaction), or other ophthalmokinetic muscle reflexes, so as to start the process of transmitting the signal backwards when it has achieved its best possible visual quality.

Obviously, this is one of the reasons why there are people who can read with ease, without getting tired, while there are others who can still read distinctly, but not with ease, as they constantly delay in the process of creating the best retinal image.

For the immediate future, what is needed is a simplified technology, able to render the cornea absolutely spherical or aspherical, without requiring for this purpose a complicated interconnection of multiple information and data obtained through topographic patterns, as well as various ablation patterns resulting from sophisticated software. The PALM Technique (see insert) could be considered as having such characteristics. PALM was developed at the University of Crete and promises such simplicity. Using a simple material as a mold, and the already long-available hard contact lens technology, any corneal surface irregularity can be rendered spherical. Future ophthalmology will not only aim at correcting refractive errors, but at perfecting the optical system of the eye. In the new era of refractive surgery, laser technology will be concerned with equipment capable of performing customized ablations, based on information obtained not only from corneal topography, but one based on systems that could:

- Analyze spherical errors dealing with the optical system of the eye as a whole.
- Make a spot-by-spot analysis of the refractive condition of the pupillary aperture.

Such systems of customized ablation will be based on analysis of chromatic and other aberrations induced by refractive errors, or probably, on the online analysis of aberrations and their simultaneous interpolation for an optimized pattern. With such equipment, modification of the cornea will not aim at the best possible optical surface of the cornea, but at the best possible optical surface offering the best optical and functional performance of the specific optical system. A correction that will include aberrations of the whole system, not only concerning the cornea, but also the lens and retinal functional topography where the final image is perceived.

Back to the future...Refractive surgery will be soon passing through the path connecting its quantitatively improving vision era with an era of qualitatively perfecting vision. We should all expect the appearance of new magnificent tools to build up this new era. Some time, however, will be spent in realizing and dealing with what our recent experiences suggest.

INDEX